3/04

SEXUAL
REVOLUTION

SEXUAL REVOLUTION

EDITED BY
Jeffery Escoffier

Photographs by Fred W. McDarrah

THUNDER'S MOUTH PRESS • NEW YORK

SEXUAL REVOLUTION

Compilation copyright © 2003 by Jeffrey Escoffier
Photographs © Fred W. McDarrah

Published by
Thunder's Mouth Press
An Imprint of Avalon Publishing Group, Incorporated
245 W. 17th St., 11th Floor
New York, NY 10011

Library of Congress Cataloging-in-Publication Data is available.

ISBN 1-56025-525-0

9 8 7 6 5 4 3 2 1

Book design by Paul Paddock
Printed in the United States of America
Distributed by Publishers Group West

CONTENTS

PART III: Changing Sex Lives

PART IV: Obscenity, Pornography and Erotica

PART VI: Thinking About Sex

Introduction

Jeffery Escoffier

Sexual intercourse began
In nineteen-sixty-three
(Which was rather late for me)—
Between the end of the Chatterly ban
And the Beatles' first LP.

—Philip Larkin

Sex, drugs and rock 'n' roll—for many, these three words sum-up the counter-culture of the sixties and seventies. Rock 'n' roll was the music of the age. Created from country music and blues, it emerged from the experience of rural blacks and whites. Marijuana and LSD were the drugs of the sixties; marijuana, long known in the urban black ghettos, was widely used by jazz musicians, the Beat generation and other bohemian circles. And sex! Well, sex had gained world-wide attention when Alfred Kinsey published his reports on sexual behavior in 1948 (Males) and 1954 (Females) which showed that Americans were more sexually unconventional that anyone would have guessed. By the mid-sixties—Philip Larkin's '1963' is almost exactly right—sex, drugs and rock 'n' roll were taken up by many in the generation born, for the most part, in the first decade after World War II.

The counter-culture was not the only thing that shaped the sexual revolution. Radical politics were often the context for new sexual experiences or sexual tensions—whether it was interracial sex, sex without marriage, or sex with someone of the same gender. With the bus boycott by African Americans in Montgomery, Alabama, a new era in American politics was launched—one that has lasted for almost fifty years; an era in which political battles for the civil rights for minorities have become a form of everyday politics. Throughout the fifties, sixties and seventies, the black civil rights movements played a leading role in redefining American politics—opening it up to racial minorities, creating new opportunities, and also serving as a role model for other identity-based social movements such as the women's, and gay and lesbian movements. The black civil rights movements and the movement against the war in Vietnam created new ways of talking about politics and new methods for organizing opposition and resistance.

The sexual revolution was also a contradictory experience. The exhilaration, the sense of freedom and the utopian impulse that underlay it is often forgotten today. Even those who contributed to it directly—hippies, rock musicians, anti-war activists, leftist revolutionaries, feminists, and lesbian and gay activists—sometimes felt that it was irrelevant, perhaps dangerous, misguided or even misogynist. But the sexual revolution shared the same sense of energy, adventure, and utopianism that the political and cultural movements did.

What "sexual revolution"means, when it began (if it did), to whom it applied, and what changes it wrought are highly contested subjects. There is some presumption that the twentieth-century experienced two sexual revolutions—one in the years during and after World War I and the second in the 1960s and 1970s. What is not clear, however, is whether or not earlier periods experienced comparable shifts in sexual attitudes and conduct. The emergence of the flapper and the "New Woman"in the 1920s signaled a challenge to the double standard and led as well to a reformulation of male gender roles. But there is no unequivocal evidence of significant changes in sexual behavior.

According to sociologists, patterns of sexual partnering underwent significant change in the 1960s, and it is this shift away from "monogamous"sexuality that is usually signified by the term "sexual revolution."However, the revolution that emerged in the sixties was as much a change in attitudes about sex as it was a significant shift in sexual conduct. Changes in the way that people thought about sexuality and gender roles stimulated new modes of behavior that were not always measured by increased sexual activity. For example, women entered marriage with greater sexual experience and confidence than women in the past. As a result, there was an increased demand for sexual satisfaction in marriage. It contributed to the growth of a market for books and magazine articles about how to improve one's sex life as well as a greater demand for marriage manuals and counselors. It may have also led to an increase in divorces thereby reinforcing the likelihood of those who were divorced having additional sexual partners in their lifetimes. These developments also challenged the double standard— which permitted men to engage in sexual activity before or outside their marriages, but harshly stigmatized women who had pre- or extramarital affairs. In ways like these the emergence of feminism and women's rights overlapped with and were intertwined with the developments later labeled "the sexual revolution."In the end, all these experiences both heightened frustrations and created greater freedom.

Before the Revolution: Rock 'n' Roll, the Beats, and Playboy

Elvis Presley, the Beat Generation and *Playboy* magazine, each was a sign that something new—something sexual—had arrived on the American scene in the 1950s. *Playboy* was one of the first. Inspired by Alfred Kinsey's 1948 report on male sexuality, Hugh Hefner founded it in 1953 when he was only 27 years old. Hefner envisioned an overtly sexual magazine that featured nude photographs of attractive young women—Marilyn Monroe was on the centerfold in the first issue. Over the course of the fifties and sixties Hefner elaborated a philosophy of the sexually active young bachelor who avoided the entanglements of marriage.

At the same time, Elvis Presley's music swept across America like wildfire—drawing together white and black audiences with an amalgam of black-inspired rhythm and blues and country western, generating tremendous excitement among teenagers. Parents reacted much more negatively, believing that Presley's gyrating hips and his overtly sexual style of performance threatened the morals they were seeking to establish in their children. To young people, his music conveyed a sense of yearning and release from a humdrum daily life. In his wake, rock n' roll emerged as the new American music—vigorously alive and full of promises of happiness created by the powerful beat and country soul.

The Beat Generation was a loose group of poets and writers who eschewed the conformist ethos of the 1950s. 'Beat' implied both poverty and beatitude. But the Beats set out on a quest for what Arthur Rimbaud called the mystical 'derangement of senses.' Drugs, sex, jazz and Zen Buddhism were the means used to achieve the Beats' other-worldly forms of enlightenment. The Beat Generation's spiritual odyssey was portrayed in Allen Ginsberg's epic poem *Howl*:

> "I saw the best minds of my generation destroyed by madness, starving hysterical naked,/dragging themselves through negro streets at dawn looking for an angry fix, angelheaded hipsters burning for the machinery of night, . . ."

The Beat Generation emerged on the national scene in 1957 with the widely-publicized censorship trial of *Howl*'s publisher, Lawrence Ferlinghetti, and the publication of Jack Kerouac's novel *On the Road*. They offered a vision of creativity and freedom outside of the conventional life of the suburb and the corporation. They were 'Holy Barbarians' who renounced ordinary success and conventional family life for a life of spiritual seeking and sensual pleasure.

The fifties and early sixties displayed many other signs of sexual openness and experiment. In popular fiction, Grace Metalious' *Peyton Place* created a tremendous furor. In eighth grade, I remember sitting in the auditorium waiting for the school day to begin, pretending to study my notebook, with *Peyton Place* held down below the sightlines of the monitors, reading 'the dirty parts' to my friends. I remember my frustration, anxiously waiting to steal the unexpurgated *Lady Chatterly's Lover* at my local drug store; I was afraid that the owner would tell my mother, in the end I settled for the expurgated edition.

The sexual revolution of 1960s and 1970s gained its momentum from the confluence of numerous social currents: demographic, cultural, technological, social and political factors all came together in the early sixties. Three developments, however, predominated: first, the intellectual and cultural influence of the sexual theories of psychoanalyst Wilhelm Reich and the survey research of biologist Alfred Kinsey; second, the expansion of sexual speech that emerged from the numerous battles fought by underground publishers, merchants of sexual fantasies, and bitter comedians who fought to include sexual expression under the First Amendment; and third, the emergence of social movements during the sixties—beginning with the black civil rights movement, the student anti-war movement, the counter-culture, all of which created new contexts for intimate relationships, up through the women's movement and the gay and lesbian movements—which fought for new sexual norms.

These three developments were not always compatible with one another—contradictions and tensions repeatedly surfaced between them. The dynamic that emerged from the struggle to publish sexually explicit images and writing for instance, reinforced a process of commercialization (and commodification) that contradicted sharply with the grassroots ideals of the women's and gay movements. Reich's stress on the heterosexual orgasm as the standard for sexual health proposed an unyielding "tyranny of the orgasm"against non-genital forms of polymorphous sexuality. The emergence of a lesbian and gay movement that stressed sexual identities gradually eroded the accent on sexual liberation. Numerous counter-currents and cross-currents among all these developments made the sexual revolution of the sixties and seventies an incoherent process; new groups and movements constantly emerged to battle repressions and intolerance previously unchallenged by the proponents of sexual revolution (for example, S & M activists) or to mount repressive measures in the name of freedom (such as the anti-porn feminists).

The Mysteries of the Orgasm: Wilhelm Reich, Alfred Kinsey and Sexual Liberation

"the search for an orgasm more apocalyptic than the one which preceded it."

—Norman Mailer, *The White Negro*

As the 1950s drew to a close, novelist Norman Mailer began work on a novel he called *The Time of Her Time* in which he sought to capture the historical moment about to emerge. The 'Time' of her 'Time' was both zeitgeist and orgasm—the Time of Coming/the Coming of her Time. "Coming out of the orgy of the war,"Mailer wrote, "our sense of sex and family was torn in two. The past did not exist for us. We had to write our way out into the unspoken territories of sex—there was so much there, it was new, and our talent depended on going to the borderland."He never completed the novel, but the excerpt that he published in *Advertisements for Myself* was a daring piece of erotic writing—in which the novel's narrator and a young woman battle for each other's soul while engaged in achieving the perfect orgasm. For Mailer the rapturous orgasm signified the battle for the political and cultural health of American life. In his controversial essay "The White Negro,"Mailer, invoking the cultural critiques of Henry Miller, D.H. Lawrence and Wilhelm Reich, lamented the absence of mercy, charity and justice in American life. Mailer believed that black culture, in contrast to mainstream white America, had preserved a certain degree of vitality because:

> The Negro had stayed alive and begun to grow by following the need of his body where he could. Knowing in the cells of his existence that life was war, nothing but war, . . . he lived in the enormous present, he subsisted for his Saturday night kicks, relinquishing the pleasures of the mind for the more obligatory pleasures of the body, and in his music he gave voice to the character and quality of his existence, to his rage and the infinite variations of joy, lust, languor, growl, cramp, pinch, scream and despair of his orgasm. For jazz is orgasm, it is the music of orgasm, good orgasm and bad, and so it spoke across a nation . . . .

Although Mailer had portrayed the orgasm as a transcendent experience, two other men in the 1930s and 1940s had acknowledged the orgasm as the peak experience of sexual life—Wilhelm Reich for whom the "unconditional"orgasm signified sexual health, and Alfred Kinsey who sought, literally, to classify and measure sexual activity by enumerating orgasms. Inventors of the sacred and the profane meanings of orgasm, Reich and Kinsey both made the orgasm the measure of sexual significance.

Once considered Freud's most brilliant protégé, Reich at the time of his death in 1957, was widely considered a crank and a fraud. Reich died of a heart attack while serving a sentence in the Federal Penitentiary in Lewisburg, Pennsylvania, for selling and leasing the Orgone Accumulator—popularly known as an "orgone box"—a booth that accumulated and focused the cosmic orgone energy in the earth's atmosphere in order to help patients achieve a complete sexual release. Throughout the sixties, in the early years of the sexual revolution, there was no more influential theorist of sexuality than Reich. Many prominent writers and intellectuals were followers of his theoretical work (Paul Goodman, Norman Mailer, radical educator A.S. Neill, therapist Fritz Perls, and psychoanalyst Robert Lindner, the author of *Rebel without a Cause*) or his therapeutic methods such as the orgone box (Saul Bellow), or like Allen Ginsberg and William Burroughs, who in their *Yage Letters* fused Reichian rhetoric with an apology for homosexuality and hallucinatory drugs (Reich disapproved of both things). Despite Reich's conservatism on certain issues (like homosexuality) and the questionable theories of cosmic orgone energy, the influence of Reich's thinking on the social and political impact of sexual repression and the importance of the orgasm was unsurpassed during the sexual revolution's early days.

Since the 1920s, Reich had explored how social institutions limited sexual fulfillment. He was committed to "sexual revolution"as the fundamental change necessary to promote mental health—by ending, among other things, the double standard as applied to women and by eliminating the deleterious impact of enforced sexual abstinence on adolescents. Reich argued that all neuroses were accompanied by a disturbance of genitality and that dammed-up sexual energy was the cause of neurotic symptoms. While he recognized that sexuality had nongenital aspects, Reich stressed the unequivocal importance of the orgasm. The capability of achieving an orgasm—the release of sexual energy—marked the difference between sickness and health, and a true orgasm resulted in the complete release of all damned-up sexual excitation through involuntary pleasurable contractions of the body. For example, the sexual abstinence imposed on adolescents led, Reich argued, to juvenile delinquency, neuroses, perversions and political apathy. Long active on the left, Reich also contended that progressive political change was doomed to failure unless it was accompanied by the abolition of sexual repression. "To define freedom is the same as to define sexual health,"he wrote. Reich's books on the relation of social institutions to sexual health—*The Sexual Revolution* (1935) and *The Mass Psychology of Fascism* (1933)—were enormously influential works in the late 1950s and early1960s.

However, at the time of Reich's emigration to the U.S. in 1939, he had begun to move away from his stress on social change and sexuality and begun to emphasize the importance of orgone energy—a visible and measurable form of energy which, he believed, circulated in the atmosphere and in the blood stream of living beings. He developed a number of scientific instruments to measure orgone energy and invented the Orgone Accumulator in order to harness orgone for therapeutic purposes.

In 1954, the Federal Food and Drug Administration filed a complaint against him for renting a fraudulent therapeutic device, the Orgone Energy Accumulator, across state lines. The Accumulator was a six-sided box, the size of an old-fashioned telephone booth, made of metal on the outside and wood on the inside. The box focused and concentrated Orgone radiation in the atmosphere. The patient had merely to sit inside and absorb the concentrated energy in order to achieve orgiastic potency. The FDA ordered many of Reich's books and all his orgone boxes seized and destroyed. Amid the bustling trucks and warehouses of New York City's meatpacking district, Federal officials confined to the flames of the public incinerator at Gansevoort and Hudson streets all the copies they had seized of Reich's *People in Trouble* and *Ether, God and the Devil: Cosmic Superimposition*—in one of the few official book burnings to take place in American history.

If, for Reich, the complete orgasm was the sign of sexual health, for Alfred Kinsey the orgasm was also the one empirically measurable unit of sexual behavior. The Kinsey Reports and the public debate that resulted from the publication of his empirical investigations of American sexual habits were the opening shots of the sexual revolution. Kinsey's two path-breaking volumes on human sexuality in 1948 (*Sexual Behavior in the Human Male*) and 1953 (*Sexual Behavior in the Human Female*) were based on the most extensive survey of sexual behavior ever undertaken. The Kinsey reports had succeeded in a "detailed mapping of a submerged continent known only from the archipelagos of exposed mountain tops."

Moral outrage and a great deal of professional hypocrisy greeted the report, but few Americans remained indifferent to the surprisingly large gap between the publicly accepted sexual norms and American's daily sexual activities. Many readers objected to Kinsey's research for its empirical, materialistic, and ostensibly value-free investigation into the subject of human sexuality. Although he never considered it as moral position, Kinsey's fundamental ethical tenet throughout his work was tolerance; in both volumes he stressed sympathetic acceptance of people as they are and repeatedly noted the limits of a person's ability to modify his or her sexual behavior. Kinsey was so struck by the extraordinary extent of individual variation in sexual behavior, he argued that any attempt to establish uniform standards of sexual behavior was both impracticable and unjust. Kinsey supplemented this theme of individual variation by stressing what Paul Robinson has called our "common deviance."He believed that his discovery of the widespread deviation from accepted sexual standards showed that attempts to regulate sexual behavior were doomed to failure and "the only proper sexual policy was no policy at all."

Kinsey's radical empiricism led him to measure sexual experience in quantitative terms as orgasms and by tabulating the number of orgasms of his interview subjects. Thus Kinsey's tolerance was, in part, a statistical concept. In his schema, heterosexual intercourse was demoted to only one of six possible forms of "sexual outlet"that also included masturbation, nocturnal emission, heterosexual petting, homosexual relations, and intercourse with animals. From this perspective the sole distinction between heterosexuals and homosexuals is that the former are sexually attracted to people of the other gender while the latter are attracted to those of the same gender.

Kinsey's findings on homosexuality were among his most controversial and widely publicized. His volume on male sexuality concluded that 37 percent of the male population of the United States had had at least one homosexual experience to orgasm between adolescence and old age. The data also seemed to suggest that many adults were neither permanently nor exclusively homosexual or heterosexual but displayed a continuum of sexual behavior. Kinsey measured this fluidity along the Kinsey scale of hetero- to homosexual behavior and fantasy which ranged from 0 (exclusively heterosexual) through 6 (exclusively homosexual). While

Kinsey's findings clearly encouraged him to reject homosexuality as a pathological syndrome, the range and fluidity of many American's sexual behavior also led him to reject the idea of a sexual identity; he believed that there were no homosexual or heterosexual persons, only heterosexual or homosexual acts.

Even before the emergence of the women's movement in the late sixties, debates about women's sexuality emerged in the wake of the 1953 *Kinsey Report* on female sexuality. Kinsey's report had revealed that women's interest in sex extended beyond an interest in reproduction. Kinsey's research dispelled a number of influential myths about women and sex, among them among psychologists that women had greater difficulty achieving orgasm. Moreover, only half of women interviewed said they had been virgins when they married and 25 percent said that they had had extra-marital affairs. It was certainly no surprise that 90 percent of men acknowledged that they routinely masturbated while only 62 percent of the women did.

Kinsey died slightly more than a year before Reich. Exhausted by the fruitless search for funding after the Rockefeller Foundation withdrew its financial support after the controversy created by Kinsey's first report and suffering from heart disease, Kinsey struggled to renew his research despite straightened circumstances. After his death, the Kinsey Institute survived on a series of modest research grants but it was never again to undertake any research on the scale of Kinsey's earlier studies. When John Gagnon and several colleagues attempted to mount a comparable survey in the 1990s, as a way of identifying sexual risk behavior in light of the AIDS epidemic, Senator Jesse Helms and conservatives in Congress scuttled the federal funding for it.

If Reich had theorized the possibility of sexual revolution and identified the orgasm as the supreme achievement of sexual liberation, and Kinsey had revealed the actual behavior of Americans by measuring the frequency of orgasms and outlets, the pioneering experimental research of William Masters and Virginia Johnson refuted once and for all the damaging misconceptions about the female orgasm and by doing so made a decisive scientific breakthrough for the sexual revolution's feminist moment. In some respects, their work exemplified the sexual egalitarianism of the sixties, not only in their working relationship, but also in the image of sexual relations that they project in their books. Both *Human Sexual Response* (1966) and *Human Sexual Inadequacy* (1970) were based on laboratory observations of sexual behavior and became the basis of a therapeutic practice devoted to sexual dysfunction. However, in the end Masters and Johnson focused almost exclusively on the quality of sexual experience within committed relationships—they made the couple rather than the unattached individual the preferred unit of analysis and therapy. They did not discuss improving the quality of sexual experience for those men and women who chose to engage in sex with casual (non-marital) sexual partners—that is so essential to the definition of the sexual revolution.

The Freedom of Sexual Speech: Obscenity, Pornography and the First Amendment

The sexual revolution of the sixties and seventies would not have taken place were it not for the battles fought over obscenity and pornography during the late fifties by pornographers, stand-up comics, and literary writers. The most embattled "pornographer" was, arguably, publisher Samuel Roth, arrested many times after 1928 for distributing works like D.H. Lawrence's *Lady Chatterly's Lover*, the *Kama Sutra* (the ancient Hindu sex manual that had been originally brought to the attention of Western readers by the explorer Sir Richard Burton), a book of Aubrey Beardsley's erotic drawings, and many other lesser known but sexually "explicit" works. In 1956, Roth, facing a twenty-six-count obscenity indictment in Federal Court, was found guilty and sentenced, at the age of 62, to five years in a penitentiary and a substantial fine. His lawyer appealed the case, and it eventually made its way to the Supreme Court. His lawyers argued the controversial literature distributed by Roth was protected by the First Amendment. The Government's attorney's had argued that "absolute freedom of speech was not what the founding fathers had in mind, at least where the interest in public morality was at stake." The Court endorsed Roth's conviction. While earlier decisions had dismissed obscenity charges against Radcliffe Hall's lesbian novel *The Well of Loneliness* and James Joyce's earthy *Ulysses*, Justice Brennan, who wrote the majority opinion in the Roth case, established a definition of obscenity—a milestone itself—which has continued to exercise a tremendous influence over legal issues of obscenity and pornography in the US: "whether to the average person, applying contemporary community standards, the dominant theme of the material taken as a whole appeals to prurient interest." Roth went to jail, but subsequently lawyers have used *Samuel Roth v. United States of America* to reshape the treatment of sexual speech. Brennan's opinion was, in fact, ambiguous. While Brennan had declared "obscenity as utterly without socially redeeming importance,"and ruled that it was not protected by the freedoms of speech and press, Brennan had also created an opening for the freedom of sexual speech when he noted that "sex and obscenity were not synonymous . . . obscene material having a tendency to excite lustful thoughts,"and that "All ideas, even ideas hateful to prevailing climate of opinion—have the full protection"of the First Amendment.

Also taking place in 1957 was the obscenity trial of San Francisco bookseller and publisher Lawrence Ferlinghetti for selling obscene literature, Allen Ginsberg's poem *Howl*. Ferlinghetti was acquitted, and the trial, in conjunction with the publication a month earlier of Jack Kerouac's *On the Road*, put the Beat Generation on the cultural map.

Just two years after *Samuel Roth v. U.S.A.*, another publisher, Barney Rosset of Grove Press, sued the United States Postal Office, which had responsibility for enforcing the Comstock Act of 1873 which banned obscene and pornographic literature from the U.S. mails. The federal judge in the case rescinded the ban against distributing *Lady Chatterly's Lover*. Almost immediately, Grove Press published the D.H. Lawrence novel, Henry Miller's *Tropic of Cancer* and many other controversial works with sexual content. Similar cases popped up around the country.

Comedian Lenny Bruce was another unlikely crusader for free speech. Bruce found himself repeatedly contesting obscenity charges. Over the course of his career, Bruce had evolved from the role of a traditional stand-up comic telling off-color jokes at strip clubs to that of a brutal and devastating social critic—and, in his case, as the relentless transgressor of the norms of public speech. Before Bruce, stand-up comics had relied on jokes and stories, but Bruce took on the sanctity of organized religion, racism, and sexual taboos. Audiences were both titillated and shocked by Bruce's opinions and his obscene language. He claimed that he was exposing social hypocrisy and challenged stereotypes by using common terms of abuse: "faggots,""niggers,"and "kikes."Bruce's shocking treatment of social issues—some of his frequent routines were: "Infidelity,""How to Relax Colored People,""Sex is Dirty?"and "Who's a Fag?'—and his use of obscene language provoked local authorities in Los Angeles, San Francisco, Chicago and New York City to arrest him for obscenity. Bruce's battle for freedom of expression led him onto the terrain established by Brennan's majority opinion in *Samuel Roth v. U.S.A.* He fought his legal battles (complicated at times by his arrests and trials for heroin possession) up until his death in 1966—when emotionally worn out and ill he died of an overdose. Ultimately Bruce won his battle—though after his death—and along with the writers like Henry Miller and publishers Samuel Roth and Barney Rosset had helped to create a space in American public life for sexually explicit speech.

The Roth decision, however, had created an enduring double bind—it continued to pose an enormous obstacle to free and honest expression of sexual thoughts by defining obscenity as "utterly without socially redeeming importance"—thus in effect, the public expression of sexual fantasies and thoughts was not protected by the First Amendment.

In the early 1960s, John Gagnon, a sociologist on the staff of the Kinsey Institute suggested to Steven Marcus, a young professor of English at Columbia University, that a study of the Institute's rich collection of Victorian pornography and the period's medical literature on sexuality might prove to be a rewarding research subject. In 1966, Marcus published the results of his research at the Kinsey Institute in his book, *The Other Victorians*. Among his most remarkable discoveries: the anonymous autobiography *My Secret Life*, a four-thousand-page eleven-volume memoir of one man's 40 year pursuit of sexual experience which included many, many permutations of heterosexual coitus, flagellation and even homosexuality and sodomy. Marcus's work inspired Grove Press, flush from the successful publication of *Lady Chatterly's Lover* and Henry Miller's novels, to embark upon a massive reprinting of Victorian pornography, much of it still in print, of which *My Secret Life* is the flagship.

The following year, in 1967, Congress set up a Commission on Pornography and Obscenity to define pornography, provide guidelines for its regulation, study its effects on its audience and assess its significance in American society. The landmark *Report of the Commission* found no evidence that exposure to explicit sexual materials led to any criminal or delinquent behavior among youth and adults. This report was later criticized by conservatives and some feminists in the eighties and was countered by a later Commission appointed by the Reagan administration.

These developments greatly expanded the degree of sexual explicitness throughout the culture. Advice books like *The Sensuous Woman* (1969), *The Sensuous Man* (1970), Nancy Friday's *My Secret Garden* (1974) and the most spectacularly successful book of them all, Alex Comfort's lavishly and explicitly illustrated volumes, *The Joy of Sex* (1972) and *More Joy: A Lovemaking Companion to the Joy of Sex* (1973), poured from the presses. Sexually explicit pulp novels like Jacqueline Susanne's *Valley of the Dolls* (1966), memoirs like Xavier Hollander's *The Happy Hooker*, and sexually explicit movies like *I Am Curious (Yellow)* (1967), *Deep Throat* (1972), *Beyond the Green Door* (1973), *The Devil in Miss Jones* (1973) attempted to satisfy the public's growing hunger for a vicarious experience of sex. *Deep Throat*, *Green Door* and *The Devil in Miss Jones* all played at mainstream movie houses, reviewed by established daily newspaper critics and were often more commercially successful than contemporary Hollywood releases. *Boys in the Sand*, the first sexually-explicit commercial gay film opened in New York City at a mainstream movie theater in 1971, even before the straight porn classics like *Deep Throat* and *The Devil in Miss Jones* were released.

By the 1970s, newspapers with names like *Screw*, offering sexual information, personal ads, and sexually explicit photos and art, were available on street corners in larger American cities. These cultural developments demonstrated an increased public interest in sex and suggested that sexual behavior was undergoing changes as well. Despite the political and cultural importance of the First Amendment battles, the legal victories often translated into phenomenal economic success for the publishers, filmmakers and distributors of sexually explicit materials. Moreover, these materials were aimed primarily at male audiences, and thus sought to satisfy many of the traditional male sexual fantasies. They tended to reinforce standardized conceptions of sexual attractiveness—contributing to enormous success of magazines like Hugh Hefner's *Playboy*, Bob Guccione's *Penthouse*, and Larry Flynt's *Hustler*. While many applauded the freedom of sexual expression, feminists and others critical of the cultural impact of sexual stereotypes were uncomfortable with the commodified and commercialized portrayal of sexuality.

The political upshot is that freedom of sexual expression is the necessary condition in the struggle for identity politics and civil rights—nevertheless this implies an odd coalition between principled first amendment activists, porn entrepreneurs, and sex radicals among feminists, gay activists, and sexual minorities.

Making the Revolution: Sex and the Radical Movements

Socialism without fucking is dull and lifeless.
—the heroine, WR: *The Mysteries of the Organism* (1971),
a film by Dusan Makavejev

The massive upheaval of the sixties and seventies took place on many fronts: cultural, political, social, and psychological. Since the fifties blacks had fought for civil rights and to transform the quality of their lives. The younger generation of whites and blacks built on the changes wrought by the civil rights movement to launch a radical political movement against the war in Vietnam and to eliminate social and economic inequities that had existed for generations. The women's movement emerged in the wake of the black civil rights and student anti-war movements. The gay and lesbian liberation movement emerged from the welter of anti-war, civil rights and women's organizing. Sexual revolution was intertwined with each of these other movements—all these movements generated cross-currents that intersected with one another. In addition, cultural and artistic movements such as rock and roll, the theater of the absurd, Pop art, Happenings, and the "new Hollywood" movies like *Easy Rider* or *Alice's Restaurant*, along with those directed by Martin Scorsese and Robert Altman, were central to the creation and dissemination of new sexual mores.

Beginning as early as 1962, Helen Gurley Brown (who later became the editor of *Cosmopolitan* magazine) in a series of magazine articles and in her book *Sex and the Single Girl* set out to attack the double standard that made it acceptable for men but not women to have sex before marriage. Barely a year later, Betty Friedan's *The Feminine Mystique* (1963) challenged the widely-held belief that women could only find fulfillment in the role of wife and mother. Friedan argued that this "feminine mystique" was deliberately promulgated in order to prevent women from competing with men for jobs, careers and public roles. Her book spurred a revival of feminism. Shortly thereafter, young women active in the political movements of the sixties—the civil rights movement, the movement against the war in Vietnam, and the New Left—formed small discussion groups, known as conscious-raising groups, to explore the everyday patterns of behavior that supported male privileges and denigrated women. "The personal is political" became the motto of the women's movement.

In a series of groundbreaking intellectual contributions, radical feminists such as Kate Millet (*Sexual Politics*, 1970) and Shulamith Firestone (*The Dialectic of Sex: The Case for Feminist Revolution*, 1970) launched a fierce intellectual attack on the patriarchal power structure. Millet took up "sexual revolution" in the broadest possible terms. Sexual revolution, in Millet's sense of the term, was the process necessary to "bring the institution of patriarchy to an end, abolishing both the ideology of male supremacy and the traditional socialization by which it is upheld in matters of status, role, and temperament." But the term, sexual revolution, also implied, she noted, the end of "traditional sexual inhibitions and taboos, particularly those that threaten patriarchal monogamous marriage: homosexuality, 'illegitimacy,' adolescent, pre- and extra-marital sexuality." Thus from its moment of inception, the feminism of the sixties and seventies emphasized a revolution in sexual behavior and attitudes—"the goal of revolution would be a permissive single standard of sexual freedom, and one uncorrupted by the crass and exploitative economic bases of traditional sexual alliances." Shulamith Firestone took up similar themes. The "dialectic of sex" like Millet's sexual revolution was the process by the "sex class system"was to be overthrown. Firestone believed that Freud had "grasped the crucial problem of modern life: Sexuality." But she viewed Freudianism as a form of misguided feminism. Thus Firestone chose not to focus of changing sexual mores—"Wilhelm Reich's *The Sexual Revolution,*" she noted in passing, "could have been written yesterday."—but on how Freudianism had undermined feminism and helped to maintain male dominance. The radical feminism that emerged from the women's involvement in the black civil rights and anti-war movements also sought ways to translate the ideas developed by feminist theorists into practical actions and cultural change.

The central ambiguity of feminism's first moment of sexual revolution never quite dissipated—many feminists believed that the tectonic shift in sexual behavior and attitudes that took place in the sixties and seventies had, in fact, failed, that it benefited men far more than women. The first issue of *Ms.* magazine featured an article entitled "The Sexual Revolution Isn't Our War" which argued that the sexual revolution was "a male invention." Many years later, in 1986, Barbara Ehrenreich, Elizabeth Hess, and Gloria Jacobs countered that persistent belief and argued, instead, that "there had been a genuine revolution in sexual attitudes" and that it had, in fact, been initiated by women.

In 1966, William Masters and Virginia Johnson published the first of their scientific studies. Their findings seemed to, once and for all, disprove Freud's theory of the vaginal orgasm and stressed the centrality of the clitoral orgasm. Feminists explored the implications of Master and Johnson's findings on female sexuality—the stress on clitoral stimulation, the possibility of multiple orgasms, and the insignificance of the penis. Feminist such as Anne Koedt, Barbara Seaman, and Alix Kates Shulman, among others, developed the feminist implications of Masters and Johnson's research. Popular sociologists, such as Vance Packard in *The Sexual Wilderness: The Contemporary Upheaval in Male-Female Relationships* (1968) deliberately explored the interplay of both feminism and sexual revolution.

The cumulative impact of the attack on the double standard, the radical feminist critique of male-female sexual relations and the renewed emphasis on the clitoral orgasm (spurred by Masters and Johnson's research) was reinforced by the growing acceptance of the birth control pill. It became much easier to engage in sex without fear of pregnancy—various sexually transmitted diseases had receded, and AIDS was as yet unknown. Thus women were able to pursue sexual experience without either the commitment or romance that had previously validated sex outside of marriage for women. Novelist and poet Erica Jong, following in the footsteps of Henry Miller, published *Fear of Flying*, a picaresque tale of Isadora Wing's quest for the "zipless fuck"—pure sex for pleasure and without commitment.

> For the true, ultimate zipless A-1 fuck, it was necessary that you never get to know the man very well. I had noticed, for example, how all my infatuations dissolved as soon as I really because friends with a man, became sympathetic to his problems, listened to him kvetch about his wife, or ex-wives, his mother, his children."

Exploring the separation of sex from romance, and probing its benefits and difficulties, seemed to be an important bridge to the social experiments of the sexual revolution—swinging, mate-swapping and communal sex.

By the late 1960s, there were also many signs that homosexuals were also engaged in the process of creating a civil rights movement, inspired, in part, by the black struggles of the sixties. Finally, in 1969, a police raid on a Greenwich Village bar the Stonewall Inn provoked a series of riots that mobilized drag queens, street hustlers, lesbians and gay men, many of whom had been politicized by the movement against the war in Viet Nam. The Stonewall riots set in motion a broad grass-roots mobilization across the country. Under the banner of the sexual revolution, the gay and lesbian movement initially stressed sexual liberation rather than the question of identity or civil rights—though both of these issues eventually emerged as significant.

From the beginning, gay activists believed that gay liberation had "ramifications and importance" beyond homosexuals themselves—as Dennis Altman, author of the pioneering *Homosexual Oppression and Liberation* (published in 1971) suggested: "not only for those of us who are homosexuals, who are finding the courage and self-assurance to come out in public, but indeed . . . for everyone else." Lesbians and gay liberationists also stressed the connection between sexual preferences and gender norms. In a forum on sexual liberation Altman went on to comment how

"our society denies the inherent bisexuality of all humans. . . .
[A]mong most people who identity themselves as heterosexual
there is a very determined and calculated attempt to deny their
homosexual component and this leads to the quite grotesque
cults of masculinity and femininity."

Gay novelist Brad Gooch called the 1970s the "Golden Age of
Promiscuity." During the 1970s gay men had developed a culture of
'easy sex'—of social spaces (bars, bathhouses, and discos) where sex
without commitment, obligation, or a long-term relationship was
possible. Many gay men pursued this kind of 'impersonal' sex as an
end in itself—for the adventure and variety of sexual experience—
rather than as a substitute for personal sex. These impersonal relationships were not seen as superficial, tawdry, depressing or
pathological, but rather as fun, enjoyable or exciting. In *The Gay
Report*, published in 1979, Karla Jay and Allen Young found that 10
percent of the men had sex daily, 60 percent had sex at least once a
week—and more than 50 percent had had at least ten different partners in the previous year. Gay men sought to create safe places where
without fear of outsiders intruding or arrest, an ample supply of
sexual partners, and a physically comfortable space they could
engage in casual sex. The gay bathhouse was a successful realization
of these social conditions.

By the late sixties, there were a growing number of communities and
other institutions that sought to establish the social conditions of sexual
freedom. The most famous of these was Sandstone—a sexual utopian
community—which was founded in the late sixties by John and Barbara
Williamson. Set in Topanga Canyon, a beautiful and isolated area of the
Malibu Mountains just outside of Los Angeles, it was dedicated to the
full and open expression of sexuality. Inhabited by a core-group of men
and women in committed heterosexual relationships, they were also
open to sex with people outside their relationships. In addition, Sandstone also had outside members who were able to visit the community
for its pool, 'ballroom' (where "balling' took place), and the parties that
took place several times a week. From 1969 to December 1973, Sandstone was a model community of sexual freedom which attracted many
prominent professionals from all over the country. Robert Rimmer,

author of *The Harrad Experiment*, a widely read sexual utopian novel, recounted how at Sandstone, he would

> . . . stand on the fireplace hearth, naked, and lecture about sexual experience. Some of those around me were actually making love while I spoke. Frequently, I would look down and notice a couple of girls sitting there with their legs open...The people who could cope with Sandstone ... were not frightened by the human body or body contact. What probably brought them there was the conscious realization that none of us gets as much sex of the kind we want as we'd like. We're constantly looking for a kind of sexual nirvana.

Other places that encouraged sexual experimentation were Esalen in Big Sur, California, the Playboy Clubs, the chain of nightclubs founded by *Playboy* magazine's Hugh Hefner.

Sex for the sake of pleasure was one of the most insistent, if often unexpressed, ideals of the sexual revolution. There have always been nightclubs and bars in sex districts—often on the margins of minority communities such as Harlem, Times Square, the South Side of Chicago, or the Tenderloin of San Francisco—that facilitated sexual contacts between men and women. But in the seventies, singles bars, where men and women could hook-up for casual sex, opened in middle-class neighborhoods. Weekly alternative newspapers sprouted in most major cities—all of which carried personal ads of people looking for sexual partners and relationships. Swinging or mate-swapping also became the practice among certain social circles where couples swapped partners among themselves. Swingers clubs were started and others took out ads in swinging and alternative publications. Within this context other kinds of sexuality also gained visibility—fetishes, S/M and trans-vestitism. The proportion of the population that participated in the new swinging and singles scene was probably small, but the scene was widely publicized in the press and popular culture. The dilemmas of sophisticated sexual experiments like swapping were satirized in movies like *Bob & Carol & Ted & Alice* (1969) and *Shampoo* (1975). Movies like *Looking for Mr. Goodbar* (1977) exploited the vulnerabilities and anxi-eties of this new trend for young women. Likewise, the movie *Cruising*

(1980) set a police thriller in a gay world of bars and clubs where men engaged in an never-ending hunt for sex.

The social movements and the many experiments in communal living, open marriage or mate swapping not only transformed sexuality, but also changed the way we understood it. The organization of new movements, the creation of sexual communities, and the exploration of new ways to relate to one another sexually demonstrated that sexual engagement and the meaning of the sex were shaped by the social context—both pleasure and danger were possible. Though each sexual experiment differed in the degree of concerted action required to undertake it as a course of action, together they demonstrated the overwhelming significance of sexual politics and social change as a factor in the sexual revolution.

What Price Revolution? The Limits of Sexual Freedom

I can't get no satisfaction
I can't get no satisfaction
'Cause I try and I try and I try and I try
I can't get no, I can't get no
　　　　　—The Rolling Stones (1965)

The very idea of 'sexual revolution' implies that sexual behavior and norms can be changed by human action. The regulation of sexuality therefore, whether it's by religion, morality, law or psychiatry, is a social construction. What historical and social processes underlie the grand narrative of the sexual revolution? What are the long-term consequences of changing the way that sex is regulated by social institutions? The sexual revolution was also a cultural revolution in which the social framework within sex took place was radically transformed—the everyday sexual scripts, the grand cultural narratives (of sex, gender, age and race) and the scientific understanding of sex were all dramatically modified. There is no grand theoretical synthesis of the process, instead theorists like Freud, Reich, Marcuse and Foucault must be put in play and questioned, so that we grasp the historical process.

Freud had believed that repression was the necessary 'price' of civilization—sexual liberation in that case implied the breakdown of society and culture. Wilhelm Reich argued that sexual repression—the "unsatisfied orgiastic longing of the masses"—was, in fact, the basis of fascism. In the long run, the sexual revolution of the sixties and seventies showed that society could co-exist with sexual freedom. The sexual revolution had failed to eliminate sexual repression—thus neither Freud (who thought that sexual liberation implied the downfall of society) nor Reich (who believed that sexual revolution would eliminate repression) had been proven right. Ironically, the sexual revolution that had begun under the aegis of Wilhelm Reich, was transformed from one in which sexuality was initially understood as 'natural,' a turbulent and volatile form of energy controlled only by social repression, to one in which sexuality was formed primarily through patterns of social interaction, discourses and cultural scenarios—exemplified by the writing of John Gagnon, William Simon and Michel Foucault that emerged during the sexual revolution's second decade.

Late in his life, Freud came to believe that perverse desires were incompatible with a stable social order because they failed to support the organization of sex for the purposes of economic discipline (the repression of sex as a distraction from work) and family formation (sex as procreation). Instead, Freud believed that sexual energies must be transformed, through repression and sublimation, into new forms of energy that are more compatible with "civilized society"such as the dedication to work and cultural production—by his account, sublimated sexuality put extraordinarily large amounts of energy at the disposal of social activities.

The sexual theories of Herbert Marcuse and Norman O. Brown were way stations on the road to this intellectual and political transformation. They both conceived of sexuality as a transcendent realm of personal freedom. Their respective books *Eros and Civilization* (Marcuse) and *Life Against Death* (Brown) offered dramatic re-interpretations of the Freudian theory of repression and society. They each attacked the tyranny of genital organization of the sexuality, with its stress on heterosexual intercourse. According to Freud, the adult's sexual development had progressed from infancy organized around oral and anal eroticism to the final adult stage of genital sexuality. In its stead, Marcuse and Brown proposed sexual liberation through the cultivation of a "polymorphous perverse" sexuality (which included oral, anal and genital eroticism) that eschewed a narrow focus on genital heterosexual intercourse. According to Marcuse, sexual liberation was achieved by exploring new permutations of sexual desires, sexual activities and gender roles—what Freud called 'perverse' sexual desires, that is, all non-reproductive forms of sexual behavior of which kissing, oral or anal sex are familiar examples. Marcuse identified the homosexual as the radical standard bearer of sex for the sake of pleasure, a form of radical hedonism that repudiates those forms of repressive sexuality organized around genital heterosexuality and sex exclusively for biological reproduction.

Marcuse also rejected Freud's conservative view of the value of sublimation. Instead, he argued for the possibility of, what he called, "non-repressive sublimation"—a form of sublimation that diverted libidinal energies to social activities without narrowly focusing on heterosexual genital sexuality and procreation. This kind of "non-repressive sublimation" would also allow for new forms of work based on non-alienated labor as well as the creation of new kinds of libidinal communities.

Both Marcuse and Norman O. Brown (who had a more mystical approach and was much less political) had an enormous influence on the early theories of sexual liberation, particularly in the gay movement and on the left. Many young people in the sixties adopted a sexual politics resembling Marcuse's as the basis for the counterculture's "radical transformation of values" and by exploring drugs, music and sex, they sought to experience, what Brown called, an "erotic sense of reality."

However, Marcuse had begun to experience serious misgivings about sexual liberation as it played out in American's advanced industrial society. He was increasingly concerned that sexual liberation was impossible. In *One-Dimensional Man*, his most influential book during the sixties, he argued that the un-sublimated (or "de-sublimated") sexuality released by the sexual revolution was channeled into commercialized forms of advertising and entertainment and into institutionalized forms of aggression, and that it was, in fact, isolated from broader forms of erotic life. Sexuality freed from the constraints of repression and sublimation was exploited by capitalist businesses which harnessed the liberated—"de-sublimated"—libidinal energies to increase productivity and to generate increased consumption through the use of sex appeal in marketing, rather than by encouraging new social forms of erotic communities or pleasant and fulfilling work environments.

Nevertheless, the process of sexual revolution during the sixties and seventies undermined many of the social structures of sexual repression and led to new social patterns, attitudes, and ways of sexually interacting—this took place both through individual actions and through those undertaken by the various social movements dedicated to sexual liberation. The Freudian tradition—both Reich and Marcuse worked in that tradition—had failed to anticipate such an historical process. Instead, John Gagnon and William Simon, two sociologists working at the Kinsey Institute in the late sixties and early seventies, developed a way of thinking that reflected the experience of the sixties and seventies. Gagnon and Simon understood sexual behavior was a process of learning, one that is possible, not because of instinctual drives or physiological requirements, but because it is embedded in complex social scripts that are specific to particular locations in culture and history. Their approach stressed the significance of individual agency and cultural symbols in the conduct of our sexual activities. They had redefined sexuality from being the combined product of biological drives and social repression into one of creative social initiative and symbolic action.

Freud and Marcuse had assumed that society regulated perverse sexual energies primarily through repression and/or sublimation, but the success of the sexual revolution had shown that Freud and Reich's repression hypothesis failed to anticipate the course of a sexual revolution. By the end of the seventies, Michel Foucault argued, like Gagnon and Simon, that the proliferation of discourses on sex—whether the theories and ideas of psychiatry, medicine or statistics, the patterns of social interaction, or popular cultural beliefs—stimulates the development of certain sexualities. In his *History of Sexuality: An Introduction*, Foucault showed that certain late-eighteenth-century and nineteenth-century discourses (such as medicine and psychiatry) articulated a series of pathological sexual stereotypes that exerted a tremendous influence up through the twentieth century: the masturbating child, the hysterical woman, the Malthusian couple (who practiced birth control), and the homosexual. Through the construction of these "identities,"society is able to govern what would otherwise be an uncontrolled underground sexuality. Thus sexual revolution and its discourses of sexual liberation, in Foucault's theory, both emancipates those who are stigmatized for their sexuality and facilitates the governing of these newly emancipated identities. It was one of Foucault's most bitter truths that every socially institutionalized form of sexual liberation only furthered disciplinary and normalizing processes that controlled sexual expression and behavior. Yet he also believed that only the active struggle for the freedom to explore "our bodies and pleasures"allows us to also resist, modify or restructure the disciplinary and normalizing mechanisms that shapes our sexuality.

The Sixties Are Gone: The Aftershocks

The '60s are gone, dope will never be as cheap, sex never as free, and the rock and roll never as great. —Abbie Hoffman

In time, the sexual revolution would provoke a profound and powerful counter-revolution—led by the religious right, one of whose fundamental goals is to turn back the sexual revolution. It spawned new organizations, elected political representatives, passed legislation, fought to defund sexually progressive programs and to fund sexually conservative programs. Battles between sexual progressives and religious conservatives continue to take place up until the present. What many commentators have called "the culture wars" are, in part, a counter-attack on the sexual revolution. The religious right continues to wage a battle against the forces—the women's movement, the gay and lesbian movement, pornography, and over the issues such as homosexuality, abortion, sex education, and non-marital sexuality that originally ignited the revolution.

The sexual revolution also encountered obstacles of another sort— sexually transmitted diseases (STD). The diseases spread by sex are numerous and ancient: gonorrhea, syphilis, genital warts, genital herpes, hepatitis B. Starting in the late seventies, there were a growing number of reports about STD—both *Time* and *Newsweek* produced cover stories on herpes, and the gay male communities were swept by waves of gonorrhea, syphilis and Hepatitis B. The discovery of an AIDS epidemic among gay men in the early eighties provoked a major crisis in sexual politics of the gay community. Medical researchers and gay leaders struggled to find ways of stopping the epidemic without completely excluding all sexual activity. Eventually a number of gay activists invented "safer sex"—in which gay men could engage in sex, using condoms, without transmitting the virus (HIV) that causes AIDS. Soon after, safer sex was adopted by public health educators and AIDS activists as the basis for HIV prevention. Safer sex and traditional public health treatment programs for the older STDs have since reduced the spread of these diseases considerably. (Escoffier 1999)

The sexual revolution is the historical culmination of processes begun long before—during World War II—and it has continued to produce significant changes in the decades that followed. The term "revolution"usually implies something that occurs rapidly and dramatically. However, the time frame of the sexual revolution is much longer: it more resembles the time frame of "the industrial revolution"—the transition from an agricultural society to one built on new technologies and industrial production). It is an immense and contradictory process, stretching out over the life span of two generations. This sexual revolution has radically altered our lives as gendered and sexual human beings.

Pure Possibility

Foreword

Erica Jong

A ll modern revolutions have begun on the printed page and these are the texts that fired the second great sexual revolution of the twentieth century, the one that began in 1967 and ended in 1975 with the close of the Viet Nam war. It dragged on for another few years through the sheer force of inertia, but when the heart went out of the antiwar movement (middle class white kids stopped being drafted), the sexual revolution sputtered too. It left its legacy to be sure, but it was officially dead by the time Ronald Reagan got elected in 1980 and ever since then we have been in a period of prolonged reaction—overreaction you might say—to the brief period of exuberant freedom called "The Sixties."

And how exuberant it was! What I remember about that sliver of time (not even a decade) is how excited we were reading these texts. One would read with a pen in hand to underline. One's heart would race, one's underwear grow wet. The word had the power to do all that. We truly believed we were on the verge of a New World. (A few bars of Dvorak here.)

Of course the Clinton years showed us that many ideals of "The Sixties" had been absorbed into the mainstream, but his impeachment reaffirmed that Puritanism in America was hardly dead, it was only playing peek-a-boo. Since Clinton's "disgrace" and the resultant triumph of the Bush-Cheney oil cartel, it has become clear how truly ephemeral "The Sixties" were.

Now, some thirty plus years later, when reading (if you can call it that) is the dull, predictable province of sausage-makers Steele, Grisham, Patterson, and various schlock romance writers who used to be paperbacked, when all but a few publishers have totally capitulated to the commodified reading tastes of Sam's Club and Costco, it is hard to even remember the rapture of those times. The word mattered. And here are the words that mattered most.

Jeffrey Escoffier has bravely assembled the texts that underlay (excuse the pun) that particular sexual revolution, the successor to the nineteen twenties' discovery of "flaming youth." This evanescent epoch, popularly called "The Sixties" (by those unborn then), actually took place in the late sixties and first half of the seventies. Like a complex nebula of fireworks, it died almost as soon as it was born. But it was enshrined in the collective memory of the media as a dazzling moment of youth and light—and almost immediately distorted into something it was not.

The media remembers it as drugs n' rock n' roll and free sex. I remember it as a time of pure possibility.

Suddenly, everything was possible. Women could be free of the prison of bourgeois marriage. Men could live their wildest fantasies. Men and women could tell each other the truth about their feelings. Sexual hypocrisy could go the way of the chastity belt. Clothes could be colorful and comfortable. Hair could go extravagantly uncoiffed. Gay people could celebrate their sexuality. Black people could love their skin and ringlets. Girls could taste their menstrual blood and discover it was, if not delicious, then at least not disgusting. Boys could admit to liking the taste of pussy. Masturbation could be celebrated as a sacrament. Pornography could be read and analyzed, watched and discussed. Fiction writers could enter the bedroom without trailing asterisks. Poets could call cocks and cunts cocks and cunts. Artists could do away with fig leaves. Musicians could experiment with different harmonies, even silences. Scientists could experiment with psychedelic drugs and learn why so many cultures had used them in religious rites throughout history. Publishers could vie with each other to publish the most far-out books—and some of them, like *The Whole Earth Catalog, Zen and the Art of Motorcycle Maintenance,* and *Fear of Flying,* could even make fortunes. Experimentation was as rampant as marijuana smoke. Even movie companies, book publishers and music companies wanted to sign radical artists. The focus group and the ubiquitous computer were yet to be widely adopted. Editors and executives actually acquired works based on their own gut feelings. Personal taste was not yet suspect.

This was not a time of groping and grabbing but of realization and recognition. The groping and grabbing were collateral. We were hoping to grope at and grab the truth. For there is no mistaking the fact that it was truth we were seeking. If this quest now seems utterly silly it is because the success of the reactionaries has been almost total.

Now that youth's search for truth has become youth's search for cynicism, it is easy to see "The Sixties" as the orgy of self-indulgence the corporate media wants to make of it. This was far, far from the truth. (Though what other point of view can you expect of corporations that make munitions, television programs and report the "news"?)

Sure, there were people even back then who commercialized and exploited the search for truth. (Remember the Woodstock festival? Remember *Deep Throat*?) And there were conscienceless thugs who made fortunes off what used to be called hard-core porn (a term that became quaint as the mass media wholly assimilated its techniques and profits). We are speaking of fallen human beings after all.

But at the base of what is called "The Sixties" there was something touchingly innocent. We wanted to penetrate the veil of human delusion. We wanted to perceive life and death plainly. We wanted to understand civilization and its discontents. We wanted to pierce the wild heart of sex. We wanted to see the world in a grain of sand and eternity in a wild flower. (It was no accident that Allen Ginsberg revered William Blake above all artists).

For "The Sixties" were, in a way, an extension of the Enlightenment. We had the same besotted belief in reason—and like all who worship reason we also sought the derangement of the senses. The Age of Reason succumbs to the Age of Romanticism. In truth the two are Siamese twins. Reason seeks its opposite in Romanticism. And Romanticism is nearly always followed by Reaction.

So here are the texts that made "The Sixties" and also doomed us to the Age of George W. Bush. Bush is as much a product of "The Sixties" as Osama bin Laden. If it were not for that dazzling breath of freedom and possibility, we would not have religious fundamentalists like these two trying to turn the world back to the Dark Ages.

Looking back on "The Sixties" now is a lot like looking back on the Weimar Republic from the vantage point of Kristallnacht. Freedom was ours once and then the Brown Shirts came and clubbed it away. We don't have to burn books any more if we can only publish sausages. We don't have to censor people if we can make them censor themselves. We don't have to fear art and music and literature. We can merely cut off its funding and send the money to the military industrial complex.

Reading these effervescent texts took me back to a time of ferment and hope. The principal feeling I had examining this expansive collection was nostalgia for all we have lost.

Above all, we have lost hope. We hoped to end all war, create a nuclear-free world, end the battle between the sexes, create equality of opportunity where there was inequality, liberate gay people from prejudice, open all the doors to people of color, allow freedom of worship of every kind except state religion and put a flower in the muzzle of each gun. Not only are we further from this than ever but our children mock these dreams as impossible. Impossible is the devil's favorite word. When the next generation despairs of all that is impossible, the Kingdom of Darkness cannot be far behind.

So go back to that time of possibility. Read Angela Carter's brilliant "Pornography in the Service of Women." Revel in Mary Jane Sherfey's exploration of female insatiability, "A Theory of Female Sexuality." (This was a text I loved when I was young). Explore Henry Miller's classic essay on obscenity from *Remember to Remember*, "Obscenity and the Law of Reflection" (one of the truest analyses of the erotic in literature ever written). Re-read Steven Marcus on Victorian Pornotopia. Study the Sigmund Freud, Wilhelm Reich, Simone de Beauvoir and Herbert Marcuse texts that started it all. Consider Reich's assertion that the "unconscious content" of "ecclesiastical, fascist and other reactionary ideologies" are "essentially defense reactions. They are formed for fear of the unconscious inferno which everyone carries within himself." Reich sees sexual liberation and progressive politics as going together—and our contemporary situation clearly proves him right. His writings influenced every avatar of sexual revolution from Simone de Beauvoir to Norman Mailer to William Burroughs and

Allen Ginsberg. His conviction that sexual repression leads to author-itarian behavior must be reevaluated in our time. Now that we have a dry drunk, born-again Christian President threatening nuclear Armageddon against the Third World, Reich's theories clearly merit a closer look. Unfortunately he has been remembered only for his unfor-tunate Orgone Box. Jeffrey Escoffier rightly revives his writings—along with Sigmund Freud's and Herbert Marcuse's. We cannot understand "The Sixties" without looking at its vast intellectual underpinnings. And some of the most important essays are here.

There is also lighter matter which remains amazingly fresh. Delight in Helen Gurley Brown's goodbye to sexless spinsterhood. Enjoy Betty Dodson's examination of self-pleasuring as the key to all good sex. Explore Nancy Friday's revelation of male and female fantasy. Follow Gay Talese to Sandstone and Timothy Leary to an LSD nirvana.

Read Bernard-Henry Levy's interview with Michel Foucault and understand how far Foucault is from what his followers have made of him. Read, if you can (for it is deliberately not written in English), the famous Masters and Johnson text that told us all about the physiology of orgasm. Read the essays by Pat Califia, Jill Johnston and others that brought gay sex out of the closet.

Not everything from that exhilarating period is here but there is enough to make the open-minded reader understand that "The Sixties" were not just about sex n' drugs n' rock n' roll. They constituted an age of innocence, exploration and possibility—possibility we desperately need now. I fervently pray that reading these exhilarating works will rekindle some of the vitality and experimentalism of that meteoric period.

Or maybe it is the hope in these pages that we need most: hope, that thing with feathers that tells us we can fly.

August 7, 2003

PART I

Recognitions

• • •

What is a sexual revolution? Fluctuations in the frequency and kind of sexual activity have taken place in many historical periods and cultures —most are local and limited to one aspect of sexual life and they do not necessarily reflect deep structural change. Shifts in sexual behavior do not leave many traces in the historical record, except for information that can be gleaned from birth and marriage records or from public pronouncements of moral guardians such as sermons, newspaper editorials, or from the writers of erotic literature. The term "revolution" often implies something that occurs rapidly and dramatically, but sexual revolution as it emerged in the sixties is based on a different model of historical change. Large-scale changes in attitudes and behavior took place over more than two decades. In addition, it radically altered the social relation in American society between sex and gender.

Throughout history, sexual behavior that took place outside of marriage or that did not lead to procreation has been either quietly tolerated or vigorously suppressed. Even in the early American colonies settled by Puritans (New England), Quakers (Pennsylvania), and Catholics (Maryland), attitudes towards sexual expression could vary significantly over time. The Puritans, in particular, had a healthy respect for the joys of marital sex, but sexual behavior also had bearing on their religious beliefs, the size of community and its ability to feed itself, and on the maintenance of family institutions and the civil order.

Alfred Kinsey's reports *Sexual Behavior in Human Male* (1948) and *Sexual Behavior in the Human Female* (1954) made Americans aware of how little they knew about people's sexual behavior. While Kinsey's research had focused on the inter-war generations, the reports came to symbolize the dramatic changes that emerged in the late 50s and early sixties in the popular consciousness and in the history of American culture. Kinsey's unpublished research showed traces of an earlier wave of sexual revolution, but these data were not published in either of the two reports.

The appearance of the banner "Sex in the U.S." on the cover of *Time* magazine (on January 24, 1964) referred to a lead article on "the second sexual revolution"—one of the first indications that a dramatic shift was taking place. Despite the nod to Wilhelm Reich and his orgone boxes, for the editors of *Time* magazine, the arrival of the "second sexual revolution" was signaled by an increase in sexually explicit culture—what they called "Spectator Sex." The magazine's editors took for granted that the twentieth-century experienced two sexual revolutions—one in the years during and after World War I, the second then beginning to emerge in the early 1960s.

The article capitalizes on the growing public interest in sex since the late forties—a flood of novels, magazine articles, and advice books dealing with sexuality had grown dramatically since the end of World War II. Novels by Henry Miller, William Burroughs, and Norman Mailer; *Playboy* magazine, and sexual explicitness in Broadway plays seemed to lead to the demise of the old religious morality that *Time* called "Puritanism." Over the next few years, articles also appeared in *America* (1965), a magazine published by the Catholic Church, and in *Ebony* (1966), a mass market magazine with a predominately African-American readership.

The cultural atmosphere of the sixties—particularly what was referred to as "the counterculture"—emerged clearly only later in the decade. The popularity of rock music, the increased use of marijuana, LSD and other drugs among youth, widespread public displays of nudity, and a new openness about sexuality contributed to the awareness of radical cultural change. Most of the sexual behavior that constitute what we call the sexual revolution refers to non-marital sexual activity. By the early sixties, shifts had begun to take place along several fronts that consolidated the sexual revolution. One of the most important was that young men and women engaged in their first acts of sexual intercourse at increasingly younger ages. The impact of earlier sexual experimentation was reinforced by the later age of marriage; thus young men and women have more time available to acquire sexual experience with partners before entering upon a long-term monogamous relationship. In addition, the growing number of marriages resulting in divorce provided another opportunity for men and women (to a lesser degree) to engage in non-monogamous sexual activity. All three of these developments allowed the generation born between 1935-1945 to experience sexual activity with a larger number of sexual partners in their lifetime than most men and women born earlier.

The Second Sexual Revolution

Time, January 24, 1964

*This **Time** magazine article was in some ways an impressively learned essay on the history of sexuality, a field of study acknowledged by few historians. What is especially interesting is that the sexual revolution of the early sixties is authoritatively identified as the second sexual revolution; the first having taken place in the years following World War I. By differentiating between a first and second sexual revolution and making the essay an example of comparative historical analysis, it suggested that there are identifiable historical conditions underlying the shift in sexual attitudes and behavior.*

The Orgone Box is a half-forgotten invention of the late Dr. Wilhelm Reich, one of Sigmund Freud's more brilliant disciples, who in his middle years turned into an almost classic specimen of the mad scientist. The device was supposed to gather, in physical form, that life force which Freud called libido and which Reich called orgone, a coinage derived from "orgasm." The narrow box, simply constructed of wood and lined with sheet metal, offered cures for almost all the ills of civilization and of the body; it was also widely believed to act, for the person sitting inside it, as a powerful sex stimulant. Hundreds of people hopefully bought it before the U.S. Government declared the device a fraud in 1954 and jailed its inventor. And yet, in a special sense, Dr. Reich may have been a prophet. For now it sometimes seems that all America is one big Orgone Box.

With today's model, it is no longer necessary to sit in cramped quarters for a specific time. Improved and enlarged to encompass the continent, the big machine works on its subjects continuously, day and night. From innumerable screens and stages, posters and pages, it flashes the larger-than-life-sized images of sex. From countless racks and shelves, it pushes the books which a few years ago were considered pornography. From myriad loudspeakers, it broadcasts the words and rhythms of pop-music erotica. And constantly, over the intellectual Muzak, comes the message that sex will save you and libido make you free.

The U.S. is still a long way from the rugged debaucheries of Restoration England or the perfumed corruption of the Gallant Century in France. But Greeks who have grown up with the memory of Aphrodite can only gape at the American goddesses, silken and seminude, in a million advertisements. Indians who have seen the temple sculptures of Konarak can only marvel at some of the illustrated matter sold in American drugstores; and Frenchmen who consider themselves the world's arbiters on the subject, can only smile at the urgency attached to it by Americans. The U.S. seems to be undergoing a revolution of mores and an erosion of morals that is turning it into what Reich called a "sex-affirming culture."

Two Generations. Men with memories ask, "What, again?" The first sexual revolution followed World War I, when flaming youth buried the Victorian era and anointed itself as the Jazz Age. In many ways it was an innocent revolution. In *This Side of Paradise,* F. Scott Fitzgerald alarmed mothers by telling them "how casually their danghters were accustomed to being kissed"; today mothers thank their stars if kissing is all their daughters are accustomed to. It was, nevertheless, a revolution that took nerve, and it was led by the daring few; today's is far more broadly based. In the 1920s, to praise sexual freedom was still outrageous; today sex is simply no longer shocking, in life or literature.

The difference between the '20s and '60s comes down, in part, to a difference between people. The rebels of the '20s had Victorian parents who laid down a Victorian law; it was something concrete and fairly well-defined to rise up against. The rebels of the '60s have parents with only the tattered remnants of a code, expressed for many of them in Ernest Hemingway's one-sentence manifesto: "What is moral is what you feel good after, and what is immoral is what you feel bad after." Adrift in a sea of permissiveness, they have little to rebel against. Parents, educators and the guardians of morality at large do pull themselves together to say "don't," but they usually sound halfhearted. Closed minds have not disappeared, but as a society, the U.S. seems to be dominated by what Congregationalist Minister and Educator Robert Elliot Fitch calls an "orgy of open-mindedness." Faith and principle are far from dead— but what stands out is an often desperate search for "new standards for a new age."

Wide-open Atmosphere. Thus everybody talks about the current sexual situation; but does everyone know what he's talking about? No new Kinsey report or Gallup poll can chart the most private—and most universal—of subjects. What people say does not necessarily reflect what they do, and what they do does not necessarily show how they feel about it. Yet out of an aggregate of words and actions, every society makes a statement about itself. Methodist Bishop Gerald Kennedy of Los Angeles sums it up: "The atmosphere is wide open. There is more promiscuity, and it is taken as a matter of course now by people. In my day they did it, but they knew it was wrong."

Publicly and dramatically, the change is evident in Spectator Sex— what may be seen and read. Thirty-five years ago, *Elmer Gantry* and *All Quiet on the Western Front* were banned in Boston; today Supreme Court decisions have had the net effect of allowing everything to be published except "hard-core pornography." It is hard to remember that as recently as 1948, in *The Naked and the Dead*, Norman Mailer felt compelled to reduce his favorite four letters to three ("fug"), or that there was ever any fuss about poor old *Lady Chatterley's Lover* and his worshipful deification of sexual organs. John O'Hara, whose writing until recently was criticized as "sex-obsessed," appears positively Platonic alongside Calder Willingham and John Updike, who describe lyrically and in detail matters that used to be mentioned even in scientific works only in Latin.

Then there is Henry Miller with his scabrous *Tropics*, and William Burroughs *Naked Lunch*, an incredible piece of hallucinatory homosexual depravity. And if these are classed as literature and are democratically available at the neighborhood drugstore, who is going to stop the cheap pornographer from putting out *Lust Hop, Lust Jungle, Lust Kicks, Lust Lover, Lust Lease, Lust Moll, Lust Team, Lust Girls,* and *Call Boy?* In girlie magazines, nudity stops only at the *mons Veneris—et quandoque ne ibi quidem.* Asks Dr. Paul Gebhard, the late Alfred Kinsey's successor at Indiana University's

Institute for Sex Research: "What do you do after you show it all? I've talked to some of the publishers, and they are a little worried."

The Next Step. The cult of pop hedonism and phony sexual sophistication grows apace. It produces such books as *Sex and the Single Man*, in which Dr. Albert Ellis, a supposedly reputable psychologist, offers crude but obvious instructions on how to seduce a girl, and the Playboy Clubs, which are designed to look wicked except that no one is supposed even to touch the "Bunnies"—creating the teasing impression of brothels without a second story. But by no means all of Spectator Sex is unpleasant. American clothes nowadays manage to be both free and attractive—necklines are down, skirts are up, ski pants are tight, girdles are out, and figures are better than ever, to which there can be very few objections.

Hollywood, of course, suggests more of morals and immorals to more people than any other single force. Gone with Marilyn Monroe is the last, and perhaps the greatest, of the sex symbols. Lesser girls in ever crasser if no more honest stories now symbolize very little except Hollywood's desire to outshock TV (easy because the living room still imposes some restraints) and outsex foreign movies (impossible). European films have the best-looking girls; they also have a natural, if sometimes amoral, attitude toward sex, somewhere between a shrug and a prayer, between desire and fatigue, which makes Hollywood eroticism seem coyly fraudulent.

As for Broadway, quite a few plays lately have opened with a couple in bed—to show right away, as Critic Walter Kerr says, that the male is not a homosexual. As another critic has seriously suggested, the next step in the theater will be to represent sexual intercourse onstage. Meanwhile, the forthcoming musical, *What Makes Sammy Run?*, at least represents how to feel about it. In a pleasant but unmistakable song, one of Sammy's girls croons, without reference to love or even to passion:

Drinks are okay, they break the ice,
Dancing this way is also nice.
But why delay the friendliest thing two people can do?
When it can be the sweetest and,
Let's face it, the completest and friendliest thing
Two people can do![1]

1. Copyright 1963 by Ervin Drake. Reprinted by permission of Harms, Inc.

The Unique Conflict. It remains for each man and woman to walk through this sexual bombardment and determine for themselves what to them seems tasteless or objectionable, entertaining or merely dull. A healthy society must assume a certain degree of immunity on the part of its people. But no one can really calculate the effect this exposure is having on individual lives and minds. Above all, it is not an isolated phenomenon. It is part and symptom of an era in which morals are widely held to be both private and relative, in which pleasure is increasingly considered an almost constitutional right rather than a privilege, in which self-denial is increasingly seen as foolishness rather than virtue. While science has reduced fear of long-dreaded earthly dangers, such as pregnancy and VD, skepticism has diminished fear of divine punishment. In short, the Puritan ethic, so long the dominant moral force in the U.S., is widely considered to be dying, if not dead, and there are few mourners.

The demise of Puritanism—whether permanent or not remains to be seen—is the latest phase in a conflict, as old as Christianity itself, between Eros and agape, between passionate love named for a pagan god and spiritual love through which man imitates God. It is a conflict unique to the Christian West. The religions of many other civilizations provide a clearly defined and positive place for sex. In the West, the tension between the two, and the general confusion about the many facets of love, leads to a kind of self-torment that, says Italian Author Leo Ferrero, "might well appear to a Chinese psychiatrist as symptomatic of insanity."

The Decline of Puritanism. Yet that "insanity" is among the great mysteries and challenges of the Christian tradition—the belief that sex is not only the force by which man perpetuates himself on God's earth but also the symbol of his fall, and that it can be sanctified only in the sacrament of marriage.

The original American Puritans understood passion as well as human frailty: in Plymouth in the 1670s, while ordinary fornicators were fined £10, those who were engaged had to pay only half the fine. But a fatal fact about Puritanism, which led to its ever-increasing narrowness and decline, was its conviction that virtue could be legislated by the community, that human perfection could be organized on earth.

What the first sexual revolution in the U.S. attacked was not original

Puritanism so much as its Victorian version—which had become a matter of prudery more than of purity, propriety more than of grace. The 19th century frantically insisted on propriety precisely because it felt its real faith and ethics disappearing. While it feared nudity like a plague, Victorian Puritanism had the effect of an all-covering gown that only inflames the imagination. By insisting on suppressing the sex instinct in everything, "the age betrayed the fact that it really saw that instinct in everything. So, too, with Sigmund Freud, Victorianism's most perfect rebel.

Romantic Revolt. Freudian psychology, or its popularized version, became one of the chief forces that combined against Puritanism. Gradually, the belief spread that repression, not license, was the great evil, and that sexual matters belonged in the realm of science, not morals. A second force was the New Woman, who swept aside the Victorian double standard, which was partly based on the almost universally held notion that women—or at any rate, ladies—did not enjoy sex. One eminent doctor said it was a "foul aspersion" on women to say they did. The celebrated 2nd century Physician Galen was (and is) often incompletely quoted to the effect that "every animal is sad after coitus." Actually, as Kinsey pointed out, he had added the qualification, "except the human female and the rooster." Siding with Galen, women claimed not only the right to work and to vote, but the even more important right to pleasure.

These two allies against Puritanism seemed to be joined by Eros in person. The cult of romantic passion, with its assertion that true love could exist only outside marriage, had first challenged Christianity in the 12th century; some consider it an uprising of the old paganism long ago, driven underground by the church. From *Tristan* on, romance shaped the great literary myths of the West and became a kind of secular religion. Christianity learned to coexist with it.

But in the early 20th century, the religion of romance appeared in a new form, and its troubadour was D. H. Lawrence. Until then, it had been tinged by the polite and melancholy suggestion that desire, not fulfillment, was the best part of love. Lawrence countered vehemently that fulfillment is everything, that sex is the one great, true thing in life. More explicitly than anyone before him, he sentimentalized the orgasm, in whose "final massive and dark collision of the blood" he saw man's apotheosis and fusion with the divine.

Beyond Prohibition. Christianity does not share this mystique of sex, insisting that the primary purpose of the sexual act as ordained by God is procreation. It never considered the flesh to be intrinsically evil. But for a thousand years, the Church was deeply influenced by the views of St. Augustine, a profligate in his youth and a moralist in middle age, who held that even within marriage, sex and its pleasures were dangerous—a necessary evil for the begetting of children. Gradually, partly under the influence of the Reformation, which denied the "higher value" of celibacy, Christianity began to move away from this austere Augustinian view, and toward an acceptance of pleasure in sex as a positive good.

In 1951, Pope Pius XII still warned against un-Christian hedonism, but reaffirmed it was right that "husband and wife shall find pleasure and happiness of mind and body." Today, says Father John Thomas, noted Roman Catholic sociologist, "what is needed is a whole new attitude by the church toward sexuality. There is in both Catholicism and Protestantism a relatively well-developed theology of sex on the negative side. Now more than prohibition is needed."

The Protestant churches have indeed gone far beyond prohibition through their wide approval of birth control not only as an aid in sensible family planning but, in the words of the Anglican bishops at the 1958 Lambeth conference, as a "gate to a new depth and joy in personal relationships between husband and wife." Ironically, it is Communism, having long ago silenced all its bold talk about "free love," which may be the most puritanical force in the world today. In *1984*, George Orwell attributed the old Victorian code to his fictional dictatorship: "goodsex" was marital intercourse without pleasure on the part of the woman, "sexcrime" was everything else.

Search for Codes. A great many Americans—probably the majority—live by the old religious morality. Or at least they try to; they may practice what Max Lerner describes as "patterned evasion," a heavy but charitable way of saying that to keep society going people must be free, up to a point, not to practice what they profess.

Many others now live by what State University of Iowa Sociologist Ira Reiss calls "permissiveness with affection." What this means to most people is that: 1) morals are a private affair; 2) being in love justifies pre-marital sex, and by implication perhaps extramarital sex; 3) nothing really is wrong as long as nobody else "gets hurt."

This happens to be reminiscent of the moral code expressed in *Memoirs of a Woman of Pleasure*, otherwise known as *Fanny Hill*, the celebrated 18th century pornographic novel now freely available in the U.S. One of the principals "considered pleasure, of one sort or another, as the universal port of destination, and every wind that blew thither a good one, provided it blew nobody any harm."

No Absolutes. One trouble with this very humane-sounding principle is that it is extremely difficult, if not impossible, to know what, in the long run, will hurt others and what won't. Thus, in spite of what may often appear to be a sincere concern for others, it remains an essentially self-centered code. In his categorical imperative, Kant set down the opposite standard, a variation of the Golden Rule: Judge your every action as if it were to become a universal principle applicable to all.

Undoubtedly, that is a difficult code to live by, and few try to. But living by a lesser code can be difficult too, as is shown by the almost frantic attempt of sociologists and psychologists to give people something to hold on to without falling back on traditional rules. Typical of many is the effort of Lester A. Kirkendall of Oregon State University, in his recent book, *Premarital Intercourse and Interpersonal Relationships:* "The moral decision will be the one which works toward the creation of trust, confidence and integrity in relationships." What such well-intentioned but tautologous and empty advice may mean in practice is suggested by one earnest teacher who praises the Kirkendall code: "Now I have an answer. I just tell the girls and boys that they have to consider both sides of the question—will sexual intercourse strengthen or weaken their relationship?"

The "relationship" ethic is well expressed by Miami Psychologist Granville Fisher, who speaks for countless colleagues when he says: "Sex is not a moral question. For answers you don't turn to a body of absolutes. The criterion should not be, 'Is it morally right or wrong,' but, 'Is it socially feasible, is it personally healthy and rewarding, will it enrich human life?' " Dr. Fisher adds, correctly, that many Protestant churchmen are beginning to feel the same way. "They are no longer shaking their finger because the boys and girls give in to natural biological urges and experiment a bit. They don't say, 'Stop, you're wrong,' but, 'Is it meaningful?' "

Methodist Bishop Kennedy condemns premarital sex "in general" but adds, "I wouldn't stand in judgment. There would be exceptions." Recently, Wally Toevs, Presbyterian pastor at the University of Colorado, more or less condoned premarital sex when there is a "covenant of intimacy." A distinguished Protestant theologian privately recommends—he doesn't believe the U.S. is ready for him to say it publicly—the idea of a trial affair for some people, a "little marriage" in preparation for the "great marriage" which is to last.

Too Much, Too Soon. From current reports on youth, "meaningful relationships" and "covenants of intimacy" are rampant. Teen-agers put great stock in staying cool. But even discounting the blasé talk, the notion is widely accepted today on the basis of Kinsey and a few smaller, more recent studies, that the vast majority of American men and at least half the women now have sexual intercourse before marriage. Dr. Graham B. Blaine Jr., psychiatrist to the Harvard and Radcliffe Health Service, estimates that within the past 15 years the number of college boys who had intercourse before graduation rose from 50% to 60%, the number of college girls from 25% to 40%. A Purdue sociologist estimates that one out of six brides is pregnant.

These figures may be flawed, and they certainly do not apply to all parts of the U.S. or to all schools. But there is almost universal agreement that youngsters are pushed toward adult behavior too soon, often by ambitious mothers who want them to be "well adjusted" and popular; hence champagne parties for teen-agers, padded brassières for twelve-year-olds, and "going steady" at ever younger ages. American youngsters tend to live as if adolescence were a last fling at life, rather than a preparation for it. Historian Arnold Toynbee, for one, considers this no laughing matter, for part of the modern West's creative energy, he believes, has sprung from the ability to postpone adolescents' "sexual awakening" to let them concentrate on the acquisition of knowledge.

Most significant of all, the age-old moral injunctions are less readily accepted by the young—partly because they sense that so many parents don't really believe in them either.

Crisis of Virginity. "Nice girls don't" is undoubtedly still the majority view, but definitely weakening, as is "No nice boy will respect you if you go to bed with him." A generation ago, college boys strayed off campus to seek out professionals; today they are generally looked down on if they can't succeed with a coed.

In a way, the situation is the logical consequence of U.S. attitudes toward youth. In other societies, the young are chaperoned and restricted because it is assumed, human nature being what it is, that if they are exposed to temptation they will give in. The U.S., on the other hand, has set the young free, given them cars, given them prosperity—and yet still expects them to follow the rules. The compromise solution to this dilemma has long been petting, or "making out," as it is now known, which the U.S. did not invent but has carried to extreme lengths.

Now there are signs of resentment against a practice that overstimulates but blocks fulfillment. The resentment, however, is taking forms that alarm many parents. In a sweeping generalization, Dr. Blaine reports that "Radcliffe girls think petting is dirty because it is teasing. They feel if you are going to do that, it is better just to have intercourse." This may apply to some, but, as Harvard's President Pusey reported in a speech last week, 80% of Radcliffe girls get degrees with honors, "so they can't do all that running around they're supposed to."

Many girls are still sincere and even lyrical about saving themselves for marriage, but it is becoming a lot harder to hold the line. There is strong pressure not only from the boys but from other girls, many of whom consider a virgin downright square. The loss of virginity, even resulting in pregnancy, is simply no longer considered an American Tragedy. Says one student of the American vernacular: "The word virgin is taking on a slightly new meaning. It seems acceptable to consider a girl a virgin if she has had experience with only her husband before marriage, or with only one or two steadies." At a girls' college in Connecticut, one coed recently wrote a poem about the typical Yale man which concluded:
And so I yield myself completely to him.
Society says I should.
Damn society!

Talk of the Pill. Some girls are bothered to the point of consulting analysts when they find that having an affair makes them uneasy; since everyone is telling them that sex is healthy, they feel guilty about feeling guilty. Some girls, says an Atlanta analyst, "are disturbed because they are no longer able to use fear of pregnancy as an excuse for chastity." In many parts of the country, physicians report the use of Saran Wrap as a male contraceptive, but such improvisation seems hardly necessary, since birth control devices of all kinds are sold freely, often at supermarkets. Parents have been known to buy diaphragms for their daughters (although in Cleveland recently, a woman was arrested for giving birth control information to her delinquent daughter).

The big new development is the oral contraceptive pill, widely used and even more widely discussed both at college and at home. A considerate boy asks a girl politely, "Are you on pills?" If not, he takes the precautions himself. Current joke definition of a good sport: A wife who keeps taking the Pill even when her husband is away.

In spite of all this, the number of illegitimate children born to teenage mothers rose from 8.4 per thousand in 1940 to 16 in 1961, in the 20-to-25 age group from 11.2 per thousand to 41.2. Some girls neglect to use contraceptives, psychologists report, because they consciously or unconsciously want a child, others resent the planned, deliberate aspect; they think it "nicer" to get carried away on the spur of the moment. College girls have been known to take up collections for a classmate who needed an abortion, and some have had one without skipping a class.

Girls Aren't Things. Still, by and large, campus sex is not casual. Boys look down on a "community chest," meaning a promiscuous girl. Sociologist David Riesman believes that, far more so than in the '20s, boys treat girls as persons rather than objects: "They sit down and really talk with them."

Not that talk is universally appreciated. When New York girls speak of a date as N.A.T.O., they mean contemptuously, "No Action, Talk Only." Some find the steady affair on the dull side. One Hunter girl told Writer Gael Greene: "Sex is so casual and taken for granted—I mean we go to dinner, we go home, get undressed like old married people, you know—and just go to bed. I mean I'm not saying I'd like to be raped on the living-room floor exactly. But I would love to just sit around on the sofa and neck."

The young seem to be earnestly trying to construct their own code and are even rediscovering for themselves some of the older verities. "They are piecing together lives which are at least as whole as their parents," says Lutheran Minister Martin Marty. They marry early—

probably too early—and they give the impression of escaping into marriage almost with a sense of relief. Often they are disappointed by what marriage brings.

Serial Polygamy. For the dominant fact about sexual mores in the U.S. remains the fragility of American marriage. The institution has never been easily sustained; "forsaking all others," in human terms, represents a belief that in an average life, loneliness is a greater threat than boredom. But the U.S. has a special concept of marriage, both Puritan and romantic. In most Eastern societies, marriages are arranged by families; the same is true in many parts of Europe, and there, even where young people are free to choose, they often choose for purely practical reasons. In arranged marriage, it is expected that love may or may not come later—and remarkably often it does. If not, it may be found outside marriage. The church, of course, does not sanction this system, but in European countries it has managed to live with it.

In the U.S., this notion is repugnant. St. Paul said that it is better to marry than to burn; except for Roman Catholics, Americans tend to believe that it is better to divorce than to burn. The European aim is to keep the family under one roof; the American aim is to provide personal happiness. Partly as a result, the U.S. has developed what sociologists call "serial polygamy," often consisting of little more than a succession of love affairs with slight legal trimmings. Cynics point out that serial polygamy was a fact even in Puritan times, when men had three or four wives because women were apt to die young; nowadays, divorce rather than death provides variety.

There is some sympathy for the European system. Says Psychiatrist Joseph Satten of the Menninger Foundation: "Fewer people feel now that infidelity demands a divorce. There is some value to this increased tolerance, because it may help keep our families together. But our society will suffer terribly if we equate freedom in sex with irresponsibility." Most Americans still feel that if the family is to be kept together, it cannot be through infidelity. There are, in fact, signs of stability in the divorce statistics, which have remained steady over the past four years.

Oh Men, Oh Women. Those marriages which do survive seem to be richer and more fun. Part of the reason may be that Americans are becoming more sophisticated and less inhibited in bed—as just about everyone is urging them to be. As respectable an authority as Robert C.

Dodds, a minister in the United Church of Christ, and General Director of Planning for the National Council of Churches, appends a chapter on sex practices to a marriage handbook, in which a physician urges couples to explore and "conjure up various positions and actions of sexual intercourse." Old taboos are slowly beginning to disappear, and while the upper and educated classes were always more adventurous in their techniques, sexual class lines show signs of fading. Reportedly declining are such prudish practices as making love with one's clothes on or in total darkness.

The long-standing cold war between men and women in the U.S. may be heading for a *détente*. While American women often still seem too strong and American men too weak, the U.S. has learned that men have the kind of women they deserve. The image of the all-devouring, all-demanding but never-giving American Bitch is virtually gone, both in life and in literature, (except possibly on Broadway, where so many plays are written by homosexuals). With the new legitimation of pleasure, the American woman increasingly tries to combine the role of wife and mistress—with the same man, that is. It may be an unattainable goal, but the attempt is fascinating and often successful.

Perhaps, American men have yet to discover that in her new and complicated role, woman must be wooed more than ever—and that wooing women is not a part-time occupation but a full-time attitude. But almost all American men have begun to accept the fact that women nowadays have to be competent and managing types—without giving up their femininity. As for the often-heard charge that American men really want mothers. Henry Miller, of all people, recently replied: "I have often wondered what is so objectionable about being mothered by the woman one loves."

Sexual Democracy. In extramarital sex, one of the chief trends is toward sexual democracy. Today's sexual adventuring seems to be among social equals, even if it means the best friend's wife or husband. The old double standard involved a reservoir of socially inferior women, some of them prostitutes, others "nice" girls but not really quite nice. The prostitutes' ranks are thinning more than ever. As for the little seamstress or shopgirl type, she hardly exists any longer; heaven and union wages protect the working girl.

Today's catalyst for sex, at least in urban communities, is the office girl, from head buyer to perky file clerk. To many men, the office remains a refuge from home, and to many girls a refuge from the eligible but sometimes dull young men they meet in the outside world. One of the difficulties of the office affair, except for those who relish intrigue for its own sake, is the problem of sheer logistics and security. Semipublic, semipermanent affairs are still not readily condoned—or perhaps even really enjoyed—in the U.S. American men seem to have decided that if there is love, only marriage will suffice in the long run, and if there is no love, only boredom can result; thus does life forever reinvent morality.

The New Sin. Some sociologists believe that the U.S. is moving toward a more Mediterranean attitude toward sex and life in general. But the U.S. still cannot relax about it the way Europe does, which accepts sex without much discussion, as it accepts bread and wine, earth and sin.

In contrast, the U.S. is forever trying to banish sin from the universe—and finding new sins to worry about. The new sex freedom in the U.S. does not necessarily set people free. Psychoanalyst Rollo May believes that it has minimized external social anxiety but increased internal tension. The great new sin today is no longer giving in to desire, he thinks, but not giving in to it fully or successfully enough. While enjoyment of sex has increased for many, the "competitive compulsion to prove oneself an acceptable sexual machine" makes many others feel neurotically guilty, hence impotent or frigid. As a fellow analylist puts it bluntly: "We are always anticipating the 21-gun salute, and worried if it doesn't happen." This preoccupation with the frequency and technique of orgasm, says May, leads to a new kind of inverted Puritanism.

If there is indeed a new Puritanism, it has its own Cotton Mather. Man, says Norman Mailer, "knows at the seed of his being that good orgasm opens his possibilities and bad orgasm imprisons him." Many people take this issue very seriously: next month, the American Association of Marriage Counselors will hold a three-day conference on the nature of orgasm.

There is also a tendency to see in sex not only personal but social salvation— the last area of freedom in an industrialized society, the last frontier. In one of the really "in" books of recent years, *Life Against*

Death, Norman O. Brown has even suggested a kind of sexual Utopia. In his vision, all repressions would be eliminated, along with civilization itself; the future would belong to sexuality, not just of the present "genital" variety, which Brown considers a form of tyranny, but the all-round, innocent sexuality a child enjoys.

Such notions mean burdening sex with too much deadly importance, suggesting an absurd vision of all those college kids making out, the clerks trying to learn the art of seduction from Dr. Albert Ellis, the young married couples in their hopeful conjugal beds—all only serving the great cause of some socio-sexual revolution.

The Supreme Act. Contemplating the situation from the vantage point of his 79 years, Historian Will Durant recently decided it was time to speak out, not only on sexual morality but on morals generally. Said he: "Most of our literature and social philosophy after 1850 was the voice of freedom against authority, of the child against the parent, of the pupil against the teacher. Through many years I shared in that individualistic revolt. I do not regret it; it is the function of youth to defend liberty and innovation, of the old to defend order and tradition, and of middle age to find a middle way. But now that I too am old, I wonder whether the battle I fought was not too completely won. Let us say humbly but publicly that we resent corruption in politics, dishonesty in business, faithlessness in marriage, pornography in literature, coarseness in language, chaos in music, meaninglessness in art."

Many Americans will share Durant's broad indignation, many will dissent from it. But one of the remarkable facts is that there is much less indignation in the churches today—at least as far as sexual morality goes. The watchword is to be positive, to stress the New Testament's values of faith, hope and charity rather than the prohibitions of the Commandments. Many sermons, if they deal with sexual transgressions at all, prefer to treat them simply as one kind of difficulty among many others. The meaning of sin in the U.S. today is no longer predominantly sexual.

Few will regret that. But many do feel the need for a reaffirmation of the spiritual meaning of sex. For the act of sex is above all the supreme act of communion between two people, as sanctified by God and celebrated by poets. "Love's mysteries in souls do grow, but yet the body is his book," wrote John Donne. And out of this connection and commitment come children, who should be a responsibility—and a joy.

When sex is pursued only for pleasure, or only for gain, or even only to fill a void in society or in the soul, it becomes elusive, impersonal, ultimately disappointing. That is what Protestant Theologian Helmut Thielicke has in mind when he warns that "a dethroned god seems to be staging his comeback in a secularized world." Eros is accorded high rank today, "a rank that comes close to the deity it once had." The spiritual danger is that Eros may leave "no room for agape, which lives not by making claims but by giving."

The Victorians, who talked a great deal about love, knew little about sex. Perhaps it is time that modern, Americans, who know a great deal about sex, once again start talking about love.

The Erotic Revolution

Lawrence Lipton

from *The Erotic Revolution*, 1965

The Erotic Revolution was probably the first book devoted to the dramatic changes in sexual mores that were taking place at the time. Based in Venice, California, Lawrence Lipton (1898-1975) was a freelance writer and journalist long associated with Beat Generation poets and writers such as Allen Ginsberg, Gregory Corso, and Lawrence Ferlinghetti. In 1959 he wrote **The Holy Barbarians**, *an in-depth portrait of Beat culture on the West Coast. In* **The Erotic Revolution** *he argued passionately for what he called "the New Morality," such as repealing the laws that penalized sex outside of marriage and legalizing contraceptives, abortion, and homosexuality. He was one of the first authors to explore infidelity, wife-swapping, and the planning of orgies.*

O f all the revolutions sweeping the world today, political, economic, social, scientific and moral, the last may prove to be the most far-reaching, the most deep-going of all. Usually referred to as the Sexual Revolution, it is actually more than a revolt against the moral code. It is a determined move on the part of millions of people to restructure the very process of the orgasm itself, a thoroughgoing change in the whole sexual economy. It could more accurately be called the Erotic Revolution.

On every hand there are evidences that the Old Morality no longer fits the needs of a society that is rapidly outgrowing such traditional categories as urban and rural which once defined their cultural patterns and moral imperatives: the rural determined by the seasonal cycle and the urban by manufacture and commerce. As the two merge each takes on some of the characteristics of the other. Mechanization and electrification have wrought revolutionary changes on the farm and in the city; automation and atomic energy are already bringing further changes, changes which affect the lifeways and the sexways of the whole population. The New Leisure which began with the eight-hour day, expanded to the five-day forty-hour week and is now being nibbled down to the thirty-five and even the thirty-hour week, is already presenting new opportunities for orgastic recharging of the life-force and experiments with new sexual relationships. Millions are already answering the question—handled so gingerly on television panel programs—what will people do with their new leisure?

Sex, as an enriching mutual experience, a therapy or a release from tensions, is already competing successfully with such highly recommended avocations as fifty-mile hikes, do-it-yourself machine tool handicrafts, and getting into bed and curling up with a good book.

The Orgastic Revolution, like all revolutions, has its false prophets, its meretricious advocates, its unsuccessful experiments, its martyrs and its casualties. In this book I propose to afford the reader a close-up view of all these aspects of the revolution. To provide perspective, I shall take a look back into the past, not with a view to finding a regressive retreat from the present, a snug harbor to crawl into, but a point of departure for the future. If we know enough about the past we may not be condemned to repeat its mistakes. We may learn how to ask the right questions.

The first manifestations of every revolution are always symptoms of the decay of the old order. Today we have passed beyond this first stage into promising new experiments in natural love, in mating, in marital relations. The sick, the neurotic, the desperate reactions to the old morality are still with us. But there are enough fresh, guilt-free, joyous new sexways to merit a careful reexamination of the subject from an affirmative point of view.

There are signs that the time is past for new patches on the old fabric of sexual morality. Or, to change the metaphor, why pour new wine into old wine skins?

To those who ask: Is this the new morality?—by which they mean the experiments, both sick and healthy, which I have alluded to and which I deal with in this book—to those who ask this question my answer is: No. Nobody knows what the new morality will be like. All we can do today is make an educated guess. In answer to a similar question, an Ohio State senior replied: "Premarital sex doesn't mean the downfall of society, at least not the kind of society that we're going to build." I would ask, "What kind of society *are* you going to build?" and the only sensible answer he could make would be: Wait and see.

One thing we can be sure of, those who, like Sociologist Ira Reiss, call for "permissiveness with affection" and defend it on the grounds that morals are a private affair, that being in love justifies premarital sex, and nothing is really wrong as long as nobody gets hurt: those who cherish such hopes will often be doomed to disappointment. Anthropology teaches us that morals have *never* been a private affair; that premarital and, for that matter, extra-marital sex can be "justified" (whatever that means—or matters) by love, by need, by custom, and even, in some cultures past and present, by law and religion; and that *no* system of morality can guarantee that "nobody gets hurt."

And that, by the way, goes far in answering the question: What would you put in place of the old morality? There is nothing that can be put in place of the old except experimenting with the new. And hoping that something humanly good will come of it. In the meantime there are some measures which I would recommend as desirable because they would help to make experiment safer and more intelligent.

> Repeal all the laws and statutes regulating premarital sex. Make legal marriage optional, as religious marriage is now optional. Those desiring contract marriage, providing for husband or wife in case the marriage fails, or for the children of such a marriage, should be able to make such contracts and seek legal adjudication in case differences arise.

> Repeal all laws making homosexuality, male or female, illegal.

> Repeal all laws making any sexual act, the so-called "unnatural" acts, illegal. Nature knows no unnatural sexual acts.

> Make all contraceptives and abortions legal everywhere and free to all who are unable to pay.

Make all forms of mating legal if there is mutual agreement between the parties concerned.

These would do for a starter. Questions like divorce, rape, psycho-neurotic sexual behavior, inheritance, and related questions like wife-swapping, infidelity, incest, and illegitimacy would appear in a new setting, if the measures I recommend were adopted, action could then be taken on them in the light of changed conditions.

The assertion that changes in the law must wait on changes in custom and consensus is only a half truth. The assertion that changes in custom must wait on changes in the law is also a half truth. The two taken together do not add up to a whole truth; neither do they add up to a whole lie. History offers abundant evidence that law and custom are *interactive*, at all times, in intricate and often unexpected ways. What is unthinkable today may be inevitable tomorrow.

Among the unthinkables is the notion that one of the inalienable rights of man is the right to probe, explore and experiment sexually and, together with others like him, male and female, establish any sexual relationships that satisfy their needs, as long as they do not attempt to force their ideas on others or interfere with the corresponding right of others to follow their own sexways.

This is not to say that in such a case there would never be any significant social conflict between individuals and groups holding views and following practices which are sharply at variance with one another. Such conflicts exist and have always existed and presumably will always continue to occur in the lifeways of every society. There are conflicts in our notions of the destiny of man and his relation to the universe, fundamental differences which cannot be logically resolved by discussion, even with the best will in the world. But despite all the bloody conflicts and persecutions of the past over such irreconcilable differences, the conviction that peaceful coexistence is desirable and possible in such matters is gaining ground.

The radically fundamental changes that have been brought about in the sciences during the last few decades, and particularly since the explosive dawn of the atomic age, are conditioning millions of people the world over to view new and shocking lifeways and sexways with more tolerance, even with humility. Admittedly, the more popular any radical social change becomes, especially in the sphere of sex and morals, the more active the reaction against it becomes. For example, television panel shows have proliferated during the last five years, sponsored by a dozen or more religious bodies on airtime donated by the networks, all of them slanted toward defending the Judeo-Christian ethical and moral code against attack from any and every quarter. In addition there are thousands of local programs broadcasting the most benighted and frequently illiterate and vulgar, television and radio sermons. Some of them are paid network shows featuring hell fire and brimstone evangelism and some are "healing" services conducted by Fundamentalist preachers who can well afford to pay for airtime out of the proceeds, "love offerings" which in some cases add up to an annual take of impressive proportions.

The ostensible purpose of these godly activities is to preach the Gospel, but anyone who can bring himself to listen to a few of them will discover that their target is moral nonconformism of any and every kind, and by moral they always mean *sexual* morality, not political corruption or lying or theft or even rape. Their targets are Freud and Darwin and modern art and art films, especially foreign art films, and novels, plays and motion pictures that deal with modern sexways in any way that might have offended the religious principles of Martin Luther, Cotton Mather or the moral criteria of the Watch and Ward Society. In short, every idea, scientific or artistic, that bears a dateline later than 1860.

On the other hand, the mass communications media are virtually closed to any outright spokesman who challenges the Judeo-Christian ethos, only to those who come on panel shows as the Devil's Advocate and put on a display of token opposition that the moderator can glibly dispose of in his summation and then pat himself—and the communications media—on the back for presenting "both sides of the question." On the other hand, script writers are sometimes able to smuggle a bit of intelligent social and moral criticism into dramatic shows and get away with it till the sponsors, the listener ratings, the censors and the indignant letter writers, organized and unorganized, catch up with them. It is characteristic of Vox Pop to regard itself as Vox Dei, which recalls H. L. Mencken's remark: "If the voice of the people is the voice of God, the *Congressional Record* is the Bible."

In a society whose real religion is neither the voice of the people nor the voice of God but Moneytheism, a theology which is summed up in the dictum, "Money talks," it is to be expected that nothing will be given wide currency in the mass communications media that challenges the prejudices of the customer or the sponsor, from whom all blessings flow. The result is that the gagged and/or "self-censored" writer, director or actor on television looks around him for others in the same predicament and little enclaves of the dissenting, disenchanted and disaffiliated are formed, secretly, to keep one another, as more than one of them has told me, "from going insane." Some of these crypto-disaffiliates are among the most active, and most intelligent and successful, experimentors of the New Morality, as we shall see when we deal with their case histories in this book.

No radical change in the lifeways or sexways of a culture are ever voted into effect or legislated into practice, but something like a plebicite does take place, a plebicite of actions rather than words. A new idea begins and its adherents proliferate almost like a biological process, by mental and emotional impregnation, by parturition and maturation. Little cells or enclaves of dissent and experimentation appear in the womb of the body politic and eventually force their way into being. The history of social change, especially in morals and sexual behavior, is the story of such enclaves.

In our own time these enclaves are of two sorts. There is the enclave that has no special home base or habitat and exists only as a kind of intellectual and spiritual brotherhood. Its members meet only by chance, at certain plays and lectures for example, or in the lobbies of art film theaters, or at social gatherings where they tend to attract one another by a kind of molecular action and huddle around a bottle in the kitchen. Such occasions often lead to the second kind of enclave, the neighborhood or suburban "set," which develops a measure of social cohesiveness and autonomy. Examples of both kinds will be presented in their proper place in this study of contemporary sexways. For the moment it will be sufficient to indicate some of the causes which give rise to this phenomenon and the marks—I was almost tempted to say "stigmata"—by which they recognize one another.

It is universally conceded by most observers who have made a study of the subject, whether they view the situation with approval or alarm, that all is not well with the sexual morality that is based on the Judeo-Christian ethos. Apostates and blasphemers appear on every hand and their defections are not limited to words; they carry their apostacy into action. Behind this dissident movement lies the growing conviction that the sexual mores, adolescent, premarital, marital and extramarital, no longer fit the conditions of modern living. The opportunities and circumstances of male and female intercourse, social and sexual, in an age of automobiles and mobile homes, bear no resemblance whatever to the close-knit family and tribal life which the Mosaic Code was designed to govern and regulate. To be sure, changes have been made in religion and law since the 15th Century B.C., changes calculated to reflect and serve changing needs and conditions, but in the last fifty years, and particularly since the Second World War, the changes have been taking place with a dizzying speed that makes adherence to the Old Morality harder than ever before in history.

In addition to the greater opportunities for social and sexual mobility there is the population explosion. This is more than a statistical fact, it is more than a question of finding food and shelter and employment for a larger number of people than have ever lived at one time on the face of the earth. It poses problems which are problems not of numbers alone, not of degree but of kind. A young man or woman free from home ties at an age that tends to grow younger as pre-school educational facilities increase and improve, and away from home influences for more of their teenage and young adult life than ever before as higher education expands and lengthens out to meet the demands of modern technology, is faced with moral problems the Mosaic and Pauline lawgivers of the Old Morality never dreamed of. Moreover, the population explosion is not uniform in its effects. Along with it there is a steady movement from the small town to the big city and now, from the big city to the suburbs. It is as if one were living in a continual earthquake of population shifts and dislocations, and stability of human relationship of every kind is difficult under such conditions.

Monogamy and the moral code governing premarital and extramarital relations were designed in the first place to fit an agricultural society which put a premium on the stability of the family farm unit organized as an on-going economic entity geared to the seasonal cycle.

Children, like wives, were valuable property, the labor source without which the family would face economic collapse or be forced to resort to border raids in search of slave labor, which could result in costly feuds and often in mutual extermination, as the early books of the Old Testament record in gruesome detail.

As industrial societies came into being the agricultural code was altered in order to adapt it to changed conditions. The alterations were made slowly, cautiously, over centuries of time, because the changeover from agriculture to an industrial and commercial economy was slow. It did not begin in England as some historians have assumed, it began with the first city-states of Asia Minor, Greece and Rome and, after a long period of conquest and consolidation, in Europe. It began when the mining and metal-working centers sprang up in Israel and Tyre and manufacturing became a way of life in the cities of the Mediterranean basin. (In the Far East it had a similar development, but that does not concern us here.)

The manufacturing and commercial societies of antiquity required the migration of workers, sometimes a forced migration, from the farm to the city. Torn from the land, from tillage and harvesting to mine, mill and hand or animal-powered industrial labor, the farmer's life-ways underwent a painfully radical change. His system of values, his familial relationships and his sexways, torn from their moorings in the seasonal cycle of religious ritual, broke down and he found himself adrift in a world which was little better than slave labor. He could no longer rely on the reassuring numinous powers of the shaman or the tribal chief. He was no longer part of an awe-inspiring seasonal cycle of death and resurrection, of rites which fructified not only the earth but rejuvenated his own sexual energies. He was no longer priest and master in his own household, with his own household gods. He was a slave to a machine, however crude it may now seem to us, a machine that had no life-renewing powers, that did not need him or his shaman or his household gods to renew and sustain its life.

He had used primitive machines on the land, to be sure, the ox-driven corn mill, the irrigation water wheel, the textile loom, the potter's wheel, but these were his own property, products of his own handicraft. He even had folk songs and folk dances which celebrated the work of these simple machines. In the city industries he was a laborer working with machines and tools that were not his own, for wages which were at or below the lowest subsistence level short of starvation, with no rights that the employer was under any obligation to respect.

To keep such a worker under control it was necessary to convince him of the evil nature of his own deepest instincts, fill him with a sense of guilt and let self-punishment do the rest. All the power and prestige of State and Church was mobilized to inculcate and enforce the process of self-denigration and psychological castration. The sexways which had formerly been regarded as sacred and vital to the very life, health and preservation of the individual and the group, were now evil, degrading, unclean, illegal, irreligious and a peril to body and soul.

History has seen many such revisions and reversals, always with the aim of diabolizing the gods and symbols of the conquered, exploited and enslaved and setting up a system of values and a code of social and sexual conduct designed to sanctify the powers and privileges of the conqueror. These conquests have not always been military. In those cases where they have been most effective and enduring they have been economic conquests of one class over another, as in the case of the urban industrial class over the agricultural population. What is significant for us here is the fact that such changes have always involved an assault upon the sexways of the vanquished in order to revise them in the interests of the conquerors.

But rarely have such repressive codes of sexual behavior gone unchallenged or unviolated. There is always an underground resistance which eventually surfaces and reasserts itself. This happens when new inventions or other influences and forces affect a realignment of political and social powers, toppling old religious institutions and the moral codes they were created to preserve. Such a change is taking place today as economic power shifts from ownership to management, as mechanization or production gives way to automation, with the resultant dislocation of skills and employment practices, and the rapid increase in leisure and living standards.

A vital factor in the picture is the decline of infant mortality and at the same time the unprecedented rise in the life span. As a consequence of these changes one-half of the population of this country today is under twenty-five years of age. At the other end of the life span, the aged are increasing in number, this at a time when the active, producing years in the work-life of the individual are shrinking at both ends of the life span. Industrial production demands greater, more complex skills, raising the educational requirements to the point where all of one's youth and young manhood are schooling years during which there is little or no income as yet to make marriage and raising a family possible without the utmost hardship.

Under such conditions it is a self-delusion to expect anything but lip service to a moral code which demands premarital continence. The very word "premarital" becomes obsolete as applied to unmarried sexual relationships.

Other factors, such as job mobility and population shift, alter marital sexways. Family ties loosen and in many cases break down completely. Sons and daughters go off at an earlier age than ever to schools which are frequently far from home. The results are a subject of wide concern today and are dealt with in this study at some length.

Another factor is the increase of women in business and industry. This, as we shall see, is not a new development. On the contrary, it is a return to what has been the normal working relationship of men and women for most of human history. The resultant sexual relationships of men and women working together on the job are similar to those which have obtained in the past under such conditions. Where they differ from those of the past the difference is easily traced to changed sexways in other human relationships. Since the co-working relationship of men and women is undoubtedly destined to be the normal one for a long time to come, it may well be that in time society will have to accept and sanction this manifestation of the New Morality.

What makes the present state of moral transition so hard to bear is the fact that so many millions of people are compelled to keep up a pretense of loyalty to religions they no longer believe in and a sexual morality they no longer respect or find it possible to live by without psychological damage to themselves and those they love.

The Old Morality dies hard. But it is later than you think. Those of us who look forward to the New Morality can take heart from the assurance, voiced by more than one wise man of the past, that no force on earth is strong enough to stop a new idea once its time has come.

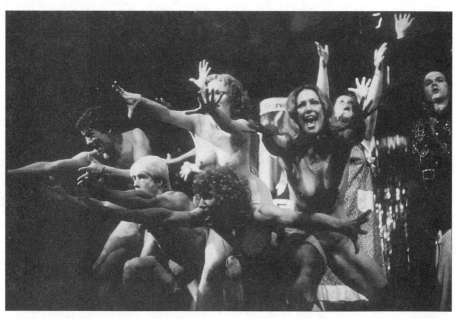

© Fred W. McDarrah

Reflections on the Revolution in Sex

Francis Canavan, S.J.

from *America*, March 6, 1965

*Both Catholic and Protestant churches had begun to examine sexual morality in light of the possibility that sex without love and sexual activity for pleasure might become the dominant new pattern of sexuality. In the Jesuit publication **America**, Father Canavan argued that the "Sexual Revolution of the 20th century" was comparable to the 18th century's French Enlightenment in its challenge to contemporary Christianity.*

Sex is here to stay. But the sexual moral standards of Christian civilization may not be. They are being attacked today as seldom before. "For the first time for centuries," said the British magazine *New Society*, in its January 24, 1963 number, "the Judeo-Christian code is under fire, not just from people who wish to break it for their own pleasure's sake, but from people who believe that it is actually wrong."

This revolt against Christianity, which is comparable to the Enlightenment in the 18th century, is the Sexual Revolution of the 20th century. It is taking place in almost every Western nation; in the United States it is already well advanced. But since the advocates of the revolution are somewhat more outspoken in Great Britain than they are here, this article will report on what they are saying in the United Kingdom rather than in the United States. No invidious comparison is intended. The Land of the Free, after all, is also the Home of the

Playboy Philosophy. In this respect, Americans have no reason to look down on anyone.

At the root of the sexual revolution is the growing awareness that modern contraceptive technology has radically separated sex from pro-creation. Reflection on this fact is leading many thoughtful persons to ask why sexual relations must be confined to marriage or even, for that matter, to the normal organs of reproduction. The contemporary pre-occupation with meaningful interpersonal relationships has only added force to this questioning.

Prof. G. M. Carstairs of Edinburgh University, raised the question in trenchant form in his series of Reith Lectures on the British Broad-casting Corporation's Home Service in November, 1962. Young people, he said, are rapidly turning British society "into one in which sexual experience, with precautions against conception, is becoming accepted as a sensible preliminary to marriage."

Among the "indications of precocious sexual behavior in our society," he mentioned "the increasing number of cases of venereal dis-ease in young people and the fact that in 1961 no less than 31 per cent of girls who married in their teens were pregnant at the time of their wedding." The professor was not alarmed, however. "The interesting thing," he remarked, "is that this premarital license has been found to be quite compatible with stable married life."

"Is chastity the supreme moral virtue?" he asked. "Surely charity, that is, consideration of and concern for others, comes first." Besides, he said, the former theological cannons of behavior are seldom taken seriously. "In their place a new concept is emerging of sexual relations as a source of pleasure, but also as a mutual encountering of personal-ities in which each explores the other and at the same time discovers new depths in himself or herself."

The distinguished literary critic, Cyril Connolly, proclaimed: "The Reith Lectures are an achievement of which our culture can be proud." Not everyone in Britain shared his jubilation, of course. Some felt more disturbed than proud. But they had even greater cause for disquiet with the publication, in February, 1963, of a booklet entitled *Towards a Quaker View of Sex*.

The authors were a group of eleven Quakers. They spoke in their own name, not in that of their denomination. Six of them, however, were Elders of the Society of Friends. The group included teachers, psychiatrists, a barrister and a housewife. All were married except one, Dr. Anna Bidder, who was a Cambridge University expert in zoology specializing in the giant squid.

Towards a Quaker View of Sex "rejects almost completely the traditional approach of the organized Christian Church to morality, with its supposition that it knows precisely what is right and what is wrong, that this distinction can be made in terms of an external pattern of behavior, and that the greatest good will come only through universal adherence to that pattern." Its own answers, it says, are "tentative and incomplete." They are certainly different from the accepted Christian norms.

The authors note "an increase in transient premarital sexual intimacies generally." They refuse to frown upon it, however, since "it is fairly common in both young men and young women with high standards of general conduct and integrity to have one or two love affairs, involving intercourse, before they find the person they will ultimately marry."

It is even more common, they say, for those who do marry each other to have intercourse before the ceremony, "This is true, probably, of a majority of young people in all classes of society, including those who often have a deep sense of responsibility."

Even after marriage, the group of Friends observe, "the sexual drive differs in strength and frequency in different individuals, and what is customary and normal in one marriage may not be so in another." In this connection, they mention the so-called "triangular situation." It "is too often thought of as a wholly destructive and irresponsible relationship," they feel. "Not sufficient recognition is given to the fact that a triangular situation can and often does arise in which all three persons behave responsibly, are deeply conscious of the difficulties and equally anxious to avoid injury to the others."

(In the second edition of their booklet; published in January, 1965, the authors reject an interpretation of this passage "in terms of an adulterous relationship being good and beneficial to all three persons concerned." But they still feel that "more often than is recognized, the three people concerned behave responsibly," etc.)

Responsibility is also the keynote of their treatment of homosexuality, which "one should no more deplore than left-handedness." They see

> no reason why the physical nature of a sexual act should be the criterion by which the question whether or not it is moral should be decided. An act which (for example) expresses true affection between two individuals and gives pleasure to them both, does not seem to us to be sinful by reason alone of the fact that it is homosexual. The same criteria seem to us to apply whether a relationship is heterosexual or homosexual.

"Homosexual affection," they explain, "can be as selfless as heterosexual affection, and therefore we cannot see that it is in some way morally worse."

It is not surprising, therefore, that these Quakers feel that Christian sexual morality up to the present has been pretty much a ghastly mistake. "The fulfillment of our nature as distinctively human beings," they say, "is through relationships that are *personal*, through the kind of friendship that is its own justification." These relations cannot be confined to marriage, even when they are sexual in nature.

This conviction leads them to criticize the Anglican theologian Sherwin Bailey. They acknowledge their indebtedness to him in general, but they state their dissent from one of the conclusions in his book, *Common Sense About Sexual Ethics.* Their complaint is this:

> He holds that to say "I love you" means nothing less than this: "I want you, just as you are, to share the whole of my life, and I ask you to take me, just as I am, to share the whole of your life." He further says that it ought never to be said unless marriage is possible, right, and at the time of speaking intended. That such a statement is unrealistic is at the root of our work. Nothing that has come to light in the course of our studies has altered the conviction that came to us when we began to examine the actual experiences of people—the conviction that love cannot be confined to a pattern.

The authors quote with approval of John Macmurray's *Reason and Emotion*, in which he says:

> Our civilization, for all its scientific and administrative capacity, has remained emotionally vulgar and primitive, unchaste in the extreme. We do not recognize this, of course, because it is simply the reflection of our inner insensibility. That insensibility is the inevitable result of a morality based upon will and reason, imposing itself upon the emotions and so destroying their integrity.

But it would be wrong to interpret the authors of *Toward a Quaker View of Sex* as being anti-moral. They themselves say, *"There must be a morality of some sort to govern sexual relationships,"* and put it in italics for emphasis. They explain the basic principle of their morality by stating that they "accept the definition of sin given by an Anglican broadcaster, as covering those actions that involve exploitation of the other person." This, they say, "is a concept of wrong doing that applies both to homosexual and heterosexual actions and to actions within marriage as well as outside it. It condemns as fundamentally immoral every sexual action that is not, as far as is humanly ascertainable, the result of a mutual decision."

On a later page they add:

> Where there is a deliberate intention to avoid responsibility and all possibility of being involved and committed, then evil creeps in and the act becomes mutual exploitation. But where there is genuine tenderness, an openness to responsibility, and the seed for commitment, God is surely not shut out. Can we say that God can enter any relationship in which there is a measure of selfless love?—and is not every generalization we make qualified by this?

The next round in Britain's controversy over sexual morality came in July, 1963. Dr. Peter Henderson, the principal medical officer of the Ministry of Education, said at a teacher's meeting:

> I do not think that it is wrong if a young man and women who are in love and who intend to get married but who put off marriage, perhaps for economic reasons, have sexual intercourse before marriage. I do not think they are unchaste or immoral. They may or may not be wise if they do so, but I cannot convince myself that they are immoral.

After *Towards a Quaker View of Sex*, Dr. Henderson's views should have seemed almost conventional. But because of his position, his words were nationally reported and stirred up considerable protest. Sir Edward Boyle, the Minister of Education, refused to repudiate Dr. Henderson. "It is not part of my function to prescribe what moral teaching could take place in the schools," he said. "The voice of conscience, not society, should guide people in their views."

A view more radical than Dr. Henderson's was expressed by Dr. Alex Comfort in his book *Sex in Society*. According to a review in the London *Daily Telegraph*: "He starts from the premise that no form of sexual behavior is sinful unless it has demonstrably bad effects, and going on from there examines such vital questions as teen-age morality, extramarital relations, and the law and deviation." Another review, in the *Sunday Times*, quotes Dr. Comfort as saying: "It is highly probable that adultery today maintains far more marriages than it destroys."

Advanced views turned up even in the Established Church of England. Canon D. A. Rhymes of Southwark Cathedral gave a sermon in March, 1963, in which he announced: "We need to replace the traditional morality based upon a code with a morality which is related to the person and the needs of the person." He also said: "Much of the prejudice against homosexuality is on the ground that it is unnatural. But unnatural to whom? Certainly not for the homosexual himself."

In September of the same year, Canon T. R. Milford published a pamphlet, *Talking of Sex*. In it he questioned the idea that marriage is essentially indissoluble and that divorce is always and in every circumstance a sin. On concubinage or triangular relationships, he quoted a group of professional people who had come to this conclusion: "We should not condemn as simply immoral those who in good faith have chosen this way. But they cannot expect approval of conduct which, taken as an example by others, would be disastrous."

Theory was reduced to practice in the fall of 1963, when the Marie Stopes Memorial Foundation started consultative sessions for young unmarried people in its Tottenham Court Road clinic in London and offered birth control appliances to some of them. The foundation was affiliated to, but not a part of, the London Federation of the Family Planning Association, whose own clinics at that time were forbidden to advise single people, even those about to marry.

In June, 1964, however, the Family Planning Association decided to encourage the setting up of youth advisory centers, at which unmarried people could get medical advice on sex problems, including advice on birth control. The decision was taken after two hours of debate. Mrs. Leah Manning expressed the majority point of view, saying: "We have to face facts; we have to realize that the practice of premarital sexual intercourse has begun to establish itself." Lady Limerick objected on the ground that the Family Planning Association would have to change its name, because it would be dishonest if the motion passed. In certain cases, she said, it would "merely be giving advice to people to help them avoid marriage."

Finally, in December, 1964, despite opposition from its Catholic members, the London County Council approved plans to assist organizations providing contraceptive advice to young unmarried persons. The *Observer* praised the move because "we must guard against the crime of producing children without parents." To clinch the argument, it added: "It is certainly easier to teach contraception than chastity."

International opinion made its impact felt in Britain with the conference of the International Planned Parenthood Federation in London in June, 1964, The *Sunday Times* reported: "There was general acceptance, among most of the representatives of 46 countries attending, of premarital intercourse (even among boys and girls in their early teens)." But attitudes still varied in different countries, they admitted. A 14-year-old girl in Stockholm did not much mind being seen abstracting a contraceptive from a slot machine. But Italy, "still under the dominating influence of the Roman Catholic Church, would appear to be one of the few European countries where a bride is still expected to be a virgin."

American attitudes were revealed by Dr. Alan F. Guttmacher, president of the Planned Parenthood Federation of America. "Parents themselves are becoming more sophisticated," he was reported as saying. "They know, for example, that their son or daughter must go to college equipped with contraceptives." But, he felt, "so long as they are taught responsibility to each other, I think some better humans may come out of this new morality."

J. Kruithof, professor of moral philosophy at the University of Brussels and Ghent, offered a philosophical analysis of the whole situation. According to the London *Times*, the Belgian professor told delegates to the conference that he believed the traditional system of morality was on the way to complete breakdown.

Traditionally, he said, sex, love, marriage and children were considered to belong together. Today, childless couples were no longer looked down on. Extramarital and premarital relationships were quite common. It was even possible that sex without love—a kind of prostitution for enjoyment rather than financial gain—might be the new pattern emerging among young people.

"We need a new code of morality," Professor Kruithof said. "This new system is in a process of formation. We are going toward a re-evaluation of the sex act."

The British Council of Churches had already reacted to this kind of challenge to Christian morality. At its half-yearly meeting in April, 1964, it decided to set up a working party charged with producing a statement of the Christian position on sexual morals in a persuasive, modern style. This was to include the Christian case for abstinence from sexual intercourse before marriage and faithfulness within marriage.

The Rev. Kenneth Greet, chairman of the Council's advisory group on sex, morality and the family, was reported the by the London *Times* as saying at the meeting that if the churches were to engage effectively in defense of Christian standards, they must listen seriously to what the most responsible of their critics were saying. Further, the positive things Christians had to say needed to be said more effectively and with a greater sense of urgency. "We must say very much more than we have said in the past about the Christian understanding of sex," he declared, "not merely in terms of procreation but in terms of rich and diversified human relationship."

The churches that form the British Council of Churches have already accepted contraception as a Christian practice. Indeed, it was the Anglican Communion that gave the lead in that direction at its Lambeth Conferences of 1930 and 1958. It would seem difficult, therefore, for the Council to defend traditional Christian standards of sexual morality in terms of the procreative purpose of sex. Whether a successful defense can be mounted "in terms of rich and diversified human relationships" alone remains to be seen. So far as this writer knows, the working party has not yet made its report.

Catholics, for their part, should not dismiss the attack on Christian sexual morality as the mouthings of a few extremists. The sexual revolution is a reality that will grow and spread as time goes by. Its advocates will become more numerous and more bold. They must be taken seriously.

One final reflection on the revolution in sex comes to mind. There are Catholics today who urge Rome to go to Lambeth and accept contraception as a means of solving problems in family life. Nothing that has been reported in this articles *proves* that these Catholics are wrong. But the arguments of the sexual revolutionists against Christian morality suggest a thought. It is this: the road to Lambeth may not end there.

The Sexual Revolution

Kermit Mehlinger, M.D.

from *Ebony*, August, 1966

There were vigorous debates among African Americans about whether or not the sexual revolution was limited to white Americans. This piece, which appeared in a magazine with a large black readership, focuses on the impact of the emerging sexual revolution on women—especially, in this article, on black middle class women. Throughout the sixties and seventies **Ebony** *published many articles on how the sexual revolution affected the relations between black men and women as well as on the sexual relations between blacks and whites.*

Birds do it, bees do it, in Boston even educated fleas do it. Let's do it-let's fall in love." These lines from the pen of the late Cole Porter come to my mind when I think of the current preoccupation with sex. Some of the "in crowd" act as if sex has replaced baseball as the favorite national pastime. I have female patients who compare notes on their "boy-watching" pursuits. There appears to be an increasing number of aggressive females who act as if "Sadie Hawkin's Day" is to be celebrated 365 days a year. The hip-gyrating "go-go" girl is a symbol of the permissive society of the sexy 60s. Rising hemlines and flamboyant "mod" styles punctuate her attire. Scanty bikinis have replaced bloomers and 20 tiny pills have given her 20 days each month to celebrate her newly acquired emancipation. It's as if she received an added dividend from the civil rights movement—sexual rights. "Incredible," she remarks. "How did it come about?" No, she didn't picket; she didn't march; she didn't sit-in; nor did she protest—

not to mention rebel. Then it must have occurred through some forces beyond her control . . . and, so it did. It happened this way. In the year 1948, a man named Kinsey published a book entitled *The Sexual Behavior of the Human Male* which was followed in 1953 by a companion edition, *The Sexual Behavior of The Human Female*. It was initially received with much indignation by the prudish, Victorian indoctrinated, anti-sex members of our society as being pornographic, non-scientific—a "dirty book" intended to appeal to sex-pots and arouse their erotic passions. Unfortunately, the Negro female wasn't accorded the dignity of a human being at that primitive age in our history. She wasn't included in the professor's studies. However, later investigators have correlated Kinsey's studies with those on the Negro woman and his results can in many instances be applied to Negro women if comparable social classes of women are investigated.

Kinsey's books eventually became best sellers as more mature members of our society realized that his contribution to the enlightenment and understanding of human sexual behavior was a monumental one. A good majority of American women discovered that they had been "talking out the corners of their mouths." If they had described their sexual practices to intimate associates, it was according to the way *they thought it should be* but not according to the way *it really was*. There was, for instance, the wide-spread belief that oral love was invented, copyrighted and used exclusively by the French people. As more information about human sexual behavior became public, many Americans found out that 50 million Frenchman can't be wrong. Even the Catholic Church recognized that there is nothing wrong with this kind of sexual conduct as long as there is mutual consent by marital partners and used as an entrée for coitus. Several decades earlier, Sigmund Freud had shocked the moralists of our society with his penetrating insight into infantile sexuality. The infant was no longer innocent and pure. He, also, had "bad" sexual feelings, to contend with during the genital phase of his development from ages three to six.

The old-fashioned girl and that "ole fashioned religion" is out. We are confronted with an enormous exploitation of sex. Conspicuous sexuality greets us from the moment we are awakened by the sensuous wails of a husky-throated blues singer to the moment we retire. Our clock radio seems to be perennially tuned to station S-E-X! And at bedtime, we are further mesmerized to the "land of nod" by sheer exhaustion from multi-channel "girl watching" around the clock. These babbling hucksters extol the merits of products from sleek limousines to exotic perfumes. Alluring close-ups of lovers in torrid embraces brighten up our TV screen. The sexual revolution is with us. The question is: are we accepting its challenge?

Yes, many Negro women are experiencing and freely expressing their changing attitudes regarding sexual values and mores. In many respects, the revolution has affected middle class Negro women more than women of the lower class. Of course, a growing number of lower class Negro women are achieving the status of middle class. Fuller participation in the cultural aspects of our society and better employment opportunities have accelerated their upward social mobility. The revolution is definitely on although there hasn't been an official proclamation.

Apparently, society's once frigid attitude towards sex has thawed and the Negro woman is now able to understand more about the unconscious motivations and drives determining her sexual behavior. She is achieving a more valid image and identification through the enhancement of her self-esteem by the thrust of the civil rights movement. In the past, her image was greatly distorted by omissions, caricatures, taboos and old wives tales that were projected onto her by white society. She was reputed to be a torrid sex-pot of animalistic abandon. She was viewed only as a three-letter word, S-E-X, all physical, without the ability to express tenderness and receive aesthetic reciprocal gratification with her mate through the more mature feeling of love. The white man projected a schizophrenic image onto her. On the one hand, she was like a jezebel, a passionate, hyper-sensuous siren—easy to "make" and responding to his overtures in a completely uninhibited, receptive manner. On the other hand, she was a grinning, roly-poly mammy, moored down to her fat bottom by the sheer weight of her ample breasts. Thus she was only to him like a vending machine with two slots. One for sexual pleasures, the other for oral (milk) pleasures. This machine was a simple device, running on instinctual energy. It lacked a governing mechanism and thus called for little maintenance. When it fouled up or became old, it was readily discarded. However, the machine wasn't just a Frankenstein. Somehow, the white man, who was so busily engrossed in the exploitation of this machine, had overlooked an ever-present concealed mechanism. We may call it the soul or, in more scientific terms, the psyche. Here there was stored the capacity to love, to be sensitive, considerate and discriminating-to interact with others in an understanding manner while at the same time while at the same time to maintain her independence, personal integrity and uniqueness. While the civil rights revolution is more of a black revolution, the sexual revolution tends to be more of a white revolution. Enlightened forces in each revolution have catalytically interacted with one another so that the white man is developing a growing awareness that his distorted sexual image of the Negro woman is a pygmalion of his own inner fabrication. Likewise, the Negro woman is achieving keener awareness of her real sexual self.

She is aware, like her white sister, that there is a general trend in our culture for accepting fuller participation by women in all echelons of society. She realizes that there are less clear-cut boundaries as to what is the male's role and the female's role in her position as worker, wife, and mother. She is struggling to accept the changing picture of woman's role as a mother and her long treasured position as the homemaker. She is working alongside men in many diverse occupational roles. The birth control pills and other "sure" contraceptive devices are freeing her from the fear of pregnancy, which is given as the second most prevalent problem among women who are impounded in the "cold war" of a conflictual, maladjusted marital relationship. In general, both males and females consider sexual maladjustment as the No. 1 problem in marriage.

The sexual revolution in some respect may be identified as a nonviolent revolution. There are fewer women identifying the bedroom as a battleground to resist sexual advances by their spouses. Their defenses have been lowered by the protection of the "pill." Lower class women, existing on a subsistence level, are not as status conscious and may not interpret "another child" as a financial and emotional burden. Ironically, their welfare dependency, with fees and allotments contingent upon family size may enable to provide more adequately for their children than a husband's income could allow if he were in the home. Fortunately, many public aid and welfare agencies are in favor of giving birth control information to indigent mothers. The sexual revolution has exerted strong pressure towards the passing of such legislation and, as a result, many lower class mothers have been taken out of the wilderness of ignorance. Since promiscuity is productive of illegitimacy, it has only taken some statistical gymnastics to "prove" that lower class women are more promiscuous than middle or upper class women. Abortion statistics enter into this juggling act too but their validity is highly questionable, since, for the most part, they are obtained from police records. But we do know that since the "pill," there is a decreasing rate of illegitimacy and recorded abortions. Thereby, we can infer that lower class women aren't' any more promiscuous than the other two classes; they are just more unprotected. In many cases, I find that many of our culturally disadvantaged mothers are frigid and experience sex more as a punishment than a pleasure because a great deal of their energy is drained away in their struggle to subsist. They have said "no" to their husbands or boyfriends on many days of the month to avoid being intimate. Ironically, but physiologically explainable, their discipline may fail because they can no longer withhold their suppressed passions that have been stirred up by repeated seductive overtures. These passions, heightened by the surge of hormones during their ovulatory period, get them into trouble if they are unprotected. Another child is conceived and prior troubles are compounded...even more trouble than before the sexual revolution. Now, they have no excuse. A positive feature of the sexual revolution, the "pill", has only made them feel the pangs of guilt and shame. They can no longer hide behind their veil of ignorance.

There are many women who were brought up in a rigid, puritanic, overly moralistic home climate where anything even suggestive of sex was equated with sin. The increasingly enlightened attitudes of society cannot alter their lifetime rigid attitudes and inflexible defenses. They may deny that such a revolution exists. If they become aware of it, they may retaliate by mobilizing their defenses and protest in a hostile, aggressive manner. They swell the ranks of the sexually fearful women who see the bedroom as a battle ground. They are unable to be passive, receptive, tender and loving towards their spouse. Instead, they are aggressive, non-receptive, cold and rejecting. A tug of war ensues from which no one emerges victorious.

The male partner's ardor has been lost in the heat of the battle. His masculine ego has been reduced to Lilliputian size by his warrior mate.

The battling spouse syndrome is in full play and the "better-half" also is humiliated—a tension ridden hysterical female trapped in a neurotic marriage that will never work. Their set reply to the question, "How do you get along sexually?" is: "He tries to *bother* me all of the time." They may reside in a ghetto kitchenette or an elegant, doorman attended high-rise apartment building. Tragically, sex to them is only seen as a malady—a chore.

The sexual revolution has resulted in a growing number of Negro women being familiar with psychiatric and social resources that deal with these problems. Women are reading Ann Landers column with its common sense advice as religiously as they read about child rearing techniques in books by Dr. Spock. Many myths and old wives tales are being questioned. They no longer believe that a teaspoon of baking soda in a glass of warm water will keep them from "getting caught." The occult stores that dispense skunk oil, goose grease and assorted fetishes for restoring "nature" are noticing diminished sales. Psychiatric jargon is becoming part of their vocabularies and many are substituting libido for nature. More and more women can define and understand the meaning of orgasm, frigidity, sterility and potency. There is also a growing awareness of their own intricate feminine biology and they have a better understanding of the rhythmicity of ovulation, menstruation, the "safe" and fertile period and the menopause.

The wide coverage of subjects on sex by our communications media has helped to neutralize many of their long-standing taboo feelings. Now sex can be discussed more intelligently with less feelings of shame and guilt. In social gatherings, it appears that many women are competing with their male companions in narrating risque jokes. The party records don't have to be played in a soundproof room and the double-meaning monologues by Redd Foxx may be programmed along with the down-to-earth humor of Moms Mabley.

Apparently, "Freedom Now" also means more freedom for the Negro woman to enjoy and understand the sexual aspects of her being. She doesn't feel that Freud was a fraud and is finding long-sought truths in his epochal writings. It's regrettable that Freud didn't have any Negro women reclining on his couch. Where could he have found a more sensitive, emotional, expressive person to help him unravel the feminine mystique?

Middle age women are also benefiting from the enlightened attitude towards sex. The long-standing myth that menopause means the end of an active, enjoyable sexual life has been dispelled. Colored women in their 50s and 60s are no longer acting as if their sex life is obsolete. They are grooming themselves fashionably and attractively. Dietary measures and exercises to keep their figures trim are being religiously adhered to by many. When they gaze at their more rapidly aging white sisters, they can be thankful that their pigmented epidermis is less prone to become wrinkled. The road to senescence is a longer one for them and to many of them, life is beginning at 50 or 60. Many of these women who have had an impoverished sexual life before reaching their menopausal years, have found out what they interpreted as "hot flushes" were instead feelings of passion from their long-surpressed sexual feelings. Some are able for the first time in their lives to be recep- tive towards their husbands and enjoy sex.

Before the sexual revolution, the majority of women kept their sexual thoughts secret; maybe, their husbands or a confidante would occasionally get a fleeting glimpse. Now and then they would mutually exchange ideas and express intimate feelings with a girlfriend. There were no real scientific guide lines. At the same time, snatches of star- tling revelations were being echoed by women who had sought the protective sanctuaries of the psychiatric couch so that they could pour out their true feelings without the fear that they would be condemned by others for telling it "like it is." The psychiatrist further helped the patient to gain awareness of deep-seated unconscious motivations and drives of which she was unaware by interpreting dreams, loose associ- ations (talking at random—without censoring thoughts) and slips of the tongue. Pandora's box was opened and many repressed demons started to come out. She began to be more aware that her sexual values, sentiments and ideas were highly colored with distortions and myths, that many truths had been omitted and many denials had been made. Initially, reports were published for medical circles only, but, with the revolution, this formerly taboo material became available to the lay public. Society began to realize that the rigid censorship of sexual information was primarily because of our own infantile fears of sex. Now society is beginning is beginning to have both macroscopic and microscopic awareness of how people behave sexually. For instance, I have seen many middle class women who are extremely neat, overly conscientious, punctilious, obsessive and compulsive about performing their household chores. You know the type: there's a place for everything and everything is in its place. Well, sex is included in this scheme of things, too. They just don't have sex; they must schedule it. Sex is doled out and dispensed like a doctor's prescription. They totally disregard the feelings of their spouses who must follow the Boy Scout motto: "Be Prepared!" If they say, "Monday, Thursday, Friday but never on Sunday," they really mean it. They have reduced their sex life to a baseball score card. But they are playing a losing game because their composite batting average is low and there is never a home run. In fact, their husbands are left helplessly stranded. Invariably, he strikes out after which they retire hurriedly to the showers chalking up another victory. But how in the world can they be the winners?

The benefits to emotional and physical well-being cannot be obtained from sexual interplay while husband and wife are on two opposing teams. They have to be on the same team—a harmonious battery of pitcher and catcher. The husband should always be the aggressive pitcher and the wife the passive receiver. Either member may be at fault and in many cases the male remains a rookie because, unfortunately, the oppressive forces of society didn't give him the opportunity to acquire the necessary growth experiences. On the other hand, women received more preferential treatment and training because, for some unexplored reason "Mr. Charlie" was more attractive to them. Thank goodness, Mr. Charlie has just about passed from the scene. Now the husband and wife team are trying hard to get rid of the mess he created. They now begin to have a better understanding of the historical truths that have contributed to the breakdown of the Negro family and the low status of the Negro male.

Today we are having increasing dialogue between male and female. The impetus of the civil right movement with stress on freedom has increased the Negro woman's awareness of the destructive impact which slavery and years of oppression and discrimination had on the Negro male's dignity. She knows that she also suffered, but in most instances, it was her man who bore the full impact of the white man's oppression.

There is a stress on freedom, but sexual freedom does not impart a license to do what one wants without self-discipline and self-restraint.

Sexual freedom is beginning to mean to many Negro women that sex is an exciting, pleasurable, physiological function and that it is not sinful to enjoy sex. A mature, mutually gratifying sexual life is essential for a successful marriage. It will give strength, happiness, affection, security and the ability to sacrifice for one's mate. Her maternal potentialities are being realized and her role as a mother is being more adequately fulfilled.

From teenagers to grandmas, women have been affected by the sexual revolution. The old kissing parlor games "Post Office" and "Spin the Bottle," have gone out of style and instead young girls from nine up are talking about going steady. Mothers and chaperones have to keep a vigilant eye on the light dimming at the pre-teen parties. Youngsters compete with one another during the hip gyrations, syncopated body vibrations and shoulder wobblings of the Watusi, twist, and frug. These youngsters are dressing as seductively as their mothers. This change is so dynamic that one authority has suggested that if Booth Tarkington were writing *Seventeen* today, he would call it *Twelve*.

Girls are menstruating a year earlier than did their grandmothers. Their sexual feelings are awakened earlier and young mothers of age 10 and 11 don't even make the newspapers anymore. Many teen-age girls have stashed in their purses alongside their compacts a dialpack of an oral contraceptive. The premium on virginity is gone with the winds. There is no less adherence to religious concepts. Many teenage girls, like their mothers, are easing their guilt of "wrong doing" by adhering to the tenets of the 11th commandment. "Thou shall not get caught."

Our chronicle of the sexual revolution and the Negro female wouldn't be complete if we didn't add some thoughts about Old Ironside, the stalwart matriarch.

Like the Rock of Gibraltar, she has maintained her position as the dominant figure in many Negro families. Matriarchy means rule of the mothers and many a present-day Negro family structure has a matriarchal pattern. Both girls and boys brought up in the matriarchal family climate find it difficult to assume a mature masculine or feminine identification. In many instances, the son will abandon any attempt to free himself from the tyrannical rule of the mother. He will simply identify with her, give up the battle, and resolve his need to be loved by becoming a homosexual. Mother's feared image has instilled in him a dread fear of all women so that he has become psychologically castrated and is unable to have genuine sexual feelings towards other women. The female child suffers also in this relationship. Her sexual identification will also be unclear as to the inherent passive-receptive role of the female and she may adopt her mother's strong, aggressive tendencies and strive to be a completely independent, competitive, aggressive female. As with her mother, every meeting with a man becomes a challenge—a clash of wills—a competitive struggle. She wants to occupy the driver's seat at any cost and do the back seat driving too. She may also take the homosexual route because her mother has taught her little or no respect for men.

The sexual revolution has had less impact on the middle class colored woman. In many instances she is more Victorian than her white puritanic sister. She is a far cry from the unrestrained, sex-loving, passionate person that white's stereotype may portray. As a result of her rigid repressions, she has the highest incidence of emotional hypertension of any racial group. She is trying too hard to conform and repress many of her justifiably hostile aggressive feelings. At all costs, she must remain unruffled, lady-like and inoffensive. Before the sexual revolution, middle class Negro women would point an accusing finger at the lower class. Allegedly, the lower class had a monopoly on deviates, nymphomaniacs, homosexuals, rapists, prostitutes and unwed mothers. We now know that perverted sexual behavior is more common in higher educated people. Lower class women have been the target projection of taboos, sexual habits and practices on part of the middle class. The middle class does not dare point an accusing finger towards the upper class for their practices. In fact, in most instances, members of the middle class have less contact with the upper class than with the lower class.

Lower class sexual behavior is more visible; there is more interaction between participants because of closer interpersonal relations, less privacy because of overcrowded living conditions and children often sleep in the same room or even in the same bed with parents. It is more prone to be of short duration (you never know who is entering or leaving), to aggressive acting-out rivalry and jealousy (closer interaction with large numbers of people). In middle class sexual behavior, on the other hand, there is less interaction, less visibility, more privacy, less interference, more time for preliminary love play, less need for vigilance. Upper class sexual behavior takes place in luxurious surroundings. There is seclusion and quiet. There is no interaction with others but there is more participation and interaction with objects (my art collection—my guns—my etchings).

The sexual revolution has played an important role in helping the Negro female achieve a more valid image and identification of her definitive role in society. The more permissive attitude of society toward sex has enabled the major social groups of our society to loosen their defenses and give up some of their distorted projections, rationalizations, myths and come to the conclusion that although there might be minor differences, Negro and white women's sexual behavior is essentially the same when equivalent class groupings are compared. The clothes that drape the human female may become obsolete, but her body with its various needs and drives has remained essentially the same since Adam and Eve. Dali and Picasso may create humanoids on canvas but any differences in the architecture of the female body exists only within man's mind.

All They Talk About Is Sex, Sex, Sex

Tom Buckley

from *The New York Times Magazine*, April 30, 1969

*After Kinsey died in 1956, the Institute for Sex Research in Bloomington, Indiana carried on the research that Kinsey had initiated. Paul Gebhard, one of Kinsey's original colleagues, was the Institute's Director and he had been joined by a number of younger ones (among them, John Gagnon and William Simon) who would continue to conduct research on sex in the Kinsey tradition. In 1969, **The New York Times Magazine** sent Tom Buckley, one of its lead reporters (he had covered the war in Vietnam from 1966-1968), to see what the Institute was up to in the early days of the sexual revolution. Buckley also checked in at the newer Reproduction Biology Research Foundation in St. Louis where its founders William Masters and Virginia Johnson were conducting their pioneering laboratory research on the human sexual response.*

The eight professional members of the staff of the Institute for Sex Research left their cloistered offices at the University of Indiana one morning not long ago and boarded a plane for St. Louis. Watteau would have painted the scene with nymphs and satyrs dancing in the departure lounge and a squadron of cupids escorting their jet.

The seven men and a woman, the institute's librarian, were embarking for Cythera, on their way to the summit conference of erotic science—the first joint meeting of the staffs of the institute and the Reproductive Biology Research Foundation, whose director, Dr. William H. Masters, and his assistant, Mrs. Virginia E. Johnson, are the authors of *Human Sexual Response*.

For a day and a half, all they talked about was sex, sex, sex. Sexual inadequacy, male and female homosexuality, college sex and high school sex, sex and the computer, even sex for the aged and infirm.

51

These are the subjects of the major studies under way at the only two centers in the country engaged in the continuing investigation of the broad range of human sexuality.

"It was just an informal get-together," said Dr. Paul Gebhard, who became director of the Institute for Sex Research after Dr. Alfred Kinsey's death in 1956. "Bill and Virginia and I are old friends, of course, but both of us have got a lot of new people who didn't know one another. We thought it would be a good idea if they got together to talk about their work."

It is a kind of sexual treadmill they are on, as busy as Norfolk bar girls when the fleet is in. The two organizations have scarcely more than 50 employees between them, only a third of them professionals, and they get by on annual budgets of about $500,000 each, derived from Federal and foundation grants, book royalties and lecture fees. Dr. Masters, who believes that overwork and mental fatigue are the greatest enemies of a successful sex life, regularly puts in six or seven long days a week. "You know doctors," he says. "They never take their own advice."

The institute and the foundation have been influential out of all proportion to their size, the public nowadays being highly interested in—not to say obsessed by—sex in all its manifestations, and fearful of missing anything new. "I sometimes think that Kinsey's greatest contribution was that he made it possible to talk about sex in the living room," Dr. Gebhard said recently in his office at Bloomington.

Sexual Behavior in the Human Male, published in 1948 by Kinsey and two colleagues, C. E. Martin and Wardell Pomeroy (both of whom have left the institute) and *Sexual Behavior in the Human Female*, brought out five years later, although flawed, cast the sunlight of rational investigation on a subject that had been kept dark and dank for centuries. The eagerness with which these volumes were read and discussed showed how hungry the public was for sexual knowledge. Inevitably, there was a strongly adverse reaction that Dr. Gebhard relates to the obscurantism of the McCarthy era. And by the middle nineteen-fifties, it had, in Dr. Gebhard's words, "very nearly put the institute out of business." The Rockefeller Institute and the Federal Government withdrew their support. Kinsey's anxiety, his frustration, and the energy he expended raising money hastened his death, Dr. Gebhard believes.

If Kinsey had not preceded him, Dr. Masters says, he could not have dreamed of undertaking in 1956 the first scientific observations and measurements of the physiology of sexual relations, gathering the data for *Human Sexual Response*, which was published in 1966. "He was the pioneer," Dr. Masters said recently, "and it was an incredible step at the time."

It is not generally known that in his later years Kinsey, dissatisfied that he had to deal, in Dr. Gebhard's words, only with reported data, began a small informal project to analyze and film mammalian and human intercourse. The study was dropped when Dr. Masters began his more detailed work. Nor are many people aware that although *Human Sexual Response* deals only with conventional coitus and masturbation Dr. Masters and Mrs. Johnson, his assistant for the last 13 years, also collected data on various forms of heterosexual intercourse and male and female homosexual acts. The material was withheld because the two researchers believed that its inclusion would make it more difficult to gain professional and public acceptance for their book, but they say that these findings will probably be published eventually.

The two organizations first approached their subject from opposite sides, as it were, Kinsey tabulating the stark facts of sexual experience such as type, frequency and age at first encounter, and Dr. Masters and Mrs. Johnson measuring blood pressure, organic changes and the like. Lately they have been working toward each other. The institute's questionnaires have been broadened to cast light on the reasons for sexual actions, and Dr. Masters and Mrs. Johnson are using their knowledge of the physiology of sex to treat—with great success, they say—the essentially emotional causes of impotence, premature ejaculation and frigidity.

"Sometimes I think time is passing us by," Dr. Gebhard said one day recently while showing me through the Indiana institute's famous library of 22,000 volumes. "We've still got things locked up here that you can buy in the campus bookstore." He laughed. "Maurice Girodias paid us a visit not long ago. I showed him our complete collection of his Olympia Press series. 'I don't even have them all myself.' he told me. We've been offered $8 each for our copies of *Captain Billy's Whiz Bang* [a magazine that was regarded as depraved beyond redemption in the nineteen-twenties because it published murky drawings of coeds in their step-ins]. We've got full files of magazines like *Nugget, Wow!* and *High Silk Stockings.* The Library of Congress won't collect them, but we think they're important social documents."

Much of the collection, hot stuff only 10 or 15 years ago, is today redolent of lavender and old lace. There are the ribald "comic books" that used to circulate in school yards at lunch time, depicting L'il Abner and other cartoon heroes in activities not necessarily undreamed of but certainly undrawn by their creators; fading daguerreotype French post-cards in which the male actors wear handlebar mustaches, and a collection of blue films dating back to the second decade of the century, many of which are somewhat less explicit than *I Am Curious (Yellow).*

Unlike the austere and humorless Dr. Kinsey, a zoologist who specialized in the life cycle of the gall wasp before he began his study of human sexuality in 1938, Dr. Gebhard is easy-going, anecdotal and not inclined to invert his glass when wine is going round. A Coloradan now 51 years old, he joined the institute in 1946, only a few months before he received his doctorate from Harvard. He estimates that he has conducted 10 per cent of the 18,000 interviews in the institute's files, and he has a connoisseur's delight in his acquaintances in the sexual half-world, ranging from Irving Klaw, an old-time pornography king who had his offices on 14th Street, to a Manhattan bootmaker named Tony who caters to the fetish trade and the imperious Monique Van Cleef, whose recent deportation brought tears to the eyes of scores of flagellants whom she had made, quite literally, her slaves.

A working lifetime spent submerged in sexuality has left its marks upon him: an air of aplomb, of amused tolerance reminiscent of say, Reginald Gardiner or George Sanders, that is also reflected in his furrowed forehead, humorous, pouchy eyes, a cosmopolitan clipped guards' mustache seldom seen in the central states and a Hapsburgian, only barely noticeable, hand tremor.

"It seems now as though it was a Golden Age when Kinsey was alive," he said. "We had only one project at a time to zero in on. Now the projects and the paperwork grow at an exponential rate."

Since 1966 the institute has been engaged in a study of homosexuality. The first phase, a survey of 480 white male homosexuals living on the Near North Side of Manhattan, has been completed. The second phase, in which 1,100 white and Negro homosexuals of both sexes and

500 nonhomosexual members of their families will be interviewed, is about to begin.

A preliminary assessment of the data collected at Chicago, not previously made public, has turned up some surprising views held by homosexuals. Asked for example, if they would take a "magic pill" that would turn them into heterosexuals, the large majority said they would not. Most say they became aware that they were sexually "different" in their early teens, although in many cases the homosexual preference did not become apperent until much later. Although many long-term homosexual relationships were found, the majority tend to engage in brief affairs and one-night stands. The number of sexual partners and the frequency of intercourse are higher than for single heterosexual males. The homosexual was also reported to be more specific in the type of partner that appeals to him—tall or short, stocky or slim, blond or dark.

The men in the survey were interviewed for about two hours each, responding to a 145-page questionnaire. On the basis of their answers, Dr. Gebhard said, many appeared to cope reasonably well with their way of life. "We look at these things in a nitty-gritty way," he said. "We ask, 'Does he have a job, social stability, love and friendship?' If he does—and more homosexuals than you might think have them—then we have to regard him as having made a pretty good adjustment."

Only a comparative few ever come to the notice of the police, he went on, and a great many successfully lead a double life, their "straight," or heterosexual, business associates and friends being unaware of their "gay," or homosexual, tastes. Few affect the blazing effeminacy or the less obvious languid mannerisms that are thought by a good many people to characterize male homosexuals: "I remember one lawyer in Chicago saying, 'For God's sake, don't let the word get around. It would be better for us if the public just continued thinking in stereotypes.' "

Kinsey's *Sexual Behavior in the Human Male* stated that 4 per cent of the country's males and 2 per cent of females were predominantly or exclusively homosexual. Dr. Gebhard believes that this figure is still substancially correct. If they *seem* to be more numerous now than when the book appeared, he suggests, it is because a significant number no longer conceal their homosexuality and have banded together into organizations such as the Mattachine Society to press for the legalization of homosexuality and the moderation of the stigma attached to it. (Although the penalties for homsexual acts conducted in private between consenting adults were removed several years ago in Britain, they are still forbidden by Federal statute and in 49 of the 50 states. The only exception is Illinois, which revised its criminal code recently. Even so, Dr. Gebhard said, Chicago is regarded as a tough place for homosexuals. Plainclothes-men are assigned to lure homosexuals into making overtures, then charge them with disorderly conduct or other offenses. This practice has been abandoned in New York.)

Another statistic that appeared in Kinsey's study of the male—that 38 per cent of all men had had at least one homosexual experience—is now thought to be far too high. The volume, which has been out of print for several years, will not be reissued, Dr. Gebhard explained, until this and other errors can be corrected. "That figure has really haunted us," he said. "What happened was that Kinsey used many prisoners for his interviews, mostly because he could have access to them. He thought their experiences were typical of the lower socio-economic group. We know now that that isn't the case at all.

"Besides, it was interpreted incorrectly," he went on. "Kinsey failed to take into account that a good deal of overt homosexuality, particularly among youngsters, has an essentially heterosexual impulse. Suppose a bunch of kids are sitting around talking about girls or looking at pictures. They get excited. . . ." He shrugged. "That certainly isn't homosexual in the true sense of the word."

Considerable disagreement has developed in recent years as to the nature of homosexuality. The traditional psychoanalytic view—that homosexuality is a pathological condition, the "mirror image" of neurosis in Freud's formulation, that has its roots in the young child's relation to his parents—is no longer accepted unquestioningly. Homosexuality may be caused in many ways, the newer theories say, even possibly by still undiscovered endocrinological or chromosomal abnormalities. Some social scientists question whether homosexuality in general can even be classified as an illness.

"Psychoanalysts never see a reasonably happy homosexual," said Dr. Martin S. Weinberg, a young sociologist on the staff of the institute who formerly taught at Rutgers. "There are probably many causes of homosexuality. For example, we know the orgasm is a powerful conditioning agent, and how many times does a pleasurable experience have to be repeated before it establishes a pattern? For some homosexuals, their sex may be pathological, just as it is with some heterosexuals."

Dr. Alan Bell, a soiologist and former Episcopal priest who heads the homosexual study, believes that such arguments are not particularly helpful. "Pathological—that's the language of the doctor, not the social scientist." What *is* important, he contends, is that homosexuals have existed in every known culture since the dawn of history, that they exist in substantial numbers now, that few are cured or changed or appear to want a cure or change and that to a considerable degree their emotional problems can be traced to their virtual exclusion from heterosexual society and the extraordinary difficulties put in the way of their achieving a measure of self-acceptance.

The removal of the taboos and penalties against homosexuality, Dr. Gebhard believes, might lead to an increase in casual homosexuality but it would sharply reduce the number of the exclusively or predominantly homosexual because fewer youngsters would feel themselves "locked into" the subculture. As Dr. D. J. West, a British psychiatrist, wrote in his recently published book *Homosexuality*: "The exclusive preference for the opposite sex is an acquired trait and involves the repression of a certain amount of homosexual feeling which is natural to a human being." Punishment for consensual homosexual acts, except those involving children, is regarded by the members of the institute staff as a hangover from medieval days.

"I remember talking to a man who had been imprisoned for a homosexual offense," Dr. Gebhard said. "There he was, able to indulge himself with hundreds of desirable partners. 'If society really wanted to cure me,' he said, 'they'd lock me up in a *women's* prison and they wouldn't let me out until the girls started looking good.' "

A great many psychoanalysts and psychiatrists would disagree vehemently with the Indiana institute's view of homosexuality. Some homosexuals themselves regard homosexuality as an affliction. In part, Dr. Gebhard agrees. His organization's studies indicate that the rate of suicide and serious neurosis is higher among homosexuals than heterosexuals. The fear of a lonely old age after a life without children is widespread. Their grasp of reality is apt to be more tenuous. A Chicago lawyer told an institute interviewer, "I've been living a lie for so long that I'm not sure any more what the truth is."

"There is no question that homosexuality is a much more difficult way of life." Dr. Gebhard said. "Life is complicated enough as it is. Anyone who can avoid it would be wise to do so."

The institute palns to publish next year a survey of sexual activity and attitudes among college students, based on interviews with 1,200 young men and women at 12 campuses around the country. The authors, Drs. John Gagnon and William Simon, who are highly regarded young sociologists, resigned from the Institute for Sex Research last year but will see the work through to completion.

Dr. Gagnon, who now teaches at the Stony Brook, L.I., campus of the State Univerity of New York, said recently that he and Dr. Simon were still putting figures through the computer, "looking at the data, turning it around, trying to see it in different ways."

"We want to be as careful as possible," he added. "Parents have enough to worry about as it is, and we don't want to cause them needless anxiety. Even if there hasn't been as much change in sexual behavior as supposed, there is a far greater potential for change than ever before. College students are certainly the most liberal segment of society, at least toward the behavior of others, and the least likely to make general moral judgments.

"What does it take to make a sexual revolution? Either an increase or a decrease in sexual activity. When women have the same attitude toward sex as men, then you might have a revolution. But do you know that 90 percent of all Americans get married? That's a higher figure than in any other Western country. Two-thirds of college girls are married within 18 months of graduation or leaving. Premarital sex is likely to be with the men they marry. That doesn't sound like a revolution. And the divorce rate has generally been steady for years."

Under a grant from the Russell Sage Foundation, the institute is also preparing to publish all 18,000 of its case histories—the raw material of its publications—for possible use by other researchers. It will preserve the anonymity of its subjects, even to the hero of *Sexual Behavior in the Human Male*, a New York lawyer who reported an average of 30 orgasms a week for 30 years. Dr. Gebhard, who interviewed him originally, saw him several years ago, and the lawyer reported that, given the inevitable encroachments of age, he was still going strong.

In other major projects, the institute is measuring the effects of sex-education courses through "before and after" interviews with elementary and high school students. Members of the upper-middle class are being asked how they learned about sex. And both the institute and the Reproduction Biology Reseach Foundation are setting up courses to train teachers for medical-school courses in sex. Such instruction was all but unheard of before the publication of *Human Sexual Response*. The confident advice that people with sexual problems see their friendly family doctor or clergyman is often ill-considered, Dr. Gebhrd and Dr. Masters agree, since neither group generally has much information on the subject. In the last few years though, more than half of the 82 medical schools in the country have begun teaching the subject—using the Masters-Johnson book as text—and the total is likely to increase.

If the quarters of the Institute for Sex Research are shabbily academic, the St. Louis offices and laboratories of the Reproductive Biology Research Foundation are dazzlingly ultramodern. It is a world of black leather, stainless steel and glowing walnut, muted telephones, silent tape recorders and machines that can analyze a blood sample in the twinkling of an eye. Dr. Masters and Mrs. Johnson are a bit dazzling, too, in their long white medical coats that glimmer and creak with starch, interweaving their friendly, earnest, well-modulated voices to answer questions. Their collaboration began when Dr. Masters decided that he could not carry out his research for *Human Sexual Response* without a female assistant, and Mrs. Johnson was one of the women who replied to his advertisement.

They complement each other. Dr. Masters, who is 52, has a face whose essential qualities have been sketched in thousands of advertisements for pharmaceuticals. He is baldish, but tan and healthily glowing. The eyes are deep-set, with a fixed, powerful gaze. The nose is straight and long, the mouth a straight, narrow line and the chin strong. Mrs. Johnson, 10 years his junior, a divorcee who, like Dr. Masters, has two teen-age children, blooms with vitality. She looks remarkably like Happy Rockefeller, and mentioned that indeed she had been mistaken for the Governor's wife at, of all places, Rockefeller University.

Unlike many scientists, they can explain their work clearly, both in technical terms and in laymen's language. The polish of their presentation is the result of hundreds of lectures before medical organizations. The talks, starting long before the book was published, were part of an attempt to gain acceptance for a project that, for all they knew, might have been turned by the hostility of the essentially conservative medical associations into an off-color joke that could have destroyed their reputations.

"You must remember that in publishing this book we were concerned primarily with acceptance," Dr. Masters said recently. "That is the reason that it wasn't written in English to start with. In fact we *rewrote* it to make the language as technical and noninflammatory as we could. In retrospect, it was probably a mistake. At the time, when all the cards were on the table and it was a matter of professional survival, we were coppering as many bets as we could. I don't think we were dodging the issue, but the one thing we could not afford was any suggestion that this was pornographic. The suggestion was never made."

Despite its almost impenetrable thicket of medical terminology, more than 250,000 copies of *Human Sexual Response* have been sold at $10 each. Other authors' paperback explanations of what Dr. Masters and Mrs. Johnson were trying to say did a great deal better. The strategy of the two researchers was proved correct, however. The book's reviews, in the lay and professional press, were overwhelmingly favorable. The propriety of their research was endorsed by the American Medical Association, an organization of such brass-bound conservativism that its approval muffled the handful of critics who asserted that human sexuality was too sensitive and sacred an activity to be subjected to the scientist's probes and that the findings were dubious because anyone who would agree to take part in the study was not normal.

The fact is that the 382 women and 312 men who took part in the research were probably a good deal closer to normal than "average" people. They were subjected to psychological screening, which eliminated 40 per cent of the volunteers. Many of the participants were drawn from Washington University, where Dr. Masters, who is still a member of the medical school faculty, began his work. He and Mrs. Johnson used male and female prostitutes at first, but found that many of the women were physiologically abnormal; the demands of their occupation had caused chronic congestion in the blood vessels of the pelvic region.

All in all, though people have been making love in the dark, scientifically speaking, since time began, *Human Sexual Response* turned out to contain few surprises and little or no information likely to cause widespread changes in sexual customs. No evidence was found to support Freud's hypothesis of two types of orgasm, vaginal and clitoral, upon which a baroque superstructure of psychoanalytical theorizing had been erected. A "sweating" effect through the walls of the vagina was found to be a source of its lubrication. (Evidence of a sperm-destroying chemical in vaginal secretions, including those of Cowper's and Bartholin's glands, was found in 41 of 382 women who took part in the research; it is being investigated in the foundation's laboratories.)

The pseudonymous authors of pornographic novels to the contrary notwithstanding, none of the women was found to discharge at climax. (The trouble with pornography, Drs. Masters and Gebhard agree, is that by providing inaccurate and exaggerated descriptions of sexual activity it fails to perform the one service it might render: instead of enlightening the inexperienced, it fills them with expectations that aren't likely to be fulfilled.) In any case, the most intense female orgasms measured were induced by masturbation.

The research also seemed to answer a question that Dr. Masters believes has bothered every man at one time or another—the size of his penis. Studies showed that while the organs of the men who took part in the study differed in size when in repose, the smaller organs showed a greater proportional increase in arousal. (Dr. Masters carefully omitted from the book any data on average dimensions to spare mini-men from a lifetime of unhappiness.) Size, the researchers concluded, doesn't matter anyhow. Their observations demonstrated conclusively that the normal vagina expands just enough to accommodate the penis, regardless of its dimensions. Nor was any correlation found between its size and the intensity and frequency of the female orgasm. "The only way it could make a difference," Dr. Masters said, "was if the woman *thought* it did."

The next work of Dr. Masters and Mrs. Johnson will be titled *Sexual Inadequacy*. They won't try to set standards of performance; each couple, they say must decide that for themselves. The book will describe the treatment they have devised for impotence, frigidity, and premature ejaculation. It involves the use of techniques that are based on their laboratory findings and on counseling sessions. Dr. Masters emphasizes that no observations or measurements of sexual intercourse are involved; they regard that phase of their work as completed.

Dr. Masters and Mrs. Johnson accept for treatment only married couples referred by physicians or psychotherapists. Each couple must agree to be available for follow-up consultations for five years. Of the 400 couples they have treated in the last 10 years, Dr. Masters says, 80 per cent have shown immediate improvement, and in all but a small number of cases there has been no relapse during the follow-up period. (On occasion, he said, eager couples have returned with Polaroid photographs of themselves to show how well they are progressing. "We tell them," he comments drily, "that we are willing to take their word for it.")

On May 1 Dr. Masters and Mrs. Johnson will begin to concentrate on writing their text. They hope to complete it in a year, in which case it will probably be published late in 1970. "We have promised Little, Brown to write it in English this time," Dr. Masters said. "I hope we can do it." Meanwhile, they have been preparing the ground, as they did with *Human Sexual Response*. They have described their method in some detail at closed meetings of physicians and allied groups, but will discuss it only in general terms with the lay press because they fear misinterpretation and sensationalized out-of-context disclosures.

On the basis of their own statements, supplemented by information gathered elsewhere, it can be said that the patients spend two weeks in St. Louis, visiting the foundation daily for varying periods except on the weekend. There are physical examinations, biochemical tests, counseling sessions and much practical advice that derives from Dr. Master's long experience as a gynecologist and obstetrician and, of course, from observations of thousands of successful instances of love-making.

"We've learned what really happens during sexual intercourse," Mrs. Johnson said, "and it's infinitely easier to treat something when you know how it should be."

The two work as a team, talking to each couple together, then man-to-man and woman-to-woman and then vise versa. "We don't to tell them why they're in St. Louis," Dr. Masters said. "They're perfectly aware of the reason. We give them some idea of why we think these distresses have developed and what we can do about it. Impotence, for example, is just as much a wife's problem as it is a husband's. There is no such thing as an uninvolved or nontraumatized partner in a marriage where there is sexual inadequacy, and that's one very important reason for the general lack of success in the separate treatment of the impotent male and the nonorgasmic female. In effect, you're simply throwing him or her back to the lions."

Nonorgasmic women are encouraged to familiarize themselves with their sexual anatomy, to caress themselves and to permit their husbands to do so. Dr. Masters has been quoted as saying that he and Mrs. Johnson have been appalled by the number of their patients who are not only unaware of the sensitivity to stimulation of the area around the clitoris but also observe taboos against touching it.

Couples who have achieved successful sexual relations have done so against the odds, the two therapists believe, since they have grown up in a culture that assigns a dishonorable role to sexual expressions. Such an inheritance makes it extremely difficult for those with sexual problems to solve them. "People must learn that they are sexual beings and learn to be comfortable with that fact," Mrs. Johnson said.

Trying to learn what to do from marriage manuals—"the 'one, two, three, kick!' approach," in Mrs. Johnson's words—can't work, they say, because such efforts become a meaningless exchange of techniques in which what should be a natural and relaxed coming together is turned into a performance in which an "A+" is awarded only if both partners reach their climax simultaneously.

"We try to tell our patients that they don't *have* to perform," Dr. Masters said. "We find, for example, that many women don't have the urge or need for orgasmic expression every time they're mounted. Does this mean she avoids intercourse? Heck, no! It's a real pleasure. She enjoys it thoroughly. She is satisfied if not satiated."

In their experience, the researchers say, primary impotence, in which the husband is never able to sustain an erection long enough to acheive penetration, is rare in marriage. Secondary impotence, which occurs after one or more successful encounters, is not. In the overwhelming number of cases, they say, the direct cause is liquor. Occasional failures to perform can be expected by anyone for a variety of reasons, fatigue and tension being the most common. But for some men failure is unacceptable. They demand the same ruthlessly efficient performance from themselves that they do from, say, their automobiles. Under this psychic burden, they tend to drink to relax but seldom stop at the one or two highballs that might help them. As a result they find themselves caught in a vicious circle of unfulfillable quotas.

Dr. Masters and Mrs. Johnson say they have found that the ability to have an erection persists more often than not into old age. What diminishes, they say, is the urge to have orgasm, and as this occurs many men lapse into sexual inactivity. Dr. Masters believes, however, that men can find pleasure in nonorgasmic sex and also give pleasure to their wives. He calls this "a new concept of sexual expression for the aging male," and it will be discussed in the forthcoming book.

Some psychoanalysts strongly oppose Dr. Master's methods, asserting that he is merely "papering over" neurotic symptoms that are certain to reassert themselves in time in what may be even more painful ways. To this, his reply is that by removing the really crushing emotional burden of sexual nonperformance he and Mrs. Johnson are enabling their patients to realize more of their human potential. In this sense, they see themselves as attacking the problem from one end while the psychotherapist is treating the underlying problems, if they persist, after functioning is restored.

A therapist who is familiar with their method attributes its success primarily to the sense of authority they bring to it. "It's magic," he said. "Let's face it, orgasms take place in the head, not in the crotch. A couple comes to St. Louis. They know they're visiting a world-famous doctor. They see this absolutely dignified man and his attractive, respectable assistant casually using what they think of as dirty words and encouraging them to do the same. Bill and Virginia are absolutely ethical and I'm sure they are just as successful as they say they are, but I don't know how many other teams could do as well."

It is an observation that Dr. Masters and Mrs. Johnson take seriously. "The point is a very fair one," Dr. Masters said recently. "We don't think this is the case, but we can't know for some time." They have trained another man and woman team to treat some of the patients at the foundation and will establish a postgraduate-level course for others. Meanwhile, they have no comparative data. In any event, they say, no informed and thorough analysis of their work can be made until they publish.

They have already blocked out the research that Dr. Masters expects will occupy him for most of the rest of his working life. A study of female homosexuality has been begun. It will relate the physiological data they accumulated during their observation and measurement of reactions to the emotional and social experience of lesbianism. "What we're trying to do is to absorb, live, learn to know the subculture," Dr. Masters said. He and Mrs. Johnson are proceeding at a leisurely pace and do not plan to publish anything on the subject until well into the nineteen-seventies. Still further in the future are additional studies of sexual activity among the aging and the development of what Dr. Masters calls "a preventative medicine approach" to sexual inadequacy.

Dr. Gebhard has raised with Dr. Masters the possibility of cooperative research on specific projects, such as their concurrent studies on homosexuality, but no decision has been made. Although such cooperation, or indeed a merger, might seem logical, both centers are anxious to maintain their hard-won independence. (Indiana University provides the institute with office space, computer time and supplies and gives faculty status to professional staff members, but does not otherwise intrude into its work. Dr. Masters set up the foundation in 1964 because he wished to be his own boss.) Meanwhile, they agree that there are more than enough aspects of sex in which ignorance and misinformation prevail to keep both organizations busy for years to come. And they applaud the fact that individual researchers are beginning to find it possible to work in this sensitive area, though for some time the institute and the foundation are likely to remain pre-eminent.

"I was driving Paul and Virginia and a car full of people out to dinner the night they were here." Dr. Masters recalled recently. "Paul said, 'Watch where you're going, Bill. If you get us all killed, there goes sex research in the United States.' "

PART II

Female Sexuality

• • •

One of the most fiercely debated questions about the sexual revolution has been whether or nor women benefited from the changes in sexual mores and behavior. There is no question that the first signs of a shift in sexual mores emerged first in the writings of Henry Miller, D.H. Lawrence and Norman Mailer, in the sexualized social commentary of comics like Lenny Bruce, and in soft-core pornography like *Playboy* magazine—all representing a male point of view.

However, the women's movement and changes in the understanding of female sexuality played a central role in the sexual revolution. The women's movement grew out of several distinct sources. Since the end of World War II married women had entered the labor force in dramatically growing numbers—and the inequities of the workplace: lower wages, limited upward mobility on the job, and the dual burden of job and domestic responsibilities underscored for many women their relative lack of income and power. Betty Friedan's *The Feminine Mystique* (1963) was a response to this development. And the National Organization of Women was a political development of this mainstream feminist perspective. Even before the appearance of Friedan's book, the growing economic independence of women had begun to encourage sexual independence as well. Helen Gurley Brown, pursuing a career in advertising, wrote *Sex and the Single Girl* which took direct aim at the sexual double standard that required women to remain virgins before their marriage while permitting men to engage in sex. *Sex and the Single Girl* was a chatty and worldly advice book; it was an unlikely manifesto of sexual adventure for the unmarried woman.

Another source of awareness grew from the experience of young women involved in the radical political movements of the late fifties and sixties—such as the black civil rights movement and in movement against the war in Vietnam. Many of the young women involved in these movements found themselves politically marginalized and under pressure to engage in sex with male activists. The disparities experienced by these politically active women made them acutely aware of the social and sexual drawbacks experienced by women. In the late 60s, many of these women formed discussion groups, political organizations, and publications to articulate their grievances.

The research of William Masters and Virginia Johnson also reinforced feminist sexual politics—their books devoted more space to discussing female sexuality (in part, because it had been much less studied) than male sexuality and debunked numerous misconceptions founded on the idea that female sexuality was strictly analogous with or a reflection of male sexuality. They characterized male sexuality as one-dimensional due to the cycle of arousal, orgasm and detumescence, whereas women were capable of sustaining a prolonged plateau of orgasmic experiences. Feminists used Masters and Johnson's findings to criticize the patterns of sexual behavior that rested on ideas of male initiative, men's greater sex drive, or their greater capacity for sexual pleasure. Masters and Johnson provided the biological evidence, feminists developed sweeping critiques of the social and cultural conventions that organized female sexual experience and repressed their sexual expression. Mary Jane Sherfey, Ann Koedt, Alix Kates Shulman, Barbara Seaman and many other feminist thinkers contributed to the growing body of literature which rested on completely new assumptions about female sexuality.

The sexual revolution was an enormous and chaotic social upheaval. It stimulated many different ways of shaping sexual lives—which in addition to new freedom from sexual repression also included forms of behavior that happened to devalue the sexual lives of others. But the sexual revolution of the sixties and seventies was, above all else, driven by the revolutions in women's sexual lives—although that does not, by any means, exclude the many other developments that favored male sexuality or various sexual minorities.

Women Alone? Oh Come Now!

Helen Gurley Brown

from *Sex and the Single Girl*, 1962

*Helen Gurley Brown was married and a successful copywriter and account executive in the advertising business when she wrote **Sex and the Single Girl**. The book offered candid advice on fashion, sex, love, career, and entertainment to the young woman who was just starting out on her career. The most controversial aspect of the book was not only its stress on the positive benefits of unmarried life, but on the importance of sex. **Sex and the Single Girl** became an instant bestseller and its success allowed Brown to leave the advertising business and write a syndicated advice column called "Woman Alone." In 1965 Brown was appointed editor-in-chief of **Cosmopolitan**, a woman's magazine that had been around since 1886. She transformed it from a foundering enterprise into a splashy and lively magazine aimed at the young single and married women who had flocked to read **Sex and the Single Girl**. She remained as the editor until she retired in 1996 after 31 years on the job.*

I married for the first time at thirty-seven. I got the man I wanted. It *could* be construed as something of a miracle considering how old *I* was and how eligible *he* was.

David is a motion picture producer, forty-four, brainy, charming and sexy. He was sought after by many a Hollywood starlet as well as some less flamboyant but more deadly types. And *I* got him! We have two Mercedes-Benzes, one hundred acres of virgin forest near San Francisco, a Mediterranean house overlooking the Pacific, a full-time maid and a good life.

I am not beautiful, or even pretty. I once had the world's worst case of acne. I am not bosomy or brilliant. I grew up in a small town. I didn't go to college. My family was, and is, desperately poor and I have always helped support them. I'm an introvert and I am sometimes mean and cranky.

But *I* don't think it's a miracle that I married my husband. I think I deserved him! For seventeen years I worked hard to become the kind of woman who might interest him. And when he finally walked into my life I was just worldly enough, relaxed enough, financially secure enough (for I also worked hard at my job) and adorned with enough glitter to attract him. He wouldn't have looked at me when I was twenty, and I wouldn't have known what to do with *him*.

There is a tidal wave of misinformation these days about how many more marriageable women there are than men (that part is true enough) and how tough is the plight of the single woman—spinster, widow, divorcee.

I think a single woman's biggest problem is coping with the people who are trying to marry her off! She is so driven by herself and her well-meaning but addlepated friends to become married that her whole existence seems to be an apology for *not* being married. Finding *him* is all she can think about or talk about when (a) she may not be psychologically ready for marriage; (b) there is no available husband for every girl at the time she wants one; and (c) her years as a single woman can be too rewarding to rush out of.

Although many's the time I was sure I would die alone in my spinster's bed, I could never bring myself to marry just to get married. If I had, I would have missed a great deal of misery along the way, no doubt, but also a great deal of fun.

I think marriage is insurance for the *worst* years of your life. During your best years you don't need a husband. You do need a man of course every step of the way, and they are often cheaper emotionally and a lot more fun by the dozen.

I believe that as many women over thirty marry out of fear of being alone someday—not necessarily now but *some* day—as for love of or compatibility with a particular man. The plan seems to be to get someone while the getting's good and by the time you lose your looks he'll be too securely glued to you to get away.

Isn't it silly? A man can leave a woman at fifty (though it may cost him some dough) as surely as you can leave dishes in the sink. He can leave any time *before* then too, and so may you leave *him* when you find your football hero developing into the town drunk. Then you have it all to do over again as if you hadn't gobbled him up in girlish haste.

How much saner and sweeter to marry when you have both jelled.

And how much safer to marry with part of the play out of his system *and yours*. It takes guts. It can be lonely out there out of step with the rest of the folks. And you may not find somebody later. But since you're not finding somebody sooner as things stand, wouldn't it be better to stop driving . . . to stop fretting . . . to start recognizing what you have *now?*

As for marrying to have children, you can have babies until you're forty or older. And if you happen to die before *they* are forty, at least you haven't lingered into their middle age to be a doddering old bore. You also avoid those tiresome years as an unpaid baby sitter.

Frankly, the magazines and their marriage statistics give me a royal pain.

There is a important truth that magazines never deal with, that single women are too brainwashed to figure out, that married women know but won't admit, that married men *and* single men endorse in a body, and that is that the single woman, far from being a creature to be pitied and patronized, is emerging as the newest glamour girl of our times.

She is engaging because she lives by her wits. She supports herself. She has had to sharpen her personality and mental resources to a glitter in order to survive in a competitive world and the sharpening looks good. Economically she is a dream. She is not a parasite, a dependent, a scrounger, a sponger or a bum. She is a giver, not a taker, a winner and not a loser.

Why else is she attractive? Because she isn't married, that's why! She is free to be The Girl in a man's life or at least his vision of The Girl, whether he is married or single himself.

When a man thinks of a married woman, no matter how lovely she is, he must inevitably picture her greeting her husband at the door with a martini or warmer welcome, fixing little children's lunches or scrubbing them down because they've fallen into a mudhole. She is somebody else's wife and somebody else's mother.

When a man thinks of a single woman, he pictures her alone in her apartment, smooth legs sheathed in pink silk Capri pants, lying tantalizingly among dozens of satin cushions, trying to read but not very successfully, for *he* is in that room—filling her thoughts, her dreams, her life.

Why else is a single woman attractive? She has more time and often more money to spend on herself. She has the extra twenty minutes to exercise every day, an hour to make up her face for their date. She has all day Saturday to whip up a silly, wonderful cotton brocade tea coat to entertain him in next day or hours to find it at a bargain sale.

Besides making herself physically more inviting, she has the freedom to furnish her mind. She can read Proust, learn Spanish, study *Time*, *Newsweek* and *The Wall Street Journal*.

Most importantly, a single woman, even if she is a file clerk, moves in the world of men. She knows their language—the language of retailing, advertising, motion pictures, exporting, shipbuilding. Her world is a far more colorful world than the one of P.T.A., Dr. Spock and the jammed clothes dryer.

A single woman never has to drudge. She can get her housework over within one good hour Saturday morning plus one other hour to iron blouses and white collars. She need never break her fingernails or her spirit waxing a playroom or cleaning out the garage.

She has more money for clothes and for trips than any but a wealthily married few.

Sex—What of It?

Theoretically a "nice" single woman has no sex life. What nonsense! She has a better sex life than most of her married friends. She need never be bored with one man per lifetime. Her choice of partners is endless and they seek *her*. They never come to her bed duty-bound. Her married friends refer to her pursuers as wolves, but actually many of them turn out to be lambs—to be shorn and worn by her.

Sex of course is more than the act of coitus. It begins with the delicious feeling of attraction between two people. It may never go further, but sex it is. And a single woman may promote the attraction, bask in the sensation, drink it like wine and pour it over her like blossoms, with never a guilty twinge. She can promise with a look, a touch, a letter or a kiss—and she doesn't have to deliver. She can be maddeningly hypocritical and, after arousing desire, insist that it be shut off by stating she wants to be chaste for the man she marries. Her pursuer may strangle her with his necktie, but he can't *argue* with her. A flirtatious married woman is expected to Go Through With Things.

Since for a female getting there is at *least* half the fun, a single woman has reason to prize the luxury of taking long, gossamer, attenuated, pulsating trips before finally arriving in bed. A married woman and her husband have precious little time and energy for romance after they've put the house, animals and children to bed. A married woman with her lover is on an even tighter schedule.

During and after an affair, a single woman suffers emotional stress. Do you think a married woman can bring one off more blissfully free of strain? (One of my close friends, married, committed suicide over a feckless lover. Another is currently in a state of fingernail-biting hysteria.) And I would rather be the other woman than the woman who watches a man *stray* from her.

Yet, while indulging her libido, which she has plenty of if she is young and healthy, it is still possible for the single woman to be a lady, to be highly respected and even envied if she is successful in her work.

I did it. So have many of my friends.

Perhaps this all sounds like bragging. I do not mean to suggest for a moment that being single is not often hell. But I do mean to suggest that it can also be quite heavenly, whether you choose *it* or it chooses *you*.

There is a catch to achieving single bliss. You have to work like a son of a bitch.

But show me the married woman who can loll about and eat cherry bonbons! Hourly she is told by every magazine she reads what she must do to keep her marriage from bursting at the seams. There is no peace for anybody married *or* single unless you do your chores. Frankly, I wouldn't want to make the choice between a married hell or a single hell. They're both hell.

However, serving time as a single woman can give you the foundation for a better marriage if you finally go that route. Funnily enough it also gives you the choice.

What then does it take for a single woman to lead the rich, full life?

Here is what it *doesn't* take.

Great beauty. A man seems not so much attracted to overwhelming beauty as he is just overwhelmed by it—at first. Then he grows accustomed to the face, fabulous as it is, and starts to explore the personality. Now the hidden assets of an *attractive* girl can be as fascinating as the dark side of the moon. Plumbing the depths of a raving beauty may be like plumbing the depths of Saran Wrap.

What it also doesn't take to collect men is money. Have you ever noticed the birds who circle around rich girls? Strictly for the aviary.

You also don't have to be Auntie Mame and electrify everybody with your high-voltage personality. Do *you* like the girl who always grabs the floor to tell what happened to *her* in the elevator? Well neither does anybody else.

And you don't have to be the fireball who organizes bowling teams, gets out the chain letters and makes certain *somebody* gives a shower for the latest bride.

What you do have to do is work with the raw material you have, namely you, and never let up.

If you would like the good single life—since the married life is not just now forthcoming—you can't afford to leave any facet of you unpolished.

You don't have to do anything brassy or show-offy or against your nature. Your most prodigious work will be on *you*—at home. (When I got married, I moved in with six-pound dumbbells, slant board, an electronic device for erasing wrinkles, several pounds of soy lecithin, powdered calcium and yeast-liver concentrate for Serenity Cocktails and enough high-powered vitamins to generate life in a statue.)

Unlike Madame Bovary you don't chase the glittering life, you lay a trap for it. You tunnel up from the bottom.

You *do* need a quiet, private, personal aggression . . . a refusal to take singleness lying down. A sweetly smiling drop-dead attitude for the marrying Sams, and that means *you too*.

You must develop style. Every girl has one . . . it's just a case of getting it out in the open, caring for it and feeding it like an orchid until it leafs out. (One girl is a long-legged, tennis-playing whiz by day, a serene pool at night for friends to drown their tensions in. Wholesomeness is her trademark. A petite brunette is gamine but serious-minded. A knockout in black jersey, she is forever promoting discussions on Stendhal or diminishing colonialism. An intellectual charmer.)

Brains are an asset but it doesn't take brainy brains like a nuclear physicist's. Whatever it is that keeps you from saying anything unkind and keeps you asking bright questions even when you don't quite understand the answers will do nicely. A lively interest in people and things (even if you aren't *that* interested) is why bosses trust you with new assignments, why men talk to you at parties . . . and sometimes ask you on to dinner.

Fashion is your powerful ally. Let the "secure" married girls eschew shortening their skirts (or lengthening them) and wear their classic cashmeres and tweeds until everybody could throw up. You be the girl other girls look at to see what America has copied from Paris.

Roommates are for sorority girls. You need an apartment alone even if it's over a garage.

Your figure can't harbor an ounce of baby fat. It never looked good on anybody but babies.

You must cook well. It will serve you faithfully.

You must have a job that interests you, at which you work hard.

I say "must" about all these things as though you were under orders. You don't have to do anything. I'm just telling you what worked for me.

I'm sure of this. You're not too fat, too thin, too tall, too small, too dumb, or too myopic to have married women gazing at you wistfully.

This then is not a study on how to get married but how to stay single—in superlative style.

The Female Orgasm

William H. Masters and Virginia Johnson

from *Human Sexual Response,* 1966

The laboratory research of William Masters and Virginia Johnson on the physiology of human sexual arousal and orgasm made a major contribution to our understanding of sex. They identified the source and significance of vaginal lubrication, measured the increases in blood pressure associated with sexual excitement, and established the basis for sex therapy. In ways that Masters and Johnson never anticipated their work had an enormous influence on the development of a new sexual politics. Their research demonstrated that women could achieve sexual fulfillment independently of sex with men, that women were capable of many more and deeper orgasms, and that men's penises (and their penis's size) were irrelevant to women's sexual gratification.

For the human female, orgasm is a psychophysiologic experience occurring within, and made meaningful by, a context of psychosocial influence. Physiologically, it is a brief episode of physical release from the vasocongestive and myotonic increment developed in response to sexual stimuli. Psychologically, it is subjective perception of a peak of physical reaction to sexual stimuli. The cycle of sexual response, with orgasm as the ultimate point in progression, generally is believed to develop from a drive of biologic-behavioral origin deeply integrated into the condition of human existence.

Where possible, material presented reflects consideration of three interacting areas of influence upon female orgasmic attainment previously recognized in attempts to understand and to interpret female sexual response: (i) physiologic (characteristic physical conditions and reactions during the peak of sex tension increment); (ii) psychologic (psychosexual orientation and receptivity to orgasmic attainment);

and (iii) sociologic (cultural, environmental, and social factors influencing orgasmic incidence or ability). The quantitative and qualitative relationship of these factors appears totally variable between one woman's orgasmic experiences, and orgasm as it occurs in other women. Only baseline physiologic reactions and occasional individually characteristic modes of expression remain consistent from orgasm to orgasm, reflecting the human female's apparent tendency toward orientation of sexual expression to psychosocial demand.

Factual data pertaining to orgasm may be more meaningful when placed in clinical context. However, in order to provide a point of departure for nonsubjective interpretation of female orgasmic response, most of the material will be related to recognizable baselines of physiologic response and psychosocial patterns of sexual expression which can be duplicated within investigative context. General impression rather than statistical data will be reflected owing to the selected quality of the population and the research atmosphere to which the female study subjects have been exposed.

Physiologic Factors of Orgasm

Female orgasmic experience can be visually identified as well as recorded by acceptable physiologic techniques. The primary requirement in objective identification of female orgasm is the knowledge that it is a total-body response with marked variation in reactive intensity and timing sequence. Previously, other observers have recognized and interpreted much of the reactive physiology of female orgasm. However, definition and correlation of these reactions into an identifying pattern of orgasm per se has not been established.

At orgasm, the grimace and contortion of a woman's face graphically express the increment of myotonic tension throughout her entire body. The muscles of the neck and the long muscles of the arms and legs usually contract into involuntary spasm. During coition in supine position the female's hands and feet voluntarily may be grasping her sexual partner. With absence of clutching interest or opportunity during coition or in solitary response to automanipulative techniques, the extremities may reflect involuntary carpopedal spasm. The striated muscles of the abdomen and the buttocks frequently are contracted voluntarily by women in conscious effort to elevate sexual tensions, particularly in an effort to break through from high plateau to orgasmic attainment.

The physiologic onset of orgasm is signaled by contractions of the target organs, starting with the orgasmic platform in the outer third of the vagina. This platform, created involuntarily by localized vasocongestion and myotonia, contracts with recordable rhythmicity as the tension increment is released. The intercontractile intervals recur at 0.8 second for the first three to six contractions, corresponding in timing sequence to the first few ejaculatory contractions (male orgasm) of the penis. The longer contractions continue, the more extended the intercontractile intervals. The number and intensity of orgasmic-platform contractions are direct measures of subjective severity and objective duration of the particular orgasmic experience. The correlation between platform contractions and subjective experience at orgasm has been corroborated by study subjects during thousands of cycles. Vaginal spasm and penile grasping reactions have been described many times in the clinical and nonprofessional literature. Orgasmic-platform contractility provides an adequate physiologic explanation for these subjective concepts.

Contractions of the orgasmic platform provide visible manifestation of female orgasmic experience. To date, the precise mechanism whereby cortical, hormonal, or any unidentified influence may activate this and other orgasmic reactions has not been determined (perhaps by creating a trigger-point level of vasocongestive and myotonic increment).

Orgasmic contractions of the uterus have been recorded by both intrauterine and abdominally placed electrodes. Both techniques indicate that uterine contractions may have onset almost simultaneously with those of the orgasmic platform, but the contractive intensity of the uterine musculature is accumulated slowly and contractions are too irregular in recurrence and duration to allow pattern definition. Uterine contractions start in the fundus and work through the midzone to terminate in the lower uterine segment. With the exception of the factor of contractile excursion (indication of intensity), physiologic tracings of uterine orgasmic contractions resemble the patterns of first-stage labor contractions. Uterine contractile intensity and duration vary widely from orgasm to orgasm. However, there is some early indication that both factors have a positive relation to the parity of the individual and the prior extent of her orgasmic experience, both incidental and cumulative.

Involuntary contractions of the external rectal sphincter also may develop during orgasm, although many women experience orgasm without evidencing sphincter contraction. When the contractions do occur, they parallel in timing sequence the initial intercontractile intervals of the orgasmic platform. The rectal-sphincter contractions usually terminate before those of the orgasmic platform.

The external urethral sphincter also may contract two or three times in an involuntary expression of orgasmic tension release. The contractions are without recordable rhythmicity and usually are confined to nulliparous premenopausal women.

The breasts evidence no specific response to the immediacy of orgasm. However, detumescence of the areolae immediately subsequent to orgasm is so rapid that its arbitrary assignment purely as a resolution-phase reaction has been cause for investigative concern. Often areolar detumescence is evident shortly after subjective report of orgasmic onset and usually develops simultaneously with the terminal contractions of the orgasmic platform. As a final stage of the rapid detumescent reaction, the areolae constrict into a corrugated state. The nipples remain erect and are turgid and quite rigid (the false-erection reaction).

Rapid detumescence of the vasocongested areolae, resulting in a constricted, corrugated appearance, occurs only with orgasm and is an obvious physical manifestation that provides for visual identification of female orgasmic experience. If orgasm does not occur areolar detumescence is a much slower process, corrugation does not develop, and the false-erection reaction of the nipples usually is reduced in intensity.

The sex flush, a maculopapular rash distributed superficially over the body surfaces, achieves its greatest intensity and its widest distribution at the moment of orgasmic expression. Subsequent to orgasmic experience, the sex flush disappears more rapidly than when resolving from plateau-phase levels of erotic tension.

From a cardiorespiratory point of view, orgasm is reflected by hyperventilation, with respiratory rates occasionally over 40 per minute. Tachycardia is a constant accompaniment of orgasmic experience, with cardiac rates running from 110 to beyond 180 beats per minute. Hypertension also is a constant finding. The systolic pressures are elevated by 30–80 mm. and diastolic pressures by 20–40 mm. Hg.

The clitoris, Bartholin's glands, and the major and minor labia are target organs for which no specific physiologic reactions to orgasmic-phase levels of sexual tension have been established.

Aside from ejaculation, there are two major areas of physiologic difference between female and male orgasmic expression. First, the female is capable of rapid return to orgasm immediately following an orgasmic experience, if restimulated before tensions have dropped below plateau-phase response levels. Second, the female is capable of maintaining an orgasmic experience for a relatively long period of time.

A rare reaction in the total of female orgasmic expression, but one that has been reduplicated in the laboratory on numerous occasions, has been termed *status orgasmus.* This physiologic state of stress is created either by a series of rapidly recurrent orgasmic experiences between which no recordable plateau-phase intervals can be demonstrated, or by a single, long-continued orgasmic episode. Subjective report, together with visual impression of involuntary variation in peripheral myotonia, suggests that the woman actually is ranging with extreme rapidity between successive orgasmic peaks and a baseline of advanced plateau-phase tension. Status orgasmus may last from 20 to more than 60 seconds. The severe tachycardia (more than 180 per minute) and the long-maintained (43 seconds), rapidly recurring contractile patterns of the orgasmic platform are identified easily.

Of interest from both physiologic and psychologic points of view is the recorded evidence of an initial involuntary spasm of the orgasmic platform, developing before the regularly recurring contractions of orgasmic expression. The study subject identified the onset of orgasm and vocalized this subjective experience before the onset of regularly recurrent contractions of the orgasmic platform. However, the initial spasm of the orgasmic platform developed parallel in timing sequence with the subjective identification of the orgasmic experience. To date, preliminary spasm of the orgasmic platform has been recorded only in situations of severe tension increment.

It is investigative impression that the inability to record initial spasm of the orgasmic platform in all orgasmic experiences well may reflect lack of effective experimental technique rather than unimpeachable physiologic fact. Subjectively, the identification of initial spasm of the orgasmic platform is a constant factor in any full orgasmic experience. The subjective and objective correlation of orgasmic experience will be discussed later in the chapter.

No preliminary spastic contraction of the uterine musculature comparable to the initial spasm of the orgasmic platform has been recorded to date. However, the work is in its infancy, and such a preliminary spasm before onset of the regular, expulsive, fundal contractions may, in fact, exist and be recorded in the future.

The subjective identification of orgasmic expression by the human female simultaneously with the initial spasm of the orgasmic platform, but 2 to 4 seconds prior to onset of its regularly recurrent contractions, draws an interesting parallel with the human male's ejaculatory experience. When the secondary organs of reproduction contract, the male feels the ejaculation coming and can no longer control it, but there still is a 2- to 4-second interval before the seminal fluid appears at the urethral meatus under the pressure developed by penile expulsive contractions. Thus the male's psychosensory expression of ejaculatory inevitability may have counterpart in the female's subjective identification of orgasmic onset. The initial spasm of the orgasmic platform, before the platform and the uterus contract with regularity, may parallel the contractions of the prostate and, questionably, contractions of the seminal vesicles before onset of the regularly recurrent expulsive contractions of the penis.

Understandably, the maximum physiologic intensity of orgasmic response subjectively reported or objectively recorded has been achieved by self-regulated mechanical or automanipulative techniques. The next highest level of erotic intensity has resulted from partner manipulation, again with established or self-regulated methods, and the lowest intensity of target-organ response was achieved during coition.

While variations in the orgasmic intensity and duration of target-organ response have been recorded and related to modes of stimulation, there have been no recorded alterations in the basic orgasmic physiology. This finding lends support, at least in part, to many earlier concepts of orgasmic response. The fundamental physiology of orgasmic response remains the same whether the mode of stimulation is heterosexual or artificial coition or mechanical or automanipulative stimulation of the clitoral area, the breast, or any other selected erogenous zone. It follows that orgasm resulting from fantasy also would produce the same basic physiologic response patterns, although a woman capable of fantasying to orgasm has not been available for inclusion in the research population. The ability of women to fantasy to orgasm has been reported by other investigators.

With the specific anatomy of orgasmic-phase physiology reasonably established, the age-bid practice of the human female of dissimulating has been made pointless. The obvious, rapid detumescence and corrugation of the areolae of the breasts and the definable contractions of the orgasmic platform in the outer third of the vagina remove any doubt as to whether the woman is pretending or experiencing orgasm. The severe vasocongestive reactions reflecting higher levels of sexual tension cannot be developed other than during involuntary response to sexual stimulation. For example, the transitory but obvious increase in nulliparous breast size, the sex flush, and the minor-labial sex skin reactions are all plateau-phase phenomena that develop only in response to effective sexual stimulation.

Psychologic Factors of Orgasm

It is well to restate from time to time the necessity for maintaining a concept of total involvement when any facet of human sexuality is to be considered. This is equally true when the study is directed to areas of psychologic influence upon orgasmic achievement.

Female orgasm, whether it is attained within the context of an interpersonal relationship (either heterosexual or homosexual) or by means of any combination of erotically stimulative activity and/or fantasy, remains a potpourri of psychophysiologic conditions and social influence. Many theoretical as well as individually graphic accounts of the female experience at orgasm have been offered in the professional literature of many disciplines and are even more widespread in general publications. This vast amount of published quasiauthority depicts both objective and subjective female reaction to orgasm with almost every possible degree of accuracy and inaccuracy.

Without referring to the prior literature, a description of subjective response to orgasmic incidence has been compiled from reports of 487 women, given in the laboratory in the immediacy of the postorgasmic period, obtained through interview only, or developed from a combination of both sources. This composite is offered as a baseline for a concept of the psychologic aspects of the human female's orgasmic experience.

The consensus drawn from the multiple descriptions has established three distinct stages of woman's subjective progression through orgasm.

Stage I

Orgasm has its onset with a sensation of suspension or stoppage. Lasting only an instant, the sensation is accompanied or followed immediately by an isolated thrust of intense sensual awareness, clitorally oriented, but radiating upward into the pelvis. Intensity ranging in degree from mild to shock level has been reported by many women within the context of their personal experience. A simultaneous loss of overall sensory acuity has been described as paralleling in degree the intensity and duration of the particular orgasmic episode. Loss of sensory acuity has been reviewed frequently in the literature.

During the first stage of subjective progression in orgasm, the sensation of intense clitoral-pelvic awareness has been described by a number of women as occurring concomitantly with a sense of bearing down or expelling. Often a feeling of receptive opening was expressed. This last sensation was reported only by parous study subjects, a small number of whom expressed some concept of having an actual fluid emission or of expending in some concrete fashion. Previous male interpretation of these subjective reports may have resulted in the erroneous but widespread concept that female ejaculation is an integral part of female orgasmic expression.

Twelve women, all of whom have delivered babies on at least one occasion without anesthesia or analgesia, reported that during the second stage of labor they experienced a grossly intensified version of the sensations identified with this first stage of subjective progression through orgasm. Reports of this concept also have appeared from time to time in the literature.

Stage II

As the second stage of subjective progression through orgasm, a sensation of "suffusion of warmth," specifically pervading the pelvic area first and then spreading progressively throughout the body, was described by almost every woman with orgasmic experience.

Stage III

Finally, as the third stage of subjective progression, a feeling of involuntary contraction with a specific focus in the vagina or lower pelvis was mentioned consistently. Frequently, the sensation was described as that of "pelvic throbbing."

Women with the facility to express sensate awareness frequently separated this final stage of subjective progression into two phases. The initial phase was expressed as contractile, followed immediately by a throbbing phase, with both sensations experienced as separate entities. The initial contractile feeling was described as localized vaginally, subsequently merging with the throbbing sensation which, though initially concentrated in the pelvis, was felt throughout the body. The "pelvic throbbing" sensation often was depicted as continuing until it became one with a sense of the pulse or heartbeat.

Only the two phases of this third stage of subjective progression during orgasm afforded positive correlation between subjective response and objective reaction. This correlation has been developed from a composite return of direct interrogation of female study subjects during investigative sessions. The phase of contractile sensation has been identified as paralleling in time sequence the recorded initial spasm of the orgasmic platform.

Regularly recurring orgasmic-platform contractions were appreciated subjectively as pulsating or throbbing sensations of the vagina. Although second-phase sensations of pulsation coincided with observable vaginal-platform contractions, consciousness of a pulsating sensation frequently continued beyond observable platform contractions. Finally this pelvic-throbbing sensation became one with a subjective awareness of tachycardia described frequently as feeling the heartbeat vaginally. Subjective awareness of orgasmic duration was somewhat dependent upon the degree of intensity of the specific orgasm.

Rectal-sphincter contraction also was described by some anatomically oriented or hypersensitive women as a specific entity during intense orgasmic response.

Observation supported by subjective report indicates that a relative norm of orgasmic intensity and duration is reflected by approximately five to eight vigorous contractions of the orgasmic platform. A level of eight to twelve contractions would be considered by observer and subject to be an intense physiologic experience. An orgasmic expression reflected by three to five contractions usually is reported by the responding female as being a "mild experience" unless the woman is postmenopausal. These physiologically recordable levels of orgasmic intensity never must be presumed arbitrarily to be a full or consistent measure of the subjective pleasure derived from individual orgasmic attainment.

Pregnancy (particularly during the second and, at times, the third trimester) has been noted to increase general sensitivity to the overall sensate effects of orgasm. To date, an increase in contractile intensity of the pregnant woman's orgasmic platform as compared to that in her nonpregnant state has not been corroborated by physiologic tracings. Orgasmic contractions of the uterus recorded during the second and third trimesters consistently have been reported as subjectively more intense sensations than those of nonpregnant response patterns. Of interest from an objective point of view is the fact that tonic spasm of the uterus develops in response to orgasmic stimulation and has been recorded during the third trimester of pregnancy.

Sociologic Factors in Orgasm

In our culture, the human female's orgasmic attainment never has achieved the undeniable status afforded the male's ejaculation. While male orgasm (ejaculation) has the reproductive role in support of its perpetual acceptance, a comparable regard for female orgasm is still in limbo. Why has female orgasmic expression not been considered to be a reinforcement of woman's role as sexual partner and reproductive necessity? Neither totem, taboo, nor religious assignment seems to account completely for the force with which female orgasmic experience often is negated as a naturally occurring psychophysiologic response.

With orgasmic physiology established, the human female now has an undeniable opportunity to develop realistically her own sexual response levels. Disseminating this information enables the male partner to contribute to this development in support of an effective sexual relationship within the marital unit. The female's age-old foible of orgasmic pretense has been predicated upon the established concept that obvious female response increases the male's subjective pleasure during coital opportunity. With need for pretense removed, a sexually responding woman can stimulate effectively the interaction upon which both the man's and woman's psychosocial requirements are culturally so dependent for orgasmic facility.

Impression formed from eleven years of controlled observation suggests that psychosocially oriented patterns of sexual expression evolve specifically in response to developing social and life cycle demands. When continuity of study-subject cooperation permitted long-range observation and interrogation, it was noted that major changes in social baseline were accompanied by actual changes in sexual expression. For the female study subjects, changes involving social or life-cycle demands frequently resulted in a reorientation of sexual focus. This was manifest in alterations in desired areas of stimulation, preferred actions of partner, and reported fantasy. Often variations in coital and masturbatory techniques were observed.

These alterations usually appeared gradually, although, depending upon the impact of the social change involved, there were occasions of sudden onset. To date, physiologically measurable intensity in orgasmic response has shown no specific parallel to onset or presence of these psychosocial influences. This may indicate that physiologic capacity, as influenced by purely biologic variations, remains a dominant factor in orgasmic intensity and facility. Reported levels of subjective pleasure in orgasm did, of course, parallel reports of desirable or undesirable social change.

It became evident that laboratory environment was not the determining factor in the success or failure of female study subjects' orgasmic attainment. Rather it was from previously established levels of sexual response that the individual female was able to cope with and adapt to a laboratory situation.

There were no particular personality trends toward high- or low-dominance individuals among the participating female research group. The women's personalities varied from the very shy through the agreeably independent, and histories reflected sexual-partner experience ranging from single to many. The ability to achieve orgasm in response to effective sexual stimulation was the only constant factor demonstrated by all active female participants. This observation might be considered to support the concept that sexual response to orgasm is the physiologic prerogative of most women, but its achievement in our culture may be more dependent upon psychosocial acceptance of sexuality than overtly aggressive behavior .

Many existing psychologic theories find support in the physiologic data emerging from this study. However, it must be recalled that these data have been presented primarily as impression, due to the selectivity of the research group and, in many instances, the absence of a statistically significant number of recorded reactions. There always is great temptation to connect theory to considered fact, when subjective reports of the research population are placed as an overlay on the observed and recorded physiologic reactions. If recall by interrogated subjects of early sexual feeling and of manipulative activity, often to a remembered peak of experience, is to be given credence, sexual response well may be viewed as an instinctual activity arising from an undifferentiated sexual state. Although molded and transmitted genetically, sexual response, in this concept, would be subject to both immediate and continued learning processes.

Unreported observations suggest that infant sexual response as an undifferentiated state is not beyond possibility. Certainly, elaboration of sexual behavior in early childhood of less restricted cultures has been reported. The development of sexual responsiveness to orgasmic level, identifiable subjectively, must be a cumulative result of interaction between the individual female's hereditary endowment and the psychosocial influence to which it is exposed. The element of time must be assumed to be a finally determining factor, as it accrues the experience of social and psychosexual maturation.

A detailed psychosocial study of the research population cannot be presented within the framework of this text. Yet neither this book nor this chapter can be considered complete without emphasizing an acute awareness of the vital, certainly the primary influence, exerted by psychosocial factors upon human sexuality, particularly that of orgasmic attainment of the female. Although the basic physiology of female orgasm never would have evolved from behavioral theory or sociologic concept, it equally is obvious that physiologic detail is of value only when considered in relation to these theories and concepts. When completed, psychosocial evaluation of the study-subject population will be published in another book.

A Theory on Female Sexuality

Mary Jane Sherfey, M.D.

from *The Journal of the American Psychoanalytical Association*, 1966

Mary Jane Sherfy was a practicing psychoanalyst who developed the radical implications for female sexuality of Masters and Johnson's pioneering research. She also developed an historical and evolutionary argument to explain why knowledge of the clitoris had been socially repressed.

No doubt the most far-reaching hypothesis extrapolated from biological data is the existence of the universal and physically normal condition of women's inability ever to reach complete sexual satiation in the presence of the most intense, repetitive orgasmic experiences, no matter how produced. Theoretically, a woman could go on having orgasms indefinitely if physical exhaustion did not intervene.

It is to be understood that repetitive orgasms leading to the satiation-in-satiation state will be most apt to occur in parous[1] and experienced women during the luteal phase[2] of the menstrual cycle. It is one of the most important ways in which the sexuality of the primate and human female differs from the primate and human male at the physical level; and this difference exists only because of the female's capacity to produce the fulminating pelvic congestion and edema. This

1. "Parous" describes women who have had at least one child.—Ed.
2. The luteal phase is the post-ovulatory phase of the menstrual cycle.—Ed.

capacity is mediated by specific hormonal combinations with high fluid-imbibing action which are found only in certain primates and, probably, a very few other mammalian species.

I must stress that this condition does not mean a woman is always consciously unsatisfied. There is a great difference between satisfaction and satiation. A woman may be emotionally satisfied to the full in the absence of *any* orgasmic expression (although such a state would rarely persist through years of frequent arousal and coitus without some kind of physical or emotional reaction formation). Satiation-in-insatiation is well illustrated by Masters' statement, "A woman *will usually* be satisfied with three to five orgasms . . ." I believe it would rarely be said, "A man will usually be satisfied with three to five ejaculations." The man *is* satisfied. The woman *usually wills* herself to be satisfied because she is simply unaware of the extent of her orgasmic capacity. However, I predict that this hypothesis will come as no great shock to many women who consciously realize, or intuitively sense, their lack of satiation.

It seems that the vast majority of cases of coital frigidity are due simply to the absence of frequent, prolonged coitus. This statement is supported by unpublished data which Masters and Johnson are now accumulating. Following this logical conclusion of their previous research, they began treating a series of couples with severe, chronic frigidity or impotence. All had received prior medical and, often, psychiatric treatment to no avail. For the women, none of whom had ever experienced orgasms after five or more years of marriage, treatment consisted of careful training of the husband to use the proper techniques essential to all women and the specific ones required by his wife. In many cases this in itself was sufficient. In the others, daily sessions were instigated of marital coitus followed by prolonged use of the artificial phallus (three to four hours or more). Thus far, with about fifty women treated, every woman but one responded within three weeks at most and usually within a few days. They began at once to experience intense, multiple orgasms; and once this capacity was achieved after the exposure to daily prolonged coitus, they were able to respond with increasing ease and rapidity so that the protracted stimulation was no longer necessary. It is too early for thorough follow-ups, but initial impressions are most favorable.

Should these preliminary findings hold, an almost total biological etiology of coital frigidity will be proved. The inordinate sexual, orgasmic capacity of the human female will fall in line with that of the other higher primates—and the magnitude of the psychological and social problems facing modern mankind is difficult to contemplate.

Historical Perspective and Cultural Dilemma

The nature of female sexuality as here presented makes it clear that, just as the vagina did not evolve for the delivery of big-headed babies, so women's inordinate orgasmic capacity did not evolve for monogamous, sedentary cultures. It is unreasonable to expect that this inordinate sexual capacity could be, even in part, given expression within the confines of our culture; and it is particularly unreasonable to expect the delayed blooming of the sexuality of many women after the age of thirty or so to find adequate avenues of satisfaction. Less than one hundred years ago, and in many places today, women regularly had their third or fourth child by the time they were eighteen or nineteen, and the life span was no more than thirty-five to forty years. It could well be that the natural synchronization of the peak periods for sexual expression in men and women has been destroyed only in recent years.

These findings give ample proof of the conclusion that neither men nor women, but especially not women, are biologically built for the single-spouse, monogamous marital structure or for the prolonged adolescence which our society can now bestow upon both of them. Generally, men have never accepted strict monogamy except in principle. Women have been forced to accept it; but not, I submit, for the reasons usually given.

The human mating system, with its permanent family and kinship ties, was absolutely essential to man's becoming—and remaining—man. In every culture studied, the crucial transition from the nomadic, hunting, and food-gathering economy to a settled, agricultural existence was the beginning of family life, modern civilization, and civilized man. In the preagricultural societies, life was precarious, population growth slow, and infanticide often essential to group survival. With the domestication of animals and the agriculture revolution, for the first time in all time, the survival of a species lay in the extended family with its private property, kinship lineages, inheritance laws, social ordinances, and, most significantly, many surviving children. Only in that carefully delineated and rigidly maintained large-family complex could the individual find sufficient security to allow his uniquely human potentialities to be developed through the long years of increasingly helpless childhood—and could populations explode into the first little villages and towns.

Many factors have been advanced to explain the rise of the patriarchal, usually polygamous, system and its concomitant ruthless subjugation of female sexuality (which necessarily subjugated her entire emotional and intellectual life). However, if the conclusions reached here are true, it is conceivable that the *forceful* suppression of women's inordinate sexual demands was a prerequisite to the dawn of every modern civilization and almost every living culture. Primitive woman's sexual drive was too strong, too susceptible to the fluctuating extremes of an impelling, aggressive eroticism to withstand the disciplined requirements of a settled family life—where many living children were necessary to a family's well-being and where paternity had become as important as maternity in maintaining family and property cohesion. For about half the time, women's erotic needs would be insatiably pursued; paternity could never be certain; and with lactation erotism, constant infant care would be out of the question.

There are many indications from the prehistory studies in the Near East that it took perhaps five thousand years or longer for the subjugation of women to take place. All relevant data from the 12,000 to 8,000 B.C. period indicate that precivilized woman enjoyed full sexual freedom and was often totally incapable of controlling her sexual drive.[3] Therefore, I

3. "Today it is unfashionable to talk about former more matriarchal orders of society. Nevertheless, there is evidence from many parts of the world that the role of women has weakened since earlier times in several sections of social structure." The evidence given here lends further support to this statement by J. Hawkes and L. Woolley. See *History of Mankind, Vol. I: Prehistory and the Beginnings of Civilization* (New York: Harper & Row, 1963). However, I must make it clear that the biological data presented support only the thesis on the intense, insatiable erotism in women. Such erotism could be contained within one or possibly several types of social structures which would have prevailed through most of the Pleistocene period.

I am indebted to Prof. Joseph Mazzeo of Columbia University for calling my attention to the fact that the first study on the existence of a pre-Neolithic matriarchal society was published in 1861: Bachofen's *Das Mutterrecht.* (Basel: B. Schwabe, 1897). Indeed, Bachofen's work remains an unsurpassed, scholarly analysis of the mythologies of the Near East, hypothesizing both a matriarchal society and the inordinate erotism of women. His entire thesis was summarily rejected by twentieth-century anthropologists for lack of objective evidence (and cultural bias). On several scores, the ancient myths have proved more accurate than the modern scientists' theories. I suspect this will be another instance in which the myths prove faithful reflections of former days.

propose that one of the reasons for the long delay between the earliest development of agriculture (c. 12,000 B.C.) and the rise of urban life and the beginning, of recorded knowledge (c. 8,000–5,000 B.C.) was the ungovernable cyclic sexual drive of women. Not until these drives were gradually brought under control by rigidly enforced social codes could family life become the stabilizing and creative crucible from which modern civilized man could emerge.

Although then (and now) couched in superstitious, religious and rationalized terms, behind the subjugation of women's sexuality lay the inexorable economics of cultural evolution which finally forced men to impose it and women to endure it. If that suppression has been, at times, unduly oppressive or cruel, I suggest the reason has been neither man's sadistic, selfish infliction of servitude upon helpless women nor women's weakness or inborn masochism. The strength of the drive determines the force required to suppress it.

The hypothesis that women possess a *biologically determined*, inordinately high, cyclic sexual drive is too significant to be accepted without confirmation from every field of science touching the subject. Assuming this analysis of the nature of women's sexuality is valid, we must ask ourselves if the basic intensity of women's sexual drive has abated appreciably as the result of the past seven thousand years of suppression (which has been, of course, only partial suppression for most of that time). Just within the very recent past, a decided lifting of the ancient social injunctions against the free expression of female sexuality has occurred. This unprecedented development is born of the scientific revolution, the product of both efficient contraceptives and the new social equality and emotional honesty sweeping across the world (an equality and honesty which owe more to the genius of Sigmund Freud than to any other single individual). It is hard to predict what will happen should this trend continue—except one thing is certain: if women's sexual drive has not abated, and they prove incapable of controlling it, thereby jeopardizing family life and child care, a return to the rigid, enforced suppression will be inevitable and mandatory. Otherwise the biological family will disappear and what other patterns of infant care and adult relationships could adequately substitute cannot now be imagined.[4]

4. On the contrary, communal family structures, with men *and* women sharing child care, are not only imaginable, but already in experimental practice.—Ed.

Should the hypothesis be true that one of the requisite cornerstones upon which all modern civilizations were founded was *coercive* suppression of women's inordinate sexuality, one looks back over the long history of women and their relationships to men, children, and society since the Neolithic revolution with a deeper, almost awesome, sense of the ironic tragedy in the triumph of the human condition.

Summary

Recent embryological research has demonstrated conclusively that the concept of the initial anatomical bi-sexuality or equipotentiality of the embryo is erroneous. All mammalian embryos, male and female, are anatomically female during the early stages of fetal life. In humans, the differentiation of the male from the female form by the action of fetal androgen begins about the sixth week of embryonic life and is completed by the end of the third month. Female structures develop autonomously without the necessity of hormonal differentiation. If the fetal gonads are removed from a genetic female before the first six weeks, she will develop into a normal female, even undergoing normal pubertal changes if, in the absence of ovaries, exogenous hormones are supplied. If the fetal gonads are similarly removed from a genetic male, he will develop into a female, also undergoing normal female pubertal changes if exogenous hormones are supplied. The probable relationship of the autonomous female anatomy to the evolution of viviparity is described.

From this surprising discovery of modern embryology and other biological data, the hypothesis is suggested that the female's relative lack of differentiating hormones during embryonic life renders her more sensitive to hormonal conditioning in later life, especially to androgens, since some embryonic and strong maternal estrogenic activity is present during embryonic life. This ready androgen responsivity provides the physiological means whereby androgen-sensitive structures could evolve to enhance the female's sexual capacity. In the primates, the marked development of the clitoral system, certain secondary sexual characteristics including skin erotism, and the extreme degree of perineal sexual edema (achieved in part by progesterone with

---

5. Estrus is that time when a female animal, because of the hormonal milieu, is capable of conception and desirous of copulation. Strictly speaking, true estrus does not occur in the human female.—Ed.

its strong androgenic properties) are combined in various species to produce an intense aggressive sexual drive and an inordinate, insatiable capacity for copulations during estrus.[5] The breeding advantage would thus go to the females with the most insatiable sexual capacity. The infrahuman female's insatiable sexual capacity could evolve only if it did not interfere with maternal care. Maternal care is insured by the existence of the extreme sexual drive only during estrus and its absence during the prolonged postpartum anestrus of these animals.

The validity of these considerations and their relevance to the human female are strongly supported by the demonstration of comparable sexual physiology and behavior in women. This has been accomplished by the research of Masters and Johnson, and a summary of their findings of the actual nature of the sexual response cycle in women is presented. Their most important observations are:

A. There is no such thing as a vaginal orgasm distinct from a clitoral orgasm. The nature of the orgasm is the same regardless of the erotogenic zone stimulated to produce it. The orgasm consists of the rhythmic contractions of the extravaginal musculature against the greatly distended circumvaginal venous plexi and vestibular bulbs surrounding the lower third of the vagina.

B. The nature of the labial-preputial-glandar mechanism which maintains continuous stimulation of the retracted clitoris during intravaginal coition has been described. By this action, clitoris, labia minora, and lower third of the vagina function as a single, smoothly integrated unit when traction is placed on the labia by the male organ during coitus. Stimulation of the clitoris is achieved by the rhythmical pulling on the edematous prepuce. Similar activation of the clitoris is achieved by preputial friction during direct clitoral area stimulation.

C. With full sexual arousal, women are normally capable of many orgasms. As many as six or more can be achieved with intravaginal coition. During clitoral area stimulation, when a woman can control her sexual tension and maintain prolonged stimulation, she may attain up to fifty or more orgasms in an hour's time.

From these observations and other biological data, especially from primatology, I have advanced four hypotheses:

1. The erotogenic potential of the clitoral glans is probably greater than that of the lower third of the vagina . . . The evolution of primate

sexuality has occurred primarily through selective adaptations of the perineal edema and the clitoral complex, not the vagina.

2. Under optimal arousal conditions, women's orgasmic potential may be similar to that of the primates described. In both, orgasms are best achieved only with the high degree of pelvic vasocongestion and edema associated with estrus in the primates and the luteal phase of the menstrual cycle in women or with prolonged, effective stimulation. Under these conditions, each orgasm tends to increase pelvic vasocongestion; thus the more orgasms achieved, the more can be achieved. Orgasmic experiences may continue until physical exhaustion intervenes.

3. In these primates and in women, an inordinate cyclic sexual capacity has thus evolved leading to the paradoxical state of sexual insatiation in the presence of the utmost sexual satiation. The value of this state for evolution is clear: with the breeding premium going to the primate females with the greatest pelvic edema, the most effective clitoral erotism, and the most aggressive sexual behavior, the satiation-in-insatiation state may have been an important factor in the adaptive radiation of the primates leading to man—and a major barrier to the evolution of modern man.

4. The rise of modern civilization, while resulting from many causes, was contingent on the suppression of the inordinate cyclic sexual drive of women because (*a*) the hyperhormonalization of the early human females associated with the hypersexual drive and the prolonged pregnancies was an important force in the escape from the strict estrus sexuality and the much more important escape from lactation asexuality. Women's uncurtailed continuous hypersexuality would drastically interfere with maternal responsibilities; and (*b*) with the rise of the settled agriculture economies, man's territorialism became expressed in property rights and kinship laws. Large families of known parentage were mandatory and could not evolve until the inordinate sexual demands of women were curbed.

Finally, the data on the embryonic female primacy and the Masters and Johnson research on the sexual cycle in women (will require amendations of psychoanalytic theory. These will be less than one might think at first sight. Other than concepts based on innate bi-sexuality, the rigid dichotomy between masculine and feminine sexual behavior, and derivative concepts of the clitoral-vaginal transfer theory, psychoanalytic theory will remain. Much of the theory concerning the "masculine" components of female sexuality will also remain but will be based on a different biological conception. Certainly, much of present and past sexual symbolism will take on richer meanings.

It is my strong conviction that these fundamental biological findings will, in fact, strengthen psychoanalytic theory and practice in the area of female sexuality. Without the erroneous biological premises, the basic sexual constitution and its many manifestations will be seen as highly moldable by hormonal influences, which in turn are so very susceptible to all those uniquely human emotional, intellectual, imaginative, and cultural forces upon which psychoanalysis has cast so much light. The power of the psychic processes will stand the stronger. Therefore it may be safely predicted that these new biological findings will not "blow away" Freud's "artificial structure of hypotheses" but will transpose it to a less artificial and more effective level.

In any event, and regardless of the validity of my own conclusions, it is my hope that this presentation of recent major contributions from biology and gynecology bearing on female sexual differentiation and adult functioning will aid in the integration of psychological and biological knowledge and will provide a firm biological foundation upon which all future theories of psychosexuality must rest.

The Myth of the Vaginal Orgasm

Anne Koedt

from *Radical Feminism*, 1970

Ann Koedt's essay was perhaps the most celebrated of the early feminist critiques of male sexuality. Like Sherfey, Koedt built on the work of Masters and Johnson to develop a powerful critique of Freud and advocated for new sexual techniques that intensified women's sexual pleasure and that suggested the irrelevance of the penis. Koedt was an early member of Students for a Democratic Society, the largest and most influential radical student organization during the sixties and a founding member of a number of radical feminist organizations.

Whenever female orgasm and frigidity are discussed, a false distinction is made between the vaginal and the clitoral orgasm. Frigidity has generally been defined by men as the failure of women to have vaginal orgasms. Actually the vagina is not a highly sensitive area and is not constructed to achieve orgasm. It is the clitoris which is the center of sexual sensitivity and which is the female equivalent of the penis.

I think this explains a great many things: First of all, the fact that the so-called frigidity rate among women is phenomenally high. Rather than tracing female frigidity to the false assumptions about female anatomy, our "experts" have declared frigidity a psychological problem of women. Those women who complained about it were recommended psychiatrists, so that they might discover their "problem"— diagnosed generally as a failure to adjust to their role as women.

The facts of female anatomy and sexual response tell a different story.

Although there are many areas for sexual arousal, there is only one area for sexual climax; that area is the clitoris. All orgasms are extensions of sensation from this area. Since the clitoris is not necessarily stimulated sufficiently in the conventional sexual positions, we are left "frigid."

Aside from physical stimulation, which is the common cause of orgasm for most people, there is also stimulation through primarily mental processes. Some women, for example, may achieve orgasm through sexual fantasies, or through fetishes. However, while the stimulation may be psychological, the orgasm manifests itself physically. Thus, while the cause is psychological, the *effect* is still physical, and the orgasm necessarily takes place in the sexual organ equipped for sexual climax—the clitoris. The orgasm experience may also differ in degree of intensity—some more localized, and some more diffuse and sensitive. But they are all clitoral orgasms. All this leads to some interesting questions about conventional sex and our role in it. Men have orgasms essentially by friction with the vagina, not the clitoral area, which is external and not able to cause friction the way penetration does. Women have thus been defined sexually in terms of what pleases men; our own biology has not been properly analyzed. Instead, we are fed the myth of the liberated woman and her vaginal orgasm—an orgasm which in fact does not exist.

What we must do is redefine our sexuality. We must discard the "normal" concepts of sex and create new guidelines which take into account mutual sexual enjoyment. While the idea of mutual enjoyment is liberally applauded in marriage manuals, it is not followed to its logical conclusion. We must begin to demand that if certain sexual positions now defined as "standard" are not mutually conducive to orgasm, they no longer be defined as standard. New techniques must be used or devised which transform this particular aspect of our current sexual exploitation.

Freud—A Father of the Vaginal Orgasm

Freud contended that the clitoral orgasm was adolescent, and that upon puberty, when women began having intercourse with men, women should transfer the center of orgasm to the vagina. The vagina, it was assumed, was able to produce a parallel, but more mature, orgasm than the clitoris. Much work was done to elaborate on this theory, but little was done to challenge the basic assumptions.

To fully appreciate this incredible invention, perhaps Freud's general attitude about women should first be recalled. Mary Ellman, in *Thinking About Women*, summed it up this way:

> Everything in Freud's patronizing and fearful attitude toward women follows from their lack of a penis, but it is only in his essay *The Psychology of Women* that Freud makes explicit . . . the deprecations of women which are implicit in his work. He then prescribes for them the abandonment of the life of the mind, which will interfere with their sexual function. When the psychoanalyzed patient is male, the analyst sets himself the task of developing the man's capacities; but with women patients, the job is to resign them to the limits of their sexuality. As Mr. Rieff puts it: For Freud, "Analysis cannot encourage in women new energies for success and achievement, but only teach them the lesson of rational resignation."

It was Freud's feelings about women's secondary and inferior relationship to men that formed the basis for his theories on female sexuality.

Once having laid down the law about the nature of our sexuality, Freud not so strangely discovered a tremendous problem of frigidity in women. His recommended cure for a woman who was frigid was psychiatric care. She was suffering from failure to mentally adjust to her "natural" role as a woman. Frank S. Caprio, a contemporary follower of these ideas, states:

> . . . whenever a woman is incapable of achieving an orgasm via coitus, provided the husband is an adequate partner, and prefers clitoral stimulation to any other form of sexual activity, she can be regarded as suffering from frigidity and requires psychiatric assistance. (*The Sexually Adequate Female*, p. 64.)

The explanation given was that women were envious of men—"renunciation of womanhood." Thus it was diagnosed as an anti-male phenomenon.

It is important to emphasize that Freud did not base his theory upon a study of woman's anatomy, but rather upon his assumptions of woman as an inferior appendage to man, and her consequent social and psychological role. In their attempts to deal with the ensuing problem of mass frigidity, Freudians created elaborate mental gymnastics. Marie Bonaparte, in *Female Sexuality*, goes so far as to suggest surgery to help women back on their rightful path. Having discovered a strange connection between the non-frigid woman and the location of the clitoris near the vagina,

> it then occurred to me that where, in certain women, this gap was excessive, and clitoridal fixation obdurate, a clitoridal-vaginal reconciliation might be effected by surgical means, which would then benefit the normal erotic function. Professor Halban, of Vienna, as much a biologist as surgeon, became interested in the problem and worked out a simple operative technique. In this, the suspensory ligament of the clitoris was severed and the clitoris secured to the underlying structures, thus fixing it in a lower position, with eventual reduction of the labia minora. (p. 148.)

But the severest damage was not in the area of surgery, where Freudians ran around absurdly trying to change female anatomy to fit their basic assumptions. The worst damage was done to the mental health of women, who either suffered silently with self-blame, or flocked to psychiatrists looking desperately for the hidden and terrible repression that had kept from them their vaginal destiny.

Lack of Evidence

One may perhaps at first claim that these are unknown and unexplored areas, but upon closer examination this is certainly not true today, nor was it true even in the past. For example, men have known that women suffered from frigidity often during intercourse. So the problem was there. Also, there is much specific evidence. Men knew that the clitoris was and is the essential organ for masturbation, whether in children or adult women. So obviously women made it clear where *they* thought their sexuality was located. Men also seem suspiciously aware of the clitoral powers during "foreplay," when they want to arouse women and produce the necessary lubrication for penetration. Foreplay is a concept created for male purposes, but works to the disadvantage of many women, since as soon as the woman is aroused the man changes to vaginal stimulation, leaving her both aroused and unsatisfied.

It has also been known that women need no anesthesia inside the vagina during surgery, thus pointing to the fact that the vagina is in fact not a highly sensitive area.

Today, with extensive knowledge of anatomy, with Kelly, Kinsey, and Masters and Johnson, to mention just a few sources, there is no ignorance on the subject. There are, however, social reasons why this knowledge has not been popularized. We are living in a male society which has not sought change in women's role.

Anatomical Evidence

Rather than starting with what women *ought* to feel, it would seem logical to start out with the anatomical facts regarding the clitoris and vagina.

The Clitoris is a small equivalent of the penis, except for the fact that the urethra does not go through it as in the man's penis. Its erection is similar to the male erection, and the head of the clitoris has the same type of structure and function as the head of the penis. G. Lombard Kelly, in *Sexual Feeling in Married Men and Women*, says:

> The head of the clitoris is also composed of erectile tissue, and it possesses a very sensitive epithelium or surface covering, supplied with special nerve endings called genital corpuscles, which are peculiarly adapted for sensory stimulation that under proper mental conditions terminates in the sexual orgasm. No other part of the female generative tract has such corpuscles. (Pocketbooks; p. 35.)

The clitoris has no other function than that of sexual pleasure.

The Vagina—Its functions are related to the reproductive function. Principally, 1) menstruation, 2) receive penis, 3) hold semen, and 4) birth passage. The interior of the vagina, which according to the defenders of the vaginally caused orgasm is the center and producer of the orgasm, is:

> like nearly all other internal body structures, poorly supplied

with end organs of touch. The internal entodermal origin of the lining of the vagina makes it similar in this respect to the rectum and other parts of the digestive tract. (Kinsey, *Sexual Behavior in the Human Female*, p. 580.)

The degree of insensitivity inside the vagina is so high that "Among the women who were tested in our gynecologic sample, less than 14% were at all conscious that they had been touched." (Kinsey, p. 580.)

Even the importance of the vagina as an *erotic* center (as opposed to an orgasmic center) has been found to be minor.

Other Areas—Labia minora and the vestibule of the vagina. These two sensitive areas may trigger off a clitoral orgasm. Because they can be effectively stimulated during "normal" coitus, though infrequently, this kind of stimulation is incorrectly thought to be vaginal orgasm. However, it is important to distinguish between areas which can stimulate the clitoris, incapable of producing the orgasm themselves, and the clitoris:

> Regardless of what means of excitation is used to bring the individual to the state of sexual climax, the sensation is perceived by the genital corpuscles and is localized where they are situated: in the head of the clitoris or penis. (Kelly, p. 49.)

Psychologically Stimulated Orgasm—Aside from the above mentioned direct and indirect stimulations of the clitoris, there is a third way an orgasm may be triggered. This is through mental (cortical) stimulation, where the imagination stimulates the brain, which in turn stimulates the genital corpuscles of the glans to set off an orgasm.

Women Who Say They Have Vaginal Orgasms

Confusion—Because of the lack of knowledge of their own anatomy, some women accept the idea that an orgasm felt during "normal" intercourse was vaginally caused. This confusion is caused by a combination of two factors. One, failing to locate the center of the orgasm, and two, by a desire to fit her experience to the male-defined idea of sexual normalcy. Considering that women know little about their anatomy, it is easy to be confused.

Deception—The vast majority of women who pretend vaginal orgasm to their men are faking it to "get the job." In a new best-selling Danish book, *I Accuse*, Mette Ejlersen specifically deals with this common problem, which she calls the "sex comedy." This comedy has many causes. First of all, the man brings a great deal of pressure to bear on the woman, because he considers his ability as a lover at stake. So as not to offend his ego, the woman will comply with the prescribed role and go through simulated ecstasy. In some of the other Danish women mentioned, women who were left frigid were turned off to sex, and pretended vaginal orgasm to hurry up the sex act. Others admitted that they had faked vaginal orgasm to catch a man. In one case, the woman pretended vaginal orgasm to get him to leave his first wife, who admitted being vaginally frigid. Later she was forced to continue the deception, since obviously she couldn't tell him to stimulate her clitorally.

Many more women were simply afraid to establish their right to equal enjoyment, seeing the sexual act as being primarily for the man's benefit, and any pleasure that the woman got as an added extra.

Other women, with just enough ego to reject the man's idea that they needed psychiatric care, refused to admit their frigidity. They wouldn't accept self-blame, but they didn't know how to solve the problem, not knowing the physiological facts about themselves. So they were left in a peculiar limbo.

Again, perhaps one of the most infuriating and damaging results of this whole charade has been that women who were perfectly healthy sexually were taught that they were not. So in addition to being sexually deprived, these women were told to blame themselves when they deserved no blame. Looking for a cure to a problem that has none can lead a woman on an endless path of self-hatred and insecurity. For she is told by her analyst that not even in her one role allowed in a male society—the role of a woman—is she successful. She is put on the defensive, with phony data as evidence that she'd better try to be even more feminine, think more feminine, and reject her envy of men. That is, shuffle even harder, baby.

Why Men Maintain the Myth

1. *Sexual Penetration is Preferred*—The best stimulant for the penis is the

woman's vagina. It supplies the necessary friction and lubrication. From a strictly technical point of view this position offers the best physical conditions, even though the man may try other positions for variation.

2. *The Invisible Woman*—One of the elements of male chauvinism is the refusal or inability to see women as total, separate human beings. Rather, men have chosen to define women only in terms of how they benefited men's lives. Sexually, a woman was not seen as an individual wanting to share equally in the sexual act, any more than she was seen as a person with independent desires when she did anything else in society. Thus, it was easy to make up what was convenient about women; for on top of that, society has been a function of male interests, and women were not organized to form even a vocal opposition to the male experts.

3. *The Penis as Epitome of Masculinity*—Men define their lives primarily in terms of masculinity. It is a universal form of ego-boosting. That is, in every society, however homogeneous (i.e., with the absence of racial, ethnic, or major economic differences) there is always a group, women, to oppress.

The essence of male chauvinism is in the psychological superiority men exercise over women. This kind of superior-inferior definition of self, rather than positive definition based upon one's own achievements and development, has of course chained victim and oppressor both. But by far the most brutalized of the two is the victim.

An analogy is racism, where the white racist compensates for his feelings of unworthiness by creating an image of the black man (it is primarily a male struggle) as biologically inferior to him. Because of his power in a white male power structure, the white man can socially enforce this mythical division.

To the extent that men try to rationalize and justify male superiority through physical differentiation, masculinity may be symbolized by being the *most* muscular, the most hairy; having the deepest voice, and the biggest penis. Women, on the other hand, are approved of (i.e., called feminine) if they are weak, petite; shave their legs; have high soft voices.

Since the clitoris is almost identical to the penis, one finds a great deal of evidence of men in various societies trying to either ignore the clitoris and emphasize the vagina (as did Freud), or, as in some places in the Mideast, actually performing clitoridectomy. Freud saw this ancient and still practiced custom as a way of further "feminizing" the female by removing this cardinal vestige of her masculinity. It should be noted also that a big clitoris is considered ugly and masculine. Some cultures engage in the practice of pouring a chemical on the clitoris to make it shrivel up into "proper" size.

It seems clear to me that men in fact fear the clitoris as a threat to masculinity.

4. *Sexually Expendable Male*—Men fear that they will become sexually expendable if the clitoris is substituted for the vagina as the center of pleasure for women. Actually this has a great deal of validity if one considers *only* the anatomy. The position of the penis inside the vagina, while perfect for reproduction, does not necessarily stimulate an orgasm in women because the clitoris is located externally and higher up. Women must rely upon indirect stimulation in the "normal" position.

Lesbian sexuality could make an excellent case, based upon anatomical data, for the extinction of the male organ. Albert Ellis says something to the effect that a man without a penis can make a woman an excellent lover.

Considering that the vagina is very desirable from a man's point of view, purely on physical grounds, one begins to see the dilemma for men. And it forces us as well to discard many "physical" arguments explaining why women go to bed with men. What is left, it seems to me, are primarily psychological reasons why women select men at the exclusion of women as sexual partners.

5. *Control of Women*—One reason given to explain the Mid-eastern practice of clitoridectomy is that it will keep the women from straying. By removing the sexual organ capable of orgasm, it must be assumed that her sexual drive will diminish. Considering how men look upon their women as property, particularly in very backward nations, we should begin to consider a great deal more why it is not in men's interest to have women totally free sexually. The double standard, as practiced for example in Latin America, is set up to keep the woman as total property of the husband, while he is free to have affairs as he wishes.

6. *Lesbianism and Bisexuality*—Aside from the strictly anatomical

reasons why women might equally seek other women as lovers, there is a fear on men's part that women will seek the company of other women on a full, human basis. The establishment of clitoral orgasm as fact would threaten the heterosexual *institution*. For it would indicate that sexual pleasure was obtainable from either men *or* women, thus making heterosexuality not an absolute, but an option. It would thus open up the whole question of *human* sexual relationships beyond the confines of the present male-female role system.

Books Mentioned in This Essay

Sexual Behavior in the Human Female, Alfred C. Kinsey, Pocketbooks, 1953.

Female Sexuality, Marie Bonaparte, Grove Press, 1953.

Sex Without Guilt, Albert Ellis, Grove Press, 1958 and 1965.

Sexual Feelings in Married Men and Women, G. Lombard Kelly, Pocketbooks, 1951 and 1965.

I Accuse (Jeg Anklager), Mette Ejlersen, Chr. Erichsens Forlag (Danish), 1968.

The Sexually Adequate Female, Frank S. Caprio, Fawcett Gold Medal Books, 1953 and 1966.

Thinking About Women, Mary Ellman, Harcourt, Brace & World, 1968.

Human Sexual Response, Masters and Johnson, Little, Brown, 1966.

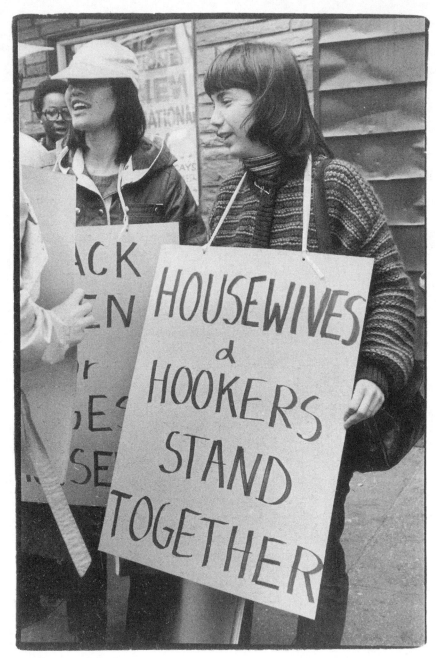

© Fred W. McDarrah

Organs and Orgasms

Alix Kate Shulman

from *Women in a Sexist Soxiety,* 1971

*A political activist in the civil rights, antiwar and women's movements of the sixties, Shulman helped to plan the famous women's liberation demonstration at the 1968 Miss America Pageant. She is the editor of a collection of Emma Goldman's writing, the author of novels (***Memoirs of an Ex-Prom Queen, Burning Questions***), a biography of Emma Goldman, memoirs (***Drinking the Rain, A Good Enough Daughter***), and several children's books. This article was originally published in one of the earliest and most influential anthologies of feminist writing. In the article Shulman explores the feminist implications of Sherfey and Koedt's arguments.*

This essay is not about love-making, a subject comprising emotional as well as anatomical considerations. Rather, it is about genital relations, and how they have adversely affected the lives of women. The myths and lies about female genital anatomy are so widespread and so harmful to women that the subject deserves an altogether separate consideration, even though it is only half the story.

Almost from the very beginning of our lives, we are all taught that the primary male sex organ is the penis, and the primary female sex organ is the vagina. These organs are supposed to define the sexes, to be the difference between boys and girls. We are taught that the reason for the differences, and the use to which the sex organs are put, has to do with making babies.

This is a lie. In our society only occasionally are those organs used to make babies. Much more often they are used to produce sexual pleasure for men, pleasure which culminates in ejaculation. The penis and the vagina together can make either babies or male orgasms; very rarely do the two together make female orgasms. Men, who have benefited greatly from both orgasms and babies, have had no reason to question the traditional definition of penis and vagina as true genital counterparts.

Women, on the other hand, have. Woman's sexual pleasure is often left out in these definitions. If people considered that the purpose of the female sex organs is to bring pleasure to *women*, then female sex would be defined by, and focused on, a different organ. Everyone would be taught from infancy that, as the primary male sex organ is the penis, so the primary female sex organ is the clitoris.

Men could never plead ignorance, as they now commonly do, if from the beginning, their sex education went something like this:

BOY: What's the difference between boys and girls?
MOTHER: Mainly their sex organs. A boy has a penis and a girl has a clitoris.
BOY: What's a clitoris?
MOTHER: It's a tiny sensistive organ on a girl's body about where a penis is on a boy's body. It feels good to touch; like your penis.
BOY: Do girls pee through their clitorises?
MOTHER: No.
BOY: What's it for?
MOTHER: For making love, for pleasure. When people love each other, one of the ways they show it is by caressing one another's bodies, including their sex organs.
BOY: How do girls pee?
MOTHER: There's an opening below the clitoris for peeing. A man uses his penis for peeing, for making love, and for starting babies. Women have three separate places for these. For peeing they have an opening into the urethra; for making love they have a clitoris; and for the first step in making babies they have a separate opening into the vagina. A lot of other organs in women and men are used in making babies too.
BOY: How are babies made? (And so on . . .)

Organs

It has long been known that the clitoris is endlessly more sensitive than the vagina, more sensitive than the penis too, if one judges by the number of nerve endings in the organs. In fact, anatomically, the clitoris and the penis have many similarities since they develop from the same cells in the female or male fetus. Yet, as Ruth Herschberger pointed out in her brilliant 1948 book on female sexuality, *Adam's Rib*, society refuses to acknowledge it: "It was quite a feat of nature to grant the small clitoris the same number of nerves as the penis. It was an even more incredible feat that society should actually have convinced the possessors of this organ that it was sexually inferior to the penis." The vagina, on the other hand, is for the most part so little sensitive that women commonly wear a diaphragm or tampon in it, and even undergo surgery on it, without feeling any sensation at all.

Despite the known anatomical facts and the experiences of many, many women, men usually insist that the vagina *is* the organ of female pleasure. Most of them insist, and probably believe, that women, like men, achieve orgasm by means of the movement of the penis back and forth into the vagina. While perpetuating this myth of vaginal primacy, from which they so readily benefit, the male "experts" make a small concession to the puzzling discrepancies in the "facts." Taking their cue from Freud, they claim that there are *two* kinds of orgasm: vaginal and clitoral. But of the two. they argue, only the vaginal kind, which is adapted to the male anatomy and suits male pleasure, is necessary, is valuable; the clitoral kind is not. Here is Freud himself:

> In the phallic phase of the girl, the clitoris is the dominant erotogenic zone. But it is not destined to remain so; with the change to femininity, the clitoris must give up to the vagina its sensitivity, and, with it, its importance, either wholly or in part. This is one of the two tasks which have to be performed in the course of the woman's development; the more fortunate man has only to continue at the time of his sexual maturity what he has already practiced during the period of early sexual expansion.

A woman who fails to transfer her sexual sensitivity from the clitoris to the vagina at puberty is, according to Freud, regressive, infantile, neurotic, hysteric, and frigid. The vaginal orgasm is supposedly mature, beautiful and good, while the clitoral orgasm is infantile, perverse, bad. A woman is frigid according to many of Freud's followers even today, if she does not have vaginal orgasms even though she may have frequent clitoral orgasms.

In their jokes and in their pornography, in their theories and in their marriage manuals, men treat the clitoris as simply one more erogenous zone like the breasts, underarms, or ears, to be used to arouse a woman sexually so that she will permit intercourse. They may remember the clitoris in foreplay, but for real sex, back to the vagina! The true center of female sexuality, the clitoris, is never identified for little girls who, when they accidentally discover they have one, often think themselves freaks to have on their bodies such a sensitive, unnamed thing. Most girls are not even told about the clitoris at puberty, when they may be instructed in the rites of feminine hygiene and intercourse. The diagrams of female genital anatomy that accompany most tampons and birth control devices usually illustrate the urinary bladder and the ovaries, but hardly ever the clitoris.

Orgasms

Women know from personal experience that there is only one kind of orgasm, no matter what name it is given, vaginal, clitoral, psychological. It is a sexual orgasm. Women know there is only one set of responses, one group of things that happen in their bodies during orgasm. It may vary in intensity from one experience to another, but for any woman who has ever masturbated, orgasm is unmistakable and certainly cannot be confused with anything else. No woman masturbating ever wonders whether or not orgasm has occurred. She has no doubts about that. When it happens, she knows it.

The recent laboratory research on female sexuality conducted by Virginia Johnson and William E. Masters confirms clinically what women know to be true from their own experience. If a woman experiences orgasm during intercourse, it is not a special kind of orgasm with a special set of physiological responses; it is like any other orgasm. Without exception, the Masters-Johnson data show that all orgasms, *no matter what kind of stimulation produces them,* result in almost identical bodily changes for all women—vaginal contractions, increase in body temperature, increase in pulse and respiration rate, and so forth. Though it is produced through the clitoris, the orgasm occurs as well in the vagina, the anus, the heart, the lungs, the skin, the head.

Given this clarity about what an orgasm feels like, why then does a woman occasionally confess she "doesn't know" whether or not she has had orgasm during intercourse? If orgasm had occurred, she would know it. Since she does not know it, it cannot have occurred. Nevertheless, since she has been taught to expect some special kind of orgasm called vaginal orgasm which can occur only during intercourse, she wonders. She can not know what such an orgasm is supposed to feel like because *there is no such thing*. The sensations of a penis in a vagina are indeed different from other sensations; accompanied by the right emotions they may be so pleasurable as to tempt a woman to hope that they can somehow qualify for that mysterious, desirable thing that has been touted as vaginal orgasm, even though they may not at all resemble the sensations she knows as orgasm. If she does not take advantage of the mystery and confusion surrounding the term to believe that perhaps she has indeed had a vaginal orgasm, she may feel compelled at least to pretend that she has. If not, she must submit to being called frigid or infantile by professional name-calling psychologists, doctors, and all who listen to them, and she must risk the displeasure and reprisal of her mate.

The truth is, there is only *one* kind of orgasm, one set of physiological responses constituting orgasm, all those Freudians to the contrary. The term "vaginal orgasm" must go. It signifies orgasm achieved by means of intercourse alone (for which no special term is necessary), or it signifies nothing at all. Some women testify to having experienced orgasm at some time in their lives through intercourse alone; some women say they have experienced orgasm through stimulation of the breasts alone, or through stimulation of the mind alone, or during dreams. Apparently orgasm can be achieved by various routes. However, the Masters-Johnson research shows, the most reliable way of regularly reaching orgasm for most women is by stimulation of the clitoris.

The clitoris may be stimulated to climax by a hand, by a tongue, or, particularly if the woman is free to move or to control the man's movements, by intercourse. No one way or combination of ways is "better" than any other, though women often prefer one way or another, finding that one way is rather more effective than another. Evidently for most women, intercourse by itself rarely results in orgasm, though vaginal stimulation may certainly make enjoyable foreplay or even afterplay. Masters and Johnson observe that the clitoris is automatically "stimulated" in intercourse since the hood covering the clitoris is pulled over the clitoris with each thrust of the penis in the vagina—much, I suppose, as a penis is automatically "stimulated" by a man's underwear whenever he takes a step. I wonder, however, if either is erotically stimulating by itself.

Reactions

The word about the clitoris has been out for a long time, and still, for political reasons, society goes on believing the old myths and enforcing a double standard of sexuality. Some societies have dealt with the facts by performing clitoridectomies—cutting off clitorises. More commonly, the facts about female sexuality are simply suppressed, ignored, or explained away. A century before Freud, for example, the learned Diderot cited women's lack of control over her senses to explain the infrequency of her orgasm during intercourse:

> There are some women who will die without ever having experienced the climax of sensual pleasures. . . . Since [women] have much less control over their senses than we, the rewards they receive from them are less certain and less prompt. Their expectations are being continually belied. With a physical structure so much the opposite of our own, the cue that sets their sensuality in play is so delicate and its source so far removed that we cannot be surprised at its not reaching fulfillment or becoming lost on the way.

Freud's ingenious formulation, though widely believed, is only one of many.

Since the Kinsey Report and the Masters-Johnson studies, it has become increasingly embarrassing to certain experts and self-styled lovers to go on ignoring the clinical facts and the testimony of women. In 1966 in an analysis of the Masters-Johnson research, Ruth and

Edward Brecher listed three myths now recognized to have been disproved by the sex research, among them the myth that women have two kinds of orgasm, one clitoral, the other vaginal. The Brechers' conclusion was that "women concerned with their failure to reach 'vaginal orgasm' can thus be reassured." But that is surely the wrong conclusion. It is not women who have been "failing" and must be "reassured." It is the male-dominated society that has been failing and must be changed. Many studies of female sexuality (95 percent of which, Masters and Johnson point out, are undertaken by men "either from the defensive point of view of personal masculine bias, or from a well-intentioned and often significant scientific position, but, because of cultural bias, without opportunity to obtain unprejudiced material") remark on the spectacularly high degree of frigidity among women. Almost all of them interpret it as a failing of women, not of men or of society, despite the intrusive fact that, as Masters and Johnson observe, "women's . . . physiological capacity for sexual response infinitely surpasses that of man."

Although Masters and Johnson share the assumptions of our male culture that woman's goal must be to reach orgasm during intercourse—even though this usually requires getting to the brink of orgasm outside intercourse—- in their newest report, *Human Sexual Inadequacy*, they examine the causes of "female sexual dysfunction" more honestly than their predecessors.

> Sociocultural influence more often than not places woman in a position in which she must adapt, sublimate, inhibit, or even distort her natural capacity to function sexually in order to fulfill her genetically assigned role [i.e., breeding]. *Herein lies a major source of woman's sexual dysfunction."*
>
> Probably hundreds of thousands of men never gain sufficient ejaculatory control to satisfy their wives sexually regardless of the duration of marriage or the frequency of natural sexual exposure.
>
> Another salient feature in the human female's disadvantaged role in coital connection is the centuries-old concept that it is woman's duty to satisfy her sexual partner. When the age-old demand for accommodation during coital connection dominates

any woman's responsivity, her own opportunites for orgasmic expression are lessened proportionately. . . . The heedless male driving for orgasm can carry along the woman already lost in high levels of sexual demand, but his chances of elevating to orgasm the woman who is trying to accommodate to the rhythm, depth, and power of his demanding pelvic thrusting are indeed poor.

The most unfortunate misconception our culture has assigned to sexual functioning is the assumption, by both men and women, that men by divine guidance and infallible instinct are able to discern exactly what a woman wants sexually and when she wants it. Probably this fallacy has interfered with natural sexual interaction as much as any other single factor.

The husband must not presume his wife's desire for a particular stimulative approach, nor must he introduce his own choice of stimuli.

But of the experts, Masters and Johnson are almost alone in not blaming women for the terrible betrayal of their sex lives.

Why? Clearly, this state of ignorance is not a result of simple unavailability of the facts. It is a manifestation of political and social choices. For, as Ann Koedt pointed out in "The Myth of the Vaginal Orgasm," "Today, with extensive knowledge of anatomy . . . there is no ignorance on the subject. There are, however, social reasons why this knowledge has not been popularized. We are living in. a male society which has not sought change in women's role." No, given our male-dominated society, the mere facts about female sexuality are not enough. The medical experts to this day find it easy to acknowledge the research evidence about the primacy of the clitoris—and *then* to dismiss its obvious meaning. Dr. Leslie H. Farber, for example, upon learning that the female orgasm is not produced by the vagina, simply throws out the importance of female orgasm. In a celebrated essay lamenting the Masters and Johnson research, Dr. Farber announced:

As far as I know little attention was paid to female orgasm before the era of sexology. Where did the sexologists find it? Did they discover or invent it? Or both? . . . My guess, which is not subject to laboratory proof, is that the female orgasm was always an occasional, though not essential, part of woman's whole sexual experience. I also suspect that it appeared with regularity or predictability only during masturbation. . . . *She was content with the mystery and variety of her difference from man, and in fact would not have had it otherwise.*

But surely, some attention was paid to female orgasm before the era of sexology, or else how could it have appeared "with regularity . . . during masturbation"? What Dr. Farber apparently means to say is that before Kinsey little attention was paid to female orgasm *by men.* Too true. Why does Dr. Farber lament the findings of the sexologists? Because look what the findings do to a man's sex life. Nowadays, while ejaculating a man must "learn to take his moment in stride, so to speak, omitting the deference these moments usually call forth and then without breaking stride get to his self-appointed and often fatiguing task of tinkering with his mate—always hopeful that his ministrations will have the appearance of affection." If a woman had to endure that attitude to reach orgasm outside of masturbation, no wonder she preferred to accept her "difference from man." As Masters and Johnson observe "epaculation . . . may provide welcome relief for the woman accepting and fulfilling a role as a sexual object."

Donald W. Hastings, reviewing medical literature dealing with masturbation, observes a double standard of sexuality (and likely its cause) which in less sensational form persists to this day.

Articles in the older literature even went so far as to advocate the following procedures for correcting female masturbation: amputation or cautery of the clitoris, . . . miniature chasity belts, sewing the vaginal lips together to put the clitoris out of reach, and even castration by surgical removal of the ovaries. [But, continues Dr. Hastings in a footnote,] there are no references in the medical literature to surgical removal of testicles or amputation of the penis to stop masturbation. One wonders what heroic measures might have been proposed for boys if women instead of men had composed the medical profession of the time.

Yes, one wonders. And one wonders what might have been defined as the major male and female sex organs, the standard sexual position, the psychic "tasks of development" as Freud called them, and in fact, masculinity and femininity themselves, if women instead of men had composed not only the medical profession, but the dominant caste in society as well.

Men do not easily give up the myths about female sexuality because, whether they are aware of it or not, men benefit from believing them. Believing in the primacy of the vagina allows them to use women for their own sexual pleasure, commandeering vaginas without considering themselves rapists. Believing in vaginal orgasm frees them of responsibility for a woman's sexual pleasure; if a woman does not reach orgasm through intercourse, it is her own psychological failing. If they give pleasure to a woman another way, they are doing her a favor. It does not occur to them that, as Ann Koedt says, "if certain sexual positions now defined as 'standard' are not mutually conducive to orgasm, they [must] no longer be defined as standard." They do not admit that, as Ti-Grace Atkinson observes in "The Institution of Sexual Intercourse," "the whole point of vaginal orgasm is that it supports the view that vaginal penetration [by a penis] is a good in and for itself." By perpetuating these myths society perpetuates the notion that women must be dependent solely on men for their sexual satisfaction and subordinate to the male interpretation of female pleasure.

The Discovery

For thousands of years men have—perhaps unconsciously—benefited from these myths and have therefore believed them, nourishing them through all the various channels of culture, despite all the evidence to the contrary. But why have women, who know from experience that the vagina is *not* the source of their sexual pleasure, and who know only one kind of orgasm, believed in these myths?

Kept apart for so long, women until recently have been under great pressure not to discuss their sexual experiences with other women, just as Masters and Johnson were under great pressure not to study sex in the laboratory. Without information many women have, from childhood on, considered their own sexual experience exceptional and themselves inadequate, if not neurotic, infantile, frigid, or simply freaks. Though each one recognized that the sex myths did not describe *her own* experience, she assumed that they did describe the experience of *other* women, about whom she had no real information. And many women secretly hoped that their own experience would some day follow suit. Now that women, the only real experts on female sexuality, are beginning to talk together and compare notes, they are discovering that their experiences are remarkably similar and that they are not freaks. In the process of exposing the myths and lies, women are discovering that it is not they who have individual sex problems; it is society that has one great big political problem.

There are actually laws on the books in most states that define as "unnatural" and therefore criminal any (sexual) position other than that of the woman on the bottom and the man on the top; laws that make oral sex a crime though for many women it is the only way of achieving orgasm with another person; laws that make homosexuality a crime, though for some people it is the only acceptable way of loving.

The pressures that have long made so many women forego orgasm during love-making and fake orgasm during intercourse are real social pressures. The explanation that it is all simply a result of ignorance, men's and women's, will not do. Hopelessly isolated from each other in their cells in a male-dominated society, even with the facts around, women have still had to fake orgasm to keep their men, to hide their imagined or imputed inadequacy, to demonstrate "love," to gain a man's approval, to boost a man's ego, or, with orgasm nowhere in sight, to get the man please to stop. But with women getting together, the day may soon be approaching when they will exert enough counterpressure to define female sexuality in their own way, and to insist that, just as male sexuality is centered not in the scrotum but in the penis, female sexuality is centered not in the vagina but in the clitoris. When that happens, perhaps it will seem as perverse for a man to ejaculate without stimulating a woman to orgasm as it is now for a woman to reach climax outside intercourse.

Think clitoris.

Is Woman Insatiable?

Barbara Seaman

from *Free and Female: The Sex Life of the Contemporary Woman*, 1972

*In her book **Free and Female**, Barbara Seaman developed the implications of Masters' and Johnson's experimental research and of the theoretical work of Mary Jane Sherfey on the female orgasm. In this chapter, Seaman explores the anthropological literature. Barbara Seaman played an increasingly important role as an activist in the women's health movement. Her 1969 book, **The Doctor's Case Against the Pill** raised serious concerns about the side effects of the oral contraceptive pill, a key factor in the sexual revolution, and led the federal Food and Drug Administration to require detailed informational inserts in the packages of oral contraceptives and other medicines. She is a founder of the National Women's Health Network.*

Did Eve come out of Adam, or did Adam come out of Eve? Which sex is primary? At first glance, this may appear to be a trivial enough question. Who cares, actually, particularly in these times when few of us take the Bible literally?

And yet the myth of creation continues to shape our lives. It is still generally assumed that the male is somehow primary, the female *his* helpmeet, *his* companion. And sexually, many women are still made to feel that men got there first with the most. We have a womb, of course, and we can grow babies, but that is a separate function, or so it seems. As far as the more strictly sexual apparatus go, it is so easy to think of ourselves as possessing "miniature" structures, derived from the male, but humbler and less magnificent. (And perhaps, the implication goes, also less responsive and less enjoyable.)

In some stunning research which had been going on for the previous fifteen years and which came to full flowering in 1957–58, embryologists established, beyond any doubt, that *all mammalian embryos are innately female.* Female development is basic and autonomous; male development is a deviation triggered by hormones. In the beginning, we were all created female.

Genetic sex is established at fertilization, of course, but during the first five or six weeks of fetal life, the influence of the sex genes have no bearing. Then, if the fetus is a normal male, his genes somehow trigger off an "androgen bath," which gradually converts his basically female structures into male structures. Should something go wrong, as occasionally happens, and the "androgen bath" not occur, or should the baby's mother be given anti-androgens, the baby, while genetically male, will look like a female at birth.[1] Only the male embryo is required to undergo a transformation of his sexual anatomy. Without androgens this cannot be achieved. The female embryo needs no such transformation. Hence, male development is now considered a *deviation* from the basic female pattern.

Dr. John Money, a Johns Hopkins University researcher, puts it like this: "Nature simply uses the rule, add androgen and get a male; do nothing and get a female."

Not surprisingly, modern biologists have recorded these facts with little fanfare or comment. It took a woman psychiatrist, Mary Jane Sherfey, to draw the logical conclusion:

"Embryologically speaking, it is correct to say that the penis is an exaggerated clitoris, the scrotum is derived from the labia majora, the original libido is feminine, etc. The reverse is true only for the reptiles. For all the mammals, modern embryology calls for an Adam-out-of-Eve myth!"[2]

It is also well established through medical statistics that the human male is far more vulnerable to a variety of diseases than is the female. Indeed, the male is "in trouble," or "endangered," comparatively speaking, from the moment he is conceived, for more males than females die in the womb, in the birth canal, and at every subsequent step along the way. It is now believed, although the whys and wherefores are not yet clear, that the greater vulnerability of the male may be

1. Anti-androgens are biochemical compounds, related to progestins. They are being used experimentally to treat sex criminals. They wipe out the effect of natural androgens.
2. Mary Jane Sherfey, "The Evolution and Nature of Female Sexuality in Relation to Psychoanalytic Theory," *Journal of the American Psychoanalytic Association,* 14:50 (1966).

related to the fact that his embryonic development is less autonomous and more chancy. There are more opportunities for things to go wrong—in his body and in the male circuits of his brain. . . . The male may be larger, on the average, and better able to lift weights, but let us not allow appearances to deceive us any longer. In many respects, including staying power, we must correctly be called the first and the stronger sex.

One writer enumerated some of the female's biological advantages: ". . . more efficient metabolism, the more specialized organs, the greater resistance to disease, the built-in immunity to certain specific ailments, the extra X chromosome, the more convoluted brain, the stronger heart, the longer life. In nature's plan, the male is but a 'glorified gonad.' The female is the species."[3]

Modern research also indicates that females are emotionally less "vulnerable" than males. Dr. Nancy Bayley, a recipient of the American Psychological Association's Distinguished Scientist Award, began a study of seventy-four babies in 1929. Dr. Bayley is still in touch with fifty-four of them, still testing and interviewing. She found that girls are more "resilient" and less susceptible to the ups and downs of the environment, perhaps because of the pattern of genes that makes one female. (We don't have different genes from men, but we have more of them because the male Y chromosome is an incomplete X.)

Dr. Bayley explained at the American Psychological Association's annual meeting in September, 1966, "The female of the species tends to return somehow to an innate potential. A boy's mental growth depends a good deal on his mother's treatment of him, but the only thing we could find to correlate with the I.Q.s of girls was the intelligence of their mothers."

Woman's sexual, reproductive and excretory organs are also better differentiated than the male's and therefore more elegant and more advanced. For example, men possess only one canal for the emission of both seminal fluid and urine, while women have separate orifices for ovum and urine. In lesser animals, a single cavity, the cloaca, is the opening for the intestinal, generative and urinary canals.

In sexual potential, as well as the other features mentioned, *woman* now appears to hold the anatomical edge. Freud called the clitoris a

---

3. Elizabeth Gould Davis, *The First Sex* (New York, G. P. Putnam's Sons, 1971), p. 329.

"stunted penis." He maintained that many of woman's sexual difficulties stemmed from the fact that her clitoris is rudimentary, vestigial, a feeble imitation of the superior male organ.[4]

But Freud was wrong on this, or certainly "superficial." For the fact is that the clitoris is merely the visible tip of a vast and complicated internal system of highly responsive sexual tissue. When you compare the penis to the entire *clitoral system*, which is hidden from the eye but which, biologically, is what the penis should be compared to, you find that woman is *more* richly endowed. During sexual excitement, the blood vessel engorgement of the male is obvious. (It's what creates his erection.) The blood vessel engorgement of the female is less obvious, being mainly subterranean, but it is probably greater. This may explain why woman takes longer to prepare for her orgasm. In Dr. Sherfey's words, ". . . the female undergoes a more generalized pelvic vasocongestive process . . . which simply takes longer to develop fully. . . . Women have a larger volume capacity of venous networks to maintain in the engorged state. . . ."[5]

It's sort of like this: It takes more furniture to fill up a large apartment than a small one. Well, we, not they, have the larger apartment. Contrary to what may meet the eye, we have *more* sexy tissues. Furthermore, *our* apartment keeps growing. The male's sexual capacity peaks in his late teens and thereafter diminishes. But in woman, sexual experience (and also pregnancy) increases her "venous bed capacity." Provided she is sexually active, her "sexy tissues" continue to enlarge and grow.

This is all so contrary to what we have been taught about "masculinity" (very sexy) and "femininity" (reserved, shy, feeble) that the mind can hardly absorb it. Nonetheless, the latest scientific evidence indicates that, sexually, the male is but a pale imitation—of *us*.

His capacity, which, compared to ours, was not much to start with,

4. As a consequence of her genital inferiority, Freud believed, woman is also morally inferior. He reasoned as follows: When the girl child discovers that she does not possess a penis, she inevitably becomes envious of the male. She rejects her mother, who also has no penis, and therefore she cannot resolve her Oedipal complex (through identification with her own sex) as successfully as her brothers can. The resolution of the Oedipal complex, in Freud's system, is necessary for the development of a sturdy conscience or superego. Because she lacks a penis, woman possesses an inadequate sense of justice, a predisposition to envy, weaker social interests and a lesser capacity for sublimation. She is also, normally and inevitably—masochistic and passive.
5. Shurfey, *op. cit.*, p. 91.

peaks at a ridiculously early age, and after that, it's downhill all the way. Our capacity continues to grow throughout much of our adult lifetime, *if* the world we inhabit and the men we consort with do not cruelly abort it.

Psychosexually, you may be entirely different from your own sister or your best friend, much more different from her than your husband is apt to be from *his* brother or *his* best friend. For, as anthropologist Lee Rainwater has written:

"Men only rarely say they are indifferent to or uninterested in sexual relations. But women present the gamut of responses, from 'If God made anything better, He kept it to Himself' to 'I would be happy if I never had to do that again; it's disgusting.'"[6]

As a twentieth-century woman, sex may be the most important thing in your life, or it may be one of the least important. Whatever it is, it's your secret. Women who are very sexy walk and talk and look like other women. And so do women who are very frigid.

You cannot tell a sexy woman by her pointy breasts, her mini-skirts, or the way she may or may not undulate her hips.

For in some cultures, and in many American subcultures, girls and women are encouraged to *look* seductive, without *feeling* sexy.

Moreover, consciously or unconsciously, many men *do not want* passionate wives. They fear that if they stimulate and please a woman, "she might get to like it too much," and then, presumably, she might be unfaithful. (Or she might be distracted from cooking and washing socks.)

Rainwater tells us that the lower-class males—in the United States, in England, in Mexico and Puerto Rico—still hold openly to the *macho* concept of masculinity where the man is insistent on taking his own pleasure without reference to the woman's needs. Sure, he may try to stimulate her when he is first courting her, but after that—no.[7]

---

6. Donald S. Marshall and Robert C. Suggs, ed., *Human Sexual Behavior* (New York, Basic Books, Inc., 1971), p. 188.

7. It is better for men if their partners are responsive. They will enjoy sex more frequently, and they will not be made victims in the kinds of punitive power games that sexually frustrated women are wont to play.

In my opinion, men have to be taught *early* through subtleties of precept probably, more than through words, that women are sexual creatures, too. The commitment to satisfy a woman must he made a very basic part of their egos or sense of sportsmanship or else they will not satisfy most of their partners, on most occasions. The model of an *obedient* wife, who never refuses sex, but who enjoys it only for the pleasure she gives her

In cultures where the men expect their wives to enjoy sex, they do, they do! as we shall see. In cultures where the men do not expect their women to enjoy sex, the women usually don't. Of course we cannot make any generalizations about our twentieth-century American males because our culture is so complex (and so confused and contradictory about sex) that our men's expectations probably run the gamut. To some, their partner's satisfaction is almost as important as their own, while to others, it hardly matters or might even *frighten* them.

Now let us look at a happy Polynesian island, Mangaia, where no woman is frigid. Dr. Donald S. Marshall, an anthropologist, has made three field trips there and has reported his findings in two books:[8]

> The Mangaian male lover aims to have his partner achieve orgasm (mene) two or three times to his once. . . . His responsibility in this matter is so ingrained into the Mangaian male that upon hearing that some American or European women cannot or do not achieve a climax, the Mangaian immediately asks (with real concern) whether this inability will not injure the married woman's health.

The seriousness which Mangaians pay to the sex education of their adolescent boys could be a lesson to us except it is difficult to imagine

husband, has much to recommend it from the male perspective. One thinks of the classic story of the Victorian bride who, on her wedding day, asked her mother for sex information. "Well, dear," her mother replied, "I've always found it helpful to lie back and think of England." No doubt this bride made an estimable wife, in her husband's view. He never dreamed that her chronic backache and fatigue or her annoying attempts to reform and refine him were probably a product of bitterness and sexual frustration.

Some British and American physicians still (as a joke!) define woman as "a constipated biped with lower back pains."

Today, in our supposedly sexy society, it has become rather common for women to fake orgasms. The woman who finds herself "faking it" is probably responding to the signals of a man who is ambivalent about feminine sexuality. He wants her to moan and groan because *Playboy* has assured him that's part of the procedure. But if her satisfaction is genuinely important to him, why isn't he taking the trouble to find out what *she* really likes? I think the reason is that he doesn't want a woman who is truly responding.

8. Marshall and Suggs, "Sexual Behavior of Mangaia," op. cit., Chapter 5. Also Donald S. Marshall, Ra'ivavae: an Expedition to the Most Fascinating and Mysterious Island in Polynesia (New York, Doubleday, 1961).

that even the most progressive school or family in the United States would be willing to experiment with a similar program.

First of all, in Marshall's words, ". . . the average Mangaian youth has fully as detailed a knowledge—perhaps more—of the gross anatomy of the penis and the vagina as does a European physician." He, the Mangaian youth, also has a *better* vocabulary, simply because a better vocabulary is available. To some extent, you can measure the importance which a certain people give to an activity just from the richness of the vocabulary they have developed to describe it. In the English and European languages we note, merely, that clitorises come in different sizes and shapes. But in Mangaia, they have specific modifying terms for different kinds of clitorises. That means, presumably, that the men pay more attention to them. Clitorises are classified by their degree of sharpness or bluntness and are also described as "projecting," "erecting" or "protruding." (The Mangaian male is equally expert on the size, shape and consistency of the mons veneris.)

The serious sex education of a Mangaian youth begins when he is circumcised, early in adolescence. The skin is cut, and the penis has "no hat," as the local expression goes.

The reason for this procedure is that the Mangaian male would not want a malodorous penis. Indeed, to suggest that he has one is practically the worst insult an enemy could deliver. After his circumcision, the youth runs into the sea, proclaiming, just as Jewish boys do at their Bar Mitzvahs, "Now I am really a man."

But here the similarity ends. The Bar Mitzvah boy must prove that he knows Hebrew. The boy in Mangaia must establish other skills:

> . . . more important than the physiological treatment . . . is the knowledge of sexual matters and the training in sexual behavior given to the youth by the circumcision expert. Not only does this detailed information concern techniques of coitus but . . . the expert teaches the youth (as the elderly woman instructs the young female) about such techniques as cunnilingus, the kissing and sucking of breasts, and a means of achieving simultaneous mutual climax, as well as how to bring the woman to climax several times before the male partner permits himself to achieve

the goal. Some of this instruction is by straightforward precept, some by the use of figurative stories.

The period of formal instruction is followed by a "practical exercise" in copulation. . . . The intercourse, often arranged by an expert, must be with an experienced woman . . . of significance to the youth is the coaching he receives in the techniques he has learned from the expert. The woman teaches him to hold back until he can achieve orgasm in unison with his partner; she teaches him the techniques involved in carrying out various acts and positions about which the expert has advised him—especially the matter of timing . . . the last day . . . is marked by a feast given for both the boy and his mentor. . . . This feast is the signal for the boy to be called a man by his people.

In Mangaia, then, a boy is a man when he has proved he can satisfy a woman. The Mangaians believe that "the orgasm must be 'learned' by a woman and that this learning process can be achieved through the efforts of 'the good young man.' " A boy is not unleashed on young girls until he has proved his skills. Should he seduce a virgin and should she not reach orgasm, he has a solemn obligation to continue "visiting her" until she does.

"There is considerable technique involved in Mangaian foreplay," Marshall reports, but performance during intercourse is considered more important.

Once penetration has been made, the male realizes that his action must be continuously kept up in order to bring his partner to climax . . . a "good man" will be able to continue his actions for fifteen to thirty minutes or more . . . the ultimate and invariable goal of the two lovers is to so match their reactions that when the male finally does permit himself to reach climax it is achieved simultaneously with the peak of his partner's pleasure . . . the really important aspect of sexual intercourse . . . is to give pleasure to his wife or woman or girl. . . . Supposedly this is what gives the male partner his own pleasure and a special thrill. . . .

In contrast, consider nineteenth-century England, where William Acton, the leading authority of his time, could declare it a "vile aspersion" to even suggest that woman has any sexual nature.[9] "The majority of women (happily for society) are not very much troubled with sexual feelings of any kind," he wrote.

Did Victorian women conform to Acton's view of them? As best we know, most of them did. Dr. Marie Nyswander tells the following story about a late friend of hers, a liberated woman in some respects (a very successful physician) who married, happily, in 1904, and reared five children. This woman had only one orgasm in her lifetime, and it was not a welcome event. When she married, the mantle of Victorianism was still very much upon her, and so although she was deeply in love with her husband, she was totally frigid. After the birth of her third child, she confessed to Dr. Nyswander, she started to experience some feelings of pleasure during intercourse. Now she had her fourth child, and intercourse was interrupted for several months. Upon resumption, the pleasure had increased enormously, and on the second time, she had a profound orgasm. Alas, Dr. Nyswander relates, her friend was very consciously frightened and very consciously ashamed. She decided never to let the experience repeat itself and was entirely successful in her resolution. Not until years later, after her husband had died, did this woman physician, who, for her time, must have been exceptionally sophisticated and knowledgeable, recognize the tragedy of her decision.[10]

Occasionally, a male from one sort of culture encounters a female from the other sort, and the outcome, if successful for the woman, is perplexing for the man. John C. Messenger, who has been performing field studies in a small and isolated Irish folk community, recently reported:

There is much evidence to indicate that the female orgasm is unknown—or at least doubted, or considered a deviant

9. Acton, a London urologist (1813–1875), was sort of the Dr. David Reuben of his day. Acton's highly influential book, published in 1857, bore the catchy title *The Functions and Disorders of the Reproductive Organs, in Childhood, Youth, Adult Age, and Advanced Life, Considered in Their Physiological, Social and Moral Relations* (London, J. Churchill, 1857).
10. Marie N. Robinson (Nyswander), *The Power of Sexual Surrender* (New York, Doubleday, 1959).

response. One middle-aged bachelor, who considers himself wise in the ways of the outside world, and has a reputation for making love to willing tourists, described one girl's violent bodily reactions to his fondling and asked for an explanation; when told the "facts of life" of what was obviously an orgasm, he admitted not realizing that women also could achieve a climax, although he was aware that some of them enjoyed kissing and being handled.[11]

The male orgasm is nowhere unknown, or doubted, or considered a deviant response. With rare exceptions (which are pathological), a sexually mature male must have an orgasm to deposit sperm. He cannot perform his part in 'reproduction without sexual pleasure. By contrast, a woman can and often does. She can ovulate monthly, get pregnant yearly, can live and die, and leave behind a huge family, without ever having an orgasm or dreaming that it is possible. Reproductively, the female orgasm is a luxury, the male orgasm a necessity.[12]

But precisely because orgasm and sperm production are intertwined, there is a natural ceiling, as well as a floor, to the number of orgasms a man can have. Women have no such limitation, which brings us to the "unmentionable" finding of modern sex research, the finding which no one likes to talk about.

In her extraordinary study, entitled *The Evolution and Nature of Female Sexuality in Relation to Psychoanalytic Theory*, Dr. Mary Jane Sherfey, recognizing the "extreme importance of cutting across the compartmentalization of knowledge," has undertaken a vast integrative effort, which explains female sexuality in terms of "physiology, anatomy, comparative embryology, endocrinology, gynecology, paleontology, evolutionary biology, population genetics, primatology, and ethology—not

11. Marshall and Suggs, "Sex and Repression in an Irish Folk Community," *op. cit.*, Chap. One.
12. This all too evident fact of life has been widely construed to mean that the male, exclusively, is and should be the initiator of sexual relations. But at the 1971 annual meeting of the American Psychological Association, Dr. Eleanor Maccoby, a professor at Stanford and editor of the highly regarded book *The Development of Sex Differences*, pointed out that, in fact, throughout the mammalian kingdom it is usually the female who initiates sex relations. The male, as it were, is always prepared, and sex relations ensue when the female signals that *she* is available. In many species, sex relations only occur at certain times in the female cycle.
Rape is exclusive to human beings.

to mention anthropology and psychiatry, the central foci upon which the rest converge."[13] She concludes that—potentially—women may well have an insatiable sex drive, like the sex drive of certain female primates who have an anatomy much like ours:

> Having no cultural restrictions, these primate females will perform coitus from twenty to fifty times a day during the peak week of estrus, usually with several series of copulation in rapid succession. If necessary, they flirt, solicit, present and stimulate the male in order to obtain successive coitions. They will "consort" with one male for several days until he is exhausted, then take up with another. They emerge from estrus totally exhausted, often with wounds from spent males who have repulsed them. I suggest that something akin to this behavior could be paralleled by the human female if her civilization allowed it.

Why hasn't civilization allowed it? Dr. Sherfey suggests that:

> The human mating system, with its permanent family and kinship ties, was absolutely essential to man's becoming—and remaining—man. . . . The forceful suppression of woman's inordinate sexual drive was a prerequisite to the dawn of every modern civilization and almost every living culture. Primitive sexual drive was too strong, too susceptible to the fluctuating extremes of an impelling, aggressive eroticism to withstand the disciplined requirements of a settled family life. . . . It could well be that the "oversexed" woman is actually exhibiting a normal sexuality—although because of it her integration into her society may leave much to be desired . . . this hypothesis will come as no great shock to many women who consciously realize or intuitively sense their lack of satiation.

In sedate, scientific language, Dr. Sherfey predicts that all hell could break loose as more and more modern women come to recognize— even to dare suspect—what a vast sexual capacity they have. "The

---

13. Sherfey, *op. cit.*, p. 30.

magnitude of the psychological and social problems facing mankind is difficult to contemplate," she observes.

Woman, it appears, has a plastic sex drive which both is and isn't designed for monogamy. At the lower limits, it can be turned off almost completely. Woman can live virtually without sexual expression if she and her lovers were reared to expect that she requires none. But sex may well be addictive in woman, and once she starts letting herself enjoy it, there may be no upper limit short of her own exhaustion.

An orgasmic woman can be emotionally satisfied with an average sex life of several copulations per week, and sometimes she can *will* herself to believe that she is physically satisfied as well. But if Dr. Sherfey is correct, such a woman is never sated—as her husband or lover is sated. At some primitive level of her being, she desires a much higher frequency than does her mate. Recent sex research suggests that the female orgasm may increase pelvic vasocongestion, which sparks a taste for further orgasm. *The more a woman does, the more she can, and the more she can, the more she wants to.* Masters and Johnson claim that they have observed females experiencing six or more orgasms during intercourse and up to fifty or more during masturbation with a vibrator.

Dr. Sherfey, who maintains that the nymphomaniac may actually be the most normal and natural of women, practices psychiatry and psychoanalysis in New York City. As an undergraduate, she studied with Dr. Alfred Kinsey at Indiana University. She received her MD degree in 1943.

Dr. Sherfey points out with some bitterness that nearly all anatomy books were written by men who tend to regard the human female as "sexually inadequate or inferior" and the clitoris as a pale imitation of the penis. Quite to the contrary, however, the external clitoris is merely the tip of the iceberg or (more accurately) the volcano. Conventional anatomy books usually ignore the internal clitoral system, as distinct from the clitoris itself.

Surprisingly, Dr. Sherfey is a Freudian. While on a superficial level she appears to disagree violently with Freud's thoughts on orgasms and female sexuality, she actually views his theories as flexible, and feels that he might have agreed with her biological updating. She quotes from his famous book *Behind the Pleasure Principle,* which was published in 1920:

> Biology is truly a land of unlimited possibilities. We may expect it to give us the most surprising information, and we cannot guess what answers it will return in a few dozen years to the questions we have put to it. They may be of a kind which will blow away the whole of our artificial structure of hypotheses.

Freud recognized that the twentieth century would bring many scientific advances. Now, as we have seen or shall see:

—Embryologists have established that females are the first sex and that the male sexual structures are merely a variation on the structures of the female.

—Sex researchers, especially Masters and Johnson, have established that the female has a sexual capacity which is at least as great as the male, and probably greater.

—Anthropologists have clarified that in some cultures, even today, the vast sexual capacity of the female is taken for granted. Their field work in primitive cultures lends extremely convincing support to the historical thesis that the forced suppression of female sexuality was somehow necessary for the development of "higher civilizations."

Does all this mean that women (under ideal conditions) actually enjoy sex more than men?

There may never be an answer because sexual experience remains so subjective and even mystical. It is one thing to take measurements in a laboratory and quite another to describe the meaning of an act. It appears that most people's most tenderly remembered sexual experiences have little to do with number of contractions, length of orgasm, or anything else of the sort. A reunion with a beloved person is, obviously, far more significant than a blast-off which is merely technically terrific.

Nonetheless, the mystical appeal of sex, crucial as it is, has been too often used in a fashion that disserves women and encourages selfish or lazy men. (Good women only care about the "closeness" and "don't really mind" if they aren't brought to climax; that sort of thing.) Therefore, if only to redress this imbalance, it should be stated here that we just might be able to have better orgasms than men. At least, we are reported to have more erogenous zones, throughout the body, and more sexy tissue in and around the pelvis. Our orgasms are longer and perhaps more complex, occupying "three stages," in Masters-Johnson terms, while the male orgasm exhausts itself in only two. Also, if a male is low on seminal fluid, his orgasms are usually less enjoyable, whereas the female has no such limitation. For whatever it's worth, she can have many more orgasms in a short period of time, and the second or third may be even better than the first. (Some males under thirty, and relatively few thereafter, can climax several times within ten or fifteen minutes. The quality invariably diminishes. But many females can climax even more times in the same period.)

Also, what the Mangaians call "knockout" orgasm and Masters and Johnson call *status orgasmus* has been observed—in islands under the sun and in sex laboratories both—in females only. This is an orgasm that seems to go on and on, the heart beating at an inordinately rapid rate.

Well, then, if women have all this sexy tissue (which grows richer and sexier with pregnancy and experience, rather as a well-chewed piece of bubble gum gets more expansive) and if we also have this impressive capacity to keep having more, and even better, orgasms, for as many minutes or hours as good stimulation abides, and if we also occasionally demonstrate a capacity for a "knockout" orgasm, which is apparently rather beyond anything the male experiences, then why do so many women not know how sexy they are?

Sherfey, as mentioned earlier, believes that males have forcibly suppressed the vast and virtually insatiable erotic potential of females. She goes so far as to suggest that "the suppression by cultural forces of woman's inordinately high sexual drive and orgasmic capacity" has been a "major preoccupation of practically every civilization." (Dr. William Simon, a former Kinsey Institute researcher, agrees with Sherfey and carries her thinking one step further. "The suppression of female sexuality has not been easily achieved," he comments. "Societies have had to work very hard at it. A similar investment in males would have paid off easier.")

Dr. Sherfey accepts J. J. Bachofen's theory of human history, which was first published in 1861. From his analysis of myths and early artifacts, Bachofen concluded that until about 8000 B.C. human societies were ruled by women.

Sherfey writes:

> There are many indications from the prehistory studies in the Near East that it took perhaps 5,000 years or longer for the subjugation of women to take place. All relevant data from the 12,000 to 8000 B.C. period indicates that the precivilized woman enjoyed full sexual freedom and was often totally incapable of controlling her sexual drive. Therefore, I propose that one of the reasons for the long delay between the earliest development of agriculture (c. 12,000 B.C.) and the rise of urban life and the beginning of recorded knowledge (c. 8000–5000 B.C.) was the ungovernable cyclic sexual drive of women. Not until these drives were gradually brought under control by rigidly enforced social codes could family life become the stabilizing and creative crucible from which modern man could emerge.

To this day, the Bachofen thesis attracts interesting and eloquent advocates. Yet most conventional historians reject it. This does not at all disturb Sherfey, for, as she points out, most conventional historians are also conventional males.

Men, however scholarly, are usually quite loath to concede any area of female equality, much less superiority, until the evidence becomes overwhelming.

Earlier we noted that there are two ways of comparing clitoris to penis. One can examine and dissect the externals only, in which case the laurels go to the penis. If, however, one adds up external *and* internal anatomy, the laurels go to the clitoris, for a more complicated and responsive venous system underlies it.

By the end of the nineteenth century dissections and studies of human anatomy were well enough advanced so that any scientist working in this area could and should have been able to note that the female clitoral system was rather impressive. Yet this anatomical evidence was given so little importance that it even failed to come to Freud's attention. Apparently, the only nineteenth-century physician who made any fuss over it was Elizabeth Blackwell (1821–1910), a staunch feminist who was the first woman to be graduated from any United States medical school.[14]

The historical evidence may still be shrouded in fog, but the scientific and anthropologic evidence has become overwhelming. Woman, while having a plastic sex drive which can be repressed more completely than the sexuality of the male, has, under optimum or natural conditions, as good as and probably a *better* sexual potential than the male. It is clear that in many cultures some social process has taken place which has curbed or muted female sexuality or—sometimes—eliminated it.

We can assume that in prehistoric days the basic family unit was probably mother and child and that it must have been a genius, let alone a "wise child," who knew his own father. Women may have sensed a glimmering of immortality, through their children, and men must have envied it.

It seems only common sense to suppose that in the interests of establishing paternity, an orderly family life, the descent of property, and so on, it was necessary to curb woman's sex drive and encourage her to be monogamous. And surely one way to do this was to make sex unsatisfactory for her. After all, we know that sex, even today, is more or less addictive in women, and the more-she-gets-the-more-she-wants. We know that there are sound biological reasons for this, for as she enjoys sex, the sexy tissues get more sexy, their vascularity increasing, and the muscles of orgasmic response being strengthened. We know that the

---

14. Dr. Blackwell, a proper Victorian, held typically repressive attitudes toward sexuality in both the female and the male. However, she hated to see the female belittled, and so she wrote:

"The chief structures of the male are external, but they are internal in the female . . . failure to recognize the equivalent value of internal with external structure has led to such crude fallacy as a comparison of the penis with such a vestige as the clitoris, whilst failing to recognize the vast amount of erectile tissue, mostly internal, which is the direct seat of special sexual spasm."

In the United States, Dr. Blackwell is best known for pioneering medical education for women and for founding the New York Infirmary for Women and Children and the Women's Medical College of the New York Infirmary. However, after returning to her native England in 1869, Blackwell wrote many books and pamphlets on sex and sex education. These were collected and published in 1902 in a three-volume book entitled *Essays in Medical Sociology* (London, E. Bell).

Blackwell recognized that women, as well as men, have orgasms or "sexual spasms," and somewhat unlike other Victorian sexologists, she held to a single standard of sexual behavior, urging men, as well as women, to save themselves for higher things.

She suspected the motives of male gynecologists, who, she suggested, did altogether too much unnecessary poking around with their speculums. ". . . this custom is a real and growing evil," she asserted.

male, whose sexual capacity peaks in his teens, is not likely to keep up with his wife's growing needs, as they mature together. And finally, we know that males in most civilized cultures have long feared sexy women, drawing a sharp division (which may be justified) between the chaste and sexless "good" woman and the unreliable woman who *likes* sex. Even today, as sophisticated as we think we are, in many of our sub-cultures the males deliberately refrain from using their best erotic techniques on their wives, in fear that their wives might get to like it. These men possess something of a sexual "repertoire" to borrow Margaret Mead's phrase, but they deliberately withhold it.

On the other hand, it seems to me implausible that it was *men only* who set out to cool and restrain the natural passions of women. A pregnant woman, a woman in labor, or a mother with a nursling at her breast is vulnerable. She cannot run as fast or as far, nor can she hunt and gather food so efficiently, nor can she hide from an enemy as quietly or as well. Surely, under primitive conditions, the survival chances of a mother and her babies were improved if she had protectors. Thus, I think we must consider the possibility that it was adaptive for woman herself to curb her own sexuality. The children of a mother who was capable of forming ties with one male probably stood a better chance of growing up. The "plastic" woman who smothered her own sexuality lost something, but gained something, too.[15]

Sherfey concludes that the ruthless suppression of female sexuality was a historical necessity:

---

15. On reviewing all that is presently known (1971) about biologically based differences between the sexes, Eleanor Maccoby finds three essentials:
    1. Males have greater physical strength, of the sort that allows them to fend off an attacker or beat up a wife.
    2. Males are more aggressive, although not necessarily more active and certainly not smarter.
    3. The childbearing and nursing functions of the female have made her dependent on men.
Today, Dr. Maccoby adds, the greater muscular strength and aggressiveness of the male are no longer assets. He need not fend off wild animals. Even in the business world, the old captains of industry who pounded the table and terrified employees have gone out of style. Today managerial decisions are made by teams and committees, and the overly aggressive executive is *unlikely* to succeed.
    Woman's biological dependence on the male is also obsolete, for she is no longer pregnant or nursing throughout most of her adult life. "Let's be realistic," Dr. Maccoby urges, "about the kinds of lives most women led until quite recently. They were pregnant or nursing most of the time, and this fostered a state of dependence which is not functional in the modern world."

Although then (and now) couched in superstitions, religious and rationalized terms, behind the subjugation of woman's sexuality lay the inexorable economics of cultural evolution which finally forced men to impose it and women to endure it. If that suppression has been, at times, unduly oppressive or cruel, I suggest the reason has been neither man's sadistic, selfish infliction of servitude upon helpless women nor women's weakness or inborn masochism. The strength of the drive determines the force required to suppress it.

But even sexy women can learn, as Sherfey points out, to *will* satisfaction. And so the wives of Mangaia, who are surely very stimulated and who, by middle age, want more sex than their husbands, nonetheless stay with their husbands because of economic and affectionate bonds. The same was true, by and large, of the sexy American women in a study I made in the spring of 1971. As one said, "When we have sex, I always want to do it again, immediately or sooner, but he can't. So I adjust to it. I'm horny the first twelve hours, but then I feel fine. The strange thing is that when we are apart from each other, he misses it more than I do. He needs sex every three days or so. I can turn off completely when there's no stimulation around, or when I am stimulated, I could just go on and on. Well, obviously I've had to adjust to his pattern. But I'm not complaining because he's good, very good."

Men may or may not have suppressed our sexuality more brutally than was necessary. On the one hand, as Sherfey points out:

Each orgasm is followed promptly by refilling of the venous erectile chambers; distention creates engorgement and edema, which creates more tissue tension, etc. The supply of blood edema fluid to the pelvis is inexhaustible. . . . *To all intents and purposes, the human female is sexually insatiable in the presence of the highest degrees of sexual satiation.*

On the other hand, as Sherfey also allows:

I must stress that this condition does not mean that a woman is always consciously unsatisfied. There is a great difference between satisfaction and satiation. A woman may be emotionally satisfied to the full in the absence of *any* orgasmic expression (although such a state would rarely persist through years of frequent arousal and coitus without some kind of physical or emotional reaction formation . . .).

The man *is* satisfied. The woman *usually wills herself* to be satisfied because she is simply unaware of the extent of her orgasmic capacity. However, I predict that this hypothesis will come as no great shock to many women who consciously realize, or intuitively sense, their lack of satiation.

Has woman's inherent drive abated in all these years? Sherfey thinks not. She believes that every girl born has the capacity to become a veritable nymphomaniac.

Even if she is right, however, I think that most of the women who opt for marriage and family life will continue, sedately and perhaps a little sadly at times, to "will themselves" satisfied. A mother's attachment to her young is very strong and not easily jeopardized.

On the other hand, there is no question that a new life-style is emerging for educated women in civilized countries. The world is pretty well filled up, and the men who rule it are coming to view babies as a threat to their own survival. The pressures on women to marry and reproduce are rapidly diminishing, at the same time as their solo economic position is improving.[16]

16. The first steps, at least, have been taken. Thanks to Congresswoman Martha Griffiths, the Civil Rights Act of 1964 prohibits job discrimination based on sex. At first the men who were charged with enforcing this law tried to make a joke of it. They wasted their time arguing over specious issues like: Would Playboy Clubs be required to hire male bunnies?

Recently, however, groups of women who were barred from job promotions because of their sex have been bringing class suits against their employers and have been winning these cases. Employers have been held liable for hefty amounts of back pay.

But overall the situation is still dismal. Teresa Levitin, of the University of Michigan's Survey Research Center, recently analyzed the income of working women. She reports: "Although we expected to discover that a woman received fewer occupational rewards than a man with equal scores on the achievement predictors, we were hardly prepared for the size of the discrepancy between observed and expected annual income. The average woman actually received $3,358 less than she should have received." In other words, it costs you an average of $3,358 a year to be a woman. Your income would have to be increased by 71 percent to bring it to the level of a man with precisely comparable qualifications.

Such discrimination is apparent in traditionally "feminine" fields, such as teaching,

A certain group of educated, independent single women in my study were sexually active beyond the wildest dreams of most wives. They didn't look like nymphomaniacs or prostitutes or loose women. Indeed, as a rule they *appeared* rather prim and ladylike.

There is no doubt that such women will increase, for, to complicate matters further, we may be very close to the day when scientists (male) will be able to grow babies in test tubes, thereby proving themselves equal to Eve and leaving woman even freer to indulge her own sexuality.

As the woman as mother becomes obsolete, perhaps packs of ravenously sexy, rapacious women will roam the world, as in some grim work of science fiction. But sufficient unto the day is the evil thereof. For now it is problem enough, convincing our husbands and lovers that we have sexual appetites, too, which may have a different rhythm from theirs but which are every bit as normal and (in an aroused woman) every bit as urgent.

There are those who deplore feminism and the "melting of the sexes," but it is difficult not to be hopeful about the situation when currently so few people are happy or sexually satisfied. As Dr. Alfred Auerback, clinical professor of psychiatry at the University of California School of Medicine in San Francisco, pointed out recently:

. . . the pattern of rearing children in this country is designed

as well as traditionally "masculine" fields. It is true that entering female teachers receive the same salaries as males, but after that, less competent men are normally promoted to higher-paying administrative jobs, over the heads of more competent and better-qualified women, according to Dr. Neal Gross of the Harvard School of Education.

It appears that few women recognize what a bargain they are to employers. Levitin notes that only 7.9 percent of the women in her sample (most of whom were, in fact, grossly underpaid) said that they *felt* discriminated against.

It is curious how job discrimination is so taken for granted in our society since, in a sense, it is economic discrimination against all groups except bachelors. Married men, as well as single and married women, are hurt by it since the more a wife earns, the more secure is her husband's economic position. Martha Griffiths tells the story of a friend of hers, a married man, who was unhappy in his job. Reviewing his problems with the Griffithses, he suddenly brightened. "I'll quit," he announced. "Harriet is making fifteen thousand dollars a year, and we won't starve while I look for another job." Where Harriet isn't making $15,000 a year, Mrs. Griffiths points out, her husband does not enjoy the same freedom.

Men and women alike may be afraid that marriage and family life will deteriorate if women gain too much economic independence, I have heard brilliant and capable women express fear that if they started to earn more than their husbands, it might ruin their marriages.

to make the male and female incompatible in terms of later intimate relationships. Boys are brought up not to show their feelings. They are not supposed to cry. They are supposed to be little men. The emphasis is on being emotionally detached, playing it cool. Sexual activity is heralded as a form of conquest. It's an activity in which you don't get emotionally involved. So the pressures are toward making the male predatory, certainly not romantic or involved.

Girls in our society are brought up to he narcissistic. They are supposed to look pretty and hence to be eventually marriageable. There is increasing pressure on them to be sexually alluring and coquettish but at the same time to hold back their feelings, not to get physically involved. They are taught to be careful about sex, to be ladylike, to protect themselves from exploitation by the male. Their attention is focused on romance, falling in love, being a wife, having children, raising a family.

In the so-called primitive societies, children are educated in the skills of pleasurable sexual activity through erotic teachings, pictures, and puberty rites. Yet in our Western culture, we have subdued overt eroticism. We imply that the biological drive is sufficient unto itself. Therefore, it is no wonder that most men assume that inserting the penis into the vagina after minimal sexual foreplay is all that is required to satisfy a female partner.

The Kinsey studies of some 20 years ago found that about 75% of men ejaculate in less than 2 minutes, many within 10 or 20 seconds after entrance into the vagina. Obviously, it's over before it's begun, and there isn't much in it for the female partner.[17]

---

17. Dr. Alfred Auerback, moderator, "Roundtable: How Can Sex Be More Pleasurable?" Medical Aspects of Human Sexuality, Vol. v, No. 9 (September, 1971).

The Zipless Fuck

Erica Jong

from *Fear of Flying*, 1973

*Erica Jong's novel **Fear of Flying** is both a novel about sex and a novel of ideas. The novel's heroine sets out on a quest to experience sex for pleasure alone—without the commitment or romance with which sex is often intertwined. Male reviewers, in particular, reacted to it violently; one man wrote that it was like being trapped in an elevator "with a woman who tells you her story . . . rapes you and stops you reaching for the emergency button." But Jong's novel was runaway bestseller, selling over six million copies in the U.S. alone and twenty million around the world.*

Five years of marriage had made me itchy for all those things: itchy for men, and itchy for solitude. Itchy for sex and itchy for the life of a recluse. I knew my itches were contradictory—and that made things even worse. I knew my itches were un-American— and that made things *still* worse. It is heresy in America to embrace any way of life except as half of a couple. Solitude is un-American. It may be condoned in a man—especially if he is a "glamorous bachelor" who "dates starlets" during a brief interval between marriages. But a woman is always presumed to be alone as a result of abandonment, not choice. And she is treated that way: as a pariah. There is simply no dignified way for a woman to live alone. Oh, she can get along financially per- haps (though not nearly as well as a man), but emotionally she is never left in peace. Her friends, her family, her fellow workers never let her forget that her husbandlessness, her childlessness—her *selfishness*, in short—is a reproach to the American way of life.

Even more to the point: the woman (unhappy though she knows her married friends to be) can never let *herself* alone. She lives as if she were constantly on the brink of some great fulfillment. As if she were waiting for Prince Charming to take her away "from all this." All what? The solitude of living inside her own soul? The certainty of being herself instead of half of something else?

My response to all this was not (not yet) to have an affair and not (not yet) to hit the open road, but to evolve my fantasy of the Zipless Fuck. The zipless fuck was more than a fuck. It was a platonic ideal. Zipless because when you came together zippers fell away like rose petals, underwear blew off in one breath like dandelion fluff. Tongues intertwined and turned liquid. Your whole soul flowed out through your tongue and into the mouth of your lover.

For the true, ultimate zipless A-1 fuck, it was necessary that you never get to know the man very well. I had noticed, for example, how all my infatuations dissolved as soon as I really became friends with a man, became sympathetic to his problems, listened to him *kvetch* about his wife, or ex-wives, his mother, his children. After that I would like him, perhaps even love him—but without passion. And it was passion that I wanted. I had also learned that a sure way to exorcise an infatuation was to write about someone, to observe his tics and twitches, to anatomize his personality in type. After that he was an insect on a pin, a newspaper clipping laminated in plastic. I might enjoy his company, even admire him at moments, but he no longer had the power to make me wake up trembling in the middle of the night. I no longer dreamed about him. He had a face.

So another condition for the zipless fuck was brevity. And anonymity made it even better.

During the time I lived in Heidelberg I commuted to Frankfurt four times a week to see my analyst. The ride took an hour each way and trains became an important part of my fantasy life. I kept meeting beautiful men on the train, men who scarcely spoke English, men whose clichés and banalities were hidden by my ignorance of French, or Italian, or even German. Much as I hate to admit it, there are *some* beautiful men in Germany.

One scenario of the zipless fuck was perhaps inspired by an Italian movie I saw years ago. As time went by, I embellished it to suit my head. It used to play over and over again as I shuttled back and forth from Heidelberg to Frankfurt, from Frankfurt to Heidelberg:

A grimy European train compartment (Second Class). The seats are leatherette and hard. There is a sliding door to the corridor outside. Olive trees rush by the window. Two Sicilian peasant women sit together on one side with a child between them. They appear to be mother and grandmother and granddaughter. Both women vie with each other to stuff the little girl's mouth with food. Across the way (in the window seat) is a pretty young widow in a heavy black veil and tight black dress which reveals her voluptuous figure. She is sweating profusely and her eyes are puffy. The middle seat is empty. The corridor seat is occupied by an enormously fat woman with a moustache. Her huge haunches cause her to occupy almost half of the vacant center seat She is reading a pulp romance in which the characters are photographed models and the dialogue appears in little puffs of smoke above their heads.

This fivesome bounces along for a while, the widow and the fat woman keeping silent, the mother and grandmother talking to the child and each other about the food. And then the train screeches to a halt in a town called (perhaps) CORLEONE. A tall languid-looking soldier, unshaven, but with a beautiful mop of hair, a cleft chin, and somewhat devilish, lazy eyes, enters the compartment, looks insolently around, sees the empty half-seat between the fat woman and the widow, and, with many flirtatious apologies, sits down. He is sweaty and disheveled but basically a gorgeous hunk of flesh, only slightly rancid from the heat. The train screeches out of the station.

Then we become aware only of the bouncing of the train and the rhythmic way the soldier's thighs are rubbing against the thighs of the widow. Of course, he is also rubbing against the haunches of the fat lady—and she is trying to move away from him—which is quite unnecessary because he is unaware of her haunches. He is watching the large gold cross between the widow's breasts swing back and forth in her deep cleavage. Bump. Pause. Bump. It hits one moist breast and then the other. It seems to hesitate in between as if paralyzed between two repelling magnets. The pit and the pendulum. He is hypnotized. She stares out the window, looking at each olive tree as if she had never seen olive trees before. He rises awkwardly, half-bows to the ladies, and struggles to open the window. When he sits down again his arm accidentally grazes the widow's belly. She appears not to notice. He rests his left hand on the seat between his thigh and hers and begins to wind rubber fingers around and under the soft flesh of her thigh. She continues staring at each olive tree as if she were God and had just made them and were wondering what to call them.

Meanwhile the enormously fat lady is packing away her pulp romance in an iridescent green plastic string bag full of smelly cheeses and blackening bananas. And the grandmother is rolling ends of salami in greasy newspaper. The mother is putting on the little girl's sweater and wiping her face with a handkerchief, lovingly moistened with maternal spittle. The train screeches to a stop in a town called (perhaps) PRIZZI, and the fat lady, the mother, the grandmother, and the little girl leave the compartment. Then the train begins to move again. The gold cross begins to bump, pause, bump between the widow's moist breasts, the fingers begin to curl under the widow's thighs, the widow continues to stare at the olive trees. Then the fingers are sliding between her thighs and they are parting her thighs, and they are moving upward into the fleshy gap between her heavy black stockings and her garters, and they are sliding up under her garters into the damp unpantied place between her legs.

The train enters a *galleria,* or tunnel, and in the semi-darkness the symbolism is consummated. There is the soldier's boot in the air and the dark walls of the tunnel and the hypnotic rocking of the train and the long high whistle as it finally emerges.

Wordlessly, she gets off at a town called, perhaps, BIVONA. She crosses the tracks, stepping carefully over them in her narrow black shoes and heavy black stockings. He stares after her as if he were Adam wondering what to name her. Then he jumps up and dashes out of the train in pursuit of her. At that very moment a long freight train pulls through the parallel track obscuring his view and blocking his way. Twenty-five freight cars later, she has vanished forever.

One scenario of the zipless fuck.

Zipless, you see, *not* because European men have button-flies rather than zipper-flies, and not because the participants are so devastatingly attractive, but because the incident has all the swift compression of a dream and is seemingly free of all remorse and guilt; because there is no talk of her late husband or of his fiancée; because there is no rationalizing; because there is no talk at *all*. The zipless fuck is absolutely pure. It is free of ulterior motives. There is no power game. The man is not "taking" and the woman is not "giving." No one is attempting to cuckold a husband or humiliate a wife. No one is trying to prove anything or get anything out of anyone. The zipless fuck is the purest thing there is. And it is rarer than the unicorn. And I have never had one.

Getting to Know Me

Betty Dodson

from Ms., August, 1974

Betty Dodson gave three groundbreaking erotic art shows in the sixties and early seventies—the shows consisted of life size images of people having sex, women masturbating, and photographs and drawings of women's genitals. In the early seventies, she organized consciousness-raising groups to encourage women to appreciate the beauty of their genitals and she challenged the widespread belief that masturbation was a substitute for 'real' sexual activity. She published her defense of masturbation in the feminist magazine Ms. and later expanded it into a book illustrated with her own drawings and paintings. Today, she is a professional sex therapist and continues to publish on a wide range of sexual issues

Masturbation has been a continuous part of my sex life since the age of five. It got me through childhood, puberty, romantic love, marriage, and it will, happily, see me through old age. I am not typical in this respect. As I have learned, very few women masturbate regularly once they're past childhood exploration, and a lot of women have no memory of even childhood masturbation.

But I am typical in most other respects—I was subjected to the same barrage of negative sexual conditioning all women get. I was made to feel ashamed and guilty about masturbation. Even as an adult, I felt that masturbating meant there was something wrong with my sex life.

Coming from the "Bible Belt" in Kansas, I knew very well where the church and moralists stood on the subject of masturbation. But even my liberal, intelligent friends put down masturbation, making clear that it was a second-rate sexual activity. If there were any touching of my genitals to be done, my beloved should do it. My only source of sex information in those days was dreary marriage manuals and random bits of psychiatry. When I finally made it to the couch, therapists were mainly Freudians and into love and marriage, which was supposed to include passionate sex. So masturbation, especially in women, was considered either compulsive or infantile behavior. Mature, good sex was vaginal and included love and a meaningful relationship with a man.

Even if masturbation was "wrong," I kept doing it. At 29, after much conflict over marriage versus art career and after several affairs that were superromantic and monogamous, I got married—just in time to escape the horrible fate of going over the hill alone. Quite typically, my marital sex soon got down to twice a month—but even then my husband would come too fast, and I wouldn't come at all. We would both be embarrassed, depressed, and silent. After he went to sleep, I would quickly and quietly masturbate under the covers. I did it without moving or breathing, feeling sick with frustration and guilt the whole time.

My marriage ended after five years of struggling to "adjust" and "work through our problems." Any possibility of substituting bridge, golf, or work for a diminished sexuality had been ruined by my moderately healthy sexual beginnings. I had a continuous reminder from my masturbation that pleasure through sexual expression could be available to me. When I got divorced, I was a 35-year-old emotional virgin facing the terrors of "dating" again.

My first postmarital affair was a turning point. Both of us sexually starved, we plunged headlong into an intense, joyful, experimental physical exchange. My lover, just out of a 17-year marriage, was overjoyed to be completely open sexually, and so was I. Our exploratory conversations quickly got onto the subject of marriage, monogamy, and sexual repression, and I was able to tell him openly and honestly about my guilt-ridden marital masturbation. And he told me about his. The "toning down" of sex that had occurred in his long marriage and the subsequent lack of sexual communication had depressed him. Sometimes he would sneak another orgasm by masturbating in the bathroom just 30 minutes after love-making. He had longed for a more experimental relationship, but his only variety came from masturbation, which would have been okay if he could have done it positively and joyfully. But, like me, he felt sick with frustration and guilty. He had begun to regard himself as a "dirty old man," and his self-esteem steadily sank.

As we shared information, I began to understand how our whole antisexual social system represses and controls us; and I was able to let go of my remaining sexual guilt. We both realized that masturbation had saved our sexual sanity—and we would never again consider it a second-rate sexual activity. It was very important for me that I had finally found someone else who had fought the same sexual battles, and who agreed with me about sex and masturbation without female-male sex-role distinction.

My art began to reflect my growing sexual affirmation. I felt so good about myself and my new sexuality that I started to transfer my discoveries in bed to the canvas. My first one-woman exhibition of erotic art was held in New York City in 1968. Naturally, the whole concept of displaying my sexuality publicly was frightening, but I had learned that the first enemy a person encounters on the path to knowledge is fear. And fear must be overcome by defying it. I had to fully feel the fear and to take the next step in learning. This understanding carried me through, but not without a lot of sweating. I had envisioned irate citizens throwing rocks, or the show getting busted for pornography, but I needn't have. The exhibition was beautiful and enormously successful. Heroic, classical figures copulating behind huge sheets of brightly colored Plexiglas. My erotic art was still art and therefore acceptable.

I decided to devote my second show to the celebration of masturbation. Getting models to pose for me was difficult—but finally, with a little help from my friends, I drew four magnificent, life-size classical nudes masturbating. Eveyone said I was nuts, that the drawings would never sell (absolutely true), but what I learned was invaluable.

The response to the drawings was fascinating and informative. I discovered that a lot of people did not know women ever masturbated ("Why should they?"), and that a vibrator pictured in one of the drawings made several men very hostile and defensive. One man remarked, "If that was my woman, she wouldn't have to use that thing." I found myself fielding hundreds of questions. Yes, I did it myself and loved it. No, you don't get warts. Yes, I use live models. Yes, the woman with the vibrator in the picture has a boyfriend—he's standing right over there. No, despite what society tells us; intercourse isn't necessarily better—it's just different. I like to do both.

I explained many times that seeking sexual gratification should be a basic drive, and that masturbation is our first explicitly sexual activity. It's the way we discover our eroticism, the way we learn to respond sexually. Sexual skill and the ability to respond are not "natural"—at least not in our society. Doing what "comes naturally" for us is to be sexually inhibited. Sex is like any other skill or art form—it has to be learned and practiced.

It is my feeling that when a woman masturbates, she learns to like her own body, to enjoy sex and orgasm, and to become proficient and independent about sex. Our society does not really approve of sexually proficient and independent women. Which gets us to the double standard—the concept that men have the social approval to be aggressive (independent) and sexually polygamous, but that women should be nonaggressive (dependent) and sexually monogamous. We become fixed in nonsexuality and a supportive role that induces us to seek security, rather than independence, new experiences, and sexual gratification.

I think that one of the best ways to make women accept and conform to this double standard is to deprive us of direct sexual self-knowledge—especially masturbation. In other words, deprive us of our own bodies and of a way of discovering and developing orgasmic response patterns. Start early. Instill the notion that female genitals are deficient and inferior and that women's main social value lies in producing babies. Avoid any information about the clitoris and life-affirming orgasm. Prohibit touching of your genitals through the suggestion of supernatural punishment. Socially ostracize nonconforming women. Sexual repression is a vital aspect of keeping us in our "proper" role.

An important part of our sexual development is learning to like and accept all of ourselves, including our genitals—to become what I call "cunt positive." Most women feel that their genitals are ugly, funny-looking, disgusting, smelly, and not at all desirable—certainly not a beautiful part of their bodies. A woman who feels this way is obviously going to have a lot of reservations about an intimate sharing with another person. We therefore need to become very aware of our genitals. We want to know how we look, smell, and taste—and how we vary.

Last year I produced a set of color slides of the genitals of twenty different women. I use the slides to create an aesthetic for female genitals in lectures and in my bodysex workshops (physical and sexual C-R groups). Because most women do not have a visual image of their own or other women's genitals, they find the slides reassuring, informative, and healing.

The slides reveal a vast range of differences and similarities in the color, texture, size, and shape of women's genitals. Women with extended inner lips who thought themselves deformed saw many other women with the same genital configuration; the brownish color of some genitals turns out to be natural and not the result of aging or childbirth. The range of differences in the distance between the clitoris and vaginal opening may explain why some women never achieve orgasm through penetration only: if the clitoris is close to the vaginal entrance, it is more likely to receive indirect stimulation with penetration. How many women are suffering or confused from this lack of fundamental information?

Although this may sound frivolous, I find that trimming or shaping the pubic hair enhances genital awareness. It gives me the chance to explore my genitals with the same kind of attention that I used to lavish on my face and hair. (I've spent much of my adult life fixated on my face and hairstyle while the rest of my body has gone unexplored.)

I now feel that masturbation is a form of meditation on self-love. When I masturbate, I create a space for myself in the very same way I would for a special lover—soft lights, candles, incense, music, colors, textures, sexual fantasies, anything that turns me on. If I use my hand, I also use oil or cream. The slippery, moist feeling of oil on my genitals is very sensuous. I use one finger or my whole hand, making circular motions, above the clitoral body, below, on top, or to the side. I experiment with several techniques—going slow, fast, soft, firm, observing the arousal potential of each. I'll lie on my stomach, side, back; put my legs up and also stretch them out. I have also experimented with watching myself in a mirror. I saw that I didn't look awful or strange— I looked sexual and wonderfully intense.

Some women achieve orgasm by pressing their thighs together and squeezing and tensing the muscles rhythmically. It is impossible for me to experience orgasm this way, as I require more direct stimulation. I have also had orgasms by letting water run on my genitals in the bathtub. The pressure can be easily controlled and water is symbolically pleasing.

For the past two years I have been experimenting with different vibrators. I have found that the vibrator gives me the strongest and most consistent form of stimulation and is especially good for women who have never experienced orgasm. It also overcomes the problem of your hand or arm getting tired while masturbating manually. Some women complain that the vibrator simply makes them go numb. Of course, if you put the vibrator directly on your clitoris and don't move either the vibrator or your body, you will numb out. I always use a bit of material between me and my vibrator—a piece of velvet, satin, fur, a towel. I move the vibrator back and forth besides rocking my pelvis forward and back and around. It's very much like dancing, and I love to masturbate with music and follow the musical buildup to orgasm.

Some women I know have put such tremendous pressure on themselves to have orgasms, that they have not developed the capacity for pleasure in the buildup of sexual tension. I encourage them to spend several self-lovemaking sessions without performance demands, just bringing themselves up slowly . . . experiencing the pleasurable sensations and the fantasies. Sometimes when I feel I'm getting close to coming, I drop back—tease and please myself. When I have an orgasm, I don't stop stimulation. I just soften up, and stay with the good feelings. I'll let the pleasure come with movement, breathing, sounds, or words. If I feel like it, I'll go on to another buildup and a second orgasm, spending at least 30 minutes to an hour. We have been conditioned to make love as though we are rushing to an appointment.

Joyful masturbation and self-love naturally flows into a sexual exchange with another person. We can give and receive love best when we feel good about ourselves. Because I am secure about my sexual response and orgasm, I feel free to stimulate my clitoris along with penetration—or to show my partner what turns me on. During oral sex, I can state my preference—giving my partner necessary feedback on what pleases me. There are many positions where I can use the vibrator while being penetrated, enhancing my partner's sensation as well. I have never met a person whom I would consider a good lover who wasn't totally turned on by any information I could give about what turned me on.

Exploring my sexual potential has taken me on many paths of learning and change. Reclaiming my body as a source of strength and pleasure has given me power over my own life and the freedom to design my sex life creatively, just like painting a picture. Self-sexuality, along with heterosexuality, homosexuality, bisexuality, and group sexuality is simply all part of human sexual behavior.

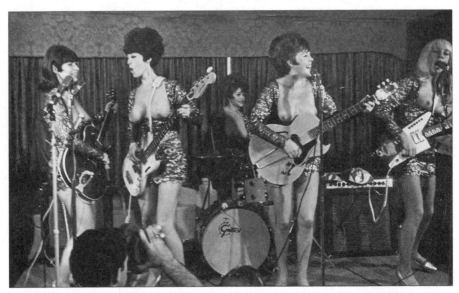

"Tell Me What You Are Thinking About," He Said.

Nancy Friday

from *My Secret Garden*, 1973

Nancy Friday's **My Secret Garden** *was the first comprehensive exploration of women's sexual fantasies. There had always been ways for men to express their sexual fantasies in the small magazines like* **Penthouse Letters** *that published advice about sex as well as erotic fiction. Friday's book had a similar appeal. Many of its female readers found it powerfully erotic in addition to pedagogic, while males were quite often shocked at the 'perversity' of some fantasies or even felt violated by some women's imagined sexual scenarios. The Prologue of the first edition was by the anonymous J. author of another bestseller,* **The Sensuous Woman.** *Like* **Fear of Flying** **My Secret Garden** *was also a runaway bestseller and it has remained in print for 30 years*

n my mind, as in our fucking, I am at the crucial point: . . . We are at this Baltimore Colt–Minnesota Viking football game, and it is very cold. Four or five of us are huddled under a big glen plaid blanket. Suddenly we jump up to watch Johnny Unitas running toward the goal. As he races down the field, we all turn as a body, wrapped in our blanket, screaming with excitement. Somehow, one of the men—I don't know who, and in my excitement I can't look—has gotten himself more closely behind me. I keep cheering, my voice an echo of his, hot on my neck. I can feel his erection through his pants as he signals me with a touch to turn my hips more directly toward him. Unitas is blocked, but all the action, thank God, is still going toward that goal and all of us keep turned to watch. Everyone is going mad. He's got his cock out now and somehow it's between my legs; he's torn a hole in my tights under my short skirt and I yell louder as the touchdown gets nearer now. We are all jumping up and down and I have to lift my leg higher, to the next step on the bleachers, to steady myself; now the man behind me can slip it in more easily. We are all leaping about, thumping one another on the back, and he puts his arm around my shoulders to keep us in rhythm. He's inside me now, shot straight up through me like a ramrod; my God, it's like he's in my throat! "All the way, Johnny! Go, go, run, run!" we scream together, louder than anyone, making them all cheer louder, the two of us leading the excitement like cheer leaders, while inside me I can feel whoever he is growing harder and harder, pushing deeper and higher into me with each jump until the cheering for Unitas becomes the rhythm of our fucking and all around us everyone is on our side, cheering us and the touchdown . . . it's hard to separate the two now. It's Unitas' last down, everything depends on him; we're racing madly, almost at our own touchdown. My excitement gets wilder, almost out of control as I scream for Unitas to make it as we do, so that we all go over the line together. And as the man behind me roars, clutching me in a spasm of pleasure, Unitas goes over and I . . .

"Tell me what you are thinking about," the man I was actually fucking said, his words as charged as the action in my mind. As I'd never stopped to think before doing anything to him in bed (we were that sure of our spontaneity and response), I didn't stop to edit my thoughts. I told him what I'd been thinking.

He got out of bed, put on his pants and went home.

Lying there among the crumpled sheets, so abruptly rejected and confused as to just why, I watched him dress. It was only imaginary, I had tried to explain; I didn't really want that other man at the football game. He was faceless! A nobody! I'd never even have had those thoughts, much less spoken them out loud, if I hadn't been so excited, if he, my real lover, hadn't aroused me to the point where I'd abandoned my whole body, all of me, even my mind. Didn't he see? He and his wonderful, passionate fucking had brought on these things and they, in turn, were making me more passionate. Why, I tried to smile, he should be proud, happy for both of us. . . .

One of the things I had always admired in my lover was the fact that he was one of the few men who understood that there could be humor and playfulness in bed. But he did not think my football fantasy was either humorous or playful. As I said, he just left.

His anger and the shame he made me feel (which writing this book has helped me to realize I still resent) was the beginning of the end for us. Until that moment his cry had always been "More!" He had convinced me that there was no sexual limit to which I could go that wouldn't excite him more; his encouragement was like the occasional flick a child gives a spinning top, making it run faster and faster, speeding me ever forward toward things I had always wanted to do, but had been too shy even to think about with anyone else. Shyness was not my style, but sexually I was still my mother's daughter. He had freed me, I felt, from this inappropriate maidenly constraint with which I could not intellectually identify, but from which I could not bodily escape. Proud of me for my efforts, he made me proud of myself, too. I loved us both.

Looking back over my shoulder now at my anything-goes lover, I can see that I was only too happily enacting *his* indirectly stated Pygmalion–D. H. Lawrence fantasies. But mine? He didn't want to hear about them. I was not to coauthor this fascinating script on How To Be Nancy, even if it was my life. I was not to act, but to be acted upon.

Where are you now, old lover of mine? If you were put off by my fantasy of "the other man," what would you have thought of the one about my Great Uncle Henry's Dalmatian dog? Or the one member of my family that you liked, Great Uncle Henry himself, as he looked in the portrait over my mother's piano, back when men wore moustaches that tickled, and women long skirts. Could you see what Great Uncle Henry was doing to me under the table? Only it wasn't me; I was disguised as a boy.

Or was I? It didn't matter. It doesn't, with fantasies. They exist only for their elasticity, their ability to instantly incorporate any new character, image or idea—or, as in dreams, to which they bear so close a relationship—to contain conflicting ideas simultaneously. They expand, heighten, distort or exaggerate reality, taking one further, faster in the direction in which the unashamed unconscious already knows it wants to go. They present the astonished self with the incredible, the opportunity to entertain the impossible.

There were others lovers, and other fantasies. But I never introduced the two again. Until I met my husband. The thing about a good man is that he brings out the best in you, desires all of you, and in seeking out your essence, not only accepts all he finds, but settles for nothing less. Bill brought my fantasies back into the open again from those depths where I had prudently decided they must live—vigorous and vivid as ever, yes, but never to be spoken aloud again. I'll never forget his reaction when timidly, vulnerable, and partially ashamed, I decided to risk telling him what I *had* been thinking.

"What an imagination!" he said, "I could never have dreamed that up. Were you really thinking *that?*"

His look of amused admiration came as a reprieve; I realized how much he loved me, and in loving me, loved anything that gave me more abundant life. My fantasies to him were a sudden unveiling of a new garden of pleasure, as yet unknown to him, into which I would invite him.

Marriage released me from many things, and led me into others. If my fantasies seemed so revealing and imaginative to Bill, why not include them in the novel I was writing? It was about a woman, of course, and there must be other readers besides my husband, men and other women too, who would be intrigued by a new approach to what goes on in a woman's mind. I did indeed devote one entire chapter in the book to a long idyllic reverie of the heroine's sexual fantasies. I thought it was the best thing in the book, the stuff of which the novels I had most admired were made. But my editor, a man, was put off. He had never read anything like it, he said (the very point of writing a novel, I thought). Her fantasies made the heroine sound like some kind of sexual freak, he said. "If she's so crazy about this guy she's with," he said, "if he's such a great fuck, then why's she thinking about all these other crazy things . . . why isn't she thinking about him?"

I could have asked him a question of my own: Why do men have sexual fantasies, too? Why do men seek prostitutes to perform certain acts when they have perfectly layable ladies at home? Why do husbands buy their wives black lace G-strings and nipple-exposing bras, except in pursuit of fantasies of their own? In Italy, men scream "Madonna mia" when they come, and it is not uncommon, we learn in *Eros Denied*, for an imaginative Englishman to pay a lady for the privilege of eating the strawberry cream puff (like Nanny used to make) she has kindly stuffed up her cunt. Why is it perfectly respectable (and continually commercial) for cartoons to dwell on the sidewalk figure of Joe Average eyeing the passing luscious blonde, while in the balloon drawn over his head he puts her through the most exotic paces? My God! Far from being thought reprehensible, this last male fantasy is thought amusing, family fun, something a father can share with his son.

Men exchange sexual fantasies in the barroom, where they are called dirty jokes; the occasional man who doesn't find them amusing is thought to be odd man out. Blue movies convulse bachelor dinners and salesmen's conventions. And when Henry Miller, D. H. Lawrence and Norman Mailer—to say nothing of Genet—put their fantasies on paper, they are recognized for what they can be: art. The sexual fantasies of men like these are called novels. Why then, I could have asked my editor, can't the sexual fantasies of women be called the same?

But I said nothing. My editor's insinuation, like my former lover's rejection, hit me where I was most sensitive: in that area where women, knowing least about each other's true sexual selves, are most vulnerable. What is it to be a woman? Was I being unfeminine? It is one thing not to have doubted the answer sufficiently to ever have asked the question of yourself at all. But it is another to know that question has suddenly been placed in someone else's mind, to be judged there in some indefinable, unknown, unimaginable competition or comparison. What indeed was it to be a woman? Unwilling to argue about it with this man's-man editor, who supposedly had his finger on the sexual pulse of the world (hadn't he, for instance, published James Jones and Mailer, and probably shared with them unpublishable sexual insights), I picked up myself, my novel, and my fantasies and went home where we were appreciated. But I shelved the book. The world wasn't ready yet for female sexual fantasy.

I was right. It wasn't a commercial idea then, even though I'm talking about four years ago and not four hundred. People said they wanted to hear from women. What were they thinking? But men didn't really want to know about some new, possibly threatening, potential in women. It would immediately pose a sexual realignment, some rethinking of the male (superior) position. And we women weren't yet ready either to share this potential, our common but unspoken knowledge, with one another.

What women needed and were waiting for was some kind of yardstick against which to measure ourselves, a sexual rule of thumb equivalent to that with which men have always provided one another. But women were the silent sex. In our desire to please our men, we had placed the sexual constraints and secrecy upon one another which men had thought necessary for their own happiness and freedom. We had imprisoned each other, betrayed our own sex and ourselves. Men had always banded together to give each other fraternal support and encouragement, opening up for themselves the greatest possible avenues for sexual adventure, variety and possibility. Not women.

For men, talking about sex, writing and speculating about it, exchanging confidences and asking each other for advice and encouragement about it, had always been socially accepted, and, in fact, a certain amount of boasting about it in the locker room is usually thought to be very much the mark of a man's man, a fine devil of a fellow. But the same culture that gave men this freedom sternly barred it to women, leaving us sexually mistrustful of each other, forcing us into patterns of deception, shame, and above all, silence.

I, myself, would probably never have decided to write this book on women's erotic fantasies if other women's voices hadn't broken that silence, giving me not just that sexual yardstick I was talking about, but also the knowledge that other women might want to hear my ideas as eagerly as I wanted to hear theirs. Suddenly, people were no longer simply *saying* they wanted to hear from women, now women were actually talking, not waiting to be asked, but sharing their experiences, their desires, thousands of women supporting each other by adding their voices, their names, their presence to the liberating forces that promised women a new shake, something "more."

Oddly enough, I think the naked power cry of Women's Lib itself was not helpful to a lot of women, certainly not to me in the work that became this book. It put too many women off. The sheer stridency of it, instead of drawing us closer together, drove us into opposing camps; those who were defying men, denying them, drew themselves up in militant ranks against those who were suddenly more afraid than ever that in sounding aggressive they would be risking rejection by their men. If sex is reduced to a test of power, what woman wants to be left all alone, all powerful, playing with herself?

But if not Women's Lib, then liberation itself was in the air. With the increasing liberation of women's bodies, our minds were being set free, too. The idea that women had sexual fantasies, the enigma of just what they might be, the prospect that the age-old question of men to women, "What are you thinking about?" might at last be answered, now suddenly fascinated editors. No longer was it a matter of the sales-minded editor deciding what a commercial gimmick it would be to publish a series of sexy novels by sexy ladies, novels that would give an odd new sales tickle to the age-old fucking scenes that had always been written by men. Now it was suddenly out of the editors' hands: Women *were* writing about sex, but it was from their point of view (women seen only as male sex fantasies no more), and it was a whole new bedroom. The realization was suddenly obvious, that with the liberation of women, men would be liberated too from all the stereotypes that made them think of women as burdens, prudes, and necessary evils, even at best something less than a man. Imagine! Talking to a woman might be more fun than a night out with the boys!

With all this in the air, it's no surprise that at first my idea fascinated everyone. "I'm thinking of doing a book about female sexual fantasies," I'd say for openers to a group of highly intelligent and articulate friends. That's all it took. All conversation would stop. Men and women both would turn to me with half-smiles of excitement. They were willing to countenance the thought, but only in generalities, I discovered.

"Oh, you mean the old rape dream?"

"You don't mean something like King Kong, do you?"

But when I would speak about fantasies with the kind of detail which in any narrative carries the feel of life and makes the verbal experience emotionally real, the ease around the restaurant table would abruptly stop. Men would become truculent and nervous (ah! my old lover—how universal you are) and their women, far from contributing fantasies of their own—an idea that might have intrigued them in the beginning—would close up like clams. If anyone spoke, it was the men:

"Why don't you collect men's fantasies?"

"Women don't need fantasies, they have us."

"Women don't have sexual fantasies."

"I can understand some old, dried-up prune that no man would want having fantasies. Some frustrated neurotic. But the ordinary, sexually satisfied woman doesn't need them."

"Who needs fantasies? What's the matter with good old-fashioned sex?"

Nothing's the matter with good old-fashioned sex. Nothing's the matter with asparagus, either. But why not have the hollandaise, too? I used to try to explain that it wasn't a question of need, that a woman is no less a woman if she doesn't fantasize. (Or that if she does, it is not necessarily a question of something lacking in the man.) But if a woman does fantasize, or wants to, then she should accept it without shame or thinking herself freaky—and so should the man. Fantasy should be thought of as an extension of one's sexuality. I think it was this idea, the notion of some unknown sexual potential in their women, the threat of the unseen, all-powerful rival, that bothered men most.

"Fantasies during sex? My wife? Why, Harriet doesn't fantasize . . ." And then he would turn to Harriet with a mixture of threat and dawning doubt, "Do you, Harriet?" Again and again I was surprised to find so many intelligent and otherwise open-minded men put off by the idea of their women having sexual thoughts, no matter how fleeting, that weren't about them.

And of course their anxiety communicated itself to their Harriets. I soon learned not to research these ideas in mixed company. Naively at first, I had believed that the presence of a husband or an accustomed lover would be reassuring and comforting. Looking back now, I can see that it had been especially naive of me to think he might be interested, too, in perhaps finding out something new in his partner's sexual life, and that if she were attacked by shyness or diffidence, he would encourage her to go on. Of course, that is not how it works.

But even talking to women alone, away from the visible anxiety the subject aroused in their men, it was difficult getting through to them, getting through the fear, not of admitting their fantasies to me, but of admitting them to themselves. It is this not-so-conscious fear of rejection that leads women to strive to change the essence of their minds by driving their fantasies down deep into their forgotten layers of mind.

I wasn't attempting to play doctor in the house to my women contributors; analyzing their fantasies was never my intention. I simply wanted to substantiate my feeling that women do fantasize and should be accepted as having the same unrealized desires and needs as men, many of which can only find release in fantasy. My belief was, and is, that given a sufficient body of such information, the woman who fantasizes will have a background against which to place herself. She will no longer have that vertiginous fright that she alone has these random, often unbidden thoughts and ideas. Eventually, then, I developed a technique to enable all but the shyest women to verbalize their fantasies. For instance, if, as in many cases, the first reaction was, "Who, me? Never!" I'd show them one or two fantasies I'd already collected from more candid women. This would allay anxiety. "I thought my ideas were wild, but I'm not half as far out as that girl." Or it would arouse a spirit of competition which is never entirely dormant among our sex: "If she thinks that fantasy she gave me to read is so sexy, wait till she reads mine."

In this way, without really working at it too hard, I had put together quite a sizeable, though amateur, collection. After all, everything to date was from women I knew, or from friends of friends who would sometimes phone or write to say they had heard of what I was doing and would like to help by being interviewed themselves. Somewhere along the way, though, I realized that if my collection of fantasies was going to be more than just a cross section of my own narrow circle of friends, I would have to reach out further. And so I placed an ad in newspapers and magazines which reached several varied audiences. The ad merely said:

FEMALE SEXUAL FANTASIES
wanted by serious female researcher.
Anonymity guaranteed. Box XYZ.

As much as I'd been encouraged by my husband and also by the spirit of the times in which we live, I think it was the letters that came that marked the turning point in my own attitude toward this work. I am no marcher, nor Red-Crosser, but some of the cries for help and sighs of relief in those letters moved me. Again and again they would start, "Thank God, I can tell these thoughts to someone; up till now I've never confided mine to a living soul. I have always been ashamed of them, feeling that other people would think them unnatural and consider me a nymphomaniac or a pervert."

I think it fair to say that I began this book out of curiosity—about myself and the odd explosive excitement/anxiety syndrome the subject set up in others; the male smugness of my rejecting lover and that know-it-all editor kept me going; but it became a serious and meaningful effort when I realized what it could mean, not only to all the sometimes lonely, sometimes joyful, usually anonymous women who were writing to me, but to the thousands and thousands who, though they were too embarrassed, isolated, or ashamed to write, might perhaps have the solitary courage to read.

Today we have a flowering of women who write explicitly and honestly about sex and about what goes on in a woman's mind and body during the act. Marvelous writers like Edna O'Brien and Doris Lessing. But even with women as outspoken as these, they feel the need for a last seventh veil to hide acknowledgement of their sexuality; what they write calls itself fiction. It is a veil I feel it would be interesting and even useful to remove as a step in the liberation of us all, women and men alike. For no man can be really free in bed with a woman who is not.

Putting this book together has been an education. Learning what other women are like, both in their fantasies and in their lives—it is sometimes difficult to separate the two—has made me gasp in disbelief; laugh out loud occasionally; blush; sigh a lot; feel a sense of outrage, envy, and a great deal of sympathy. I find my own fantasies are funnier than some, less poetic than others, more startling than a good number—but they are my own. Naturally, my best fantasies, my favorites of the moment—numbers 1, 2, and 3 on my private hit parade—are not included here. One thing I've learned about fantasies: they're fun to share, but once shared, half their magic, their ineluctable power, is gone. They are sea pebbles upon which the waters have dried. Is that a mystery? So are we all.

Uses of the Erotic: The Erotic as Power*

Audre Lorde

Keynote, Conference on Women's History, 1978

Raised in Harlem, Lorde was a novelist, poet, and essayist. Her work explored the terrain where black culture, sexuality and feminism come together. She was author of **Zami: A New Spelling of My Name**, *a profoundly original autobiography that Lorde herself characterized as a "biomythography." Lorde's essay on the erotic grew out the early feminist debates on the importance of sexual freedom for women's liberation. One of the leading questions that Lorde addresses is whether or not pornography was, in fact, sexually oppressive. Lorde concludes that the acknowledgement of woman's erotic desire is a profoundly political act.*

There are many kinds of power, used and unused, acknowledged or otherwise. The erotic is a resource within each of us that lies in a deeply female and spiritual plane, firmly rooted in the power of our unexpressed or unrecognized feeling. In order to perpetuate itself, every oppression must corrupt or distort those various sources of power within the culture of the oppressed that can provide energy for change. For women, this has meant a suppression of the erotic as a considered source of power and information within our lives.

We have been taught to suspect this resource, vilified, abused, and devalued within western society. On the one hand, the superficially erotic has been encouraged as a sign of female inferiority; on the other hand, women have been made to suffer and to feel both contemptible and suspect by virtue of its existence.

It is a short step from there to the false belief that only by the

*Paper delivered at the Fourth Berkshire Conference on the History of Women, Mount Holyoke College, August 25, 1978.

suppression of the erotic within our lives and consciousness can women be truly strong. But that strength is illusory, for it is fashioned within the context of male models of power.

As women, we have come to distrust that power which rises from our deepest and nonrational knowledge. We have been warned against it all our lives by the male world, which values this depth of feeling enough to keep women around in order to exercise it in the service of men, but which fears this same depth too much to examine the possibilities of it within themselves. So women are maintained at a distant/inferior position to be psychically milked, much the same way ants maintain colonies of aphids to provide a life-giving substance for their masters.

But the erotic offers a well of replenishing and provocative force to the woman who does not fear its revelation, nor succumb to the belief that sensation is enough.

The erotic has often been misnamed by men and used against women. It has been made into the confused, the trivial, the psychotic, the plasticized sensation. For this reason, we have often turned away from the exploration and consideration of the erotic as a source of power and information, confusing it with its opposite, the pornographic. But pornography is a direct denial of the power of the erotic, for it represents the suppression of true feeling. Pornography emphasizes sensation without feeling.

The erotic is a measure between the beginnings of our sense of self and the chaos of our strongest feelings. It is an internal sense of satisfaction to which, once we have experienced it, we know we can aspire. For having experienced the fullness of this depth of feeling and recognizing its power, in honor and self-respect we can require no less of ourselves.

It is never easy to demand the most from ourselves, from our lives, from our work. To encourage excellence is to go beyond the encouraged mediocrity of our society is to encourage excellence. But giving in to the fear of feeling and working to capacity is a luxury only the unintentional can afford, and the unintentional are those who do not wish to guide their own destinies.

This internal requirement toward excellence which we learn from the erotic must not be misconstrued as demanding the impossible from ourselves nor from others. Such a demand incapacitates everyone in the process. For the erotic is not a question only of what we do; it is a question of how acutely and fully we can feel in the doing. Once we know the extent to which we are capable of feeling that sense of satisfaction and completion, we can then observe which of our various life endeavors bring us closest to that fullness.

The aim of each thing which we do is to make our lives and the lives of our children richer and more possible. Within the celebration of the erotic in all our endeavors, my work becomes a conscious decision—a longed-for bed which I enter gratefully and from which I rise up empowered.

Of course, women so empowered are dangerous. So we are taught to separate the erotic demand from most vital areas of our lives other than sex. And the lack of concern for the erotic root and satisfactions of our work is felt in our disaffection from so much of what we do. For instance, how often do we truly love our work even at its most difficult?

The principal horror of any system which defines the good in terms of profit rather than in terms of human need, or which defines human need to the exclusion of the psychic and emotional components of that need—the principal horror of such a system is that it robs our work of its erotic value, its erotic power and life appeal and fulfillment. Such a system reduces work to a travesty of necessities, a duty by which we earn bread or oblivion for ourselves and those we love. But this is tantamount to blinding a painter and then telling her to improve her work, and to enjoy the act of painting. It is not only next to impossible, it is also profoundly cruel.

As women, we need to examine the ways in which our world can be truly different. I am speaking here of the necessity for reassessing the quality of all the aspects of our lives and of our work, and of how we move toward and through them.

The very word *erotic* comes from the Greek word *eros*, the personification of love in all its aspects—born of Chaos, and personifying creative power and harmony. When I speak of the erotic, then, I speak of it as an assertion of the lifeforce of women; of that creative energy empowered, the knowledge and use of which we are now reclaiming in our language, our history, our dancing, our loving, our work, our lives.

There are frequent attempts to equate pornography and eroticism, two diametrically opposed uses of the sexual. Because of these attempts, it has become fashionable to separate the spiritual (psychic and emotional) from the political, to see them as contradictory or antithetical. "What do you mean, a poetic revolutionary, a meditating gunrunner?" In the same way, we have attempted to separate the spiritual and the erotic, thereby reducing the spiritual to a world of flattened affect, a world of the ascetic who aspires to feel nothing. But nothing is farther from the truth. For the ascetic position is one of the highest fear, the gravest immobility. The severe abstinence of the ascetic becomes the ruling obsession. And it is one not of self-discipline but of self-abnegation.

The dichotomy between the spiritual and the political is also false, resulting from an incomplete attention to our erotic knowledge. For the bridge which connects them is formed by the erotic—the sensual—those physical, emotional, and psychic expressions of what is deepest and strongest and richest within each of us, being shared: the passions of love, in its deepest meanings.

Beyond the superficial, the considered phrase, "It feels right to me," acknowledges the strength of the erotic into a true knowledge, for what that means is the first and most powerful guiding light toward any understanding. And understanding is a handmaiden which can only wait upon, or clarify, that knowledge, deeply born. The erotic is the nurturer or nursemaid of all our deepest knowledge.

The erotic functions for me in several ways, and the first is in providing the power which comes from sharing deeply any pursuit with another person. The sharing of joy, whether physical, emotional, psychic, or intellectual, forms a bridge between the sharers which can be the basis for understanding much of what is not shared between them, and lessens the threat of their difference.

Another important way in which the erotic connection functions is the open and fearless underlining of my capacity for joy. In the way my body stretches to music and opens into response, hearkening to its deepest rhythms, so every level upon which I sense also opens to the erotically satisfying experience, whether it is dancing, building a bookcase, writing a poem, examining an idea.

That self-connection shared is a measure of the joy which I know myself to be capable of feeling, a reminder of my capacity for feeling. And that deep and irreplaceable knowledge of my capacity for joy comes to demand from all of my life that it be lived within the knowledge that such satisfaction is possible, and does not have to be called *marriage*, nor *god*, nor *an afterlife*. This is one reason why the erotic is so feared, and so often relegated to the bedroom alone, when it is recognized at all. For once we begin to feel deeply all the aspects of our lives, we begin to demand from ourselves and from our life-pursuits that they feel in accordance with that joy which we know ourselves to be capable of. Our erotic knowledge empowers us, becomes a lens through which we scrutinize all aspects of our existence, forcing us to evaluate those aspects honestly in terms of their relative meaning within our lives. And this is a grave responsibility, projected from within each of us, not to settle for the convenient, the shoddy, the conventionally expected, nor the merely safe.

During World War II, we bought sealed plastic packets of white, uncolored margarine, with a tiny, intense pellet of yellow coloring perched like a topaz just inside the clear skin of the bag. We would leave the margarine out for a while to soften, and then we would pinch the little pellet to break it inside the bag, releasing the rich yellowness into the soft pale mass of margarine. Then taking it carefully between our fingers, we would knead it gently back and forth, over and over, until the color had spread throughout the whole pound bag of margarine, thoroughly coloring it.

I find the erotic such a kernel within myself. When released from its intense and constrained pellet, it flows through and colors my life with a kind of energy that heightens and sensitizes and strengthens all my experience.

We have been raised to fear the *yes* within ourselves, our deepest cravings. But, once recognized, those which do not enhance our future lose their power and can be altered. The fear of our desires keeps them suspect and indiscriminately powerful, for to suppress any truth is to give it strength beyond endurance. The fear that we cannot grow beyond whatever distortions we may find within ourselves keeps us docile and loyal and obedient, externally defined, and leads us to accept many facets of our oppression as women.

When we live outside ourselves, and by that I mean on external directives only rather than from our internal knowledge and needs, when we live away from those erotic guides from within ourselves, then our lives are limited by external and alien forms, and we conform to the needs of a structure that is not based on human need, let alone an individual's. But when we begin to live from within outward, in touch with the power of the erotic within ourselves, and allowing that power to inform and illuminate our actions upon the world around us, then we begin to be responsible to ourselves in the deepest sense. For as we begin to recognize our deepest feelings, we begin to give up, of necessity, being satisfied with suffering and self-negation, and with the numbness which so often seems like their only alternative in our society. Our acts against oppression become integral with self, motivated and empowered from within.

In touch with the erotic, I become less willing to accept powerlessness, or those other supplied states of being which are not native to me, such as resignation, despair, self-effacement, depression, self-denial.

And yes, there is a hierarchy. There is a difference between painting a back fence and writing a poem, but only one of quantity. And there is, for me, no difference between writing a good poem and moving into sunlight against the body of a woman I love.

This brings me to the last consideration of the erotic. To share the power of each other's feelings is different from using another's feelings as we would use a kleenex. When we look the other way from our experience, erotic or otherwise, we use rather than share the feelings of those others who participate in the experience with us. And use without consent of the used is abuse.

In order to be utilized, our erotic feelings must be recognized. The need for sharing deep feeling is a human need. But within the european-american tradition, this need is satisfied by certain proscribed erotic comings-together. These occasions are almost always characterized by a simultaneous looking away, a pretense of calling them something else, whether a religion, a fit, mob violence, or even playing doctor. And this misnaming of the need and the deed give rise to that distortion which results in pornography and obscenity—the abuse of feeling.

When we look away from the importance of the erotic in the development and sustenance of our power, or when we look away from ourselves as we satisfy our erotic needs in concert with others, we use each other as objects of satisfaction rather than share our joy in the satisfying, rather than make connection with our similarities and our differences. To refuse to be conscious of what we are feeling at any time, however comfortable that might seem, is to deny a large part of the experience, and to allow ourselves to be reduced to the pornographic, the abused, and the absurd.

The erotic cannot be felt secondhand. As a Black lesbian feminist, I have a particular feeling, knowledge, and understanding for those sisters with whom I have danced hard, played, or even fought. This deep participation has often been the forerunner for joint concerted actions not possible before.

But this erotic charge is not easily shared by women who continue to operate under an exclusively european-american male tradition. I know it was not available to me when I was trying to adapt my consciousness to this mode of living and sensation.

Only now, I find more and more women-identified women brave enough to risk sharing the erotic's electrical charge without having to look away, and without distorting the enormously powerful and creative nature of that exchange. Recognizing the power of the erotic within our lives can give us the energy to pursue genuine change within our world, rather than merely settling for a shift of characters in the same weary drama.

For not only do we touch our most profoundly creative source, but we do that which is female and self-affirming in the face of a racist, patriarchal, and anti-erotic society.

PART III

Changing Sex Lives

A revolution in sexual behavior and mores is bound to have impact on many social institutions and other aspects of community life—courtship, marriage, parenting, cohabitation, and divorce are only the most obvious. The sexual revolution inspired many experiments in daily living such as open marriage, mate-swapping and ménage a trois. But it also inspired larger-scale experiments like communal living or the planning of orgies as well as the establishment of commercial sex clubs—Plato's Retreat in New York being among the most famous. The sexual revolution also opened up new sexual possibilities and gender roles for individuals, including bisexuality, homosexuality, S/M (sado-masochism), and transsexuality. Communities were organized around these new sexualities and gender possibilities.

The changing social environment presented more and more sexual opportunities—what were once temptations, soon became everyday possibilities. The institution of marriage was in a mounting crisis—by 1960 approximately half of all marriages had ended in divorce. The growing influence of the idea of sex for pleasure rather than exclusively for procreation, and the availability of an easy and efficient means of birth control with the Pill reduced the appeal of monogamous marriage as an institution with a monopoly of sex. The attack on the double standard—by which it was acceptable for men to have sexual relationships either before or during of marriage, but stigmatized women who did—reinforced the ability of women to engage in a greater range of sexual activities. In this context, there were few guidelines to help both women and men negotiate their sexual relationships.

Many women viewed marriage as the stronghold of male domination, supported by various economic factors: the income inequalities which favored men over women, the limited employment opportunities for women, and other institutionalized benefits. Nevertheless, both men and women in their struggles with one another sought to reshape marriage, to explore new sexual territories, or even to create new institutions that allowed for new ways of relating to one another—open marriage, wife swapping, swinging, and communal sex allowed for men and women to forge new kinds of sex lives.

These developments intensified the struggle between the sexes—the benefits of sexual revolution seem to move back and forth between men and women depending on the context of their sexual experiences. And these developments took decidedly different turns within different regions, social classes, and race and ethnic groups. Blue collar white women and men experienced the struggle between the sexes very differently than middle class men and women, black women and men also had different sexual legacies within which their sexual conflicts took place.

The sexual revolution also generated cross-currents with other movements and communities. The black civil rights movement and racial conflict dominated the American political landscape in the sixties and seventies and those social struggles overlapped with those of the sexual revolution. Sexual tensions between the sexes and between blacks and whites had simmered below the surface in the early civil rights struggles. Throughout the sixties, journalists, sociologists and psychologists in publications like *Ebony* and the *Black Scholar* explored many of aspects of the sexual revolution. In addition, beliefs in the hyper-sexuality of blacks—a legacy of traditional racist attitudes—continued to circulate in American society in both negative and positives versions. In his famous essay "The White Negro" Norman Mailer mythologized black sexuality—as superior, more natural, and with greater potential for orgiastic potency. Writers responded to these sexual beliefs—critically (Frantz Fanon, James Baldwin) as well as positively (Eldridge Cleaver) more often in terms of race than explicit sexuality.

America's Best Kept Secret

Lawrence Lipton

from *The Erotic Revolution*, 1965

*When Lipton published **The Erotic Revolution** in 1965, he believed that the sexual revolution was moving ahead at full throttle—it was the secret that everyone knew but no one talked about—a growing minority had already broken with what he called the "Old Morality." The New Sexual Morality was changing the way people lived, how they conducted courtship, marriage, and divorce. Nevertheless, toward the end of his book, Lipton concluded that the sexual revolution offered no guarantee of success—the era's sexual experiments would have both successes and failures.*

I t is a paradox of history that the best kept secret is the secret everybody knows and nobody is talking about. I am not referring to the sexual revolution, which is universally acknowledged and widely discussed. What I am referring to is the extent to which the beginnings of a new morality have already made their appearance in our culture. The breakdown of the Old Morality is no longer a secret, but the New Morality which is replacing it is *not* being discussed. When it is discussed, it is discussed in the kind of double-talk which characterizes polite conversation, or passes for "professional responsibility" in the mass communications media and the social sciences.

It is in the nature of every important change in the sexways of a culture that it does not easily lend itself to statistical measurement. This is especially true in a culture like that of the U.S., where nearly every departure from the mores of the society is sinful or illegal and is threatened with serious social and economic penalties. It is not a subject that lends itself to the questionnaire method or the usual analytical procedures of statistical social studies. Suitable procedures could conceivably be devised but the prevailing tendency among sociologists, psychiatrists, social workers and sexologists, official, academic and even in most cases private, is to confine themselves to the negative aspects of the sexual revolution, the breakdowns, the tragedies and the casualties, and ignore or gloss over the successful examples of sexual experimentation, lest they appear to condone or recommend them. They are under professional constraint, and in the case of legal and governmental officials actually under oath, to treat all departures from "official" morality as deviations from the "normal" and/or violations of law and custom. Any *affirmative* treatment of the new morality is avoided and when it cannot be completely ignored it is treated with equivocation and double-talk.

The more successful the new sexways appear to be the more carefully they are hedged in with cautions and disclaimers, so that their quality as well as their numerical incidence is clouded with doubt and becomes, in effect, a conspiracy of silence. This conspiracy of silence, then, conceals not only the statistical extent to which the new morality is in one form or another a matter of everyday practice in the U.S. today, but it also conceals the fact that what is taking place is not only a revolution *against the traditional morality* but also a revolution *in favor of wholly new concepts of the function of sex* in society.

Thousands of case histories have been researched and published to illustrate the dangers, penalties and pitfalls of any deviation from the prevailing sexual morality. Admittedly there are dangers, penalties and pitfalls, but what is missing from these case histories is, in nearly every case, the compensating values of such deviant behavior. Even in the darkest days of Victorian Puritanism there was always present the sly innuendo that "wild oats" were sometimes worth sowing and that "forbidden fruits" were sweetest. Today we have passed beyond such corny sentimentalities to the point where the sowing and gathering begin to take on the proportions of radically new forms of sexual relationships which are too attractive and widespread in practice to be properly called wild or forbidden. Yet there is little in contemporary sexology to indicate that the newly emerging sexways which are only hinted at in their case histories, have in them elements of life-enhancing, health-restoring qualities which make the risk of social and legal penalties worth taking. Otherwise, how shall we account for the widespread character of such deviations from law and morals?

In an effort to redress the balance, I propose to begin by affirming the life-enriching qualities of the New Morality. There are elements in the new sexways which are more viable in the context of life today than are the old sexways of the Judeo-Christian ethos. Moreover, they are beginning to reveal a superior understanding of the very nature and function of the orgasm itself. My first emphasis, therefore, will be on the positive, affirmative aspects of the new sexways as revealed in the experiences and opinions of people, young, middle aged and aging, who have gone beyond complaining and protesting and are actually testing out in their lives the theories and practices of what I prefer to call the Erotic Revolution.

The Ice Is Thin All Over

What broke the ice for Fred and Susan was the example of their next door neighbors and friends Doris and Jerry. Long before their neighborliness had progressed beyond a passing nod or an over-the-fence greeting Fred and Susan got to hear a good deal about Doris and Jerry. They couldn't *help* hearing it. It wafted over to their ears on warm summer nights. It could even be heard at times through closed windows and locked doors in midwinter. Usually late at night and sometimes on Sundays at almost any hour of the day. What they heard was the neighborly sound of middle class married America enjoying wedded bliss.

Fred and Susan congratulated themselves that their own married life was free from the noisy quarrels and squabbles of their neighbors. Theirs was a happy marriage. No violent episodes, no doors slamming, no dishes flying. Sex wasn't what it used to be but, "Is it ever," they asked one another, "after five years of marriage?" The occasional brush-fire warfare next door, they decided, was the exception. Their own married life was more like the normal middle class American home, neither hell nor paradise but something more like—what? Purgatory? Because, despite their constant mutual reassurances, something *was* missing, something *had* gone out of it. They both suspected what it was but they couldn't bring themselves to speak of it to one another.

It was too painful, too fraught with peril, to face with any degree of candor, even in the privacy of one's own thoughts.

Fred remembered having once, long ago, anticipated such a state of affairs. He had told himself at the time that when marital sex began to pall for him, as he suspected it was doing for long-married people he knew, it would be because sex was no longer a tormenting necessity. After a few years of marriage, he told himself, sex would not seem so important to him, his interest in other women would gradually subside and finally fade into a nostalgic memory of his youth. It was the natural thing and he would find it fairly easy to go along with the ways of nature. In a vague way he even looked forward to that time with an anticipated feeling of relief. A man who had benefited by a good upbringing and had normal instincts and practical ambitions in life shouldn't expect or desire to be the slave of his passions all his life long. After a few years of married life he should, in all decency, be content to settle down and be sensible about sex.

Yet here he was, after five years of marriage, casting a hot, speculative eye in the direction of every personable young woman he met who showed any promise of availability. Once, when desire was matched with opportunity and the young woman gave every indication of welcoming his amorous intentions, he backed away, awkwardly. And spent the next few days—and nights—cursing and congratulating himself by turns. It was good to know it *could* still happen, that he hadn't completely lost his male allure, but it was also good to know that he had reached the point in his life where he could control himself in such a situation. Was this what they meant by maturity? Was this the virtue of fidelity in marriage, knowing he *could* and wouldn't? The feeling of righteousness this experience gave him was almost enough to compensate for the frustration.

Almost, but not quite. When the same thing happened again on another occasion he found the feeling of virtuous pride beginning to pall on him. Instead of congratulating himself on his self-control he felt more like a fool and ended up alternating for days between quiet desperation and impotent rage. Desperation because he could no longer reconcile his sexual desires with his inbred, inbuilt moral scruples, or even keep them in balance any more. And rage because he felt himself on the verge of a decision on a problem that he thought he had solved or would never have to solve because, with time and maturity of character, it would somehow solve itself. Rage because he felt helpless in the presence of forces within himself that he thought he would never have to face, which all his training had not prepared him to face.

As for Susan, she was conscious of the crisis in their marital sex life even before Fred was, as she later found out. Trained from young girlhood to take a passive role and let, first her father and later her husband, make all the decisions, she had fallen into a passive but receptive role in the marital sex relationship. When Fred's sexual demands began to taper off she took this to be the moral and therefore the natural way. The idea of ever straying off the reservation might be something to laugh about with friends now and then after a few drinks but if anyone had suggested seriously in those days that she had secret sexual longings for any other man she would have denied it with indignation. The very thought of such a thing was repulsive to her. It had taken the better part of their first year of marriage for Susan to enjoy the sexual act with her husband without feelings of guilt and restraining inhibitions. She had expected that love and the sanctions of marriage would liberate her from the fears and restraints that made a nightmare out of her premarital sexual relations with Fred—if relations was the right word for it, since it was all so awkward and guilt-ridden for both of them. In fact, she wasn't even sure that she had really come to orgasm once in the two years of what they later, laughingly but wryly, referred to as their engagement. And no wonder, it was all so furtive and inconvenient, since both of them were still living at home with their families and everything had to be hit and run and catch as catch can.

In short, it was an average, normal middle class American courtship. And now it was an average, normal middle class American marriage. It might have gone on like this for who knows how long if it hadn't been for the fire. A short circuit in the wiring or something set fire to the house next door and they offered Doris and Jerry the spare bedroom while the repairs were being made. It was the neighborly thing to do. It solved a temporary housing problem for Doris and Jerry, but it also, as it turned out, solved some other problems—for Fred and Susan as well as for Doris and Jerry. Propinquity led to more and more intimate conversation, man to man and woman to woman and, finally, to a candid four-way exchange of experiences and views on the problems of marriage and sex.

It was Jerry who broke the ice. He and his wife must have been aware that their loud bickering had been overheard many times by Fred and Susan. Instead of pretending the neighbors were deaf, which is the make-believe etiquette of nice people in a nice city or suburban neighborhood, Jerry came right out with it. It was a good marriage, he said, as good as any marriage they knew of among their friends and acquaintances, but he and Doris had reached the point where they just couldn't seem to help flaring up at one another on the slightest excuse. It was never over anything really important. Things like that they could talk over calmly and come to a sensible decision about. It was the trifles, the little irritations of living together.

Now, talking it over for the first time with someone else, it dawned on Jerry that the real reason for the bickering and fault-finding was a gnawing feeling in his guts that his life was in a rut, that he was missing out on something, he didn't know what. Of course he suspected all along, but he hated to admit it to himself, that dissatisfaction with the way his sex life with Doris was going lately was at the bottom of it. That he was taking it out on Doris in all kinds of petty ways simply because he couldn't bring himself to face the sex problem, much less discuss it with Doris. The arguments and mutual recriminations were all just a cover-up.

Once Jerry broke the ice and started talking, Doris spoke up. It was astonishing how close her story was to Jerry's and all four had a good laugh together when it struck them that here were two people living together in marriage for four years, thinking and suspecting and worrying about the same thing and never being able to talk about it with one another till the accident of a fire brought them into close contact with a next door neighbor. It came as news to Jerry that Doris had secretly consulted a psychoanalyst about it and stopped going after a few visits because it was beginning to look like one of those long-drawn-out and prohibitively expensive analyses. Besides, she explained, all that probing about father and mother images and sibling rivalries and early masturbation fantasies were not turning up anything that wasn't disappointingly and monotonously normal and offered no promise of a clue to her present problem. She was sure that whatever it was, it was something of much more recent origin, something simpler and more commonplace, than young daughter fantasies to murder her mother and screw her father or take her brother away from his girl friend and go to bed with him.

The idea had also occurred to her that she might consult a marriage counsellor but all those she had read in books, heard about or listened to on television sounded too much like preachers or social workers. Not that sex wasn't mentioned often enough but never in a way that suggested anything she and Jerry weren't doing already—the little thoughtful attentions, remembering anniversaries, things like that, and all those hazy generalities about making marital sex more exciting, more meaningful, always too piously evasive or too disgustingly medical.

A woman she met in the public library asked her if she had read Dr. Kinsey's *Sexual Behavior in the Human Female*. Thinking he might be something like a Dr. Spock for married grownups, she drew the book from the library after several impatient weeks on the waiting list. The title puzzled her. Sexual behavior in the human female—it sounded a little like those animal books written by hunters, travelers and popular scientists—*The Behavior of the Great Apes in Their Native Habitat*. Her heart sank when she leafed through it and found that it was heavily loaded with scientific-looking statistical tables, charts and graphs, like a government report on traffic patterns or air pollution. She managed to find a few passages that seemed to have some bearing on her problem and underlined them in pencil. When the conversations with Fred and Susan reached the point where they could discuss things like this with some degree of frankness, Doris went to the library and drew the book out again in order to discuss the marked passages with them.

Incidence and Frequency of Orgasm. The married female reaches orgasm in only a portion of her coitus, and some 10 per cent of all the females in the available sample had never reached orgasm at any time, in any of their marital coitus (Table 113, Figure 61). Some 75 per cent had responded to orgasm at least once in their coitus within the first year of marriage. The accumulative incidence curve had ultimately risen to 90 per cent by the time the females had been married some twenty years.[1]

1. Alfred C. Kinsty, Wardell D. Pomroy, et al., *Sexual Behavior in the Human Female* (Philadelphia, 1953), p. 352.

The reading of this passage had a further liberating effect on their conversation, if only because of the explosion of laughter that followed it. The closing sentence, especially—only fifteen or sixteen years to go to their 90 per cent incidence curve, whatever that was. Laughter was followed by a higher incidence of candid confession than they had been able to manage before. Compared with Dr. Kinsey's classified, graphed, tabled and averaged-out human females Susan was able to assert, with a high degree of certainty, that she was evidently a prodigy of orgasmic incidence during the first year of marriage, and Fred backed up her claim—"unless she's an acting genius—or a damn good faker."

Doris confessed herself surprised. She had underlined the passage as a mildly comforting reassurance to herself that her own experience during the first years of marital sex was at least not far from the national average. The next marked passage she produced a mixed reaction.

Apparent Aging Effect in Incidence and Frequency. It must be emphasized that these declines in the incidences and frequencies of marital coitus, and of coitus to the point of orgasm, do not provide any evidence that the female ages in her sexual capacities . . . the steady decline in the incidences and frequencies of marital coitus, from the younger to the older age groups, must be the product of aging processes in the male (see our 1948: 253–257). There is little evidence of any aging in the sexual capacities of the female until late in her life (Chapter 18, Figures 143–150).[2]

The men looked at one another with quizzical smiles and shrugged; the women looked at one another, then at their men and all four burst into laughter again. Could this be a true picture of the marital sex experience of most American families? they asked one another. If so, it was a pretty discouraging picture and, if male and female differed so radically in their sexual needs and capacities through the years, well, no wonder two out of three marriages ended in divorce. But was divorce and remarriage any solution at all? Wouldn't the same disparity between the sexes be just as disastrous in the second marriage, or the third, or the fourth?

Clearly, marriage itself was no solution of the problem. At least not

2. Ibid., p353.

as marriage was practiced normally, observing all the social, religious, legal and moral rules. It was the rules that *created* the problem.

That last thought was left hanging in the air between them and it was still there when Jerry and Doris moved back into their newly repaired and refurnished house. Not till then did it dawn on them that in the few weeks they were boarding with Fred and Susan they had not had a single one of their petty fault-finding arguments and their sex life had never been better. They gave a house-warming party for their friends, inviting Fred and Susan, of course, and discovered they now had little in common with their old friends. There was so much they couldn't talk about any more with them, and found themselves huddling in the kitchen with Fred and Susan and making whispered conversation with them. Everybody else seemed suddenly strait-laced, stodgy and hypocritical. After that the two couples started double-dating, for all the world like youngsters discovering sex for the first time, first between themselves and gradually, exploratively crossing over and breaking through the marital barrier. They took in the small night clubs in parts of town where they wouldn't have dared to go before, alone, listening to jazz music and blues singers, learning to breathe freely for the first time in a frankly erotic atmosphere among young people who thought nothing of cross-overs and breakthroughs, whether of early training, religious dogmas, or skin pigmentation, learning to swing with the liberating rhythms of the music and the frank sexuality of the dancing.

They read books on the art of sex, tried out everything at least once, and became conscious of pleasures and possibilities they never dreamed they would ever experience, or even tolerate in others, let alone practice themselves. Since both Susan and Doris had been using contraceptive pills for some time, there was little fear on this score. Both women were good looking and about the same age, and so were the men, so it wasn't a case of "rather fight than switch." They were careful to keep their interrelationship strictly to themselves and made no effort to win over anybody else to their new sexways. They did not go around trying to break up homes. It was as private an affair as any monogamous marriage is, except that it was a foursome instead of a twosome.

The case of Fred, Susan, Doris and Jerry represents only one kind of experiment in the New Morality. It is a breakthrough in the sense that it cuts across the bounds of exclusiveness set up by the religion, laws, mores and customs of Judeo-Christian society. It is, in fact, only a variation on conventional marriage and not a very radical variation, at that. Yet, whether it is illegal, and whether or not there are specific laws prohibiting it, the police have arrested and charged people living under such arrangements and the courts have applied any statute they could find—from disorderly conduct to adultery—to punish them. Where it involves families with children the charges also include contributing to the delinquency of minors.

In the case I have described no children were involved. "Plenty of time to think about that," was the way both couples put it. "Why be in a hurry to add to the population explosion. Let's live a while first," sums up their point of view in the matter. What will happen to the arrangement if one or both couples decide to raise a family only the future can tell. There are those who have faced this question and I shall have occasion to discuss their cases later. Here it is sufficient to note that the men and women involved found in this trans-marital arrangement a workable solution for problems which had plagued them. Their lives were happier and richer.

I do not present it here as a solution for all marital problems. Nor do I claim for it that it insures the participants against sexual satiety, stalemate, infelicity or any of the usual hazards of marriage. But, far from destroying their marriages it has, so far at least, preserved and prolonged them. It is not a case of switching mates. (We shall discuss that subject too in its proper place.) Both couples continue to live together, but, by their own account, more happily and with less friction or boredom, than formerly. Both were, by current standards, love matches and both couples insist that they love their mates and have no thought of separation or divorce. On the contrary, they insist that much has been added to their marriage and nothing has been taken away from it, that they love one another, if anything, more than ever before.

It is also worthy of note, I think, that new sexways brought with them, in this case, new interests in reading, in the arts, even in home decor, all in the direction of more modern, more liberal views and tastes. The drab walls of their living rooms have been brightened up in the best contemporary taste and the expensively framed conventional chromos have been tossed out in the trash and replaced by inexpensive modern originals picked up at the annual outdoor show. Their television viewing is on a higher level than before and they are frequently seen as an inseparable foursome at lectures and concerts they shunned in the past as over their heads or "too far out" for them.

This has completely changed their circle of friends, all in a like direction, from the conventional, well-meaning but mediocre "steady crowd" of the past to a new circle of friends who know how to make intelligent conversation, hold their liquor well, and show a decent respect for other peoples' opinions, lifeways and sexways. If they suspect (as they undoubtedly do) that there is more than meets the eye in the relationship of our inseparable foursome, they refrain from prying or spying and expect the same respect for their own privacy.

Both couples in this case were probably headed for the divorce courts. Luckily there was someone prepared to make a move out of the dilemma and the accident of a fire afforded him the opportunity. Once Jerry broke the ice it was sink or swim and, in this case, all parties concerned were able to swim. Their experience is far from unique. Judging by the divorce statistics there are millions of American families on the verge of divorce. For the old sexways, the traditional morality of monogamous marriage, are in an advanced state of decay. The ice is thin all over.

Exploring the New Freedom

Gay Talese

from *Thy Neighbor's Wife*, 1980

*Best-selling author and former **New York Times** journalist, Gay Talese spent much of the seventies conducting the research on the sexual revolution for his book **Thy Neighbor's Wife**. He also became a participant in the sexual revolution, working in massage parlors, going to Playboy Clubs and nudist colonies, and becoming a regular member of Sandstone, a sexual community nestled in the Malibu hills just outside of Los Angeles. Talese devoted a large portion of his book to the story of Sandstone. In this selection Talese profiles John and Barbara Williamson, Sandstone's founders.*

B arbara Cramer had first met John Williamson while attempting to sell a group-insurance policy to the Los Angeles electronics firm where he worked as the general manager. He was remote, almost rude to her after she had arrived; having forgotten about their appointment, and irritated that she could not reschedule it for the following day, he relegated her to the reception room for a long wait before finally admitting her into the grim, sparsely furnished office where he sat behind a steel gray desk, chain smoking and barely attentive, as she proceeded to explain the particulars of the policy.

It was early afternoon and, despite his aloofness, she was very relaxed and confident. She had driven here from a pleasant motel [tryst] and she had also enjoyed the ride later alone through the Valley, humming in the car to music from the radio, her body still refreshed from the shower. She often found automobile driving a sensual experience, an opportunity to be briefly removed from other people to ponder private thoughts while moving with music over smooth wide roads, and she had no doubt that thousands of other Californians also sought daily solace and the benefits of self-reflection from behind the windshields of their cars—Los Angeles was a city of motorized meditators, of interior travelers fantasizing along freeways, and the blissful mood that had encapsulated her on this sunny afternoon could not be disturbed by the ungracious atmosphere of Williamson's office.

If anything, she was merely curious about this man who seemed to be trying hard to create the impression that he did not care what impression he was creating. His office was so conspicuously austere as to suggest that he had carefully arranged it. Instead of personal mementos or photographs on his desk, there were two ashtrays filled to the brim with his cigarette butts. There was no rug on the floor, the chairs were uncomfortable. The gray office walls were completely bare except for the one large picture behind his desk that showed two empty roads extending through a desert and converging in the distance, going nowhere. His replies to most of her questions were monosyllabic; his comments were always brief, his attitude indifferent. And yet she sensed that close to his surface there was an almost desperate need. He was perhaps a man who had built a wall hoping that someone would climb it.

When she had finished explaining about the policy, he abruptly stood, signifying that their meeting was over. He said that if she would leave the documents he would study them and telephone her within the week with his reaction. After a week had passed and he had not contacted her, she called him asking if he would have lunch with her. He said that he was not interested in lunch; instead he proposed that they have dinner. She accepted and, contrary to her expectations, she had a delightful evening.

They dined at an oriental restaurant in the Hollywood Hills, later going to a nightclub. They drank a good deal, spoke easily and openly about their private lives, and she could not believe that this interesting, soft-spoken man was the same disgruntled individual that she had met in the office. Either he had a dual personality or she had merely encountered him on an unusually bad day. Now she sensed that he was completely relaxed with her; he seemed to be compatible with her background: They were both country people living in the nation's largest city, they were exiles from white rural poverty trying to succeed in corporationland without the usual credentials and connections— although Williamson acknowledged during the evening that he was about to quit his firm to begin a smaller business of his own. While Barbara quickly saw that he would now be of no use to her in pushing her insurance policy with his colleagues, she did not really care. Her interest in him was suddenly strictly personal, and when they left the club together, arm in arm, he impulsively suggested on this Friday evening that they go away for the weekend.

She agreed, and three hours later, somewhat fatigued but still exuberant, they were in San Francisco, standing in front of a hotel registration desk.

"Two rooms," Williamson announced to the clerk, who, after looking at the couple, asked, "Why two rooms?"

"Because," Williamson said, "we're two people."

Sleeping separately the first night was a decision that Barbara found very romantic, and it was one of several small and pleasant surprises that would make John Williamson more intriguing to her. They abstained from sex on the second night, too, and when they finally did make love, after they had returned to Los Angeles and spent the evening in her apartment, it was an exciting culmination to a weekend of deepening familiarity and intensified desire.

His effect upon her was immediate and agreeably bewildering. With him she felt oddly coy, unaggressive, feminine, yet no less liberated. She felt as free as ever to pursue her whims and aspirations, and she knew from their conversations that he perceived and admired her independent spirit and style, and that it had been his awareness of these qualities that had quietly attracted him to her, despite his curtness, during their first meeting. Submissive and dependent women did not appeal to him, he told her, nor did the double standard that exists between the sexes, nor the conventional roles that predominate in nearly all marriages, including his own failed marriage. If he married again, he told Barbara, he wanted not a subservient wife but a strong equal partner in a relationship that would be advanced and adventurous.

As Barbara spent more time with him in Los Angeles, seeing him nearly every evening and sometimes visiting his bachelor apartment in Van Nuys, she gradually realized that the many books he owned dealing with psychology, anthropology, and sexuality represented not only intellectual curiosity on his part but also a growing professional interest.

John Williamson's career ambitions seemed to be shifting from mechanical engineering to sensual engineering, from the wonders of electronics to the dynamics of cupidity, and although his concerns were with contemporary society, his knowledge extended back to ancient times and early religions, to the first prophets and heretics, the scientists and dissenters of the Middle Ages as well as the free-thinkers and founders of rural utopias in the industrial age. He was particularly interested in the work of the controversial Austrian psychiatrist Wilhelm Reich, who was opposed to the double standard between the sexes but recognized it, and the general repression of women, as society's venal way of preserving the family unit that it considered necessary for the maintenance of a strong government. In a male-dominated world, Reich suggested, there was an "economic interest" in the continued role of women as "the provider of children for the state" and the performer of household chores without pay. "Owing to the economic dependence of the woman on the man and her lesser gratification in the processes of production," Reich once observed, "marriage is a protective institution for her, but at the same time she is exploited in it."

The average woman's early social conditioning was described by Reich as "sex-negating" or at best "sex-tolerating"; but in view of the conservative morality advocated by governments and religious institutions, this sexual passivity made women more faithful wives if not more daring lovers. Men meanwhile indulged their unfulfilled lust in what Reich called "mercenary sexuality" with prostitutes, mistresses, or other women that respectable society held in low esteem. Largely from the lower classes, these women were the sexual servants in a system that scorned them and punished them, but could not eliminate them because, as Reich wrote: "Adultery and prostitution are part and parcel of the double sexual morality which allows the man, in marriage as well as before, what the woman, for economic reasons, must be denied."

While Reich himself did not personally favor prostitution or promiscuity, he did not believe that the law should seek to prevent acts of sexuality between consenting adults, including homosexuals, nor would he restrain expressions of sexual love between adolescents. "The statement is made," he wrote, "that the abstinence of adolescents is necessary in the interest of social and cultural achievement. This statement is based on Freud's theory that the social and cultural achievements of man derive their energy from sexual energies which were diverted from their original goal to a 'higher' goal. This theory is known as that of 'sublimation.' . . . It is argued that sexual intercourse of youth would decrease their achievements. The fact is—and all modern sexologists agree on this—that all adolescents masturbate. That alone disposes of that argument. For, could we assume that sexual intercourse would interfere with social achievement while masturbation does not?"

Throughout his professional career, which began in the 1920s when he worked as a clinical assistant to Freud in Vienna, Wilhelm Reich's daring defense of sexual pleasure brought misery to his life and would finally lead him into the American prison where he died in 1957. Departing from Freud's exclusively verbal analysis, Reich studied the body as well as the mind, and he concluded after years of clinical observation and social work that signs of disturbed behavior could be detected in a patient's musculature, the slope of his posture, the shape of his jaw and mouth, his tight muscles, rigid bones, and other physical traits of a defensive or inhibiting nature. Reich identified this body rigidity as "armor."

He believed that all people existed, behind varying layers of armor which, like the archaeological layers of the earth itself, reflected the historical events and turbulence of a lifetime. An individual's armor that had been developed to resist pain and rejection might also block a capacity for pleasure and achievement, and feelings too deeply trapped might be released only by acts of self-destruction or harm to others. Reich was convinced that sexual deprivation and frustration motivated much of the world's chaos and warfare—the 1960s' slogan of the Vietnamese war protestors, "Make Love, Not War," reechoed a Reichian theme—and he blamed the antisexual moralism of religious homes and schools, along with the "reactionary ideology" of governments, for their part in producing citizens who feared responsibility and savored authority.

Reich further believed that people who cannot achieve sexual gratification in their own lives tended to regard expressions of sexuality in society as vile and degrading, which were the symptoms of Comstock and other censors, and Reich also suggested that the religious tradition of sex as evil had its origin in the somatic condition of its celibate leaders and early Christian martyrs. People who deny the body can more readily develop concepts of "perfection" and "purity" in the soul, and Reich deduced that the energies of mystical feelings are "sexual excitations which have changed their content and goal," adding that the God-fixation declined in people who had found bliss in sex.

Such sexually satisfied people possessed what Reich called "genital character," and he considered it the goal of his therapy to achieve this in his patients because it penetrated the armor and converted the energy that nourished neurotic numbness and destruction into channels of tenderness and love that released all "damned-up sexual excitation." An individual with genital character, according to Reich, was fully in contact with his body, his drives, his environment—he possessed "orgastic potency," the capacity to "surrender to the flow of energy in the orgasm without any inhibitions . . . free of anxiety and unpleasure and unaccompanied by phantasies"; and while genital character alone would not assure enduring contentment, the individual at least would not be blocked or diverted by destructive or irrational emotion or by exaggerated respect for institutions that were not life-enhancing.

Partly because Reich suggested healthy sexual intercourse as an antidote to many ailments, his critics often saw him as espousing nothing but pleasure, whereas in fact Reich claimed that his purpose was to allow his patients to feel pain as well as pleasure. "Pleasure and *joie de vivre*," he wrote, "are inconceivable without fight, without painful experiences and without unpleasurable struggling with oneself"; although he asserted that the capacity to give love and gain happiness is compatible with "the capacity of tolerating unpleasure and pain without fleeing disillusioned into a state of rigidity."

Reich assuredly did not believe, as did many therapists who had followed Freud, that culture thrived on sexual repression, nor would he quietly condone what he saw as a church-state alliance that sought to control the masses by denigrating the joys of the flesh while presumably uplifting the spirit. Control, not morality, was the central issue, as Reich perceived it; organized religion, which in Christian countries fostered among the faithful such traits as obedience and acceptance of the status quo, strived for conformity, and its efforts were endorsed by governments that passed illiberal sex laws that reinforced feelings of anxiety and guilt among those lawful God-fearing people who sometimes indulged in unsanctioned sex. These laws also gave governments additional weapons with which to embarrass, harass, or to imprison for their sexual behavior certain radical individuals or groups that it considered politically threatening or otherwise offensive. The writer Ayn Rand went even further than Reich in suggesting that at times a government hoped that citizens would disobey the law so that it could exercise its prerogative to punish: "Who wants a nation of law-abiding citizens?" asks a government official in Rand's novel *Atlas Shrugged*; "What's there in that for anyone? . . . Just pass the kind of laws that can neither be observed nor enforced nor objectively interpreted—and you create a nation of lawbreakers and then you cash in on guilt. . . . The only power any government has is the power to crack down on criminals."

Among those upon whom it cracked down, making him a martyr of the sexual revolution, was Wilhelm Reich, whose words and ideas aroused conflict in every country in which he lived and worked. As a Communist in Germany, Reich was expelled from the party for his writings on sexual permissiveness and "counterrevolutionary" thinking, while the Nazis denounced him as a "Jewish pornographer." In Denmark the attacks on him by orthodox psychiatrists in 1933 hastened his departure for Sweden, but the hostility he encountered there led him in 1934 to Norway. In 1939, after two years of adverse publicity in the Norwegian press, he left for the United States, where he resumed his psychiatric practice in New York, trained other psychiatrists, and lectured at the New School for Social Research. In 1941, a week after the raid on Pearl Harbor, the FBI, which had a dossier on Reich as a possible enemy alien, held him on Ellis Island for three weeks before releasing him.

After the war, following the publication of magazine articles that acerbically reported his claim to have discovered "orgone energy"—a primal force found in the living organism and in the atmosphere that could be absorbed by a patient sitting in one of Reich's "orgone boxes," which resembled telephone booths—he came under investigation by the Food and Drug Administration. Ignoring the fact that his patients, before using the boxes, had signed affidavits stating that they knew the treatments were experimental and guaranteed no cures—although there was often hope on their part that the energy might cure everything from impotence to cancer—the FDA proceeded to prohibit the orgone box as a fraud, and it also banned all of Reich's books containing his sociopolitical theories on health and sex.

In the McCarthy atmosphere of the early 1950s, few people were eager to defend Reich's civil liberties, and he did not help his own cause by ignoring a court date and writing instead to the judge saying that the courtroom was an inappropriate place for adjudicating questions of science. Sentenced in 1956 to a two-year term for contempt of court as well as for violation of the Food and Drug Act, Reich was sent to the federal penitentiary at Lewisburg, Pennsylvania (where the prison population would soon include Samuel Roth, following his 1956 obscenity conviction); but after Reich had served eight months, he suffered a fatal heart attack.

The death of Wilhelm Reich in November 1957 was not considered major news by the media—his brief obituary appeared near the bottom of page 31 in the New York *Times* of November 5—and, except for dissenting academics and Reichian therapists and young Americans who identified with the "beat" movement (Kerouac, Burroughs, and Ginsberg were adherents of Reich), relatively few people were interested in the underground copies of his work that the FDA had banned and, in many instances, had burned.

But all this was changed by the mid-1960s, as biographies and articles about Reich by former colleagues and friends, as well as the legal reissue of his books—including *The Mass Psychology of Fascism*, *Character Analysis*, and *The Sexual Revolution*—found a receptive audience among college students and activists who, through him, understood more clearly the connection between sex and politics.

Had Reich lived long enough to witness the radical sixties, he undoubtedly would have seen much that would have confirmed for him his predictions made long ago that society was "awakening from a sleep of thousands of years" and was about to celebrate an epochal event "without parades, uniforms, drums or cannon salutes" that was no less than a revolution of the senses. The churches and governments were gradually losing control over people's bodies and minds, and while Reich conceded that the shifting process would initially produce confrontations, clashes, and grotesque behavior, the final result, he believed, would be a healthier, more sex-affirmative and open society.

The Berkeley Free Speech Movement in 1965, which forged its slogan with the initials of a four-letter word ("Freedom Under Clark Kerr"), as well as the civil rights protests in the South and the subsequent antiwar demonstrations and marches on Washington—the sit-ins, teach-ins, love-ins—all were manifestations of a new generation that was less sexually repressed than its ancestors and also less willing to respect political authority and social tradition, color barriers and draft boards, deans and priests. It possessed more of what Reich called "genital character" and less of what another Freudian radical, Géza Róheim, called "sphincter morality."

But while the blasphemous, braless, peace-beaded young counter-culturalists received most of the attention in the media during the sixties, multitudes of quiet middle-class married people were also involved in this quest for free expression and more control over their own bodies. Like the draft-age demonstrators who defied the law in refusing to risk their bodies in Vietnam, churchgoing women disobeyed their religion in preventing the birth of unwanted children through abortion or various forms of birth control. A reported 6 million women, many of them practicing Catholics, were using the Pill in 1967; and in this time of topless bars, miniskirts, and long-haired lawyers and businessmen it seemed clear that the governing forces of society had limited influence over what clothes should be worn or how the hair should be shorn. Pubic hair made its film debut in Michelangelo Antonioni's *Blow-Up*, and penis-shaped plastic body vibrators for women were displayed for sale in drugstore windows in many cities, although the New York *Times* censored them from its advertising columns.

The sexual satisfaction of the body—pleasure, not procreation—was generally accepted now in the middle class as the primary purpose of coitus, and in an attempt to more fully comprehend and rectify unresponsiveness among pleasure-seeking patients, the Masters and Johnson researchers in St. Louis pioneered in the use of an eight-inch plastic phallic "coition machine," employed a number of former prostitutes among its co-experimenters, and later also provided "surrogate wives" as sex partners for dysfunctional men.

A lawsuit against the Masters and Johnson center by a husband of one of the surrogates, as well as snide speculation in public print about the performance of the machine, contributed to the researchers' decision to eliminate these features from their laboratory work, although female surrogates would continue to find employment at several other sex-therapy clinics that would be established around the nation as a result of Masters and Johnson's fame and success. At some of these clinics, couples would be tutored in the art of giving erotic massages and would also be shown instructional films on fellatio, cunnilingus, and the joys of mutual masturbation that were more sexually explicit than what was passing for pornography in theaters on Forty-second Street.

The number of mate-swappers in America, most of them middle-class married people with children, were now estimated by some swing-trade periodicals to exceed 1 million couples; and in a speech to the American Psychological Association, Dr. Albert Ellis, a psychologist and author, said that marriages can sometimes be helped by "healthy adultery." Group nudity could also be personally beneficial, according to psychologist Abraham M. Maslow, who believed that nudist camps or parks might be places where people can emerge from hiding behind their clothes and armor, and become more self-accepting, revealing, and honest.

Mixed nude bathing and massage became popular during the sixties at such "growth centers" as the Esalen Institute in Northern

California, a lush retreat nestled in rocky cliffs overlooking the Pacific where the spirit of Reich seemed alive in the faculty that supervised dozens of sensuous seminars attended by thousands of predominantly middle-class couples that made Esalen a million-dollar-a-year enterprise. Most of the new forms of therapy that had been at least partly inspired by Reich's work—bioenergetics, encounter, sensitivity training, primal therapy, rolfing, massage—were available at Esalen, where the most prominent therapist was Dr. Frederick S. Perls, a German refugee who had been one of Reich's patients in Europe before the war.

Like Reich, Perls had become dissatisfied with Freud's "talking cure" as well as with many of Freud's rigid practitioners who, in Perls's view, were "beset with taboos"—it was as if "Viennese hypocritical Catholics had invaded the Jewish science"—and Perls's therapy emphasized instead new methods for achieving freer body movement, more awareness, fuller expressiveness, and "life feeling." Too many people were obsessed with their heads and were alienated from their bodies, Perls believed, adding: "We have to lose our minds and come to our senses."

Much of what was being advocated at Esalen and elsewhere was in harmony with John Williamson's own attitude, although he wanted to go further than Reich's followers in altering the sociopolitical system through sexual experimentation—he hoped to soon establish his idealized community for couples wishing to demolish the double standard, to liberate women from their submissive roles, and to create a sexually free and trusting atmosphere in which, there would be no need for possessiveness, jealousy, guilt, or lying. Now was the perfect time for such a venture, Williamson felt; society was in turmoil, and people were responsive to new ideas, particularly in California, where so many national trends and styles had started.

If successful, his project could be financially profitable—like Esalen, or the Synanon drug program founded by a onetime alcoholic; or at least heavily funded and solvent, like the Kinsey Institute and the Masters and Johnson clinic—as well as becoming a contributing force toward a healthier, more egalitarian society. But first he had to organize his core group, those intimates who would help him initiate the process and ultimately serve as the "instruments for change" in other people's lives. He already had several candidates in mind, people he had befriended since moving to California three years ago. Most of them were in their late twenties or early thirties, were employed in large corporations, were divorced or unhappily married, were restless and searching. Several of the men were engineers, conservative individuals whose livelihood was linked to the fortunes of the defense industry in California but who admitted to extreme boredom with their work and home lives and seemed ready for radical alternatives.

Among the women Williamson had in mind were Arlene Gough, with whom he had enjoyed a brief affair after meeting her at Hughes Aircraft, and with whom he was still friendly. He was also close to two other women who worked at his electronics firm, one of them an extremely attractive individual who had been an airlines stewardess. But the woman he considered most essential to his program—which he would call Project Synergy—was Barbara Cramer.

In the months he had spent with her since their trip to San Francisco, he gradually realized that she already possessed many of the qualities that undoubtedly would be the goals of women in Project Synergy: She was professionally successful, independent, and self-assured, was sexually liberated and aggressive when it suited her, and was not intimidated by the possibility of rejection. In some ways she reminded him of Dagny Taggart, the heroine in *Atlas Shrugged*, although Barbara Cramer was thankfully not a female elitist and would therefore serve as a more representative role model to the young middle-class women that Williamson hoped would be drawn into Project Synergy. He saw Barbara as the prototype of the new woman of the changing middle class; and, in a synergistic sense, she ideally suited him—her assets complemented his deficiencies, and vice versa. She was verbal and active while he was theoretical and introspective; she was more direct and efficient if less calculating and visionary. She did not procrastinate, she knew what she wanted. She had already decided, at twenty-seven, that she would never have children, being aggrieved by recollections of her hapless mother and other child-rearing women she had known since leaving rural Missouri. But Barbara nonetheless wanted to become more feminine than she was, more gentle and sensitive, and she also admitted to

Williamson that she sometimes felt sexually attracted to certain women. Williamson urged her not to repress this, but to explore it in the interest of greater self-awareness; and shortly after their marriage in the summer of 1966—a conventional act that they both agreed would create a socially acceptable facade for their unconventional life-style—John Williamson decided to fully test Barbara's tolerance of sexual variety within their marriage.

Hours before they were to leave Los Angeles for a restful weekend at Lake Arrowhead, he informed her that they would be accompanied in the car by a young woman from his office named Carol, the former airline stewardess that he had dated prior to his meeting Barbara. When Barbara seemed unenthusiastic, he assured her that Carol was very feminine and charming, adding that it would be both beneficial and enjoyable for Barbara to have her as a friend.

Barbara had heard him discuss Carol before, always fondly but never hinting that he was still seriously involved with her, if he ever was; and Barbara imagined Carol to be, like the receptionist she was, a lovely frontispiece for a faceless corporation, a naïve young individual who had found a father figure in John and had, like so many other women, been drawn to him because, unlike so many men, he would *listen* to a woman, would really listen to what she was trying to say.

Late that afternoon after she had met Carol, Barbara amended some of her assumptions about her. A tall, angular blonde with dark eyes and a graceful body, Carol seemed hardly naïve and quite composed, although there was nothing haughty or affected in her manner. She appeared to be genuinely happy to meet Barbara, and remarked on how impressed she had been by John's description of Barbara's career; as they rode in the car toward Lake Arrowhead, Carol was careful to include Barbara in all the conversations with John about their office and their mutual friends.

Still, despite these efforts, Barbara felt uneasy with Carol, and she recognized this as characteristic of the way she had nearly always felt toward women in social situations; though she privately was attracted to them, she could not easily relate to them, having had limited experience with her own sex during her tomboy adolescence and the years that followed. The one time that she had cultivated a female friendship with her schoolmate Frances, it had ended sadly and bitterly, and Barbara still could not explain her own strange, hostile reaction to Frances after Frances had announced that she was getting married and moved out of their apartment.

Barbara also felt somewhat disconcerted in the car because she sensed that she was the odd woman in this threesome with Carol and John, and that they had arranged this weekend behind her back. Barbara had pondered her husband's intentions as soon as he had mentioned that Carol would be joining them, and she now anticipated being put in the position of possibly having to accept or reject Carol as a bed partner with John at Lake Arrowhead, or perhaps being left with the choice of remaining on the sidelines while her husband embraced Carol as a way of proving, as he often said he could, that wholesome, open sex with friends need not disturb the deeper meaning of marriage.

When they arrived at the lake, it was early evening and Barbara was relieved to discover that their cabin had two private bedrooms. But before they unpacked their luggage, John suggested that they quickly go out to dinner before the restaurant closed. After a few drinks, a good meal, and much amiable conversation and laughter, Barbara felt more at ease; but later, on returning to the cabin, she saw Carol and John place their luggage in the same bedroom, and soon they began to casually undress.

Barbara remained in the living room, stunned, silent, waiting for an explanation that was not forthcoming. Too proud to reveal her discomfort, too shocked to even think clearly, she sat on the couch staring at the open door of the bedroom. She heard them hanging their clothes in the closet, speaking softly. The open door was no doubt John's way of saying that she was welcome to join them, but he would not be coaxing her, the decision would be entirely her own.

It was confusing, harsh, and frightening, and all the earlier talk on John's part since their marriage about the merits of open sexuality did not now alleviate Barbara's uncertainty; it was one thing to agree with John's theories and quite another to employ them in moments like this, with a woman she had just met, and the longer

Barbara hesitated the more she knew that she was unable or unwilling to move toward the door.

She felt numb, dizzy, and it took all her resources to stand and walk into the other bedroom. She closed the door. It was after midnight and she was very tired and cold. She realized that she had left her suitcase in the living room but she did not want to get it. Slowly undressing and folding her clothes over the back of a chair, she got into bed and tried to sleep; but she remained tearfully awake until dawn, hearing the sounds of their lovemaking.

The next day, shortly before noon, she was awakened by the soft touch of her husband and his gentle kiss. Carol was smiling behind him, holding a breakfast tray, and soon they both were sitting on the bed, stroking her and comforting her as if she were a young girl recovering from an illness. Barbara felt strange and embarrassed. John said that he loved her and needed her; Barbara, forcing a smile, did not reply. He suggested that after breakfast they all go swimming and skiing on the lake, but Barbara said that she preferred remaining in bed a while longer, and told them to go on ahead, she would join them.

She spent part of the afternoon in the cabin, then took a long walk in the sun and crisp air, regaining her composure. She was not angry with John or Carol, though she conceded that this weekend surely was the beginning of a new phase in her marriage; but instead of feeling panicked or threatened, she felt oddly contented and free. Her husband had freed her of certain indefinable fears and romantic illusions about sex and body pleasure, as distinguished from the meaning of marital love. Her awareness that her husband had been sexually engaged the previous night with another woman was, after she had recovered from the shock, not really so shocking; and when John had announced his love for her in front of Carol this morning, Barbara believed him, for now there was no reason for lying. Their relationship had become more honest and open, had expanded not only for him but for her. She knew that now she could do as she wished, with whomever she pleased, without risking his rancor, or so she assumed. His railing against covert adultery and senseless sexual possessiveness and jealousy had culminated last night in a defiant act against a centuries-old tradition of propriety and deceit, and she admitted to being both stunned and stimulated by what had just transpired in her life. She was married to an uncommon man, mysterious, unboring, unpredictable, a quiet man who said he loved her and needed her.

Soothed by the walk, she returned to the cabin, took a bath, and changed her clothes; then she left for the restaurant-bar looking for John and Carol. John smiled and waved as he saw her, and both stood to embrace her as she arrived, and Barbara soon felt almost as comfortable with Carol as she did with her husband. Though the bar was crowded and noisy, there was a special warmth among the three of them as they sat drinking and talking, and the dinner with wine that followed in the restaurant represented to Barbara an almost celebratory conclusion to all the preceding hours of anguish and anxiety; and the last thing she expected at this time was that the complexity of her life would be compounded.

Shortly before eleven o'clock, at the end of dinner, she was surprised by the sudden arrival at their table of a man to whom she had been attracted in the past. The man was a friend of her husband's named David Schwind, an engineer; about thirty years of age, he was one of the few men her husband knew in Los Angeles who had not been married at least once. Barbara had met him earlier in the year while water-skiing with John and others at Pine Flat Lake, near Fresno, and she had then been drawn to his strong but delicate features, his athletic body, and his somewhat shy, aloof manner. David Schwind was employed at Douglas Aircraft, and John had seen signs of his mechanical skill during the weekend when David had quickly repaired the motor of a malfunctioning skiboat. Since then, in various ways, John had recruited David's friendship, taking him to lunch, seeing him socially after work. Now at Lake Arrowhead, as David joined their table and sat next to Barbara, unannounced but obviously expected by her unsurprised husband, Barbara had no doubt that David's presence was attributable to a telephone call made by John earlier in the day. While the purpose of this visit was not entirely clear to her, it was a foregone conclusion on her part, knowing her husband, that it had a purpose, and would in time clearly reveal itself.

In the meantime, in a mood of blithe resignation, Barbara ordered another drink and responded amiably toward David, although she detected within him a certain discomfort and reticence. Sipping his drink, saying very little, listening absently while John and Carol did most of the talking, of which little could be heard over this increasingly noisy Saturday night crowd, David Schwind seemed to be debating within himself the wisdom of being where he was. A half hour later, after John had paid the bill and rose to leave, David reacted by suggesting that perhaps he should be on his way; but John urged that he return with them to the cabin, and Barbara smiled at David in a way she hoped was reassuring.

It was well past midnight as they returned; and, after they had sat for a while in the living room, Barbara volunteered to make a pot of coffee and asked David if he would mind igniting the small stove in the corner. While waiting for the water to boil, Barbara and David stood talking together, soon becoming so engrossed in one another that they were unaware of the fact that John and Carol had quietly left the room. When David turned and noticed the unoccupied sofa, he seemed startled.

"Where's John?" he asked.

Seeing that the bedroom door was closed, Barbara replied with newfound nonchalance, "He's with Carol." As David looked at her quizzically, she hastily added, "It's okay. There's nothing to worry about."

"But shouldn't I be going?"

"No, please don't," she said quickly. "I'd like you to stay." She moved closer to him, put her arms around him, and told him that her husband was counting on his staying overnight, and so was she. After reaching behind him to switch off the living room lights she took his hand and led him into her bedroom. She closed the door and immediately began to remove her clothes.

Making love to David that night, and again at dawn, was for Barbara a source of great release and unabashed pleasure; and far from having any misgivings about it, or feeling romantically detached from her husband, she felt quite the opposite. She believed that she had now achieved a new level of emotional intimacy with John, and that they had both shared during the night, in different rooms with different people, a gift of loving trust.

Instead of loving him less after sleeping with another man, she was sure that she loved him more; and when she got up for breakfast, leaving David asleep beside her, she was greeted in the living room by her husband's approving smile and kiss.

Open Marriages

Nena O'Neill and George O'Neill

from *Beyond Monogamy*, 1974

Many feminists and proponents of sexual liberation believed that the monogamous marriage was an oppressive or patriarchal institution that must be overthrown. One alternative to the traditional marriage was the open marriage in which each member of the couple could have sexual partners outside the marriage—some estimates put the numbers of such couples at 15% (married) and 30% (cohabiting) by the end of the seventies. In the article reprinted here, Nena and George O'Neil, both anthropologists, examine the dynamics of heterosexual couples in open relationships during the late sixties and early seventies.

In the wake of increasing dissatisfaction with the prevailing pattern of traditional monogamous marriage and the vague but general discontent with our impersonal and fragmented existence, a number of alternative marriage styles have begun to emerge. These experimentations vary from those involving more than three persons in the basic pattern—including group marriage, communal life-styles, and polygamous patterns (more often triadic and more often polygynous than polyandrous)—to modifications in the basic one-to-one monogamous configuration. The latter group may be divided into those which are nonmarriage relationships (still monogamous but extralegal) and those which represent innovations, changes, deletions, and additions to the standard expectations for those legally married. These modifications may include such items as separate domiciles, extramarital sexual relations in group or partner-exchange contexts, and reversal of traditional role patterns (i.e., woman provides, man housekeeps). None of these patterns is particularly new in transcultural contexts since all have occurred elsewhere in other societies at one time or another. However, their proliferation and the motives which have impelled men and women in our society increasingly to seek innovations in our marriage style deserve closer scrutiny.

It is not enough to say that we live in a pluralistic society and that these alternate patterns for marriage have appeared in response to the changes in our society and the development of different life-styles. Even though one can foresee a future in which there will be a range of marriage patterns to choose from, the questions still remain: Why have so many experimental forms appeared? And more important, what are the personal motivations for seeking these innovative styles? Compendiums of sociological explanations have seemed somehow to pass over the personal dimensions involved. Yet these questions are exceedingly important for the future, especially since that future will affect our styles of child-rearing and thus the perpetuation of those values we deem most humanistic and worthy of saving. Even if experimental family forms are excluded, Sussman has pointed out that some children already live in variant forms of the traditional nuclear family during their formative stages. Under these conditions some changes in our value system are to be expected. The questions are, Which values and how many changes?

With the above questions in mind we began to explore contemporary marriage in 1967. During the four years of our research we interviewed approximately four hundred persons. Our informant-respondents were seventeen to seventy-five years of age and urban and suburban middle class in orientation and occupation; approximately 75% were married or had been married. Thirty interviews, both formal and informal, with professional therapists and marriage counselors supplemented these data. The interviews included individual and couple in-depth sessions and short mini-interviews in a variety of social settings. While some topical and background questions were used (i.e., "What is your age, occupation, marital status, etc.?" and "What do you think the ingredients of a good marriage are?"), the interviews were primarily open-ended and exploratory in nature, focusing on eliciting information through face-to-face encounters about values, feelings, and attitudes toward marriage and what changes were perceived as necessary for improvement.

Our interviews began first with those who were involved in experimental structures and in the greatest variations from the norm in traditional marriage. We felt that these innovators would have greater insight because they had already opted for change and would perhaps be more articulate and perceptive about why they had chosen change. We then moved on to the divorced, the nonmarrieds,[1] the singles, the young, and both those who were disillusioned and those who were contented with traditional monogamous marriage. As research was carried out in a primarily middle-class settling, Cuber and Harroff's delineations of types of marriage relationships (i.e., conflict-habituated, devitalized, passive-congenial, the vital, and the total) gained increasing validity. During our research in the anthropological literature we found that little attention had been given to the interpersonal dimensions of marriage or to the interrelation of the intrapsychic and ideological aspects of marriage. However, we did feel that the anthropological perspective gave a holistic approach to the problems of contemporary marriage that we considered valuable. In fact one of the major causes of confusion for many married couples was the persistence of traditional cultural ideologies and prescriptions for marriage behavior in the face of changing needs, changing value orientations, and changing behavior in marriage.

The Problem

As our exploratory insights to the problems evolved, we became increasingly convinced that the central problem in contemporary marriage was relationship. The attempt to solve the problem by moving

1. The term "nonmarrieds" applies to those relationships which involve some commitment but which are not legalized. They can range in time from a few months to a lifetime. The participants can be never-marrieds, formerly-marrieds, those still married but separated, or any combination thereof. The difficulties in comprehensive terminology for emerging relationships of varying degrees of commitment are apparent. "Premarital" is an accurate term for only a portion of these relationships since some never intend to marry the nonmarriage partner or the relationship is frequently considered only a temporary plateau before each has the sustaining personal resources to move on to another level (possibly marriage) or another relationship. The word "cohabitation" is also misleading as a coverall term for these relationships. Since cohabitation implies both a shared domicile and sex without legal marriage, it did not apply to some relationships encountered, e.g., a couple who did not share a domicile but did form a cohesive unit insofar as they shared all their spare time, vacations, and sex and presented themselves as a couple in social situations. Therefore, the term "nonmarrieds" is suggested.

into group and communal situations did not seem to mitigate the problems we discovered in interpersonal relationship. With the breakdown of many external supports for traditional marriage, the pressures on the interpersonal husband-and-wife relationship became intensified. There was an increasing need for that relationship to provide more fulfillment and benefits on both a personal and interpersonal level. Problems in marriage were manifested by the inability of the majority of individuals to find in the marital relationship both intimacy and opportunity for developing their personal potential. Our understanding of the problem concluded in addition that

1) marital partners and those contemplating marriage expressed a need for intimacy and growth in a relationship where they could actualize their individual potential without destroying the relationship.

2) most people did not have the skills in relating and in communicating which would allow for growth in a noncritical atmosphere. The typical dyadic marital role relationships had already been precut for them, locking them into a negative involuted feedback system. This was their perception of their situation as well, although not with the same terminology.

3) many of the innovations and experimental forms, although not all of them, nor all of the people involved in them, were a reflection and indication of this lack of skills in interpersonal relations.

4) other important impediments to growth were the unrealistic expectations and myths stemming from the traditional marriage format of the past, overriding emotional dependencies, and possessive jealousy.

As observers and researchers we had two options available to us: (1) reporting the alternate marriage and relationship styles with their attendant disillusionments and problems or (2) choosing a less orthodox path in utilizing our research. The presentation and analysis of data may benefit policy makers, academicians, and the counseling professions, but such analysis offers little to the individual in the way of ameliorating the problems he faces. Despite the fact that some have already opted for change on an individual basis or in group contexts, the bulk of the population remains, along with the innovators, unaware of the problem in its larger cultural and anthropological framework. Therefore, we chose to utilize our research in another manner.

The Action Model

The concept of open marriage, which is outlined elsewhere in detail, is primarily based on the expression of desires for change and the perceived routes to change drawn from our interviews conducted over a period of four years and upon our observations of actual changes taking place in many relationships. The research we conducted was utilized to create a model for change. In so doing we have stepped beyond the role of objective researcher reporting data and findings into the realm of what can be termed "action anthropology." By this we mean delineating a model for change that places the problem areas in their present and past cultural contexts and presents various available options for change in marital behavior and attitudes. An attempt has been made to present the traditional marital configuration in its societal setting and to delineate the cultural imperatives and values implicit in these imperatives for examination by those involved in marriage relationships. The first purpose, then, was to make it possible for individuals to become aware of the idealized precepts of the institution of marriage and the forces influencing their attitude toward and their behavior in marriage. Without an awareness of former expectations and present conditions, they cannot perceive the pathways to change. It is to be fully understood that some will choose to remain within traditional marriage, where the perimeters and dimensions are defined for them by the norms. But for those who feel a need for change, awareness and insight are necessary first steps to determining or discovering what pathways are available. The second objective was to outline those options for change in marital interaction which we had found in our research.

Action anthropology, defined elsewhere in traditional anthropological contexts by Peattie and Piddington, is a variation on the theme of action research. In the past, action research has been directed toward finding solutions to organizational or social problems. The flow has been from the institutional level down to the individual in effecting change. More recently it has been recognized that individuals can initiate measures for change and thus reverse the flow to effect change on the institutional level. Weinberg has noted that we are a problem-solving, action-oriented society; he continues:

> On this action level, society and the person are both symbolic systems with varying capacities for solving problems. Both society and the person can respond to problems in terms of their knowledge and their capacity for decision making and executive knowledge. Both can communicate, plan, and implement programs to solve problems. . . . The individual deliberates about alternatives before selecting a problem-solving response.

Today, the orientation toward methods of change must begin with the individual. The need for a measure of self-determination is paramount. Yet the individual is frequently overlooked as a primary force for change, and the assumption is made that his behavior is shaped by impinging social forces in the environment and that he neither has sufficient knowledge and perspective to perceive these forces nor is adequately equipped to institute directive and self-motivated change. This attitude underestimates the individual. Our sample encompassed a broad range of middle-class informant-respondents. The majority expressed a desire for some feeling of self-determination and autonomy in their lives and marriage behavior. Many had already instituted it. Furthermore, most had a knowledge of what the problem areas were in marriage. We offer one quote from an interview with a twenty-three-year-old single woman, who was at that time in a non-marriage relationship with a young man and seriously contemplating marriage:

> I don't want to say yes, yes we are going to be in love forever. It's like saying, yes, yes you know the ocean—and the next wave is going to look like this one, but I *can* say it is worth the risk *if* I feel I can do something about it. I want to be understanding, and start out with the attitude of well, it ain't going to be bliss but if I do my homework I stand a very good chance, and knowing what the chances are and stepping into it with your eyes open, you got a chance of making your marriage work . . .

and there is a lot more homework to do today because people have to make decisions they never had to make before in marriage, but those marriages will be better for it. . . . It's not I'm doing this because I've got to do it, it's doing this because I *chose* to do it, and that's what it is, man is a thinking animal, therefore I am. Once you get down to this kind of foundation and you can build, you know, "well begun is half done."

While our model is directed to the individual, we are well aware that many structural and institutional changes must of necessity also occur.

The Open Marriage Model

Open marriage is presented as a model with a twofold purpose:

1) to provide insights for individuals concerning the past patterns of traditional marriage, which we have termed *closed marriage*. As a closed systems model, traditional marriage was perceived as presenting few options for choice or change.
2) to provide guidelines, based on an open systems model, for developing an intimate marital relationship that provides for growth for both partners in the context of a one-to-one relationship. This does imply some degree of mutuality. It does not imply that growth will always be bilateral but rather that there will be supportive assistance and tolerance during unilateral growth. Shostrom and Kavanaugh (1971) have delineated a rhythmic-relationship which exemplifies this pattern.

The guidelines have been designed in answer to the needs expressed by the majority of our informant-respondents for a relationship which could offer them more dimensions for growth together than either could attain singly. The principle through which this mutually augmenting growth occurs is *synergy.* Many couples found that this synergistic self-actualizing mode of relating became possible only through the revision and deletion of some of the unrealistic expectations of closed marriage.

Open marriage thus can be defined as a relationship in which the partners are committed to their own and to each other's growth. It is an honest and open relationship of intimacy and self-disclosure based on the equal freedom and identity of both partners. Supportive caring and increasing security in individual identities make possible the sharing of self-growth with a meaningful other who encourages and anticipates his own and his mate's growth. It is a relationship that is flexible enough to allow for change and that is constantly being renegotiated in the light of changing needs, consensus in decision-making, acceptance and encouragement of individual growth, and openness to new possibilities *for* growth. Obviously, following this model often involves a departure, sometimes radical, from rigid conformity to the established husband-wife roles and is not easy to effect.

In brief, the guidelines are: living for now, realistic expectations, privacy, role flexibility, open and honest communication, open companionship, equality, identity, and trust. The first step requires each partner to reassess the actual or prospective marital relationship in order to clarify and determine both individual and mutual expectations. Couples in today's society are not educated for marriage or in the requisites of a good human relationship, nor are they aware of the psychological and myriad other commitments that the typical marriage contract implies. The expectations of closed marriage—the major one being that one partner will be able to fulfill all of the other's needs (emotional, social, sexual, economic, intellectual, and otherwise)—present obstacles to growth and attitudes that foster conflict between partners. Awareness of these expectations and a realignment more in accord with a realistic appraisal of their capabilities are fundamental to instituting change and to solving their problems in relationship.

Living for now involves relating to the present rather than to the past or to future goals which are frequently materialistic and concrete rather than emotional and intellectual in nature. The granting of time off, or *privacy,* can be used for examination of the self and for psychic regeneration. A way out of what many marital partners conceive of as the role-bind involves working toward a greater *role flexibility* by exchanging roles and role-associated tasks either on a temporary or part-time basis and utilizing role reversal as a device for understanding the self and the position of the other partner. *Open and honest communication* is perhaps the most important element in an open relationship. The lack of communication skills creates a formidable barrier between husband and wife; yet these skills are the most important in sustaining a vital relationship, promoting understanding, and increasing knowledge of self. *Open companionship* involves relating to others, including the opposite sex, outside the primary unit of husband and wife, as an auxiliary avenue for growth. *Equality* involves relating to the mate as a peer in terms of ways to achieve stature rather than in terms of the status attached to the traditional husband and wife roles. *Identity* involves the development of the individual through interaction with his mate and others, through actualizing his own potentials and through building toward autonomy and personal responsibility. *Trust*, growing through the utilization of these other guidelines and based on mutuality and respect for each other's integrity, creates the climate for growth. Liking, sexual intimacy, and love grow through the exercise of these elements.

The system of guidelines for open marriage can be seen as an expanding spiral of evolving steps in complexity and depth in the marital relationship. The model begins with the self and the premise that internal communication is necessary to attain disclosure of inner feelings to one's self and subsequently to one's mate. Once open and honest communication is established with the mate, in addition to feedback from the mate, the partner's relationship can evolve through the guidelines with multilevel feedback reinforcing each phase. The system operates through the principle of synergy, a concept drawn from medicine and chemistry and first utilized by Benedict in cultural, and later by Maslow in interpersonal, contexts. In open marriage, the concept of *synergic build-up* is defined as a mutually augmenting growth system. Synergy means that two partners in marriage can accomplish more personal *and* interpersonal growth together than they could separately and without the loss of their individual identities. Synergic build-up is the positive augmenting feedback that can enhance mutual growth and dynamism in the man-woman relationship.

While only a limited few may be able to utilize all these guidelines in their totality and simultaneously, open marriage can best be considered a *resource mosaic* from which couples can draw according to their needs and their readiness for change in any one area.

The majority of our sample had already explored the possibilities for change in some of the areas covered by the guidelines. Many of them required only a change in attitude, while they acknowledged behavioral changes as difficult. The two areas of greatest difficulty were the conflicts arising from changing man-woman and husband-wife roles and the problems encountered in self-development.

The question of marital and extramarital sexual behavior, while ever present, did not seem to be the central problem with which they were coping. While marital sex sometimes posed problems, many felt the emphasis on sexual adjustment, as presented in published manuals and in the media, was exaggerated. Although many felt that they could not cope with sexual jealousy in terms of extramarital sex, they were on the verge of deciding that sex per se was not the central problem in their marriage. Numerous couples had already effected some degree of sexual latitude in their own relationships. Some had done so with tacit knowledge but without verbalized agreement. Others had done so in various types of consensual arrangements, including individual contexts, group sex, and partner exchange. While some benefits were noted for those involved in extramarital relationships which included sex, it was observed that by and large these experiences did not occur in a context where the marital partners were developing their primary marriage relationship sufficiently for this activity to count as a growth experience. Frequently this involvement became an avenue of escape, intensified conflicts, and actually obscured problems in the primary relationship. For some, however, it did become a means of revealing other problem areas in the marriage and for achieving greater understanding.

Underlying the marital couple's explorations into any area of non-conformity, whether it was extramarital sex or the equally important area of changes in typical role behavior (i.e., male-female, man-woman, husband-wife), was the central problem of relationship.[2] That

2. Concerning these two areas of change, the authors are least optimistic about the movement into group marriage and communal living situations which involve random or structured sexual intimacy among many. No true group marriage, as it is being explored in our society with an equal valence of roles and sexual sharing among all partners, has existed, according to the anthropological literature. Among all societies where larger family structures exist, they are maintained by elaborate kinship ties and other supportive structures interwoven with the institutional framework of the society; thus, goals are integrated for the group or extended family. Certainly, communal or community situations where the goals are banding together to share economic, child care or recreational activities have many advantages and, it is hoped, will increase. But when couples and individuals in groups are pressed into situations of total intimacy—including the sexual dimension—for which they have not been prepared emotionally either by training or by conditioning, the strain of the multistranded relationships tends to fragment the group. The goals of cooperation and support are difficult to maintain under the pressure of emotional conflicts which are intensified by prescriptions for sexual intimacy.

is, How can the marital partners relate in terms of their changing needs and those of society in a mutually beneficial fashion? Open marriage presents some of the elements in interpersonal relationships that allow for change, for increasing responsibility for the self and for others, and for increased understanding between husband and wife.

Most people enter marriage without preparation for this long-term intimacy and without preparation to meet changes in themselves and in society. Education for the marriage relationship in all its ramifications, from the relational and sexual aspects, through child-rearing, and on to the mature years when the children are grown, is notably absent. Skills for communication,[3] self-discovery, problem-solving, and relating in intimacy can be learned. Such skills do not demand therapy or deep introspection, for knowledge of self will evolve in progression if the skills are learned and if motivation for change follows the insights gained.

The open marriage model offers insights and learning guides for developing more intimate and understanding marital relationships. An open relationship in marriage, as well as in any interpersonal matrix, involves becoming a more open person. Since the open-minded personality is one which can perceive options and alternatives and make decisions about the paths to change, efforts to help the marital couple in perception and skills should increase their ability to solve many problems in marriage. However, it will not be easy for most couples. Emotional maturity, and the development of responsibility and confident identity, cannot emerge overnight. But standing still or merely exploring experimental *structural* forms without attention to the interpersonal factors seems to increase the number of problems in marriage and decrease the benefits to be gained from it. Open marriage is not intended to solve marital problems, but by using the open marriage model, the couple will at least be substituting problems which promote growth and learning for problems which are currently insoluble.

Implications

It is in the arena of interpersonal relations that marriage and the family will have to find new meaning and gain greater strength, no matter

3. An excellent example of a program in which these skills are taught is the four-session format developed by the Minnesota Couples Communications Program.

what the configuration of the sociocultural framework may be. Children cannot be taught the value of supportive love and caring, responsibility, problem-solving, or decision-making skills unless the parents have first developed these qualities in their own relationship. The inadequacy of our organized institutions to instill these values and skills is only too apparent. Therefore, intimate, long-term relationships such as those of marriage and the family must provide them, and to do this, they must be more rewarding and fulfilling for their members and there must be feedback and caring for each other's welfare.

Focusing on the methods for achieving a rewarding one-to-one relationship provides something that individuals can deal with and work with on a self-determining level. By encouraging personal responsibility, self-growth, and bonding through the synergic relationship, the basic unit of husband and wife should become more rewarding and offer more avenues for fulfillment.

Building from within strengthens the individual, the couple, and then the family unit, and thus the entire social structure, since the fundamental unit of society is the family. Whatever form the family unit may take, its strength will still depend on the rewards gained from interpersonal relationships. It is in this sense that the individual, and the married couple, can become not only a fulcrum for change but also a key factor leading to the strengthening of the social structure. Thus both family and society can be better equipped to cope with accelerating technological and cultural change. It is hoped that open families can evolve to an open society and eventually to an open world.

The Myth of Black Sexual Superiority: A Re-Examination

Robert Staples

from *The Black Scholar*, April 1978

Throughout the sixties and seventies, many black intellectuals claimed that the sexual revolution was irrelevant to African Americans. Robert Staples has written extensively on the black family and sexuality—here he revisits an earlier article, written ten years before, on the American myth that blacks are sexually more liberated than whites. The essay examines the patterns of sexual behavior in the black community and the impact, if any, of what Staples calls the "white sexual revolution."

Over ten years ago this writer raised the question: Are blacks sexually superior? My answer at that time was "if sexual superiority means to enjoy the pleasures of sexual congress without feelings of guilt and fear, freed from the restraints of white puritanism, the answer must be in the affirmative."[1] In the intervening decade, there has been a dramatic increase in the frequency with which most white Americans engage in various sexual activities and in the number of persons who include formerly rare or forbidden techniques in their sexual repertoires.[2] These changes have given rise to the need to re-examine the question of black sexual superiority in light of what is regarded as the white sexual revolution.

A review of the past record of white beliefs about black sexuality casts in bold relief the view that "for the majority of white men, the Negro represents the sexual instinct (in its raw state)."[3] As long ago as the sixteenth century Englishmen were imputing to Africans an unrestrained lustfulness and describing them as "large" propagators and "hot constitution'd ladies." Certainly, in comparison to European dictums about chastity being the best state for men and their *norms* that women should not enjoy sex under any circumstances, Africans represented the sexuality of beasts and the bestiality of sex.[4] History, however, tells us that Europeans were not always a puritanical culture.[5] Some claim that the beginning of human society (i.e. white society) was characterized by unrestrained sexual relations between man and woman, father and daughter, mother and son. Only with the development of private property, when men needed proof of paternity in order to will their resources to the right heir, was sexual exclusivity for women only, brought into existence and mostly among the propertied classes.[6]

Within the African continent, at least South of the Sahara, their view, in general, of sex was directed toward both physiological and psychological adjustment. Tribal values on sexual behavior were strongly woven into their social structure and the first instinctive manifestations of sexuality were conditioned by their mores and environment. Public rituals often existed to confirm the appropriate sexual elements and remove the improper ones. Whereas Europeans saw sex as inherently sinful, the African ethos was that breaches of Tribal sexual law are offenses against individuals and social groups, not against God. The African was concerned with crime and not with Sin. Conversely, it is impossible to generalize about African sexual permissiveness since there were large numbers of them who imposed harsh penalties on women who did not enter the conjugal state as virgins as well as many who allowed youth to satisfy sexual desires before marriage.[7]

It was with these diverse sexual values that Africans were brought to this country as slaves. There is sufficient evidence in the form of slave narratives, the slaveholders' own records and the considerably lighter hue of Afro-Americans, that those Tribal norms were contravened on a massive scale, whenever possible and by bondsman, overseer and slave master alike. However, within the slave quarters there were boundaries imposed on sexual activity among its inhabitants. A relationship between one man and a woman was respected and whenever possible they confined their sexual relationships to each other.[8]

● ● ●

After slavery ended Afro-Americans probably did have a more permissive sexual code than many Euro-Americans, but that fact has to be placed in the proper historical context. In accordance with Freudian theory, we can assume that the sexual drive exists in all individuals and has to be expressed in some form.[9] Historically, males in this culture have been allowed unrestrained libidinal expression. It is women on which the greatest restraints have been placed and bourgeois women at that. Even among working class white women the norm of chastity has been honored more in the breach than in its observance. A major reason for the class difference is the greater use of economic resources by the bourgeois male to exact sexual chastity from the women in his class. Where there is no exchange value of sex for material reward, the libido thrives in a more liberated way.[10]

Thus, because the black masses enjoyed a more healthy sexual equality than was possible for whites in the post-bellum era, a more permissive sexual code developed. Moreover, some of the controls on Euro-American sexuality did not exist in the same degree among Afro-Americans. The puritanical exhortations of organized religion served to effectively check much of the Euro-American's sexuality while the black church functioned more as a tension-reducing institution and eschewed monitoring the moral standards of its parishioners. Black males did not classify women into bad and good groups on that basis of their virginal status. White men did make these distinctions and women were eligible for the respectability of marriage according to their classification in one group or the other. During an epoch in which the majority of white women were economically dependent on their men this was an effective censor of their sexuality. Black women, in the main, were more economically and psychologically independent.[11]

One sees the operant effects of class as a differentiator of sexual expression by looking at variations in the black community itself. While the black bourgeoisie has, until recently, represented only a small segment of the total black community, its sexual values and behavior were often a reflection of the white bourgeoisie. Fairly conservative sexual attitudes were typical of middle-class blacks as were premarital chastity and female frigidity. Many bourgeois Afro-American males preferred that their wives stay at home rather than work. Frazier once observed that "there is much irregularity in this class. The importance of sex to this class is indicated by their extreme sensitivity to any charge that Negros are more free or more easy in their sexual behavior than whites."[12] In its most extreme manifestation their sexual conservatism was reflected in the en-loco-parentis stance of black colleges. In the 1920s Fisk University had printed regulations that "it was forbidden for two students of the opposite sex to meet each other without the presence and permission of the Dean of Women or of a teacher." A girl and boy could be sent home for walking together in broad daylight.[13]

This is not to say that there were no moral parameters among the black working class nor that all of their sexual values and behavior are healthy. In particular, we have to re-examine the stereotype of black sexual superiority as it relates to fulfilling the needs of both men and women. Furthermore, sexual competency must be defined as more than the physical fusion of bodies and consummation of the act of intercourse. We must also consider the psychological properties of the sex act, its misuse by both participants and how open blacks are to its total dimension as well as alternative sexual life styles. In part, this re-examination is forced by the new realities facing the black community and our increasing awareness that any sexual act that is biologically possible may have a socially redeeming value.

No matter how positive the eventual outcome of black working class sexual socialization, the process by which they acquire their sexual values leaves much to be desired. From the limited data on the subject, it is apparent that black parents are not the source of sex education for most black youth. The majority of them, in fact, receive their initial knowledge of sex from peers and other sources. And, much of that information is fragmented and inaccurate.[14] While it is often assumed that blacks are much earlier exposed to sex than whites, the Kinsey group found that whites tend to learn about menstruation, fertilization, pregnancy, abortion, and condoms at slightly younger ages than blacks. Furthermore, white males experienced their first ejaculation from any source earlier than black males and among females the black woman reported experiencing less nudity in their childhood homes than their white counterpart.[15]

More important than the age at which they acquire their sexual education is what many young black men learn. To wit, it is a well for-mulated system for manipulating and controlling women. Early in the life cycle they realize that money and women are the two most highly valued objects that one can gain in our system. As Hammond reports, women can supply one with money or what it can buy as well as a means of satisfying his sexual desires. Hence, a competitive system emerges among men to make as many sexual conquests as possible. It is a dog-eat-dog system whereby the man with the best rap, clothes or style wins—with women as the spoils.[16] Lost in this struggle for one-upsmanship is a feeling of relatedness toward women and an articu-lated awareness of their human qualities.

A most blatant indicator of the woman qua property ideology among many black men is the violence that often accompanies the sexual con-quest. Witness, for instance, the common and legendary practice of "taking pussy." The strongarming of black women into sexual submis-sion is pervasive in the sexual histories collected by this writer, and it is not a practice confined to working-class blacks but equally repre-sented among the bourgeoisie. While white men have always been able to use their superior economic resources to compel sexual sub-mission from white women, there is increasing evidence that black men are not reluctant to use the perquisites of high office or wealth to accomplish the same end.[17] Small wonder, then, that the black women in Johnson's college sample reported more negative feelings on the day following their first premarital sexual experience from their white counterparts.[18]

Although we recognize that much of blacks' sexual behavior is a function of forces beyond their control (i.e., white racism and internal colonialism) there must be some accountability for these individual actions. In every study comparing black and white sexuality the greatest conflict between values and feelings exists among sex roles—not racial groups. Black and white men are much more untied in the meaning of sex than are black men and black women. Men of both races are sim-ilar in the very selfish peer-oriented nature of their sexual behavior. If this self-indulgent pattern should continue we might take heed of this warning from the National Black Feminist Alliance that "we must, together, as a people, work to eliminate racism from without the black community which is trying to destroy us as an entire people but we must remember that sexism is destroying and crippling us from within."[19]

Of course, the misuse of sex is not confined to men. In this capitalistic society sex is frequently part of a profit and loss system rather than the genuine sharing of minds and bodies. There is no dearth of black women who have used sex as a punishment, a tease, or as currency. While much of male sexual jealousy is unwarranted and reflects their view of women as property, women aid in the development of this destructive emotion by the cunning ploy of keeping a partner wondering whether there is any infidelity or not. The emerging practice of women enjoying male companionship with men who are labeled as "friends" has done nothing to arrest male tendencies toward sexual jealousy.

However, the lion's share of the burden for our sex role conflict must be placed upon black males. While some black women give as much as they get, the system inherently favors men. With an effective sex ratio of three black women to every male, the females have little, if any, bargaining power, where men have such a larger number of women from which to choose.[20] In a sense, black women often find themselves in the position of sexually auditioning for a meaningful relationship. After a number of tryouts, they may find a black male who is willing to make a commitment to them.

We should not be deluded, the sexual revolution and its rhetoric notwithstanding, into believing that black women have been able to totally separate sex from love and commitment. The contemporary rhetoric of black female sexual liberation we hear may be best explained by their need for avoiding cognitive dissonance. When there is an incompatibility between an act and a belief system, the individual must reduce the dissonance by altering her behavior or beliefs. Consequently, black women who, of necessity, are sexually active develop liberal views about their sexuality. But, this psychological compartmentalization has its limitations. Within their liberal sexual activity most black women are bargaining for a stable relationship. And, they are doing so with a group that is very low on commitment as a priority in their scheme of things.

The onset of the liberated black female sexuality would have been a godsend had black men attempted to understand the nature of female sexuality. Once the gates were open to the female orifice, the legacy of the past too took hold as the man's response. Lovemaking was conceptualized as a physical act with male satisfaction as its ultimate end. Hence, we find black women decrying the fact that tenderness, communication, and emotion is not attendant to the act of sexual intercourse. Too often the male never reveals his naked emotions to his partner because he views such an act as a sign of weakness. When tenderness or affection is expressed, women complain, it is only in the context of a prelude to sexual activity.

Many black women have come to find that the sexual revolution wasn't their war. Obviously, the strict double standard no longer exists but it has been supplanted by more arbitrary male standards about how sexually liberated women can be. A women who proclaims "extreme" sexual liberation still finds herself ranked as less than desirable for the position of wife or even stable companion. In a recent study of male sexuality, a pair of researchers found that many young men still adhere to the old traditional values. A large number of them wanted their wives to be virgins.[21] While those were white men, Johnson found in her study of black males that they were more likely to have a double standard than white males in the same sample.[22] This could, of course, mean that black men do not want a women who is as sexually active as they. It still presages that the sexually liberated black women may not be among the chosen.

Even black women who accept this handicap often find less than fulfillment in their sexual efforts. Lack of tender foreplay and other insensitivities is an oft-expressed grievance. Failure to achieve orgasm is frequently attributed to his refusal to use any technique other than penile penetration and thrusts. Although clitoral stimulation or oral manipulation may be necessary to help her achieve orgasm, many black men have strong taboo against such practices. In one of the few studies on the subject, Hunt found that only 35 percent of single black males vs. 72 percent of white males had participated in cunnilingus in the last year. Moreover, 48 percent of single black women had engaged in fellatio—indicating that many black men believe it is better to receive than give.[23]

The aforementioned turn of events would have less import if not for the changing realities of the black community. As of 1976, the majority of black women between the ages of 20-45 are not married and living with a spouse.[24] Reasons for this unprecedented situation range from the serious shortage of black males to the increasing disenchantment with marriage as an institution. Whatever the reason, it is clear that this situation requires some rethinking of old values and practices. Many black women will acquire extensive sexual experience because they realize it is impractical to wait for the elusive goal of marriage. The changing definition of sex roles will also impact on the sexual assertiveness of women and the expectations of male sexual perform-ance. Black[s] will have to be open to the variety of sexual expressions if their needs are to be filled in the context at the new black reality.

Whereas moral boundaries will have to be expanded to accommo-date the new reality, some parameters must be maintained in order to preserve the Black Family. One of them may be an off-limits rule on those blacks that are currently married. Currently, it has become fash-ionable for sexually liberated black women to include married men as sexual partners. Such extra-marital relationships might be acceptable if they remained merely physical relationships but they run the constant danger of becoming emotional ones and serve to disrupt existing mar-riages. In 1975, 26.6 percent of the black population between the ages of 25 and 54 were divorced compared to only 8.4 of similar whites.[25] Some of this statistical racial disparity may be attributed to the pressure exerted by single black women entangled with married men. The same parameters should be applied to married women but they are generally less accessible, and for different reasons, than male spouses.

The continuing shortage of black men will still pose a dilemma for many black women. A common suggestion made mostly by men, is that they should be willing to share their men (i.e. polygamy).[26] Such multiple relationships could be viable if men were also willing to share and if women who had internalized values of monogamy could accept such an arrangement. In most cases they can not, especially when the sharing must be acknowledged and agreed upon. The de facto sharing that now exists has been responsible for its share of heartbreaks, jeal-ousy, violence, and mental anguish.

It is incumbent upon us to leave as open as possible the options avail-able to black women. One of them may be interracial relationships if they find a suitable partner and can withstand the stresses inherent in such an arrangement. Another is homosexuality. While the black community has never been as harshly repressive of the black homosexual as in white society, there has never been full acceptance either. Those who are willing to accept any of the above options should be aware of the pitfalls contained within them. White males, for instance, represent no improvement over black males, but their numbers are larger and college-educated black women will be able to find a mate of equal status. At the same time, it means, in many cases, virtual isolation from family and friends. Moreover, the same conflicts that characterize black marriages will prevail along with the inexorable pressures exerted on such unions.[27]

Living a gay lifestyle is still fraught with danger, especially for women who are already oppressed on the basis of gender. In the case of black women, it would be a triple minority status. Gay relationships are also rife with the problems that typify heterosexual unions. In many cases gays complain of being unable to find a meaningful relationship, of sexual jealousy, personality conflicts and the like. It is only by considering this as well as other possibilities that black women in the existentialist sense can find themselves as the subject, not the object of their social world.

Concomitant with the sexual revolution and the new reality, blacks must be accepting of the right of women to choose whether they wish to bear children or not. That means making available safe contraceptives and access to abortions on demand. Considering the unsafe nature of many female contraceptives, it also indicates greater male responsibility for birth control. The male virility cult must be abandoned for male willingness to use condoms or undergo a vasectomy after siring a reasonable number of children. Since some black women may be in the single state for perpetuity they may choose to adopt a child or have one out-of-wedlock. Such an alternative should be permissible within the expanded moral boundaries necessary to confront our new reality.

None of this critical analysis of black sexuality should be allowed to overshadow the positive aspects of their sexual life. In the main blacks continue to engage in and enjoy their sexual encounters. Part of the problem arises from the conflict of traditional values with new realities. And, for the bourgeoisie, they were not black values. This does not mean that the black sexual experience has been a bleak or negative one. For the most part sex has been the one haven they have had from the daily oppression of white racism. With all its intrusions, the internal colonial order did not enter their bedrooms.

It is not the sexual revolution but the new black reality that commands our attention. For the first time in our history the majority of black women, and large numbers of men, are and will remain unmarried. Perforce, their sexuality must be harnessed in such a way as to promote the meeting of this universal human need. Sex should be used as a means of communication not as an instrument of domination and control. The time for game playing is over. Both men and women must cultivate modalities of healthy sexual expressions which will preserve their basic integrity and humanity. As for the question of black sexual superiority, we do not need the label of sexually superior any more than we have heretofore needed the appellation of mentally inferiority. Above all, we need a sexual ethos that will contribute to our unity as a people and that value system must serve all of the black community.

• • •

1. Robert Staples, "The Mystique of Black Sexuality." *Liberator* 7 (March, 1967), p. 10.

2. Morton Hunt, *Sexual Behavior in the 1970's* (Chicago: Playboy Press, 1974).

3. Frantz Fanon, *Black Skin, White Masks* (New York: Grove Press, 1967), p. 177.

4. Winthrop D. Jordan, B*lack over White: American Attitudes Toward the Negro, 1550-1812* (Chapel Hill: University of North Carolina Press, 1968), pp. 34-35.

5. G. Rattray Taylor, *Sex in History* (New York: Ballantine Books, 1954).

6. Frederich Engels, *The Origin of the Family, Private Property and the State* (Chicago: Charles H. Kerr, 1902).

7. Boris De Rachewiltz, *Black Eros: Sexual Customs of Africa from Prehistory to the Present Day* (New York: Lyle Stuart, 1964).

8. Eugene Genovese, *Roll, Jordan, Roll* (New York: Random House, 1975), pp. 458-475.

9. Sigmund Freud, *The Basic Writings of Sigmund Freud*, trans. by A. A. Bril (New York: Modern Library, 1938).

10. Reiche Reimut, *Sexuality and The Class Struggle* (Germany: NLB, 1970).

11. C. F. Robert Staples, *The Black Woman in America: Sex, Marriage and the Family* (Chicago: Nelson- Hall, 1973).

12. E. Franklin Frazier, "Sex Life of the African and American Negro" in A. Ellig and A. Abaranel, eds., *The Encyclopedia of Sexual Behavior* (New York: Hawthorne Books, 1961), pp. 769-75.

13. Raymond Walters, *The New Negro on Campus* (Princeton, N.J.: Princeton University Press, 1975), p. 37.

14. John F. Kantner and Melvin Zelnik, "Contraception and Pregnancy: Experience of Young Unmarried Women in the United States," *Family Planning Perspectives* 4 (October, 1972), p. 9-17.

15. Alan P. Bell, "Black Sexuality, Fact and Fancy," in R. Staples, ed., *The Black Family: Essays and Studies,* Vol. II (Belmont: Wadsworth, 1978), pp. 77-79.

16. Boone F. Hammond, "The Contest System: A Survival Technique," Masters Essay, Washington University, 1965.

17. Robert Staples, *Race and Family Violence: The Internal Colonialism Perspective in Crime and Its Impact on the Black Community* (L. Gary and L. Brown, eds.) (Washington, D.C.: The Institute For Urban Affairs and Research, 1976), pp. 85-96.

18. Leanor B. Johnson, "Sexual Behavior of Southern Blacks" in *The Black Family: Essays and Studies,* Vol. II., op. cit., pp. 80-92.

19. Statement of The National Black Feminist Organization, 1973.

20. Current Population Reports, *Population Estimates and Projections,* Series P-25, No. 643. (U.S. Government Printing Office, 1977). The real sex ration is actually closer to 85:100. My effective sex ratio only includes men available and compatible to most black women.

21. Anthony Pietropinto and Jacqueline Simenauer, *Beyond The Male Myth* (Quadrangle, 1977).

22. Johnson, op. cit.

23. Hunt, op. cit., p. 198.

24. U.S. Bureau of the Census, *Marital Status and Living Arrangements,* Series P-20, No. 306. (Washington, D.C.: U.S. Government Printing Office, 1977).

25. Ibid.

26. C.F. Joseph Scott, "Polygamy: A Futuristic Family Arrangement for African Americans," *Black Books Bulletin,* Summer 1976.

27. David Heer, "The Prevalence of Black-White Marriage in the United States, 1960 and 1970," *Journal of Marriage and Family* 36 (May, 1974), pp. 246-59.

Styling, Profiling, and Pretending: The Games Before the Fall

Gloria I. Joseph

from *Common Differences: Conflicts in Black & White Feminist Perspectives*, 1981

Gloria Joseph and Jill Lewis' book, **Common Differences,** *is a pioneering examination of the ways in which race and sexuality affect women's lives. In this chapter, Gloria Joseph takes a close look at the impact of feminism and the sexual revolution on African Americans during the late seventies. Joseph discusses the sexual relationships between black women and black men in the historical context shaped by the political and cultural developments of the twentieth century.*

The Afro-American culture with all its unique features of caring, sharing, kinship networks, upward mobility aspirations, and color caste complexes interacts with and reacts to a racially and economically oppressive environment. This "double consciousness" (Afro-American culture and Western society), these two warring souls in every Black female and male body, become further compounded and complex as women's consciousness comes to the fore. In any discussion about Blacks—and Black female and male relationships are no exception—we must never lose sight of these actualities. However, these facts must not be allowed to become excuses for any and all apolitical, irresponsible behaviors on the part of Black women or men, such as Black fratricide or poverty pimping. Nor must Black women and men unwittingly enter the game of blaming the victim. Put in other words, Black men must not put a heavy blame trip on Black women, and Black women must not put a heavy, accusatory putdown on Black men. What is needed is an honest—a putting-aside-pride-and-frail-ego honest—assessment of the reality of the conditions that surround and exist for and between Black females and males. Knowing and facing one's reality is a first step, a necessary first step in any struggle. "Our reality, like all other realities, has positive aspects and negative aspects, has strengths and weaknesses . . . Man is part of reality, Reality exists independent of man's will . . . those who lead the struggle must never confuse what they have in their head with reality."[1]

It is a political reality that Black people in America are victims of institutional racism and economic oppression. To put it simply, Blacks who imagine they have escaped these oppressions have been psychologically duped. They have bought into the media's massive and successful efforts to promote and popularize the mistaken belief that inequality and racism are social ills of the past. The media cite evidence of Black professionals in the high-income brackets, token Federal appointees, and local politicians to accommodate the belief that the system is no longer racist. The problem of racism was supposedly solved in the Sixties; therefore, Blacks who don't make it have no one to blame but themselves. This, of course, is not true. The record from the Seventies clearly shows that conditions for Blacks have worsened.

In this chapter we are concerned with the realities of the sexual relationships between Black women and Black men, emphasizing Black women's sexual attitudes and behaviors. In so doing we must keep in mind that there is no monolithic group of Black women or Black men. Their conditions and situations vary according to income levels, careers, regions, age, education, and early life experiences. We are interested in the underlying commonalities that exist despite societal forces and circumstantial differences which have had substantial effects on the lives of Black women (and men).

Initially, there are several undeniable facts about Black women's lives that must be recognized and acknowledged. Their lives have been characterized by: (1) high achievement and outstanding accomplishment by a few; (2) an unending cycle of poverty for the vast majority; (3) always defining themselves and their womanhood in terms of their connection with Black men; (4) strong feeling of autonomy and independence.

In her book *Of Woman Born*, Adrienne Rich wrote, "What we bring to childbirth is nothing less than our entire socialization as women."[2] Similarly, a Black woman's sexuality is nothing less than her entire socialization as a Black female. The sexual socialization of the Black female is largely determined by her early childhood and adolescent upbringing, the influences of family, school, and religion intertwined with the roles played by culture and society. Of course, her socioeconomic class, religion, geographical region, and sense of self-esteem influence the child-raising practice to which she is subjected, as well as the ways in which resisting or succumbing to the cultural and societal pressures are enacted. These considerations remind us once again that Black female sexuality cannot be viewed through "monolithic lenses."

An analysis of the role of socialization in the Black woman's sexuality is necessarily complex. The early life experience of the female is a good starting point in examining the configuration of Black female sexuality. The "puritanical" upbringing of Black women is said to be a key cause for the problems that Black females experiences as they approach womanhood. This puritanical upbringing is said to be responsible for the attitudes among young girls that sex is dirty, that it is not a subject for polite conversation, that masturbation is unnatural, and that sex will get you in trouble.

This explanation must be juxtaposed to the realities of families that view the role of sex in a more celebratory fashion. In these homes there are various messages that say sex is desirable, sex is satisfying, sex is "good", and everyone gets involved, sooner or later. The popular songs that are heard and sung in homes and on the streets, the jokes and innuendoes, the signifying and sounding in conversations, are all fraught with sexual tones. In overcrowded dwellings it is impossible to keep sexual relations a secret. In homes at the lower socioeconomic levels, attitudes toward having babies—a most direct connection to the sex act—are an indication of the family's and community's feelings about sexual relations. Carol Stack, in her book *All Our Kin*, points out that:

> Unlike many other societies, Black women in The Flats feel few if any restrictions about childbearing. Unmarried Black women, young and old, are eligible to bear children, and frequently women bearing their first child are quite young. A girl who gives birth as a teen-ager frequently does not raise and nurture her

first born child. While she may share the same room and house-hold with her baby, her mother's sister, or her older sister will care for the child and become the child's "mamma". People show pride in all their kin, and particularly new babies born into the kinship network. Mothers encourage sons to have babies, and even more important, men coax their "old ladies" to have their babies.[4]

Puritanical attitudes exist in many homes, but in many other homes the attitude is not definitely puritanical. What is common and true in most homes is that regardless of whether sex is an open or discreet issue, Black women do not receive necessary and accurate information about sexual matters. Young Black girls pick up a lot of misinformation from the streets and from their female and male peer groups. Beauty parlors long have been a stronghold for the dissemination of facts about men and about women's involvements with men. Young ears always have strained to pick up some information about sexual mat-ters. The adult women's talk would sometimes be guarded so that the young female would not get the full picture, and other times the adult's intent was to deliberately give messages to the young sisters. Com-ments about mistreatment from men, the sweetness of men, two-timing men and faithful women are topics that typically elicit animated conversations.

The following scenario illustrates how one young female receives messages about men and sex. An older woman enters the beauty shop, and her response to the welcoming greetings of the beautician is an unenthusiastic, half-hearted, semi-articulated utterance. Another cus-tomer and good friend says, "Hmm, what's the matter with you? Didn't you get any last night?" Or she might say, "Girl, you acting like you just lost your ole man. What's happening?" Men and sex are viewed as necessities for feeling good and/or causes for feeling bad. Either way, the female is a reflection of the male. The ambivalence seen throughout male/female relationships is again apparent.

The important roles of music and dance in Black culture have a his-torically been influential in the sexual socialization of young Black females. Traditionally music—spirituals, gospel, blues, and jazz—has figured prominently in the lives of Black folks. The blues dealt with the real stuff: there's no escaping from the hard, bitter, day-to-day struggles.

Female blues singers were unique in recording Black women's history and struggles via song. The topics and words in their songs, combined with their personalized and expressive deliveries, created an idiom that has helped Black women remember the past and live the present. The sexual content of the songs reflects themes and delivers messages about: the nature of and ways to deal with two-timing men; men mistreating women; cheating women; women longing for their men and willing to pay any price to be with their men; men who can't quite measure up sexually; the hardships associated with being a poor Black woman; and the glorification of sex. The titles of the following songs reflect these themes: "Mean Mistreater Blues" by Memphis Minnie; "All Fed Up" and "Ain't No Fool" by Big Mama Thornton; "Yellow Dog Blues" by Lizzie Miles; "Tricks Ain't Walkin' No More" by Bessie Jackson; and "Empty Bed Blues" by Bessie Smith.

Bessie Smith, the legendary Bessie Smith, the Empress of the Blues, made a historical contribution to the sexual lives of Black women. Michele Russell made this point succinctly:

Bessie Smith redefined our time. In a deliberate inversion of the Puritanism of the Protestant ethic, she articulated, as clearly as anyone before or since, how fundamental sexuality was to survival. Where work was often the death of us, sex brought us back to life. It was better than food, and sometimes a necessary substitute.

For Bessie Smith, Black women in American culture were no longer to be regarded only as sexual objects. She made us sexual subjects, the first step in taking control. She transformed our collective shame at being rape victims, treated like dogs or worse, the meat dogs eat, by emphasizing the value of our allure. In so doing, she humanized sexuality for Black women.[5]

Bessie Smith's songs about those house rent parties and buffet flats gave graphic accounts of entertainment and sex as a part of economic, spiritual, and emotional survival. The musical talents of Black women blues singers were as outstanding as were the social commentaries in their songs. House rent parties and buffet flats were common in Black urban areas and offered pleasures that were not restricted to sex, such as card playing, eating, drinking, and gambling, but sex was certainly a dominant part of the scene. In a 1971 interview with Chris Albertson, Ruby Smith (Bessie's niece by marriage, who traveled with her) described a buffet flat located in Detroit.

Ruby Smith:

> . . . faggots dressed like women there it wasn't against the law, you know—that Detroit was a real open town for everybody in that town. Bessie and us all, went to a party. Some woman there had a buffet flat.

Bessie Smith paid tribute to this establishment in her recording "Soft Pedal Blues":

> There's a lady in our neighborhood who runs a buffet flat,
> and when she gives a party she know just where she's at,
> She gave a dance last Friday night, it was to last till one,
> But when the time was almost up, the fun had just begun.

> Albertson: What's a buffet flat?
> Ruby Smith: A buffet flat is nothing but faggots and, and, uh, bull dykers and—open house—everything goes on in that house . . .
> Albertson: A gay place?
> Ruby Smith: A very gay place.
> Albertson: Strictly for faggots and bull dykes?
> Ruby Smith: -Everything! Everything that was in the life, everybody that's in the life. . . . Buffet means everything—everything goes on. They had a faggot there that was so great people used to come there just to watch him make love to another man. That's right, he was real great, he'd give him a tongue bath and everything. People used to pay good just to see him come there and see him do his act . . . [6]

A graphic reflection of the urban phenomenon of the poor, the house rent party, is heard in Bessie Smith's rendition of "Gimme a Pigfoot (and a Bottle of Beer)." Her candor is amazing as she sings of "reefers and a gang of gin, lay me cause I'm in my sin," and "Check all your razors and your guns, we gonna be wrestling when the wagon comes." Fats Waller, in his recording of the "The Joint is Jumpin," makes similar references. A police whistle sounds as an indication that the joint (house, not marijuana) is being raided. References are made to "sissies switching around," and he warns "Don't give your right names!" At parties and performances Bessie Jackson (Lucille Bogan) sang "Bulldyke Woman's Blues" and Al Miller and his Swing Stompers did "Ain't That a Mess" (a song about all kinds of incestual relations in one family). These songs were sung without compunction. But it must be remembered that this was before the current women's liberation and gay activist movements, and they were recorded in a milieu that regarded homosexuality as a simple fact of life (during the Twenties and Thirties).

Women blues singers from the past to the present—Ida Cox, Mamie Smith, Ma Rainey, Bessie Smith, Bessie Jackson, Billie Holiday, Dinah Washington, early recordings of Lena Horne, Esther Phillips, Aretha Franklin, Nina Simone—where heard in the home of Blacks. Hence young females have listened to and identified with the women in the songs for generations. The younger females observed that the behavior of adult females frequently paralleled the behavior of the women described in the songs. The idea and image of men and sex being integral to and necessary for life became firmly embedded and eventually internalized in their minds. The similarity in the sentiments expressed in the songs remains relatively unchanged from generation to generation. View the following lyrics.

> People have different blues and think they're mighty sad/But blues about a man is the worst I ever had . . .
>
> —Ma Rainey (1920s)

> The blues ain't nothing but a woman crying for her man/When she wants some lovin'. I'm sure all you women will understand . . .
>
> —Dinah Washington (1950s)

> Don't send me no doctor to fill me up with all those pills/Got me a man named Dr. Feelgood/Takes care of all my pains and ills . . .
>
> —Aretha Franklin (1960s)

• • •

Among the Black youth of today, house rent parties are not even a memory, but the youth of today still party. They eat, drink, smoke, and dance. The Mess Around and Black Bottom (dances) have been replaced with the Gring (1950s), the Funky Chicken (1960s), and the Freak, the Rock, and the Dog (1970s). Generation upon generation apply different names to the sexual gyrations, with the implicative term "dry fuck" remaining unchanged.

Music—live entertainment, radio, and records—continues to provide the rhythms for the latest dance steps while lyrics continue to pour out sentiments about the material conditions of life for Black people and the personal problems and crises that exist between men and women. However, the message and meanings in the songs are no longer so astute in portraying social conditions within a political context. Commercial recording industries, with their number one goal being profit at any cost, did not allow music by, for, and about Blacks to retain its authenticity. Companies were established to record Black music. That music, one of the few areas where Blacks presented their own definitions, was violated and exploited.

> "Classic blues became a women-oriented idiom which often capitalized on lyrics that were explicit in their sexual connotations. Although the records were aimed toward the race market and were heavily purchased by Blacks, they were bought by Whites, too. The image of the Black woman is thus again projected as in the bordellos and previously on plantations as a sex object, alluring and suggestive. Though her own feelings of depressions, misery and heartbreak were aimed toward her Black men, she was being exploited by Whites for economic reasons and purposes."[7]

Black music today is heavily exploited by the White record industry. Popular Black artists, females and males, may attempt to produce songs that can be identified with various segments of the Black population and with a resistance to and struggle against oppressive conditions. However, recording corporations mainly produce a music whose role as a social conditioner is more of a sexual stimulant than anything else.

The role of religion figures prominently in the sexual socialization of most Black women. The rich gospel life with its Baptists moans, sanctified bounce, and spirited strutting was and is as rich emotional part of certain Black women's upbringing as blues and jazz was to other young women. In the "puritanical" homes, sex was spoken of as "sinful," and "nice, decent" girls didn't attend functions that featured "sinful ways."

The messages from their mothers and older females about the sinfulness of sex, though not totally unheeded, did not stop the young girls from engaging in sexual explorations with young males at church-related events and activities (Sunday school, church outings, etc.). Here again one sees the ambivalence: an unmarried teenage mother's baby would be welcomed and handled by all the women parishioners, including the minister's wife—that is, sex was "sinful," yet the product of "sinfulness" was welcomed.

It is interesting to note the results of a comparative study of premarital coitus, religion, and the southern Black. Data was gathered from a southern Black college, a Midwestern White university, and a Swedish university. Church attendance was a factor considered in the comparisons since, in previous studies, the researchers had found religion to be a most important factor operating to restrict variant sexual activity. They cited Kinsey, who reported little difference among the denominations, but considerable difference between the religiously active or devout on the one hand, and those less active or devout on the other. The former showed up with lower rates on virtually every type of disapproved sexual behavior that Kinsey studied, and this was especially true of premarital sex.[8] This relationship did not hold for the data gathered in the study of the southern Blacks. The conclusions reached were: religiosity as measured by church attendance had more effect in controlling premarital sex among the Whites than among the Blacks in the samples.[9] (As a matter of fact, for the Blacks in three of the four comparisons, coitus incidence is greater for the frequent church attenders, contrary to expectations.)

The conclusion in the study is in harmony with a similar conclusion reached by Reiss and based upon analysis of attitudinal data. For the Blacks in his sample, Reiss found little difference between frequent and infrequent church attenders in the acceptance of premarital coitus. In contrast with White society, he explained, Black communities generally have lacked strong ecclesiastical authority over sex, with their churches serving more as a source of tension reduction than as enforcers of a puritanical code of ethics.[10]

In a curious light it can be said that historically religious expressions and sexual expressions played similar roles in the survival experiences of Blacks. Religion, it is often said, provided a source of hope, and escape from the horrendous realities of slave and post-slave life. It offered faith as a healer, a balm, that renewed the spirit and soul, enabling the worshippers to continue with their daily hardships. At the end of grueling and bitter work weeks, thousands of Black folks have historically flocked to churches to have heart and soul restored and replenished, to experience joy and pleasure, religious fervor and zeal, which frequently culminated in "gettin' happy" or "gettin' in the spirit." Also on weekends, thousands of Blacks headed for the Chicken Shack, the Bucket of Blood, or Lil's Bar, or would go stompin at the Savoy, or doing the do at Minton's Play House, or boogeying at Rockland Palace or the Audubon. These places, too, served as meeting grounds where spirits were elevated and restored, the soul was replenished and hopes ran high. Joy and pleasure were experienced through dancing and other sexual expressions and encounters, which frequently resulted in deliciously heightened emotions. Opiates of the masses? Or survival activities? It has often been said that religious leaders could lead their flock to the sea or off a mountaintop. Great blues or rhythm-and-blues singers could also lead their audiences dancing and swinging to whatever destination they chose.

Young black females growing up in homes with strong or weak religious influence, Catholic or Holy Roller, were cognizant of an ambiguity associated with sex. Sex was a sort of a "desirable no-no," an "attractive nuisance." How this ambiguity was resolved was largely dependent on what was learned from messages and behaviors of significant persons in the families and from the community and peer ethos. This included information about heterosexuality and homosexuality. For example, young girls were aware of the admiration bestowed on the minister by adult females. They were also aware that occasionally the ministers had a sexual preference for younger boys.

Homosexuality among men in Black communities was considered a dubious distinction. (This, too, is prior to the gay activist movement and does not apply to those in the "fast life"—entertainers, celebrities, etc., during the Forties through the Seventies.) The male homosexual was not categorically ostracized, nor did he become totally invisible. The extent of derisions and/or acceptance depended to a great extent on how he manifested his homosexuality. Those who were extremely flamboyant in mannerism or dress were targeted for taunts ridicule, and occasional physical abuse. Those homosexuals who went about their business without an ostentatious display of what was considered to be female characteristics and behaviors, and who were discreet in their sexual encounters, were more or less "tolerated" and "accepted". The popular explanation was that these men acting sort of "sissyish" were "mama's boys" who had never grown out of that stage (whatever that stage was supposed to be)—that they had never been able to "cut their mothers' apron strings." The attitude toward male homosexuals reflected a curious tendency to recognize and even overemphasize a positive quality in spite of the gayness. For example, a male who acted kind of "sissyish" was also a *good* cook or a *good* artist or a *good* hair-dresser. Young males, however, were warned by their families to "stay away' from Mr. So-and-so. The young males implicitly understood that the reason for staying away from Mr. So-and-so was because he might "do something funny" to them—and this something funny was con-nected with sex. It is important to note here that, with males, sex was a very definite part of the definition of being homosexual.

A curious combination of intrigue and fear concerning male homo-sexuals developed in the mind of young Black males. At later stages of development it was uncommon for groups of gangs of young Black males (ages thirteen to seventeen) to extort money form the local neighborhood homosexuals. On ore more of the group members would volunteer or would be elected or designated to become sexually involved with the older man for a monetary reward. The money would be used for alcoholic beverages, drugs, or food, or put to whatever use was deemed necessary and desirable by the group. The prevailing atti-tude surrounding involvement with a homosexual adult male was, "it's no big deal. You just let him get his rocks off for a while, and then you get paid for doing nothing. It's a quick way to make some dough."

If the youth was passive rather than active in the sex act, that kept him "honest" and "innocent" of being homosexual. In cases were the young male was the active participant, he maintained his maleness, or macho-ness, with his peers on the grounds that he was playing the male role.

In the case of the young male being passive, and analogy can be made to male/female, active/passive roles in heterosexual sex. The young male is playing the role of the female. He can "just be there while the older male gets his pleasure. Being used is equated with female in the sex act. The young males, however, demand and receive pay. If the female demands and receives pay, she is labeled a whore. The double standard is working and, what's more, the young males are being socialized to view females as sexual objects that provide the sources for their pleasures. As they grow older, they learn from females and occasionally are informed by older men that women can and do play active roles in the sex act and also can show them a trick or two or three.

The fact and idea of homosexuality among women as an issue in the sexual socialization of Black women is a story with silences and denials as its most salient features. Female homosexuals (the term "lesbian" was not a popular one prior to the current gay activist movement) were viewed as "something that wasn't supposed to be." Lesbianism was considered "unnatural." The female homosexual was seen as a "man" and it was said "it's not natural for a woman to be a man!" The expression "to be a man" is key to comprehending the attitude toward female homosexuals in Black culture. The female homosexual was spoken of as if a biological condition existed. "Now, a woman is not supposed to be a man, and anyone who was what they weren't supposed to be was a sort of freak, and oddity, going against 'nature.' " Consequently, that person was to be pitied and one felt ashamed of or for "it" (her). "It" was an embarrassment. In Black communities, homosexuals were referred to as "it," not "he" or "she."

On the one hand, female homosexuals were denied "existence" by the community's refusal to openly acknowledge their lifestyle. On the other hand, when references were made to female homosexuals, it was mostly in terms of an image of woman as man. The predominant image was of a rough, tough-looking woman with short hair, wearing men's clothing and shoes, capable of drinking and swearing "like a man." It was said that lesbians "acted like men" and were "capable of cutting with razors"; one kept one's distance from these women. Young Black females in beauty parlors would hear remarks being made about "bulldaggers" or funny women." The victims were so designated largely on the basis of superficial appearances. "You could tell one of them by the way they looked."

An interesting and important point to mention is that the dominant theme of ideas expressed about female homosexuals did not relate to their sexual encounters. Certainly a percentage of the Black female homosexuals had sexual involvements with women (some had involvements with men), and somewhere in the recess of the mind of adult Black women there was an awareness of this fact. The question of why they chose to emphasize the so-called "unnaturalness" of these women and to downplay the sexual preference, since sexual contact between Black women was and is a reality, calls for further research and analysis, What we are concerned with here are the attitudes transmitted to the young Black females concerning sexual patterns and values.

The types of messages that young females received about homosexual females seldom included explicit factual information. The primary message was simply to "stay away from them." (The denial of their existence was so thorough that older women were essentially in the ludicrous position of warning young females and something that didn't exist.) The combination of the mystery and denial surrounding the Black female homosexual created an indigestible image for young Black women. This resulted in their being grossly ignorant about homosexuality and fearful of the "bulldagger," which in reality was little less than the stereotypical image of a crude male. As previously sated, explicit connections between sexual relationships and female homosexuality were rarely mentioned in the presence of young girls. The idea of a female wanting to define and express herself along non-heterosexual lines was not considered. The concept of a patriarchal society, wherein women were oppressed and therefore would logically want to break out of old patterns, was not considered as part of the psychological composition of the female homosexual. The image excluded having any mental process other than the desire to be like a man. The concept that young Black females developed concerning female homosexuality was an image of a man-woman—that is, a mannish, rough, tough, heavyset, tall or super-athletic-looking female. Central to this idea is the fact that there is a prohibition against usurping the prerogatives or the appearance of the male.

The present-day, highly discussed homophobia in Black communities must be regarded in the context of this background. Young Black females—whether they are on college campuses, on city streets, in Westchester suburbs, in Manhattan penthouses—who react negatively to lesbianism are reacting to a set of ideas and notions that differ markedly form the concepts and ideologies that surround the progressive-minded, politically astute, White and Black lesbian cultures. Present-day political lesbians speak of a feminist/lesbian politics and ideology. They are redefining women's lives in light of a raised consciousness which enables women to see their roles as women under patriarchy as oppressive and therefore to see a need for radical change. What the Black community and, in particular, Black males are reacting to are a combination of facts, myths, and old notions coupled with a resistance to change. Black feminists and/or lesbians are seen as identifying with White culture, despite references in many accounts of life in African cultures to women identifying with or relating to other women. The resentment is partially located in the "fact" that Black women are identifying with White. (The attitude is that, regardless of what benefits it may bring, "White" behavior is not for Black women.) There is also resentment of the idea of Black women becoming lesbian because of the old highly negative image of female homosexuality is still actively asserting itself.

Furthermore, the open association of sex with lesbians is a reckoning that cannot be denied today. When one recalls the belief that same-sex erotic love has its locus in the "unnatural," it can be seen that the idea of Black lesbianism is a highly unpalatable one for the Black community. There is a reluctance to seriously address the inequalities and exploitative practices that exist in Black female/male sexual relationships, as well as a resistance—indeed, a refusal—to consider lesbianism as a sexual politic. To do so might readily and logically result in Black males being displaced as number one on the sex scene. Black males fear another rejection of them, this time by lesbians. Consequently, they defensively focus on attacking those aspects female homosexuality (lesbianism) that they know will ensure support from the overwhelming majority of the Black community. They focus on the myths: (1) it's unnatural for a woman to "be like a man"; (2) lesbians *hate* men, but black men and women need to work in concert against racism. Here they are using the myth of lesbians as men-haters in conjunction with a positive truism; this serves the purposes of further alienating lesbians (and heterosexual Blacks); (3) lesbians really want and need a man, but since the couldn't get one, are competing against men, and if they succeed, our race will suffer from lack of reproduction (chauvinistic thinking and gross ignorance about who wants and can have babies).

On another level, homophobia in Black communities can be analyzed in terms of psychological defense mechanisms. This is particularly applicable to Black males. It would seem logical that since Blacks are racially oppressed, oppression for other reasons could be understood by them. Yet, there is an extremely hostile homophobic reaction, particularly among black males. The issue of lesbianism is used as a red herring to avoid reexamining and redefining Black female/male relationships. Many Black males refrain from examining lesbian politics in fear of having to relinquish some of their treasured male privileges. A reaction to lesbianism on this level represents a form of homophobic attitude. Black males who may be progressive-minded, extremely intelligent, very astute, and articulate become emotionally blind, irrationally stubborn, unnecessarily hostile, and downright reactionary when it comes to the topic lesbianism. They will cling to a stereotypical definition of female homosexuality rather than considering and accepting a current, enlightened definition.

For example, the definition of lesbianism that follows can hardly be interpreted as being a disruptive or damaging factor in Black communities. "Lesbianism—an intimate relationship between women on the conscious level, elements of this intimate relationship being: sensitivity, spiritual nurturing, validation of self, emotional and psychological growth. Expression of physical love may or may not be a part of the relationship."[11]

However, the idea of a proliferation of Black women adhering to such a definition would cause much consternation, confusion, and anxiety among most black males. They would interpret it, and rightly so, as meaning that Black women no longer were concentrating primarily on defending and nurturing the male ego. They would also feel that they were being rejected as Numero Uno in the love lives of Black women. In actuality the Black woman who rediscovers her womanhood—"colored girls who no longer consider suicide because the rainbow is enough"—will be better able to develop strong female/male relationships.

It is unwise to talk about the Black community as homophobic unless the homophobia is analyzed within the socio-psychological context Black dynamics. As has been reiterated, the Afro-American culture and the societal pressures of racial and economic oppressions have indeed constituted a society with two distinct cultures—one White and one Black. Therefore, a phenomenon that appears to be similar for both racial groups requires a historical analysis in order to attain an accurate and valid perspective. Black maleness and White maleness have similarities and differences. It is the differences that are critical in discussing Black males and females and their relations, of which lesbianism is a part.

There unquestionably is a strong negative reaction to Black lesbians within the Black community. However, the reason for this must be analyzed within the historical framework of interracial sexual attitudes. This will enable a strategy to be devised that will deal with the causes of the problem as well as with the manifestations of the problem. This is not to say that reactionary behaviors such as name calling, physical attacks, and sexual harassment stemming from homophobia can be sanctioned. By no stretch of the imagination can cruel, insensitive, ignorant, violent behavior be justified. There are a growing number of Black lesbians whose voices are being heard on the Black political scene. Their roles will be incorporated into the sexual socialization of young Black females.

An analysis of Black feminism, such as "A Black Feminist Statement," which was produced by the Combahee River Collective, unmistakably reveals a political, scholarly, and progressive-minded perspective which, not surprisingly, is threatening to those males who fear and resent giving up some male privilege and having to rethink their attitudes and behavior toward women and child raising. The following passage comes from "A Black Feminist Statement" and is taken from the section on "What We Believe":

. . . Although we are feminists and lesbians, we feel solidarity with progressive Black men and do not advocate the fractionalization that white women who are separatists demand. Our situation as Black people necessitates that we have solidarity around the fact of race, which white women of course do not need to have with white men, unless it is their negative solidarity as racial oppressors. We struggle together with Black men against racism, while we also struggle with Black men about sexism.

We realize that the liberation of all oppressed peoples necessitates the destruction of the political-economic systems of capitalism and imperialism, as well as patriarchy. We are socialists because we believe that work must be organized for the collective benefit of those who do the work and create the products and not for the profit of the bosses. Material resources must be equally distributed among those who create these resources. We are not convinced, however, that a socialist revolution that is not also a feminist and anti-racist revolution will guarantee our liberation. We have arrived at the necessity of developing an understanding of class relationships that takes into account the specific class position of Black women who are generally marginal in the labor force, while at this particular time some of us are temporarily viewed as doubly desirable tokens at white-collar and professional levels. Although we are in essential agreement with Marx's theory as it applied to the very specific economic relationships he analyzed, we know that this analysis must be extended further in order for us to understand our specific economic situation as Black women.[12]

In looking again at the sexual socialization of Black females prior to the influence of the current women's movement and the gay activist movement, consideration must be given to those post-adolescent females who felt sexually inclined toward other females while growing up, yet preferred the company of males to females after adolescence. It is known that a society develops and produces the types of individuals it needs and feels are necessary for the maintenance of that society at a particular time in history. So it can be speculated that the Black community did not nurture female relations that exceeded the prescribed lines for female friendships. There is a strong history of friendships between women—women gathering together in beauty parlors, women meeting in the kitchen over a cup of tea, coffee, or soup; women talking on the stoops; and women congregating at church meetings. However, these relationships are considered as platonic: loving but not sexual, affectionate but one doesn't fondle.

In an interview, Adrienne Rich talks about unconsummated relationships and the need to reevaluate the meaning of intense, yet supposedly non-erotic, connections between women. She asserts: "We need a lot more documentation about what actually happened. I think we can also imagine it because we know it happened. We know it happened. We know it out of our own lives."[13] The question must be raised as to what happens when there is the desire on the part of women to love sexually, to fondle, to caress, and to send inordinate amounts of time together. The close childhood friendships with holding hands and later walking arm in arm and staying overnight at one another's homes, the close-knit adult friendships—both must be channeled along purely platonic lines in order to be "acceptable" and "respectable." The erotic feelings and expressions have had to be "put on hold" or indulged in and not named.

The young Black female enters adulthood with a fixed idea about homosexuality. That fixed idea does not give her latitude for expressing her sexuality along any other lines than heterosexual ones. The concept of heterosexuality (forced as it is) is easily incorporated, given the Black female's background of her linkage with men, and the messages she received about men and sex: men are the barometer for good times, happiness, glad times, sad times, troubled times; the other half of a partnership; the ones women can't live with and can't live without; the sharers of hard times and the good life—the vicissitudes of life. She has been socialized to believe that sex is equated with man, not woman—not even a woman who "looks like [is] a man."

Black heterosexual males and females must become knowledgeable about the concept of lesbianism as a political measure, as a force against sexual oppression. Lesbians should not be viewed as being "sick," simply because they are not. Wife-beating, battered women, child abuse, the proliferation of pornography involving the young and innocent, enslaving young women (and men) in prostitution—these horrendous corruptions, heinous crimes, and inexcusable behaviors do not generate the phobic, hostile reaction that lesbianism does. The question must be raised: Does heterosexuality exempt behavior from being viewed as "sick," "abnormal," and an object of derision to the Black population?

An understanding of lesbian politics will help all Blacks feel less defensive. Black lesbians and all other thoughtful Blacks must continue to define and clarify the lesbian position in terms of a serious politic that deals with patriarchy under capitalism, racism, and classism.

Myths and stereotypes other than those related to homosexuality also play an insidious role in the young Black female's sexual socialization. Black mothers frequently overreact in response to the old myths and stereotypes about Black women being licentious, loose, immoral, and promiscuous. This overreaction takes the form of the mother being doubly strict with the rules of behavior she sets for her daughters in their dress and deportment. There may be an excessive concern about looking "decent" in public to offset stereotypes. Again, it must be emphasized that there is no monolithic Black female group. There are prostitutes among Black women, but the reason has absolutely nothing to do with a gene for licentiousness or any other such irrational explanation. . . .

Present-day society still reinforces certain myths about Black women. The young Black female experiences directly, indirectly, and vicariously hostility, violence, and sexual abuse, which are the symptoms of economic, sexual, and racial oppressions. The battered woman, childhood sexual abuse, incest, sexual harassment and extortion, rape, unwanted pregnancies, butchered abortions—these become part of her socialization as a female and, as such, influence and affect her adult sexual attitudes and behaviors. . . .

The knowledge of Black male oppression does not seem to seriously interfere with the sexual intimacy among Black men and women. The reasons for this are manifold. The word oppression may be somewhat inappropriate, since its popular usage implies systematic overpowering or imposition by abuse of power and authority, and in the case of Black men and women such domination/overpowering is not automatically transferred to other areas of social living. In addition, there are numerous Black women who neither act nor feel oppressed or over-powered in their intimate sexual relations with men. What cannot be denied is the fact that, as was pointed out by one of the women in the group, Black men in general place their number-one claim to man-hood in the locale of the groin palace, the home of the dick.

The growing awareness that their roles as women in Black society are in need of some revising was apparent in their discussion. The emer-gence of a different attitude toward males, one that is more demanding of equality in sexual and social areas, is addressed more specifically in the following discussion among four Black women: Dot, age 25, college graduate, social worker for Welfare Depart-ment, separated; Jean, age 35, two years of college, clerical worker, married; Betty, age 28 high school graduate, beautician, serial monogamy, no marriage; Sadie age 40, dietician in a public school, twice married now single.

DOT: I have just entered a new phase in my attitude toward sex. Between the media and the way I was socialized I came to look at sex as a romantic ideal. Now that's all different.

JEAN: How's that?

DOT: The way I see sex now it—it's politics, it's cash, its eco-nomics. I'm at the point where I see it as an exchange, but not a romantic exchange.

JEAN: I'm afraid I'm beginning to hear you.

DOT: In other words, no more sex in exchange for sex alone. Because the way I feel, he's getting and I'm giving! He's feeling "good" and I'm feeling tired and used.

SADIE: So you mean you're going to use sex specifically as a means to obtain other things?

DOT: Well yes, and its not my idealistic view, I wasn't raised like that, but I've become that way.

JEAN: When did get you rid of your idealistic views?

DOT: Well, within the last three relationships I had. The past three years.

BETTY: That sounds kind of interesting.

DOT: Yeah, I would say that from my experiences I've adopted this view. Not from what Mom and Dad taught me, but from the politics that males and females play. Sexual politics. You know, I got taken off. I was trying to be nice you know, romance and all that ha-di-ha-di-da.

JEAN: When you say "sexual politics," just what do you mean?

DOT: Sexual politics between a man and a woman. Games.

JEAN: Games, huh?

DOT: Yeah, X and Y, me and him, racking up points or trying to rack up points against one another.

BETTY: And who came out ahead?

DOT: Well, the last three—*they* came out on top

Betty: They *did* you in?

DOT: Did me in! But no more. It's an exchange from now on, but on my terms!

JEAN: And what are those?

DOT: I love to have the pleasure of sex, but he's got to give me something first. I have to put it on that level because when I was giving out of my heart, I didn't get nothing in return. I was giving but I didn't get.

BETTY: I hear you. I hear you.

DOT: And I don't necessarily like that policy, but I can't just, you know, be used for the American dream of romance.

BETTY: That's right. I'm with you sister!

DOT: Sex is pleasurable. It's pleasurable. But it ain't gonna be only pleasurable. It's gonna be pleasurable and something else. Dig it. Just being pleasurable ain't enough. Those days are over for me. 'Cause it can be pleasurable and I still ain't got no food in the 'fridge. That does not add up. Economics, you know. You've got to look at everything these days in those terms. The thing of it is that I don't like being like that 'cause I really care. It's like splitting myself, I feel like I'm splitting myself, you know.

JEAN: Well, tell me this now. If you go out with a guy and he really appeals to you, would you want to go to bed with him because he's him? No economics attached.

DOT: Well, I don't know.

BETTY (*laughing*): You could be persuaded.

DOT: Yeah, but I mean, you know, that does not necessarily excite me anymore. That kind of just physical stuff. It's gotta be more that just you look good, or when you talk your words come out a certain way.

BETTY: But you *could* be persuaded

DOT: Yeah, well, I could be persuaded. But I find it very, very difficult to get down and stay on the sexual level alone.

BETTY: I prefer flirting. Holding hands, walking through the park. That's physical and could be considered sexual.

DOT: I don't consider that sexual at all! That's kid stuff!

SADIE: It really doesn't pay to be involved with men just to be involved. The way men are, I don't trust them no more. You know. (*Agreement expressed from others.*)

DOT: And they lie about everything. Generally.

SADIE: That's why you can't trust them. You know, it takes a while for men to be truthful.

JEAN: You all sure are putting down the Black men when you say those things.

DOT: No, I just don't want to operate with him at *his* level. Lying and cheating. They can't understand *why* we as women want to do the things we may be into—like health awareness. Abortion rights.

JEAN: Let's be more positive and analytical. Men are important in our lives right?

BETTY: Oh, that's obvious.

SADIE: It's not so obvious to me anymore.

DOT: There's a lot of things that I like about them and a lot of tings that I don't like about them.

SADIE: It's what I don't like about them that I feel needs to be changed.

BETTY: You think you can change a man?

SADIE: No, but if we change, they'll *have* to change.

JEAN: I like the idea of meeting a man, starting a relationship and both of us going forward with it.

BETTY: I enjoy a man's company. It's fun. I like the physical difference I like the mental and emotional difference.

SADIE: Too often all you get is mental and emotional *stress*!

JEAN: Yeah, but we women still put up with them.

SADIE: I'm at the point now where I don't accept the man's role as the way it's been defined. You know, I don't believe in double standards where they hogwashed me all my life. Don't expect of me what you can't expect of yourself. Forget the double standards. Do you hear what I'm saying?

DOT: All I'm trying to say is I don't like the idea of men being able to do, like Momma used to say, "Well, a man can go and get drunk and . . ." Did your Momma ever used to tell you that? "He can get drunk and lay in the gutter and the next day he gets home and puts on his suit and he's still a man. But if a woman does it, she's a slut and all that." I don't think that should be. If she wants to lay in the gutter, you know, she should be able to get up, just like a man, get up the next day and go on about her business. And nobody say nothing except, "Sally was laying in the gutter yesterday." Or, "John was laying in the gutter the day before." You know. It's not so much a male/female thing as they make it.

BETTY: Maybe you should check out that gutter.

DOT: Yeah, you know. Check out the people that's in it.

Betty: Take me to the gutter and drop me off. That's cool. I'll lay in there myself. It might be cool. Everybody has to have a thing.

DOT: But my main concern is where his head is, how he acts, you know. What are his beliefs, what kind of culture does he come from? Is it on the map? (*laughter*)

SADIE: And where you come from sometimes also determines the kind of sexual activities you get involved with.

DOT: Right. If you don't have communication somebody who may seem nice and do all these things that you want, then when it comes time for the sexual they may be very cold, or the may be very macho. You know, they may be very quiet, and you like a screamer.

BETTY: That's the cutest thing. Being in bed and trying to explain like, "Ah . . .sweetheart, you know, that wasn't getting it. (*laughter*) Like you're trying to ram my, you know, my gizzards through my elbow. Don't do it like that. Have a little tenderness." You know a lot of men have to learn that it's not so much the heavy jamming as the communication involved. And so, you know it would be easier to get together sexually if your communication is in "synch." And then bring that communication right on outside with you—to the kitchen after you done finished with the bedroom.

JEAN: Establishing that communication can be a trip. Sometimes it hardly seems worth the bother.

DOT: Well, they're going to bother you anyway. Virtually not a day goes by when they don't bother me, you know. Also contact with men helps me to write good poetry—to bother with them also helps me to be creative about dealing with them. And so since they are here, they have to be dealt with. 'Cause you know, we can't leave them alone. They couldn't survive and where would we be?

SADIE: In my last relationship I was making an effort to do right. I suggested that we compromise on certain things. Not always do things his way. Well, he thought I was trying to prove something to him. He got an attitude. I said, "Let's deal with things like two adults. I'll give some leeway on some things and you on others," because he might be more cool in some areas, and I might be a little more cool in another. But we're going to do tings fifty-fifty, I said. You know, like if you want me to massage your feet, you've go to bathe me too. I'll lotion you down one night, you lotion me down the next night. Why I always got to be lotioning you down? Goddammit, you know, I work too. When I want to get lotioned down I got to go to a masseuse. I got to lotion you down, take a course on how to do it, to please you. Well, the upshot of it all was he split.

BETTY: Well, you know, it takes a lot of doing to get a man to accept a fifty-fifty relationship. You have to do it in a way so that you don't intimidate him because he is emotionally weaker than we are. He doesn't want to admit it, but he is. So we have to carry a lot of the weight in the relationship.

JEAN: But you know, women carry the heaviest burdens, and for years we have been putting up with an unequal exchange. And we continue to up with them in the same old ways.

BETTY: It's not so much of a burden. I don't look at is so much as a burden. 'Cause I ain't going to let nothing be no burden, now. If you have to be a burden, go on your way! But we have to work it out together because we're in a tough situation together. It's a tough struggle for all Black people.

DOT: If it was all women, you'd have to put up with the same thing.

JEAN: No, you can't say that. It wouldn't be the same with women. Since women carry the burdens, you'd have all burden carriers. There would be more sharing of loads. What do you get in exchange for the heavy load you're carrying?

DOT: I see it more as a mission than a burden.

JEAN: Okay. We can call it a mission.

BETTY: Yeah, it's a mission and a challenge. It's a mission and a challenge just like everything else. Black men represent our mission and our challenge. Because I think if Black men and Black women—and this is my one political reality of the day—if we don't somehow soon get together it will be catastrophic. I feel that one of the personal satisfactions in dealing with Black men is reinforcement as a person. You know, trying to do what's supposed to be the correct thing to do as an individual. Now I can say that I get my reinforcement as a woman by sticking by Black men.

SADIE: It's never been easy for Black women. It's been real difficult. It's my nationalism coming out now. I'm for helping all of us Black people get together. And it's also a learning experience, I would say. A learning experience in working toward a closer perfection of unity.

BETTY: I get a lot of nationalistic satisfaction, too. You know, it's somewhat of a burden, but it's with him. It ain't with White Joe Blow over there. It's with *him*. So we'll know that the species will continue and you get some personal satisfaction out of knowing that. Not necessarily as a woman, but as a person dealing with another person and coming to some compromise together.

DOT: Yeah, I *used* to feel strong about the continuation of our nationalism. About his Blackness.

JEAN: What do you mean *his* Blackness?

DOT: I mean the fact that Black men have been fucked over and are fucked up and we can't desert them. I wouldn't go out with a White man. I'm just going to make the Black man pay a price. No one gets a free lunch anymore.

JEAN: *You* may not go out with a White man, but they damn sure go out with White women.

BETTY: That's why I like the fact that we are maintaining the Black family. I feel very strongly about that. I'm doing my little piece by sticking with Black men.

SADIE: Maintaining the Black family?

BETTY: Black male and female relationships—yes, yes, the Black family. That's the mission. Besides you get personal gratification, you know, the fact that I made the effort within the Black family structure. You know what I'm saying? 'Cause I wouldn't want to go through that mission with another woman.

JEAN: But you already do.

BETTY: I wouldn't want to in the same sense!

JEAN: You're in a household family structure with women and they constitute a major part of the Black family.

BETTY: I mean just pertaining to Black male and female relationships. Hey! My mother and father, case in point. They've been together for thirty-two years and they're always constantly accentuating one another. Mom carried the heavier burden, but my father hung in there. They maintained their relationships with all their burdens.

JEAN: Okay, okay. I hear all these reasons for maintaining relationships with our Black men—like personal gratification, a learning experience for working toward unity, and maintaining the Black family, but on a really personal and intimate level, what do you receive from the relationship?

DOT: We receive *nothing!* (*laughter*) We receive nothing!

BETTY: (*in mock tones*): We got nothin'. You know (*in a loud tone*) to all you Black men out there in the sound of my voice, if you're in the sound of my voice put your hand on the radio. *We got nothing!* (*laughter*)

DOT: You give me that call to arms and watch some bitch come and hit them with a frying pan, and pick up her thirty-eight with her other hand, you know, in a southward direction, and let 'em have it. Years of reparation are due. Oh, God, (*laughter*) we can't let them die like that. We just can't.

SADIE: Now let's get back to Jean's question. I must say that I did get certain satisfaction from both my marriages, but sexual intimacy wasn't the main source of my satisfaction.

BETTY: Let me say this. I like to fuck as much as anybody, and as long as Black men are around there will be fucking.

DOT: If you're going to fuck anyway, why fuck for free? It's a physical need, so you might as well go and get some like I already said in the beginning, get something else with it! Just a commitment to him ain't enough.

JEAN: It's only a physical need because you and society *made* it a physical need. People are conditioned to want sex.

DOT: Getting horny and wanting a man is natural! You must have been conditioned to think that it's *not* natural.

JEAN: Feeling horny may be natural, but *wanting a man* is conditioning! And that's a fact!

SADIE: Dot, at one time I thought the same way you did, now I'm beginning to wonder what it really was that gave me satisfaction, pleasure, in those relationships. What was it, really?

BETTY: Listen, you all. I got to say this—the dick is good! (*laughter*) The dick *is* good. And for me, I'm just the sweetest he done had. I know this is the sweetest thing he ever done had. So if I don't get something for it, he'd probably think I'd give it up to anybody free. I don't want him to think that. Shit! So I just collect a little rent and get me some threads now and then, you know, it's like that.

DOT: It does make you feel good.

BETTY: Oh, when you be coming ain't nothing like coming! It's the best.

DOT: It's nice, it's good exercise. You can run track, but it just ain't the same thing. I think sexual intercourse is the best relaxer around other than the sauna. 'Cause if I can't get no sex, ain't nobody giving up no money. I go to the sauna and exercise and come home and masturbate and feel real good.

JEAN: But you'd rather have the man!

DOT: If there's a choice, yes. But sometimes you don't even want the damn choice for the hassle. It ain't worth the hassle. And it's not like you can say after you've had intercourse, "Okay, get up and go home. I came already, did you come? Now you can get up and go home. I've got some work to do." You can't do that.

BETTY: Personally I prefer a small dick.

JEAN: Size isn't supposed to matter.

SADIE: You couldn't prove it by barber or beauty shop talk.

DOT: Now you know what's a real joke, an embarrassment? A big two hundred and fifty pound dude with a three-inch peter. Peter is dick's little brother, you know. And you're supposed to act like it's all right.

BETTY: Well, you have got more chance to get clitoral stimulation with somebody with a small penis usually. For my build anyway.

SADIE: My final comment is, we got some problems to work out. You hear me, women? (*Doing take-off on Betty*) "Listen all you Black women out there in the sound of my voice. If you're in the sound of my voice, put your hands together and listen. We Black women have to consider some serious changes in our relationships with Black men, because we've had enough! And we know they can do better! Amen." (*Group laughter and approval*)

The Black women's comments reflect an experienced view of the effects of institutionalized heterosexuality on their relationships with men. The direct sexual feelings expressed would be termed lewd, dirty, unnecessary, or shameful only if viewed from lifeless Puritanism of Anglo-Saxon Protestant ethics. The remarks of the women also represent a focus on both the precarious sexual relationship between Black men and women and the strong counterforce of uninhibited and unrestricted joy to be found in sex. The women are direct and explicit in expressing their feelings. At times they seem to vacillate; such is the actual case. There are serious problematic aspects in their relationships with men and, in trying to think through their problems and develop new strategies and tactics, there are uncertainties in their decisions, unsure and compromising behaviors. The reality of Black females linking their existence to males as part of their socialization process was unmistakably reflected in their conversation. Equally represented was a showing of their independent spirit. What was likewise obvious was the infiltration of consumerism with sex as a commodity. We can thus see how people can be molded by environmental factors that override customs, beliefs, and behaviors that at one time were hard and fast enforcers of moral, spiritual, and emotional boundaries.

The conversation also revealed an openness and willingness on the part of the women to talk about their dissatisfactions, likes, and desires about sexual relations. Heretofore many Black women were fearful of losing their man if they did not please him sexually, so they did not disclose dissatisfaction. Black women understand that the Black male has had little opportunity for economic advancement. They have therefore provided ego gratification to the male in the area of sexual relations. In attempting not to further damage the male ego, women sacrificed their feelings. In the long run, this created more problems for both partners.

What must not be overlooked in the four women's conversation is the fact that Black women as well as Black men truly enjoy sex and view orgasm as the ultimate in pleasure. This is a positive factor and should be used as a reward or a lure. Females should not withhold sex if he doesn't behave, or promise him some if he acts right. Males should not feel that they are holding all the aces in the deck and if she doesn't conform to his desires, he'll just keep withholding those aces or play them elsewhere.

In their conversation, these Black women are not only questioning their insights on their own sexuality, they are simultaneously trying to historically analyze and assess the realities of the conditions that have contributed to the present state of affairs between Black Women and Black Men. The orientation toward males as part of the sexual socialization of Black women is a cause of ambivalence. The manner in which the Black woman defines her womanhood is central to a discussion of the attitudes toward Black males produced by the sexual socialization process of Black females.

A California study which had Black female graduate students for its subjects dramatizes how socialization processes account for the Black woman defining herself as an independent being, while simultaneously always defining herself in relation to "man." The following passage describes the women in this study collectively.

> . . . During most of the formative years, she [the daughter] had observed her mother [or the adult female of the house] leave home for work. It was at the outside employment that many hours of the mother's day were spent. With increasing awareness, the child [student] realized that her mother's outside employment had a

meaning of its own. She had another life, which was somewhat independent of but co-existed with their family life. Concurrent with the mother's maintenance of her job was also these manifested concerns for the man of their house. Given her mother's model of an outside independent life, integrated with an actualized concern and relation to her man, the student matured assuming no inherent contradictions between these two entities. Consequently the Black woman was defined as having a "life of her own" and also as "always" being in relation to man.[18]

The following passage demonstrates the formation of female attitudes that carry over into adult years. The family's concern for the welfare of the adult male is geographically articulated.

. . . Whether a father, stepfather, grandfather, or mother's boyfriend, he was a focus of consideration in determining to "cook pork chops instead of liver, 'cause he like 'em," or not to "put too much starch in that shirt, 'cause he don't want no stiff collas," or to "clean your room, 'cause he'll have a fit if he see it filthy." Likewise it was the man who could also alter many previous decisions: "You can't bring your friends over this evening 'cause he's comin'." It was this kind of emphasis within her family background that the Black female graduate student more than likely formed her definition of "Black woman" in relation to man.[19]

Another example of attitudes expressed by older females that contribute to the formation of attitudes toward males can be seen in the following passage from *All Our Kin*. Pride in sons and brothers is demonstrated. The setting is a very economically deprived household, but the sentiments hold true for millions of Black families.

. . . Alberta introduced me to her nineteen-year-old son, she pointed to him and said, "He's a daddy and his baby is four months old." Then she pointed to her twenty-two-year-old son, Mac, and said, "He's a daddy three times over." Mac smiled and said, "I'm no daddy," and his friends in the kitchen said, "Maybe going on four times, Mac." Alberta said, "Yes you are, admit it, boy!" At that point Mac's grandmother rolled back in her rocker and said, "I'm a grandmother many times over and it makes me proud," and Alberta joined her, "Yes, and I'm a grandmother many times over." A friend of Alberta's told me later that Alberta wants her sons to have babies because she thinks it will make them more responsible. Although she does not usually like the women her sons go with, claiming they are "no-good trash," she accepts the babies and asks to care for them whenever she has a chance.20

Females have to learn at early ages (12-13) to cope with young males who emulate older Black males in their attempts at sexual conquests. Thus, the styling, profiling, and pretending begins on the part of both females and males. The young males preen, prance, profile, sweet talk, Bogart, or otherwise participate in the illusionary eroticism and conspicuous paraphernalia of romantic love. The females overdress, underdress, feign attitudes, fight other females over males, and "fall in love" with "tight pants," "pretty eyes," "attention being showered on them," "recognition," peer understanding," and "comfort contact." Once the male sexual conquest is made—or, on some occasions, the female seduction—lack of information about sexual matters frequently results in unwanted pregnancies. The sex act itself often becomes a perfunctory act. The ambivalence surrounding the sex act is particularly complex for the young female. She hears about the joys and "goodness" of sex from adult women, songs, and literature, and she also dreads/fears getting pregnant or losing her virginity. She soon realizes the games, "sexual politics," that are going on.

An older woman, middle-class, age 35, put it this way:

Sisters have been socialized to believe that involvement with males is a real true relationship—a sincere commitment. The brothers, on the other hand, know that they have to "rap" to get over. So they bring wine, flowers, pizza. "If I make her *think* I care, I can get over." [So they imagine.]

"Getting over" means initially the fuck and then the repetition of it whenever the male feels like it. It is a "false" relationship in the sense that the play is to *get over*, not to establish a true relationship. (As Dot said in the conversation, "The sexual politics, the games, it splits me in two.") It is an exchange of services. For the female the game-playing is face-saving. If she gives in without the "games," she is considered a whore. Males play all sorts of games to keep the female believing that she is the one. For example, when they go away they will remind themselves to call So-and-so at a certain time to demonstrate how much they care. Notes for a trip: blue suit, shoe brush, *call Millie*, Brut, toothbrush, *call Marie*, comb, deodorant, *call Sally.* She is just another item that is needed for his care. He may make the call in between fucking rounds, but that doesn't matter. The female will feel cared for. Of course, there are occasions when the females discover the game and resort to some form of violence in retaliation—a slashed waterbed, cut-up suits, a smashed-in car window. But usually the male "gets over" for quite a while.

These games allow the woman to feel that she is not totally unrespected. She can point out to others and to herself, "See, he brings me flowers and records, pizza"—and, later in the game, groceries. Of equal concern is the situation when the male "talks politics"—that is, he is politically serious—and you have an intellectual relationship that doesn't necessitate his bringing flowers. Well, it is not considered disreputable to have this type of open relationship. But if a male starts talking *sex* right away, with no raping or presents, it's not considered respectable. So in most cases, games are played to keep the image of respectability (an important necessity for the woman) and games are played to keep women on the string (an important notion for men). It may take three weeks or more or less for the fuck to be achieved—then good-bye. Conquest is the thing. Black women feel, in many cases, that they "need" a man and it is "unnatural not to have a man." They can "only go so long without one." Should the games be stopped and the women simply say, "I'm in this for a good screw just like you, so let's stop with the games," we would have a new situation. But the male trip is so ingrained and the female role is so ingrained that it is very, very difficult for both parties to change. (Sadies's statement during the conversation, "If we change, they'll have to change," is instructive here.)

Black women are faced with a reality today that demands changes ranging from a slight shift in posture to a complete about-face as they come to grips with their sexuality and relationships with Black men. The women's movement has provided a renewed interest and impetus for Black women to formally organize around issues of feminism and sexual equality, and to informally voice their opinions and attitudes about Black female and male relationships with far less reluctance than in the past. Sex for procreation still has importance for both Black females and males, but the idea of choice is equally as important. When to have children and how many to have are decisions that females figure in more prominently than in the past. A major reality that Black women face is the shortage of Black males. "Black women 25 years old and over are more than twice as likely as white women to remain never married. The situation grows far more grave among the college-educated where—within the urban population 19 to 44 years old—for every 100 males there are 54 extra females without a mate or forced to share somebody else's."[21] It is a well known fact that there are more Black males in jails than in colleges. Drugs, war casualties, interracial marriages and homosexuality increase the scarcity of available males.

The Eighties offer the Black women the challenge of taking a giant step into a region called "her own rights" without divorcing herself from Black culture, which embodies care, concern, and nurturance for the Black community. She must do so without negating her own sexuality, which in many instances she must redefine for herself. She must come into her own being, in relationships with and to men, but ones that do not disallow her personal freedoms, personal happiness, and the opportunity to pursue her personal and private aspirations.

In the Eighties the challenge to the Black women is not to negate or neglect Black men, but to define herself in terms of her needs, her desires, and her psychological and emotional makeup. Her expressions of sexuality are indeed a very personal matter, and unless her sexuality is inextricably connected to a politic of liberating options, it need not to be the most salient aspect of her personality or person. That is to say, whether a woman defines herself as a traditional wife in a monogamous marriage, a lesbian, a celibate, a polygamous wife or a single woman, those decisions in and of themselves tell us very little about her political aspirations or political commitments or ideology. They simply tell us who she may or may not be sleeping with. In the case of traditional monogamy, we would know in general terms that she is in a situation with male dominance as a given. So it is incumbent upon Black women to start defining themselves in terms of a politic that may or may not incorporate their sexual preference.

A woman's sexuality and sexual preference should be a complement to her well-being, not the locus of her well-being. It is neither the dessert not the main course. It could be either, or it could be neither. Black women need to learn to deal with their sexuality. The old notions and myths and stereotypes must be done away with analytically and systematically. Women always have gained strength and support from other women; this practice should be embellished and drawn upon to help women further their self-development. Woman's support groups, organized and run in constructive ways, can provide an excellent source of new ideas while helping to break down old barriers and reestablish warm, rewarding female friendships. A compassionate, erudite, introspective analysis of the relationship between sexuality and politics is needed. As Black women, we have for years been strong and indestructible, as Mari Evans so eloquently put it in her classic poem, "I am a Black Woman":

> . . . I
> am a black woman
> tall as a cypress
> strong
> beyond all definition still
> defying place
> and time
> and circumstance
>   assailed
>   impervious
>   indestructible
> Look
>   on me and be
> renewed.[23]

The Eighties find the Black woman still strong, still defying definition and time. She is faced, however, with a complicated new set of circumstances, as previously examined: the woman's movement, the shortage of Black males, and an America whose corporations are reaping bigger and better profits while the deleterious effects of racism and economic oppression go on, unabated and worsening. The Eighties will be the time for Black women to be renewed as well as to provide the model, symbol, and image for others who seek their own renewal.

1. Carolyn M. Rodgers, *How I Got Ovah*. Garden City: Doubleday & Co. Inc., 1968, p. 15.

2. Amilcar Cabral, "Guardian Voices of Revolution," *The Guardian*, January 1980, p. 17.

3. Adrienne Rich, *Of Woman Born*. New York: W.W. Norton & Co., 1976, p. 182.

4. Carol Stack, *All Our Kin*. Harper/Colophon Books, 1974, p. 47.

5. Michelle Russell, "Slave Codes & Linear Notes," *The Radical Teacher*, March 1977, p. 2.

6. *AC-DC Blues* (Gay Jazz Reissues), ST-106, Stash Records, Inc., P.O. Box 390, Brooklyn, NY 11215

7. Sharon Harley and Rosalyn Terborg-Penn, Daphne Duval, "Black Women in the Blues Tradition," *The Afro-American Woman-Struggles* and Images, p. 71.

8. Harold T. Christensen and Leanor B. Johnson, "Premarital Coitus and the Southern Black: A Comparative View," 1980, unpublished paper, p. 2.

9. Ibid., p. 3.

10. Ibid., p. 4.

11. Nacemah Shabazz, "Homophobia: Myth and Reality," *Heresies*, Vol. 2, No. 4, Winter 1979. New York: Heresies Collective, Inc., 1979.

12. Zillah Eisenstein, ed. *Capitalist Patriarchy and the Case for Socialist Feminism*. New York: Monthly Review Press, 1978.

13. Barbara Smith, "Toward a Black Feminist Criticism," in *In the Memory and Spirit of Frances, Zora and Lorraine*, ed. Juliette Bowles. Washington, D.C.: The Institute for the Arts and Humanities, Howard University, 1979, p. 39.

14. Herbert G. Gutman, *The Black Family in Slavery and Freedom*, 1750-1925. New York: Vantage Books, 1977, pp. 61-62.

15. Ibid.

16. Ibid., p. 63.

17. Bessie Head, *The Collector of Treasures*. London: Heinemann, 1977, p. 39.

18. Jualynne Dodson, "To Define Black Womanhood." Georgia: The Institute of the Black World, p. 17.

19. Ibid, p. 19.

20. Carol Stack, *All Our Kin*. New York: Harper/Colophon Books, 1974, p. 120.

21. "Where Have All of the Black Males Gone?" *Black Male/Female Relationships*, Vol. 1, June-July 1979. San Francisco, California: Black Think Tank, Inc., p. 5.

23. Mari Evans, *I am a Black Woman*. New York: William Morrow & Company, 1970.

Eulenspiegel? What's That?

Ron Tyson

The Eulenspiegel Society Sexual Minorities Report,

PRO-ME-THEE-US, 1973

S/M, which stands for sadomasochism, is a complex erotic practice which plays with roles of dominance and submission as well as with the giving and receiving of pain for erotic gratification. It was hailed as the "last taboo" to be liberated by the sexual revolution. In 1973, the Eulenspiegel Society was founded by Pat Bond and others to create a forum for discussion and to defend S/M and it rights as a erotic minority.

Any social revolution (and there's nothing more social than sex), sooner or later, arrives at a stage where it becomes necessary to clarify the ideals and principles behind it. Throughout the sexual revolution in this country, much credit must be given to the many publications and organizations who have had the guts to speak out and fight for sexual freedom in our society. Special merit should be granted those few pioneers such as *Playboy*, *Screw* and the Gay and Women's Liberation movements, who have had to place their figurative heads into the civil and moral noose to obtain the comparatively vast amount of sexual freedom we enjoy today. Unfortunately, as history has proven, revolutions have a tendency, not to change, but to exchange one set of values and principles for another. This is at best only a slight improvement.

These same pioneers, who have fought so long and hard for everyone's right to enjoy sexual freedom, also feel that they have the right to draw lines and limits regarding what kind of sex everyone should have. They'll acknowledge the fact that there are sexual variants who dance to a different piper. At the same time, they'll make it quite clear that they consider such things as perversions, or sick, and they will not hesitate to downgrade or put them down at every opportunity. *Playboy* and similar magazines will fight over your right to have oral or anal sex provided it is done on a higher plane with taste and distinction. *Screw* and the other undergrounds will take you on a four letter orgy of sex saying 'anything goes' but drawing lines and putting down the 'weirdo' views. The liberation movements will fight tooth and nail for your right to be different, as long as it is their kind of different. Yet, all of these pioneers are self-proclaimed champions of sexual freedom.

According to our Declaration of Independence everyone has an 'inalienable right to life, liberty and the pursuit of happiness'. Our main concern is with the last since sexual freedom can certainly be considered a large part in the 'pursuit of happiness'.

Logic dictates that in the pursuit of sexual happiness, the only limits or boundaries—civil, moral or religious—should be when the rights of one individual overlap, intrude on or deny those of another. Inflicting force, pain or other indignities upon another human being, without their consent, SHOULD be considered legally and morally wrong. Yet, what about those to whom such actions become, not a violation of their rights, but a requirement for their happiness? Who has the right to point at a 'rape' scene which is mutually agreeable and satisfying to both participants, and claim it is immoral? Who has the right to brand or label 'perverted', the basic drives in people to give and receive pain and suffering or groove on the touch, taste, smell or feel of leather, rubber, metal, silks, furs, stained panties, tickling, old saddle shoes or their own hand? Who has the right to deny the abortion of an unwanted fetus? Who has the right to add frustrations and hangups onto a growing child by forcing him to wait till he's eighteen or twenty-one before he can legally relieve the natural urges and drives he's had since he was anywhere from five to twelve years old? The answer to all of the above questions is—NOBODY has such a right. Between mutually agreeable participants, NOBODY has the right to set limits or even infer that their sexual 'pursuit of happiness' be kept within understood boundaries.

The purpose, aim and goal of this paper is threefold. First, to communicate and explain our sexual variations to each other and the general public. Second, to show that there is no such thing as sexual perversion—only variation. Third, to fight for the rights of mutually agreeable participants to indulge in their pursuit of sexual happiness in ANY WAY they see fit, regardless of sex, age or method. While our approach will heavily emphasize the S/M or Dominant/Submissive aspect of sex, all variations are welcomed (and not just by lip service).

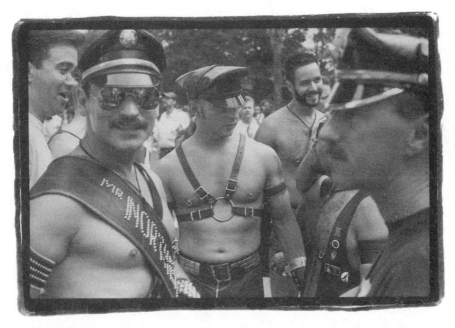

© Fred W. McDarrah

The Leather Menace:
Comments on Politics and S/M

Gayle Rubin

from *Coming to Power*, 1981

During the end of the seventies, S/M became the focus of political attacks by feminists and conservatives as one of the excesses of the sexual revolution. Gayle Rubin, anthropologist, feminist theorist and sex radical, examines the political debates on S/M that emerged within feminism and shows that S/M is a crucial issue for a liberated sexual politics.

Since Christianity upped the ante and concentrated on sexual behavior as the root of virtue, everything pertaining to sex has been a "special case" in our culture, evoking peculiarly inconsistent attitudes.

—Susan Sontag[1]

I.

I t is difficult to simply discuss the politics of sadomasochism when the politics of sex in general are so depressingly muddled. In part, this is due to the residue of at least a century of social conflict over sex during which conservative positions have dominated the terms of discussion as well as the outcome of many discrete struggles. It is important to know and to remember that in the United States and Britain, there were extensive and successful morality campaigns in the late nineteenth and early twentieth centuries. Social movements against prostitution, obscenity, contraception, abortion, and masturbation were able to establish state policies, social practices, and deeply entrenched ideologies which still affect the shape of our sexual experience and our ability to think about it. In the United States, the long term agenda of the conservative right has helped to maintain deep reservoirs of ignorance and sexual bigotry by its unrelenting opposition to sex research and sex education. More recently, the right has been spectacularly successful in tapping these pools of erotophobia in its accession to state power. The right will now use its hegemony over the state apparatus to renew and deepen its hold over erotic behavior.

Even the elementary bourgeois freedoms have never been secured in the realm of sexuality. There is, for instance, no freedom of sexual speech. Explicit talk about sex has been a glaring exception to first amendment protection since the Comstock Act was passed in 1871. Although there have been many skirmishes to establish exactly where the line will be drawn or how strongly it will be enforced, it remains true that it is still illegal in this country to produce (or show or sell) images, objects, or writing which have no other purpose than sexual arousal. One may embroider for relaxation, play baseball for the thrill, or collect stamps merely for their beauty. But sex itself is not a legitimate activity or goal. It must have some "higher" purpose. If possible, this purpose should be reproductive. Failing that, an artistic, scientific, or literary aim will do. Minimally, sex should at least be the expression of a close personal relationship.

In contrast to the politics of class, race, ethnicity, and gender, the politics of sex are relatively underdeveloped. Sexual liberals are defensive, and sexual radicals almost non-existent. Sex politics are kept far to the right by many forces, among them a frequent recourse to terror. Our sexual system contains a vast vague pool of nameless horror. Like Lovecraft's pits where unmentionable creatures perform unspeakable acts, this place of fear is rarely specified but always avoided. This reservoir of terror has several effects on our ability to deal with sex politically. It makes the whole subject touchy and volatile. It makes sex-baiting painfully easy. It provides a constant supply of demons and boogiemen with which otherwise rational people can be stampeded.

In the United States throughout the twentieth century, there have been periodic sex scares. In the late 1940's and early 1950's, the Cold War was inaugurated with a wave of domestic repression. Along with anti-communism, loyalty oaths, and the post-war reconstruction of gender roles and the family, there was a paroxysm of sex terrorism whose most overt symptom was a savage repression against homosexuals. Gay people were purged from government positions, expelled from schools, and fired from jobs (including academic jobs with tenure). Newspapers carried screaming headlines as police rounded up suspected perverts and gay bars were raided. Government agencies, legislative bodies, and grand juries held hearings and investigated the "sex deviate problem." The FBI conducted surveillance of gay people. All of these activities were both justified by, and contributed to, the construct of the homosexual as a social menace.

The repression of gay people during the Cold War has been absent from histories of the period, and the abuses suffered by homosexuals during the 1950's have never been questioned. The anti-gay repression was seen as a hygenic measure since gay life was depicted as seedy, dangerous, degraded, and scary. The impact of the repression was in fact to degrade the quality of gay life and raise the costs of being sexually different. During the 1950's, the Communist Party was just as apt to purge homosexuals as the state department. The ACLU refused to defend homosexuals who were being persecuted. The entire political spectrum, from protestant republicans to godless communists, accepted more or less the same analysis of homosexuals as scum. This period is an object lesson in the mechanics of sexual witch hunting and needs to be better known.[2]

It should be fairly obvious that the late 1970's and early 1980's are similar in many ways to the period in which the Cold War began. For whatever reason, military build-up, family reconstruction, anti-communism, and enforced sexual conformity all go together in the right wing program. But we are not simply repeating history. Among other important differences, the positions of target sexual populations have changed dramatically. The gay community is under attack and is vulnerable, but it is simply too large and too well-organized to be attacked with the impunity of the 1950's. Instead of a few tiny organizations whose names, like the Mattachine Society, gave no indications of their focus, there are now hundreds of explicitly gay political organizations. More importantly, there is an effective and extensive gay press which can document and publicize the war against homosexuals. Gay people enjoy some political legitimacy and support in the non-gay population. This does not imply complacency. The Jewish community in pre-WW II Poland was large, literate, and possessed a thriving press and was nevertheless wiped out by the Nazis. But it does mean that people know what is going on and can mount some resistance. It means that it is more difficult and politically expensive to conduct anti-gay persecution.

It is the erotic communities which are smaller, more stigmatized, and less organized which are subject to virtually unrestrained attack. Just as the political mobilization of black people has been emulated by other racial and ethnic groups, the mobilization of homosexuals has provided a repertoire of ideology and organizational technology to other erotic populations. It is these smaller, more underground groups who enjoy even fewer legal rights and less social acceptance who are bearing the brunt of current sexual repression. Moreover, these communities, particularly boy-lovers and sadomasochists, are being used as wedges against the larger gay community.

It lies well outside the scope of this essay to fully analyze the issues of cross-generational sex. But thus far, it has been the most strategically located, so a few comments are in order. In the United States, gay lovers of youth have been *the* front line of the right's battle against the gay community which has been picking up steam since the spring of 1977.[3] Lovers of youth enjoy virtually no legal protection, because any sexual contact between an adult and a minor is illegal. This means that a fully consensual love affair is, in the eyes of the law, indistinguishable from a rape. Moreover, sentences for consensual sex with a minor are usually longer and harsher than sentences for violent rape of adult women, assault and battery, or even murder. Secondly, lovers of youth are the cheapest targets for inflammatory rhetoric. Very little public education has occurred to dislodge the stereotypes which depict adult-youth relationships in the ugliest possible terms. These images of drooling old sickies corrupting or harming sweet innocent children can be relied upon to drum up public hysteria. Such stereotypes have also been used to quash any discussion of the way in which statutory rape laws function, not so much to protect young people from abuse, as to prevent them from acquiring sexual knowledge and experience.

Sex between people of different ages is not an exclusively gay phenomenon. On the contrary, all statistics on cross-generational sex indicate that the majority of instances, and the vast majority of non-consensual incidents, are heterosexual (older male, younger female). Nevertheless, most of the media coverage and legal attention has been directed at gay men. Each time another gay person is arrested for an age offense, the ensuing headlines serve to reinforce the stereotype that it is primarily a gay practice.

This claustrophobic and demonic discourse, the illegality of the sexual practices, and the ease with which the issue can be used to smear other gay people have made boy-lovers the favored target of state repression. The community of men engaged in cross-generational sex has been under seige for over four years and has been subjected to the kinds of police activity and media propaganda that were directed at homosexuals in the 1950's. Recently, NAMBLA, the North American Man/Boy Love Association, has had the dubious honor of becoming the first gay civil rights organization directly attacked by the government in the current wave of repression against dissenting sexuality. Sadly, this community has been treated by the left and the women's movement in much the same way that homosexuals were treated by so-called progressives in the 1950's. The gay movement has been repeatedly baited on this issue. When homosexuals are all accused of being "child molesters," it is legitimate to deny that all, or even a large percentage of, gay people engage in cross-generational sex. But it is crucial to add that not all adults who do have sex with minors are molesting or harming them. All too often, homosexuals have defended themselves against the accusation of child stealing by joining with the general condemnation of all adult-youth sex and by perpetuating the myths about it. Many lesbians have been doubly baited, dissassociating themselves from the practice but accepting stereotypes not only that all lovers of youth are rapists, but also that gay men tend to be lovers of youth.

Sadomasochism is the other sexual practice which to date has been used with great success to attack the gay community, and at greatest cost to those who actually practice it. Unlike sex between adults and minors, S/M is not, per se, illegal. Nevertheless there are a variety of laws which have been interpreted to apply to S/M sexual encounters and social events. It is easy to bend the applicability of existing laws because S/M is so stereotyped and stigmatized, and thus shocking and frightening. The shock value of S/M has been mercilessly exploited by both media and police.

In 1976, Los Angeles police used an obscure nineteenth century anti-slavery statute to raid a slave auction held in a gay bathhouse. The next morning, four-inch headlines screamed, "POLICE FREE GAY SLAVES." The slaves were, of course, volunteers, and proceeds from the auction were to benefit gay charities. The event was about as sinister as a Lions Club rummage sale. But sixty-five uniformed officers, two helicopters, a dozen vehicles, at least two phone taps, several weeks of surveillance of the staff of a local gay magazine, and over $100,000 were expended to bust the party and arrest some forty people. Once arrested, they were detained for many hours in handcuffs, not allowed to go to the bathroom, and subjected to full strip searches. It is only the moral stupidity induced by anti-S/M attitudes that could make anyone think that the volunteer slaves had been rescued, or that the tender mercies of the L.A.P.D. were preferable to those of their intended Masters. The statute used was actually an anti-prostitution law aimed at forcible prostitution. All charges under that statute were dropped, but four of the principals were charged with felony pandering and eventually bargained guilty pleas to misdemeanors.

S/M sex has occasionally been prosecuted under assault laws. Since assault is a felony, the state can press charges without a complaint from or even over the objections of the "victim." Once a sexual activity is construed as assault, the involvement of the partner is irrelevant, since one cannot legally consent to an assault. Since few judges or jurors can imagine why anyone would do S/M, it is easy to obtain convictions and brutal sentences. In a recent case in Massachusetts, Kenneth Appleby was sentenced to ten years in prison for hitting his lover lightly with a riding crop in the context of a consensual S/M relationship.[4] The Appleby case has some murky elements, but it sets a frightening precedent. It could happen that an S/M couple is making love. Police, perhaps called by neighbors alarmed by the noise, or perhaps looking for an excuse to arrest one of the parties, break in on the scene. They arrest the top and charge her (or him) with assault. The bottom could protest that they were only making love as her or his lover is hauled off to jail. If the couple is gay or otherwise unmarried, the submissive could even be subpoenaed and forced to testify against her or his partner in court. While the protests of the bottom might not save the top from prison, they might be used as evidence to declare the bottom mentally incompetent. Again, only the distortions of anti-S/M bigotry could locate the abuse of power in this scenario within the S/M relationship rather than with outsiders who interfere with it.

The legal vulnerability of S/M is best demonstrated by a string of police actions in Canada. In December, 1978, Toronto police raided a local leather oriented gay bath, the Barracks. They charged several men under the bawdy house laws and confiscated lots of sex toys, including dildos, butt plugs, leather harnesses, whips, etc. The bawdy house laws were originally passed as anti-prostitution measures. No prostitution was alleged to have occurred at the Barracks. But the law contains a vague phrase referring to a "place where indecent acts take place." The police were arguing that S/M sex is indecent and that any place where it occurs is a bawdy house. While this interpretation has not been clearly upheld in court, the arrests and trials have continued and generated much havoc in the interim.

Press coverage of the Barracks raid was sensationalistic. The news media jumped at the opportunity to show, in loving detail, the confiscated equipment. The Toronto gay community protested the nature of the charges, the raid, and the press coverage. A defense committee was formed.

In June of 1979, one of the members of the defense committee was arrested for "keeping a common bawdy house" in his own home. Again, no prostitution was alleged. Their redefinition of a bawdy house as a place where indecent acts took place, and of S/M sex as indecent, enabled police to bring the charges based on the man's S/M playroom. His toys, equipment, even his leather jacket and hat were confiscated as evidence, along with membership lists of the Barracks defense committee and the gay caucus of a political party.

In February, 1981, the four major gay baths in Toronto were hit with a massive raid. Over three hundred men were charged under the same bawdy house laws and hauled out into the winter snow in their towels. The Barracks was raided a second time, but the other three baths catered to a mainstream gay clientele. Having first redefined the bawdy house laws with regard to gay S/M, the police were now expanding their application to cover ordinary gay sex. This neatly circumvented Canada's consenting adults law and provoked a gay riot.

On April 14 of this year, the scope of the crackdown expanded again. Robert Montgomery, who runs a small business making custom leather gear and sex toys, was charged with fifteen separate offenses. In addition to the now obligatory bawdy house laws, relating to his apartment, several changes were brought having to do with making, selling, distributing, and possessing to distribute obscene material. The obscene material in question included the leather items and sex toys. In effect, the Canadian police have now reclassified sex toys and leather gear as pornography, and therefore prosecutable under the porn laws.

The reason behind Montgomery's arrest became clear a week later. Six men who own or have interests in gay baths in Toronto were charged with an array of offenses including keeping a common bawdy house, distribution and sale of obscene matter, and conspiracy to live off the proceeds of crime. The men charged were prominent gay businessmen, lawyers, and gay political activists, including George Hislop, a gay political official. The charges against them relied upon the whole carefully constructed edifice of redefined sex laws which the police had been building for three years. Any gay bath can be prosecuted as a bawdy house. Sex toys, leather items, enema bags, dildos, and even lubricants can be treated as contraband. In this case, the obscenity charges were related to the sale of sex equipment (including some items made by Montgomery) in shops at the baths. If these charges stick, anyone who owns or has an interest in a gay bath or sex related business can be prosecuted for conspiracy to live off the proceeds of crime.

On May 30, the gay baths were raided in Edmonton. On June 12, two men were convicted in the original Barracks case, and on June 16, the last two gay baths in Toronto were raided. What has happened very clearly in Canada is that S/M has been used to set several legal precedents which are now being used to decimate mainstream gay institutions and the bastions of mainstream gay political and economic power. Police have used the media, and manipulated sexual prejudice and ignorance, to criminalize whole categories of erotic behavior without a single new law being passed.

Nothing quite so blatant has happened yet in the United States, but we already have similar laws on the books. In California, for instance, a bawdy house is defined as a place resorted to for "purposes of prostitution *or lewdness*" (my emphasis). There is also a clause which prohibits keeping a house "for purposes of assignation." Given the current sexual climate in the U.S., whose congress has just allocated some twenty million dollars to promote teenage chastity, it does not seem farfetched to imagine people getting arrested for having assignations in their own living rooms. It takes even less foresight to predict that the next few years will see a rash of morality campaigns to exterminate vulnerable sexual populations. There are many signs that S/M is on the verge of becoming a direct target of such a campaign.

Police already harass the institutions of the leather community with a great deal of impunity. In San Francisco, the vice squad and the ABC (Alcoholic Beverage Commission) have either warned, raided, brought suspension proceedings against, or revoked the licenses of virtually every leather bar within the last five years. No other group of gay bars, let alone heterosexual drinking establishments, has faced anything like this kind of concerted enforcement of the liquor laws since 1970. This unrelenting harassment of the leather bars has not raised a peep of protest from the rest of the city's gay community. In fact, from reading the local gay press, it would be difficult to even know that it was taking place. By contrast, when mainstream gay institutions like the Jaguar bookstore have been hassled, both press coverage and gay community support have been extensive.[5]

Meanwhile, the straight media have discovered that they can bait homosexuals, smear sadomasochists, and increase their circulation or ratings all at once. The infamous CBS "documentary" *Gay Power, Gay Politics,* used S/M to question the credibility of gay political aspirations. The program implied that if gay people are allowed to acquire significant political power, S/M will be rampant, and people will be killed doing it. This analysis rested on three completely phony connections.

The program gave the false impression that S/M is especially prevalent in San Francisco, and that this high level of S/M activity results from gay political clout. The New York based reporters failed to mention that almost every major city has an S/M population, that San Francisco's is not particularly large, and that S/M institutions are more numerous and developed in New York, a city that has failed to pass a gay rights ordinance, than in San Francisco, one which has.

Secondly, the program gave the false impression that S/M is a specifically gay (male) practice. The reporters failed to mention that most sadomasochists are heterosexual and that most gay men do not practice S/M. In fact, most of the S/M section of the program was filmed at the Chateau, a heterosexually oriented establishment.

Thirdly, S/M was presented as a dangerous and often lethal activity.

Most of the evidence for this assertion consisted of the reporter, George Crile, asking leading questions in order to get his interviewees to confirm his prejudices.[6] At one point, Crile told a story about a place "where they have a gynecological table . . . with a doctor and a nurse on hand to sew people up."[7] There is no such place in San Francisco, although there are certainly people who do have sex on surplus hospital equipment, and some establishments have physicians on call. This is a rather responsible attitude, since health problems can occur during sexual activities, just as they can during sports events, academic lectures, or at the opera. Yet it was presented in a completely sinister light.

Crile interviewed Dr. Boyd Stephens, the San Francisco coroner, who estimated that ten percent of the homicides in San Francisco were gay related and that some were S/M related. Dr. Stephens later told reporter Randy Alfred that the ten percent figure included the killing of homosexuals by heterosexuals. Alfred points out that this percentage is about the same, or less than, the percentage of homosexuals in the population of San Francisco.[8] On another occasion, Dr. Stephens estimated that about ten percent of the city's homicides were *sex* related (given the amount of sex which takes place, it would appear to have a remarkable safety record). Yet the coroner has been widely misquoted (*Time Magazine, Peoria Journal Star,* and several different times in the *San Francisco Chronicle*) as the source of a completely fabricated statistic that ten percent of San Francisco's homicides are related to S/M.

After *Gay Power, Gay Politics* was aired, KPIX, the local CBS affiliate, presented a panel of local gay figures to respond. Most of them were successfully baited on the issue of S/M, hastening to disassociate themselves from it without challenging the distorted picture of S/M itself. Harry Britt, gay member of the board of supervisors, was the only panelist who criticized the coverage of S/M as well as the coverage of homosexuality. The CBS special has been widely rapped for its reporting on homosexuality. But its coverage of S/M has escaped scrutiny and has set a new low standard for the treatment of S/M in the media.

In March, 1981, KPIX ran a four part series on S/M on the 11 o'clock news. Called *Love and Pain,* the series used sensationalized facts, unsubstantiated claims, and a half-digested version of the anti-porn movement's analysis to present S/M as a public menace. The program repeatedly equated S/M with violence, called sex toys dangerous weapons, and made a wild claim that the city's emergency rooms were inundated with injuries caused by S/M activity.

Injuries and accidents do occur in the course of sexual activity, and S/M is not exempt. But by and large, S/M, particularly when practiced by people in touch with S/M communities, has a safety record most sports teams would envy. Among the people I know, there are more health problems caused by softball or long distance running than by whipping, bondage, or fist-fucking. The S/M community is obsessed with safety and has an elaborate folk technology of methods to maximize sensation and minimize danger. These techniques are transmitted largely by older or more experienced members to neophytes. S/M oppression renders this transmission difficult. Scaring people away from the community puts people in some real danger of trying things they do not know how to do.

A point of competition among tops, sadists, dominants, Mistresses, and Masters is over who is the safest (as well as the hottest, the most imaginative, and the most proficient). People who do not play safely—tops who get too drunk, bottoms who are too reckless—are identified and others are warned of them. Reputations in a small, gossip-ridden community are always fragile, so there is in fact a good deal of social control over patterns of play. People who are scared into viewing this community as dangerous are outside the protection it actually affords.

No community can completely protect its members from accidents or from people who are, for whatever reason, actually violent or dangerous. The S/M community has its criminals, just like any other. It is just as concerned that they be apprehended and put out of commission. But far more people end up in the hospital as a result of playing sports, driving cars, or being pregnant than from having S/M sex. One of the biggest sources of injury in San Francisco right now is queer-bashing, fed in part by anti-S/M hysteria. One of the worst things that I have heard of happening to an S/M person occurred when a gay man who was leaving a leather bar was assaulted by a gang of bashers. He suffered serious head injuries and the loss of an eye.

The idea that S/M is dangerous is self-perpetuating. A friend of mine died recently. He had a heart attack while he was having sex in his lovingly built playroom. When the police saw the S/M equipment they threatened to charge his lover with manslaughter. They notified the press, which aired lurid stories of "ritual sadomasochistic death." When the death was ruled accidental, the stories were quietly pulled, but no retraction or followup appeared to correct the lingering impression that S/M had caused the death. When men have coronaries while fucking their wives, the papers do not print stories implying that intercourse leads to death. Nor are their widows threatened with criminal charges. The only reason to link my friend's death to his sexual orientation was the preconception that S/M leads to death. That preconception generated the news stories. The news stories reinforce the preconception. Many people will have their prejudices about S/M corroborated by these ill-conceived "news" reports.

Besides promulgating the idea that S/M is dangerous to its practitioners, the KPIX program also alleged that S/M is harmful to those who do not do it. The program argued that S/M imagery in the media is a kind of miasma from which no one can escape. Therefore, S/M was "corroding the fabric of society," it was affecting everyone, and something ought to be done about it. Historically, crackdowns on activities which primarily affect those who are involved in them are rationalized on the basis of some similarly flimsy connection with social decay. Notions that marijuana, prostitution, or homosexuality by some vague mechanism lead to violent crime, disease, or creeping communism are used to rationalize punitive social or legal action against otherwise innocuous activities.

Love and Pain did not call for new laws to make S/M activity criminal. But the reporter, Gregg Risch, did propose that parents who do S/M be relieved of the custody of their children. The program did a whole segment on a woman who is living with her lover and her two-year-old child in a rural S/M community in Mendocino County. The reporter interviewed the child's grandmother, who was horrified and wanted to take the child. He also interviewed a shrink who pontificated that the child might be damaged by exposure to its mother's sexual orientation. He called for the Mendocino County authorities to come in and take the kid away from its mother.

Custody law is one of the places where sex dissenters of all sorts are viciously punished for being different. Lesbians and gay men are not the only groups whose rights to keep or raise offspring are drastically limited. The state may come in and snatch the children of prostitutes, swingers, or even "promiscuous" women. Society has a great deal of power to insure that sex dissenters are separated from young people, their own children as well as the next generation of sex perverts. A rough rule of sexual sociology is that the more stigmatized the sexuality, the higher the barriers are to finding one's way into that community, and the older people are when they finally get over them.

Risch expressed a great deal of dismay that so many S/M people were of child rearing age. All that this means is that the S/M community is full of adults—hardly cause for alarm. He did concede that S/M people might be allowed to keep their children if they were careful to hide their sexuality from them. But he felt that out of the closet sado-masochists should relinquish their offspring. One of the functions of custody law and practice is to reproduce conventional values. When lesbian mothers are granted custody on the condition that they do not live with their lovers, when swingers are forbidden to swing, when S/M people are required to hide, it is clear that sex dissenters are being denied the right to raise their children according to their value system. This insures that even if perverts have and keep their children, those kids will be inculcated with the dominant social mythology about sex.

In the wake of both *Gay Power, Gay Politics,* and *Love and Pain,* local news coverage of S/M has gotten worse. Less than two weeks after the KPIX series, the *San Francisco Chronicle* reported that the coroner had been conducting workshops on S/M safety, and that there was an "alarming increase in injuries and deaths from sado-masochistic sex."[9] Again, the phony statistic was quoted that ten percent of the city's homicides were S/M related. Dr. Stephens, the coroner, is currently suing the paper for libel. Aside from the inaccuracies of the article, it is true that the coroner has displayed a remarkable professionalism in dealing with the minority sexual populations of San Francisco. He has taken the trouble to learn about these communities, has displayed good judgment in dealing with them, and has earned their respect. For his trouble and his professionalism, he was given harsh treatment in the press and was chastized by Mayor Feinstein, who was quoted as saying, "It is my belief that S&M is dangerous to society and I'm not eager to have it attracted to San Francisco."[10]

In July of 1981, a large area burned south of Market Street, and press coverage was entirely sensational. The fire started on the site of a former gay and leather oriented bathhouse, the Barracks. The Barracks has been closed for years and the building was being remodeled as a hotel. But the press reported that the fire started in a "gay bathhouse." The area which burned is in the midst of the leather bars, so many gay men and S/M people lived on the street. But the neighborhood is mixed. There were old people, artists, Filipinos, and a good assortment of low income families living there as well. The largest single group of fire victims consisted of over twenty displaced children. Yet the media portrayed the fire as a gay and S/M event, as if the sexual orientation of some of the victims had somehow caused it.

One of the buildings that burned belonged to a man who manufactures Rush, a brand of poppers. The fire department suspected that Rush had caused or fed the fire and was searching for large quantities of it. No Rush was ever found. The fire department also hypothesized that since S/M people were known to live on the alley, that there might be bodies of slaves chained to their beds in the rubble. No bodies were ever found.

Media coverage of the fire promulgated the image that masochists are completely helpless, that they spend their time chained in their quarters, and that in the event of an emergency, they are simply abandoned by their callous keepers. Buried far back in the news reports on the third day were comments by neighborhood residents who pointed out that if anyone had been in bondage when the fire broke out, their lover or trick or friend would have done everything to save them. If a parent fails to save a child caught in a fire, no one assumes that families cause death. Had anyone been accidentally burned anywhere in proximity to S/M equipment or space, the tragedy would have been interpreted as sinister evidence that S/M people are inhuman monsters. Coverage of the fire was premised on the idea that S/M people do not care about one another. The straight media simply did not report on the human dimensions of a great community crisis.[11]

The papers did not mention, for instance, that the initial relief effort was run out of the Folsom Street Hotel, a fuck palace catering to the gay male leather community. They did not report that the Hothouse, a leather oriented bathhouse, immediately held a benefit for the victims. No whisper hit the papers that every South of Market bar and bath contributed some kind of aid and that all the leather bars became dropoff points for donations of food, clothing, and equipment for the fire victims, gay and straight. The *Chronicle* ran a picture of a burned out S/M playroom next to the story about how there might be dead slaves lying in the ruins. It did not report that an auction of used jockstraps was held at the Gold Coast, a leather bar, to raise money for the homeless.

All of this slanted media coverage is constructing a new demonization of S/M and probably heralds a campaign to clean it up. It is very similar to what happened to homosexuals in the 1950's. There were already plenty of antigay ideas, structures, and practices. But during a decade of headlines, arrests, investigations, and legislation, those pre-existing elements of homophobia were reconstituted into a new and more virulent ideology that homosexuality was an active menace which needed to be actively combated. Currently, there are already plenty of anti-S/M ideas, structures, and practices. But these are being drawn into the creation of a new ideological construct that will call for a more active extermination campaign against S/M. It is likely that many sadomasochists will be arrested and incarcerated for such heinous thought crimes as wanting to be tied up when they come.

The form such campaigns often take is that police use old laws, as they have done in Canada, to make a few spectacular arrests. The media cover the arrests the way they covered the fire, or my friend's death, and turn tragedy into an excuse to further harass the victims and their community. At some point, there will be an outcry for new laws to give police more power to deal with and control the "menace." These new laws will give police more summary powers against the target population and will lead to more arrests, more headlines, and more laws, until either the S/M community finds a way to stop the onslaught or until the repression runs out of steam.

Already, in the wake of the fire, a San Francisco supervisor considered introducing legislation to ban the sale of S/M equipment in the city. Many "feminist" anti-porn groups would support legislation against S/M material on other grounds. If our reading material and sexual technology were contraband, our community could be decimated by the police. And this kind of campaign, like those against homosexuals thirty years ago, will be seen as a hygenic measure, supported by conservatives and radicals alike. It will scapegoat a bunch of people whose only crime is exotic sexual tastes. And while all of this has been taking shape, what has the women's movement been doing? Why, it has been conducting a purge against its own rather tiny S/M population. The rhetoric of this purge is what most feminists think of as the "politics of S/M".

II.

Homosexuality is a response—consciously or not—to a male supremacist society. Because it is a response to oppressive institutions and oppressive relationships it is not necessarily a progressive response or one that challenges the power of the monopoly capitalist. We see that the pressures that capitalist society puts on each individual are tremendous . . . Today people are grasping at all kinds of straws, at exotic religious sects, mysticism, sex orgies, Trotskyism, etc.

Revolutionary Union[12]

While gay people can be anti-imperialists we feel that they cannot be Communists. To be a Communist, we must accept and welcome struggle in all facets of our lives, personal as well as political. We cannot struggle with male supremacy in the factory and not struggle at home. We feel that the best way to struggle out such contradictions in our personal lives is in stable monogamous relation between men and women . . . Because homosexuals do not carry the struggle between men and women into their most personal relationships, they are not prepared, in principle, for the arduous task of class transformation.

Revolutionary Union

I see sadomasochism as resulting in part from the internalization of heterosexual dominant-submissive role playing. I see sadomasochism among lesbians as involving in addition an internalization of the homophobic heterosexual view of lesbians. Defending such behavior as healthy and compatible with feminism, even proselytizing in favor of it is about the most contrafeminist anti-political and bourgeois stance that I can imagine.

Diana Russell[13]

> Sadomasochistic activity between/among lesbians is an out-
> come and perpetuation of patriarchal sadistic and masochistic
> culture.
>
> ry[14]

> The fact is, the whole culture is S/M, we're all sadomasochists.
> The people in SAMOIS, or gay people who wear leather, have a
> more severe form of the disease.
>
> Susan Griffin[15]

> SAMOIS is entitled to exist as a group devoted to S/M, but why
> should we let them get away with calling themselves lesbian-
> feminist?
>
> tacie dejanikus[16]

The first time I came out was over a decade ago, when I realized, at the age of twenty, that I was a lesbian. I had to come out again, several years later, as a sadomasochist. The similarities and differences between these two experiences have been most instructive. On both occasions, I spent several months thinking that I must be the only one on earth, and was pleasantly surprised to discover there were large numbers of women who shared my predilections. Both debuts were fraught with tension and excitement. But the second coming out was considerably more difficult than the first.

I came out as a lesbian just when a bad discourse on homosexuality, the product of the anti-gay wars of the 1950's, was coming apart. I did not experience the full force of homophobia. On the contrary, to be a baby dyke in 1970 was to feel great moral self-confidence. One could luxuriate in the knowledge that not only was one not a slimy pervert, but one's sexuality was especially blessed on political grounds. As a result, I never quite understood the experience of being gay in the face of unrelenting contempt.

When I came out as an S/M person, I got an unexpected lesson in how my gay ancestors must have felt. My youth as a sadomasochist has been spent at a time when, as part of a more general reconsolidation of anti-sex and anti-gay ideology, a new demonization of S/M is taking shape. This is happening in the society at large and in the women's movement. It is a long way from 1970 to watch the images of your love turning uglier by the day, to fear being arrested, and to wonder how bad it will get. It is especially depressing if a once progressive movement in which you have spent your entire adult life is leading the assault. The experience of being a feminist sadomasochist in 1980 is similar to that of being a communist homosexual in 1950. When left ideology condemed homosexuality as bourgeois decadence, many homosexuals were forced out of progressive political organizations. A few of them founded the Mattachine Society. Now that large parts of the feminist movement have similarly defined S/M as an evil product of patriarchy, it has become increasingly difficult for those of us who are feminists to maintain our membership in the women's community.

Some feminist bookstores have refused to carry SAMOIS publications or books having a positive attitude toward S/M. Some stores which do carry such material have it shelved obscurely, or have put up cards warning customers against the contents. One store has even prepared a packet of anti-S/M readings which are included with any purchase of pro-S/M books. "Sadomasochistic" is routinely used as an epithet. A group is putting out a book called *Against Sadomasochism*, the advertising for which has promised a response to the "threat" posed by the existence of SAMOIS. The flyer for the book expresses horror that some of us have actually been "invited speakers at university classes" and that there has been an effort to "normalize sadomasochism."

I used to read the feminist press with enthusiasm. Now I dread each new issue of my favorite periodicals wondering what vile picture of my sexuality will appear this month. Papers and journals are reluctant to print pro-S/M articles, and usually only do so if accompanied by reams of disclaimer and at least one anti-S/M essay. However, essays that trash S/M are not held until the magazine can solicit a positive viewpoint.

Recently the Women's Building in San Francisco decided that SAMOIS cannot rent space in the building. Among the stated purposes of the building are a commitment to end oppression based on sexual orientation and a promise to respect the diversity of individual women. The Women's Building has a very open policy. Mixed groups, men's groups, community groups, non-feminist groups, and private parties regularly rent space. The building has frequently rented space for weddings. It is a sad commentary on the state of feminism that heterosexual weddings, sanctioned by religion and enforced by the state, are less controversial than the activities of a bunch of lesbian sex perverts.[17]

In 1980, the National Organization of Women passed a misleadingly labeled resolution on "lesbian and gay rights." What this resolution actually did was condemn S/M, cross-generational sex, pornography, and public sex. The resolution denied that these were issues of sexual or affectional preference and declared NOW's intention to disassociate itself from any gay or lesbian group that did not accept these definitions of sexual preference. When there was an attempt ten years ago to purge NOW of lesbian members, NOW was not stampeded into denying the legitimacy of gay rights. The campaign against the leather menace has succeeded where the attack on the lavender menace failed. It has put NOW on record as opposing sexual freedom and the civil rights of erotic minorities.

There are many reasons why S/M has become such a *bête noire* in the women's movement, and most originate outside of feminism. With the glaring exception of monogamous lesbianism, the women's movement usually reflects the sexual prejudices prevailing in society. Feminists have no monopoly on anti-S/M attitudes. The medical and psychiatric establishments have moved somewhat on homosexuality, but on virtually every other sexual variation they hold barely modified 19th century views. The psychiatric theories of sex in turn reflect the sexual hierarchies which exist in society. Another general rule of sexual sociology is that the more persecuted a sexuality, the worse its reputation.

A second force for which the women's movement is not responsible is the state of sex research and sex education. While the movement has a lamentable tendency to adopt some of the worst elements of sex research, the field as a whole is underdeveloped. Sex is so loaded and controversial in western culture that research on it is loaded and controversial. Sex research is inscribed within the power relations that organize sexual behavior. Challenging those power relations with new data or original hypotheses brings one into conflict with deeply held folk theories of sex.

The sex field also reflects its marginality. Whereas almost every institution of higher learning has a department of psychology, there are virtually no departments of sexology. There are fewer than a dozen academic sites in the United States where sex research is conducted.

There are few courses taught on sex at the college level, and pre-college sex education is still tenuous. Knowledge of sex is restricted. Getting into the Institute for Sex Research is like getting into Fort Knox. Almost every library has its sexual materials in a locked case, or a special collection, or oddly catalogued. The younger one is, the harder it is to have access to information about sex. The systematic restraints on curiosity about sex maintain sexual ignorance, and where people are ignorant, they are manipulable.

There are other reasons for the controversy over S/M which are more intrinsic to the women's movement and its history. One of these is the confusion between sexual orientation and political belief which originated in the idea that feminism is the theory, lesbianism is the practice. There are elements of truth in the idea that being a lesbian brings one into conflict with some basic elements of gender hierarchy. But like many good ideas, this insight has been overused and over-applied. It has made it difficult to accept that there are heterosexuals who are feminists, and that there are lesbians who are not. It has actually inhibited the development of lesbian politics and consciousness. It has led to the belief that lesbianism is only justified politically insofar as it is feminist. This in turn has encouraged feminist lesbians to look down on non-movement dykes. It has led feminist lesbians to identify more with the feminist movement than with the lesbian community. It has encouraged many women who are not sexually attracted to women to consider themselves lesbians. It has prevented the lesbian movement from asserting that our lust for women is justified whether or not it derives from feminist political ideology. It has generated a lesbian politic that seems ashamed of lesbian desire. It has made feminism into a closet in which lesbian sexuality is unacknowledged.[18]

If feminist politics entail or require particular sexual positions or forms of erotic behavior, then it follows that other kinds of sexual activity are specifically anti-feminist. Given prevailing ideas of appropriate feminist sexual behavior, S/M appears to be the mirror opposite. It is dark and polarized, extreme and ritualized, and above all, it celebrates difference and power. If S/M is understood as the dark opposite of happy and healthy lesbianism, accepting that happy and healthy lesbians also do S/M would threaten the logic of the belief system out of which this opposition was generated. But this analysis is not based on the realities of sexual behavior. It is predicated on a limited notion of the symbolic valences of both lesbianism and S/M. Torn from real social context, sexual differences can symbolize all kinds of other differences, including political ones. Thus, to some people, homosexuality is fascist, and to others it is communist. Lesbianism has been understood as narcissism and self worship, or as an inevitably unfulfilled yearning. To many right wingers, gayness in any form symbolizes the decline and fall of empires.

There is nothing inherently feminist or non-feminist about S/M. Sadomasochists, like lesbians, gay men, heterosexuals, etc., may be anarchists, fascists, democrats, republicans, communists, feminists, gay liberationists, or sexual reactionaries. The idea that there is an automatic correspondence between sexual preference and political belief is long overdue to be jettisoned.

This does not mean that sexual behavior should not be evaluated. How people treat each other in sexual contexts is important. But this is not the same issue as passing judgment on what are essentially cultural differences in sexual behavior. There are plenty of lesbian relationships which are long term and monogamous, in which both partners switch roles or do the same thing, in which all touching is gentle, but in which the partners are mean and nasty to each other. The idea that lesbianism, especially when practiced by feminists, is a superior form of sex often leads people to ignore the actual interpersonal dynamics. Conversely, the idea that S/M is warped leads to an inability to perceive love, friendship, and affection among S/M people. S/M partners may occupy polarized roles, the touching may be rough, and yet they may treat each other with respect and affection. In all sexualities, there is a range of how people act toward one another. Ranking different sexualities from best to worst simply substitutes for exercising judgment about specific situations.

The ease with which S/M has come to symbolize the feminist equivalent of the Anti-Christ has been exacerbated by some long term changes in feminist ideology. Few women in the movement seem to realize that what currently passes for radical feminism has a tangential relationship with the initial premises of the women's movement. Assumptions which now pass as dogma would have horrified activists in 1970. In many respects, the women's movement, like the society at large, has quietly shifted to the right.

Feminists in 1970 were angry because women, the things women did, and female personality traits were devalued. But we were also enraged at the restrictions placed on female behavior. Women were not supposed to engage in a range of activities considered masculine. A woman who wanted to fix cars, get laid, ride a motorcycle, play sports, or get a Ph.D. could expect criticism from the society and support from the women's movement. The term "male identified" meant that a woman lacked consciousness of female oppression.

By 1980, the term "male identified" had lost that meaning (lack of political consciousness) and has become synonymous with "masculine." Now, women who do masculine things are accused of imitating men not only by family, church, and the media, but by the feminist movement.[19] Much contemporary feminist ideology is that everything female—persons, activities, values, personality characteristics—is good, whereas anything pertaining to males is bad. By this analysis, the task of feminism is to replace male values with female ones, to substitute female culture for male culture. This line of thinking does not encourage women to try to gain access to male activities, privileges, and territories. Instead, it implies that a good feminist wants nothing to do with "male" activities. All of this celebration of femininity tends to reinforce traditional gender roles and values of appropriate female behavior. It is not all that different from the sex role segregation against which early feminists revolted. I, for one, did not join the women's movement to be told how to be a good girl. There are many labels for this brand of feminism, but my preferred term is "femininism."[20]

Femininism has become especially powerful with regard to issues of sexuality and issues of violence, which it not surprisingly links together. Sexuality is seen as a male value and activity. The femininist view of sex is that it is something that good/nice women do not especially like. In this view, sex is not a motivating force in female behavior. Women have sex as an expression of intimacy, but orgasm is seen as a male goal. The idea that sexuality is most often something men impose upon women leads to the equation of sex with violence, and the conflation of sex with rape. These were the sexual theories I was taught growing up. I never expected to have them rammed down my throat by the women's movement. Man the Id and Woman the Chaste are Victorian ideas, not feminist ones.[21]

The re-emphasis on feminine values, especially sexual chastity, has led to a shift in the mode of argument for feminist goals. Instead of arguing for justice or social equality, much feminist polemic now claims a female moral superiority. It is argued that we should have more, or total, power in society because we are more equipped for it, mainly by virtue of our role in reproduction, than men. I did not join the women's movement to have my status depend on my ability to bear children.

I fear that the women's movement is repeating the worst errors of a century ago. The nineteenth century feminist movement began as a radical critique of women's role and status. But it became increasingly conservative and similarly shifted the burden of its argument onto a reconstituted femininity in the form of alleged female moral superiority. Much of the nineteenth century movement degenerated into a variety of morality crusades, with conservative feminists pursuing what they took to be women's agenda in anti-prostitution, anti-masturbation, anti-obscenity, and anti-vice campaigns. It will be an historical tragedy of almost unthinkable dimensions if the revived feminist movement dissipates into a series of campaigns against recreational sex, popular music, and sexually explicit materials. But this appears to be the direction in which feminism is moving.[22]

By a series of accidents, and through the mediating issue of pornography, S/M has become a challenge to this entire political tendency, which has ridden to power by manipulating women's fears around sex and around violence. Therefore, when feminists argue about S/M, there is much more at stake than sexual practice. Some women are arguing for the logical coherence of their political beliefs. Others of us are arguing that political theory about sex is due for a major overhaul based on a more sophisticated sociology of sex. But what often seems most at stake is the shape of feminist ideology and the future direction of the movement. There are ways of understanding S/M which are compatible with "femininism" and its attendent political programs. When these become more articulated (and they will, in the not too distant future), S/M will seem to be less of a threat to the hegemonic ideology of the women's movement. But for now, the fight over S/M has been the locus of a struggle over deep political differences in the women's movement.

Given the immense symbolic load that S/M has acquired, it is not surprising that it is difficult for participants in this debate to absorb information about S/M that would make these arguments difficult to sustain. Nevertheless, the picture of S/M which is assumed in the current diatribes has almost no relationship to the actual experience of anyone involved in it.

III.

. . . for "consent" to be a meaningful criteria all the parties involved must have some measure of real choices. Women, for instance, have been "consenting" to marriage for centuries. Women in China had "consented" to the footbinding of their own daughters. This is coerced-consent, and it hardly constitutes freedom. The most "heavy" masochist, who gives his hands and feet to be shackled to some rack, who offers his body to be gang-banged, fist-fucked, and pissed upon—he "consents," but if he has so internalized society's hatred of him as to offer his own body for a beating, then his "consent" is merely a conditioned reflex.

letter to *Gay Community News*[23]

Coming out has several meanings. Sometimes it refers to the point at which a person realizes that they are gay or have some other variant sexuality. Coming out in this sense is a form of self recognition. Another meaning of coming out is that of public declaration, of being willing to let other people know about it. In yet another sense, coming out is a kind of journey people take from the straight world where they start into the gay or other variant world they want to occupy. Most of us are born into and raised by straight families, educated in straight schools, and socialized by straight peer groups. Our upbringing does not provide us with the social skills, information, or routes of access into non-conventional sexual lifestyles. We must find our way into those social spaces where we can meet partners, find friends, get validation, and participate in a community life which does not presuppose that we are straight. Sometimes this journey is fairly short, from the suburbs of large cities to the gay bars downtown. In small towns, it usually means finding an underground network or building a more public community. Often it means migrating from middle America to a bigger city, such as New York, Los Angeles, Chicago, or San Francisco. A classic account of this kind of coming out is the fifties pulp novel, *I am a Woman*.[24] Laura, the heroine, suffers vague malaise in the midwest, so she takes a bus to New York City. Eventually, she stumbles into a lesbian bar in Greenwich Village. She instantly realizes who she is, that there are others like her, and that this is home. She finds a lover, develops a gay identity, and becomes an adult, functioning lesbian.

This kind of migratory behavior is characteristic of sexual minorities. There are many barriers to the process. These include the marginality of dissenting sexual communities, the amount of legal apparatus built to control them, the social penalties to which their members are subject, and the unrelenting propaganda that portrays them as dangerous, sleazy, horrid places full of dreadful people and unspecified pitfalls. It is extraordinary that young perverts, like salmon swimming upstream, continually and in great numbers make this journey. Much of the politics of sex consists of battles to determine the costs of belonging to such communities and how difficult it will be to get into them.

I came out as a lesbian in a small college town that had no visible lesbian community. A group of us formed a radical lesbian feminist group which eventually grew into a fairly large, albeit young, public lesbian community. The nearest pre-movement lesbian community was thirty miles away, where there were actually a couple of lesbian bars. There was one mostly male gay bar called the Flame. I had heard for years that it was the kind of place you wanted to stay away from. There were vague implications that if you went there, something bad would happen. But it was the only gay bar in town, and I was drawn to it. I finally screwed up my courage and walked in. The minute I got past the front door I relaxed. It was full of very innocuous looking gay men and a couple of lesbians. I instantly realized that these were my people, and that I was one of the people I had been warned against.

Before I walked into the Flame, I still thought that gay people were rare and scarce. Going through that door was like going through the looking glass. On the other side of that taboo entrance is not a place of terror, but a huge, populous, prosperous, bustling world of homosex-uals. What is most incredible about the whole experience is that so large a part of reality could have been kept so invisible to my entire generation. It is as if one grew up under the impression that there were no Italians, or Jews, or Chinese in the United States.

Seven years later, I was again sweating in front of another tabooed threshold. This time it was the door to the Pleasure Chest in New York City. I must have walked up and down Seventh Avenue twenty times before I finally got a friend to go in with me. It took a little longer to get used to the S/M world than to the gay world. But by now I feel as at home in leather bars and sex toy shops as I do in lesbian bars and gay restaurants. Instead of the monsters and slimy perverts I had been led to expect, I found another hidden community. The S/M commu-nity is not as large as the gay community, but it is complex, populated, and quite civilized. Most parts of the S/M community take a respon-sible attitude to newcomers, teaching them how to do S/M safely, S/M etiquette, and acquired wisdom. Preconceived chimeras disappear in the face of actual social practice. I had been worried that my eroticism would require that I give up control over my life or become some kind of mindless nebbish. One of the first lessons I learned was that you can do S/M by agreement *and* it can still be a turn-on. There is a lot of sep-aration between the straight, gay, and lesbian S/M communities. But there is also pan-S/M consciousness. As one wise woman who has been doing this for many years has said, "Leather is thicker than blood."

The largest sub-population of sadomasochists is probably the het-erosexuals. Of these, most appear to be male submissive/female domi-nant. Much of the straight S/M world revolves around professional female dominants and their submissive clients. There are also some straight or predominantly straight social clubs and political organiza-tions through which heterosexual sadomasochists can meet one another. In the last few years, the straight S/M community in New York City began to have regular nights at a bar. And even more recently, an S/M sex club opened which has a predominantly heterosexual clientele.

I should point out that contrary to much of what is said about straight S/M in the feminist press, heterosexual S/M is *not* standard heterosexuality. Straight S/M is stigmatized and persecuted. Whatever the metaphoric similarities between standard sex and S/M, once someone starts to use whips, ropes, and all the theatre, they are considered to be perverts, not normal. The relationship between heterosexual S/M and "normal" heterosexuality is at most like the relationship between high school faggots and the high school football team. There is some overlap of personnel. But for the most part all that fanny-patting and even an occasional blow-job does not make the jocks into fags. And the former would rather beat up the latter than accompany them to the nearest gay bar.

Gay male sadomasochists are less numerous than heterosexuals, but they are much better organized. Gay men have developed an elaborate technology for building public institutions for sexual outlaws. When the gay male leather community emerged, it followed the organizational patterns of the larger homosexual community. The first gay male leather bar opened in New York in 1955. The first one in San Francisco opened about five years later. There was a population explosion of leather bars along with gay bars in general (including lesbian bars) around 1970. In San Francisco today, there are five to ten leather bars and about five baths or sex clubs that cater to the gay male leather community. There are also several social or charitable organizations, motorcycle clubs, a performance space, assorted shops, and a couple of restaurants for the South of Market crowd. Although leather styles were faddish in the larger gay community for a couple of years, and leather/macho has replaced drag queen fluff as the dominant gay stereotype, the leather community is a distinct subgroup. The average gay man is not into leather or S/M. But the average gay man is probably more aware of sexual diversity and erotic possibilities than most heterosexuals or lesbians.

Lesbian social organization is smaller scale but similar to gay male. Bars have been for many years the most important public community space. Since 1970, feminist political organizations and cultural institutions have provided another major context for lesbian social life. Unlike gay men, lesbians have not yet developed more specialized sexual sub-groups. There are lesbians who do everything that gay men and heterosexuals do. There are girl-lovers, sadomasochists, and fetishists (probably for flannel shirts, hiking boots, cats, softball uniforms, alfalfa sprouts, and feminist tracts). There are many transvestites and transsexuals (especially female to male). But lesbian sexual diversity is relatively unnoticed, unconscious, and unorganized.

When I came out as a lesbian sadomasochist, there was no place to go. A notice I put up in my local feminist bookstore was torn down. It took months of painstaking detective work to track down other women who were into S/M. There was no public lesbian S/M community to find, so I had to help build one. At least in San Francisco, there is now a visible, accessible avenue for lesbians to find their way into an S/M context. SAMOIS is a motley collection. We have lots of refugees from Lesbian Nation, a good number of bar dykes, and many women who work in the sex industry. It is clear in retrospect that what has happened in the last three years or so is another mass coming out. There are now about as many sadomasochists in most lesbian communities as there were radical feminist lesbians in 1970. There would be groups like SAMOIS in virtually every lesbian community in the U.S. if the costs of coming out were not so excruciating. It takes someone being willing to put out the word and serve as a focus for other dyke perverts to start coming out of the woodwork. But most women have watched SAMOIS get trashed and are afraid to be treated the same way.

My second coming out has been much more difficult than the first. The S/M community is even more underground and harder to find than the lesbian community. The routes of access to it are even more hidden. The aura of terror is more intense. The social penalties, the stigma, and the lack of legitimacy are even greater. I have rarely worked so hard or displayed such independence of mind as when I came out as an S/M person. I had to reject virtually everything I had been told about it. Having struggled this hard to assume a stigmatized identity (one "they taught me to despise"), I find the idea that I have been brainwashed infuriating and ludicrous. A sadist is likely to be regarded as a dangerous character. A top is vulnerable to legal prosecution. In the current debate on S/M, a top risks having their testimony dismissed. A masochist has more credibility in defending S/M. But a masochist risks being held in contempt. I am in much less danger of being treated badly by tops or sadists than by the people who want to protect me from them.

It is an unfortunate habit of sexual thought that people so readily assume that something they would not like would be equally unpleasant to someone else. I hate to run. I might someday change my mind, but at this point it would take a lot of coercion to get me to run around the block, let alone for five miles. This does not mean that my friends who run in marathons are sick, brainwashed, or at gunpoint.

People who are not into anal sex find it incomprehensible that anyone else could enjoy it. People who gag at oral sex are baffled that anyone else would actually enjoy sucking cock or eating pussy. But the fact remains that there are uncountable hordes for whom oral sex or anal sex are exquisitely delightful. Sexual diversity exists, not everyone likes to do the same things, and people who have different sexual preferences are not sick, stupid, warped, brainwashed, under duress, dupes of the patriarchy, products of bourgeois decadence, or refugees from bad child-rearing practices. The habit of explaining away sexual variation by putting it down needs to be broken.

The idea that masochists are victims of sadists underlies much of the debate on S/M. But tops and bottoms are not two discrete populations. Some individuals have strong and consistent preferences for one role or the other. Most S/M people have done both, and many change with different partners, at different times, or according to situation or whim.

Nor are the social relations between tops and bottoms similar to the social relations between men and women, blacks and whites, straights and queers. Sadists do not systematically oppress masochists. Of course, class privilege, race, and gender do not disappear when people enter the S/M world. The social power individuals bring to the S/M community affects their ability to negotiate within it, whether as tops or bottoms. But class, race, and gender neither determine nor correspond to the roles adopted for S/M play. The oppression which is connected to S/M comes from a society bent on keeping people from engaging in non-conventional sex and which punishes them when they do.

The silliest arguments about S/M have been those which claim that it is impossible that people really consent to do it. The issue of consent has been clouded by an overly hasty application of Marxian critiques of bourgeois contract theory to sex law and practice. Marxists argue that just because someone voluntarily enters into an agreement to do something, does not mean that they have not been coerced by forces impinging on the decision. This is a useful distinction since social relations of class, gender, race, and so forth in fact do limit the scope of possible decisions which can be made. So do the social relations of sexuality, but not by forcing people to be perverts.

In sex law, consent is what distinguishes sex from rape. But consent is a privilege which is not enjoyed equally by all sexualities. Although it varies according to state, most sexual activity is illegal. The fewest restrictions apply to adult heterosexuality. But adult incest is illegal in most states, and adultery in many. In some states, sodomy laws even apply to heterosexuals, who may be prosecuted for oral or anal sex. Homosexuality is much more restricted than heterosexuality. Except for the states which have passed consenting adult statutes decriminalizing homosexuality, it is still illegal to have gay sex. Before 1976, a gay person in California did not have the legal right to have oral sex with their lover, and could be prosecuted for doing it. Minors have no right at all to consent to sex, although it is usually only adult partners who are prosecuted. But sexually active youth can be sent to juvenile homes and are subject to other penalties.

In addition to clearly defined legal restrictions, sex laws are unequally enforced. And in addition to the activities of police, forces like religion, medicine, media, education, family, and the state all function to pressure people to be married, heterosexual, monogamous, and conventional. One may more reasonably ask if anyone truly "consents" to be straight in any way. Coercion does occur among perverts, as it does in all sexual contexts. One still needs to distinguish rape and abuse from consensual situations. But the overwhelming coercion with regard to S/M is the way in which people are prevented from doing it. We are fighting for the freedom to consent to our sexuality without interference, and without penalty.

IV.

We are sworn that no boy or girl, approaching the maelstrom of deviation, need make that crossing alone, afraid, or in the dark ever again.

The Mattachine Society, 1951[25]

Current radical (mostly feminist) writing on S/M is a hopeless muddle of bad assumptions, inaccurate information, and a thickheaded refusal to accept evidence which contravenes preconceptions. It needs to be taken apart point by point. But prejudice is like a hydra. As soon as one avenue of sexual bigotry is blocked, alternative channels are developed.

Ultimately, acceptance is gained by political power as much as by rational argument. Bigotry against S/M will flourish until it is more expensive to maintain than to abandon. Like the social discourse on homosexuality, this discourse on S/M sets up phony issues and poses phony questions. At some point, we need to step out of this framework and develop an alternative way to think about sexuality and understand its politics.

Minority sexual communities are like religious heretics. We are persecuted by the state, the mental health establishment, social welfare agencies, and the media. When you are a sex pervert, the institutions of society do not work for you, and often work against you. Sexual dissenters face an endless stream of propaganda which rationalizes abuses against them, attempts to impair their self esteem, and exhorts them to recant.

In addition to social hierarchies of class, race, gender, and ethnicity, there is a heirarchy based on sexual behavior. The most blessed form of sexual contact is heterosexual, married, monogamous, and reproductive. Unions that are unmarried, non-monagamous, non-reproductive, involve more than two partners, are homosexual, or which involve kink or fetish, are judged as inferior and punished accordingly. This hierarchy has rarely been challenged since its emergence, except by the gay movement. But it is a domain of social life in which great power is exercised. The "lower" sexual orders are human fodder for the prisons and the mental institutions.

It is time that radicals and progressives, feminists and leftists, recognize this hierarchy for the oppressive structure that it is instead of reproducing it within their own ideologies. Sex is one of the few areas in which cultural imperialism is taken as a radical stance. Neither the therapeutic professions, the women's movement, nor the left have been able to digest the concept of benign sexual variation. The idea that there is one best way to do sex afflicts radical as well as conservative thought on the subject. Cultural relativism is not the same thing as liberalism.

One of the sad things about the current debates on sex in the women's movement is that they are so stupid and regressive. Once the impulse to purge all sex freaks from feminist organizations passes, we will still have to face more intelligent arguments. Among them will be a kind of neo-Reichian position which is pro-sex but which understands the more stigmatized sexualities and practices (pornography, S/M, fetishism) as symptoms of sexual repression. Unlike Reich, the neo-Reichian position may accept homosexuality as a healthy or natural eroticism.

What is exciting is that sex—not just gender, not just homosexuality—has finally been posed as a political question. Rethinking sexual politics has generated some of the most creative political discourse since 1970. The sexual outlaws—boy-lovers, sadomasochists, prostitutes, and trans-people, among others—have an especially rich knowledge of the pre-vailing system of sexual hierarchy and of how sexual controls are exercised. These populations of erotic dissidents have a great deal to contribute to the reviving radical debate on sexuality.

The real danger is not that S/M lesbians will be made uncomfortable in the women's movement. The real danger is that the right, the reli-gious fanatics, and the right-controlled state will eat us all alive. It is sad to be having to fight to maintain one's membership in the women's movement when it is so imperative to create broad based coalitions against fascism. The level of internal strife around S/M should be reserved for more genuine threats to feminist goals. If we survive long enough, feminists and other progressives will eventually stop fearing sexual diversity and begin to learn from it.

Author's Note

I have benefited immensely from innumerable conversations about sex, politics, and S/M with Pat Califia. The work that Allan Berube, John D'Emilio, and Daniel Tsang have done to exhume the story of gay persecution in the fifties has taught me how sex repression works. My sense of the politics of sex in the nineteenth century evolved during conversations with Ellen Dubois, Mary Ryan, and Martha Vicinus. My sense of the context for the politics of sex during the Cold War is largely due to input from Lynn Eden. Conversations with Jeff Escoffier and Amber Hollibaugh have sparked many lines of thought about the social relations of sexuality. I have been taught much of the recent history and many of the fine points of S/M by I.B., Camilla Decarnin, Jim Kane, Jason Klein, Terry Kolb, the Illus-trious Mistress LaLash, Steve McEachern, Bob Milne, Cynthia Slater,

Sam Steward, Louis Weingarden, and Doric Wilson. While responsibility for the opinions expressed in this essay is mine, I want to express my thanks to all these individuals for their insights, their information, and their generosity.

This essay has been revised somewhat for the second edition of *Coming To Power.*

1. *Styles of Radical Will*, 1969, New York, Farrar, Straus, and Giroux, page 46.
2. I am indebted to Allan Berube, John D'Emilio, and Daniel Tsang for much of what I know about it. Each of them has generously shared their research in progress. For published sources, see the following: John D'Emilio, "Dreams Deferred," three parts, *The Body Politic*, November 1978, December/January 1978/1979, and February 1979; John D'Emilio, "Gay Politics, Gay Community: The San Francisco Experience," *Socialist Review*. January/February 1981; Allan Berube, "Behind the Spectre of San Francisco," The Body Politic, April 1981; Jonathan Katz, *Gay American History*, 1976, New York, Thomas Crowell, pages 91–119, and 406–420. See also John Gerassi, *The Boys of Boise*, 1966, New York, Collier.
3. For further details, see Pat Califia, "The Age of Consent," two parts, *The Advocate*, October 16 and October 30, 1980; Mitzel, *The Boston Sex Scandal*, 1980, Boston, Glad Day Books; Roger Moody, *Indecent Assault*, 1980, London, Word Is Out.
4. Meanwhile, Dan White got seven years for the coldblooded murder of two public officials, one of them gay, and Ronald Crumpley was acquitted of the murder of two gay men (and the wounding of several others) by reason of insanity.
5. Lest I be misunderstood, the point is not that the Jaguar should not be supported. It should. But the contrast in community response to the troubles of the Jaguar and the troubles of the Bootcamp was stunning.
6. Randy Alfred, text of complaint against *Gay Power, Gay Politics*, lodged with the National News Council, July 10, 1980, page 4.
7. Alfred, page 5.
8. Alfred, page 5.
9. Pearl Stewart. "Safety Workshops for S.F. Masochists," *San Francisco Chronicle*, March 12, 1981.
10. Marshall Kilduff, "Angry Mayor Cuts Off Coroner's S&M Classes," *San Francisco Chronicle*, March 14, 1981.
11. San Francisco Chronicle. July 11–July 14, 1981.
12. Revolutionary Union, statement *On Homosexuality*, 1976. Note that the statement was referring to both lesbians and gay men.
13. "Sadomasochism as a Contra-feminist Activity," *Plexus*, November 1980.
14. ry, "S/M Keeps Lesbians Bound to the Patriarchy," *Lesbian Insider/Insighter/Inciter*, July 1981.
15. M.A. Karr, "Susan Griffin," *The Advocate*, March 20, 1980.
16. tacie dejanikus, "Our Legacy," *Off Our Backs*, November 1980.
17. Correspondence and other documentation of the interactions between SAMOIS and various feminist institutions (including the Women's Building and *Off Our Backs*) are on file at the Lesbian Herstory Archives in New York City.

18. The phenomenon of feminism as a closet for lesbianism is discussed by Chris Bearchell in "The Cloak of Feminism," *The Body Politic*, June 1979, p. 20.

19. I should add that the term has also simply become an all purpose insult whose meaning is simply that the speaker does not approve of the person or activity to which it is applied.

20. An excellent historical study of some of these shifts in feminist ideology can be found in Alice Echols, "Cultural Feminism: Feminist Capitalism and the Anti-Pornography Movement," unpublished manuscript, June 1981, Women's Studies Program, University of Michigan.

21. There is a certain amount of bad faith around sex in all this. There is plenty of sex in the women's movement, and most feminists are just as obsessed with it as anyone else. But it has gotten hard to call things by their real names, or acknowledge lust as an end in itself. There is rampant euphemism, and a self-centered notion that "feminist sex" is a higher form of erotic expression. And the boundaries of what can be "feminist sex" shrink by the day.

22. Among the histories which shed light on the relationship between nineteenth century feminism and various sexual populations and issues are these: Linda Gordon, *Woman's Body, Woman's Right*, 1976, New York, Penguin; Judith Walkowitz, *Prostitution and Victorian Society*, 1980, New York, Cambridge; Judith Walkowitz, "The Politics of Prostitution," *Signs*, Autumn, 1980; and Jeffrey Weeks, *Coming Out: Homosexual Politics in Britain, from the Nineteenth Century to the Present*, 1977, New York, Quartet.

23. Neil Glickman, "Letter to the Editor," *Gay Community News*, August 22, 1981.

24. Ann Bannon, 1959, Greenwich, Connecticut, Fawcett Publications.

25. Cited in John D'Emilio, "Radical Beginnings, 1950–51," *The Body Politic*, November, 1978, p. 24.

Millbrook '66: On Sex, Consciousness, and LSD

Timothy Leary

from *The Delicious Grace of Moving One's Hand*, 1999

One of the most important recreational drugs of the sixties was LSD—it was considered a consciousness expanding drug. Timothy Leary, who had conducted research on LSD at Harvard, became the prophet of the psychedelic experience as a religious one. For Leary, sexual ecstasy while using LSD is a transcendental experience with spiritual significance—a merging and a surrender of the limits of the personal ego.

U p to this moment, I've had 311 psychedelic sessions. I was thirty-nine when I had my first psychedelic experience. At that time, I was a middle-aged man involved in the middle-aged process of dying. My joy in life, my sensual openness, my creativity were all sliding downhill. Since that time, six years ago, my life has been reviewed in almost every dimension. Most of my colleagues at the University of California and at Harvard, of course, feel that I've become an eccentric and a kook. I would estimate that fewer than 15 percent of my professional colleagues understand and support what I'm doing. The ones who do, as you might expect, tend to be among the younger psychologists. If you know a person's age, you know what he's going to think and feel about LSD. Psychedelic drugs are the medium of the young. As you move up the age scale into the thirties, forties and fifties, fewer and fewer people are open to the possibilities that these chemicals offer.

To the person over thirty-five or forty, the word "drug" means one of two things: doctor-disease or dope fiend-crime. Nothing you can say to a person who has this neurological fix on the word "drug" is going to change his mind. He's frozen like a Pavlovian dog to this conditioned reflex. To people under twenty-five, on the other hand, the word "drug" refers to a wide range of mind benders running from alcohol, energizers, and stupefiers to marijuana and other psychedelic drugs. To middle-aged America, it may be synonymous with instant insanity, but to most Americans under twenty-five, the psychedelic drug means ecstasy, sensual unfolding, religious experience, revelation, illumination, contact with nature. There's hardly a teenager or young person in the United States today who doesn't know at least one young person who has had a good experience with marijuana or LSD. The horizons of the current younger generation, in terms of expanded consciousness, are light years beyond those of their parents. The breakthrough has occurred; there's no going back. The psychedelic battle is won.

None of us yet knows exactly how LSD can be used for the growth and benefit of the human being. It is a powerful releaser of energy as yet not fully understood. But when I'm confronted with the possibility that a fifteen-year-old or a fifty-year-old is going to use a new form of energy that he doesn't understand, I'll back the fifteen-year-old every time. Why? Because a fifteen-year-old is going to use a new form of energy to have fun, intensify sensation, to make love, for curiosity, for personal growth. Many fifty-year-olds have lost their curiosity, have lost their ability to make love, have dulled their openness to new sensations, and would use any form of new energy for power, control, and warfare. So it doesn't concern me at all that young people are taking time out from the educational and occupational assembly lines to experiment with consciousness, to dabble with new forms of experience and artistic expression. The present generation under the age of twenty-five is the wisest and holiest generation that the human race has ever seen. And, by God, instead of lamenting, derogating, and imprisoning them, we should support them, listen to them, and turn on with them.

Throughout human history, humans who have wanted to expand their consciousness, to find deeper meaning inside themselves, have been able to do it if they were willing to commit the time and energy to do so. In other times and countries, men would walk barefooted

2,000 miles to find spiritual teachers who would turn them on to Buddha, Mohammed, or Ramakrishna.

If we're speaking in a general way, what happens to everyone on LSD is the experience of incredible acceleration and intensification of all senses and all mental processes—which can be very confusing if you're not prepared for it. Around a thousand million signals fire off in your brain every second; during any second in an LSD session, you find yourself tuned in on thousands of these messages that ordinarily you don't register consciously. And you may be getting an incredible number of simultaneous messages from different parts of your body. Since you're not used to this, it can lead to incredible ecstasy or it can lead to confusion. Some people are freaked by this Niagara of sensory input. Instead of having just one or two or three things happening in tidy sequence, you're suddenly flooded by hundreds of lights and colors and sensations and images, and you can get quite lost. . . .

You sense a strange powerful force beginning to unloose and radiate through your body. In normal perception, we are aware of static symbols. But as the LSD effect takes hold, everything begins to move, and this relentless, impersonal, slowly swelling movement will continue through the several hours of the session. It's as though for all of your normal waking life you have been caught in a still photograph, in an awkward, stereotyped posture; suddenly the show comes alive, balloons out to several dimensions and becomes irradiated with color and energy.

LSD and the Senses

The first thing you notice is an incredible enhancement of sensory awareness. Take the sense of sight. LSD vision is to normal vision as normal vision is to the picture on a badly tuned television set. Under LSD, it's as though you have microscopes up to your eyes, in which you see jewel-like, radiant details of anything your eye falls upon. You are really seeing for the first time—not static, symbolic perception of learned things, but patterns of light bouncing off the objects around you and hurtling at the speed of light into the mosaic or rods and cones in the retina of your eye. Everything seems alive. Everything is alive beaming diamond-bright light waves into your retina.

Ordinarily we hear just isolated sounds: the rings of a telephone, the sound of somebody's words. But when you turn on with LSD, the organ of Corti in your inner ear becomes a trembling membrane seething with tattoos of sound waves. The vibrations seem to penetrate deep inside you, swell and burst there. You hear one note of a Bach sonata, and it hangs there, glittering, pulsating, for an endless length of time, while you slowly orbit around it. Then, hundreds of years later, comes the second note of the sonata, and again, for hundreds of years, you slowly drift around the two notes, observing the harmony and the discords, and reflecting on the history of music.

When your nervous system is turned on with LSD, and all the wires are flashing, the senses begin to overlap and merge. You not only hear but see the music emerging from the speaker system, like dancing particles, like squirming curls of toothpaste. You actually see the sound in multicolored patterns while you're hearing it. At the same time, you are the sound, you are the note, you are the string of the violin or the piano. And every one of your organs is pulsating, and having orgasms in rhythm with it.

Taste is intensified, too, although normally you wouldn't feel like eating during an LSD session, any more than you feel like eating when you take your first solo at the controls of a supersonic jet. Although if you eat after a session, there is an appreciation of all the particular qualities of food—its texture and resiliency and viscosity—such as we are not conscious of in a normal state of awareness.

As for smell, this is one of the most overwhelming aspects of an LSD experience. It seems as though for the first time you are breathing life, and you remember with amusement and distaste that plastic, odorless, artificial gas that you used to consider air. During the LSD experience, you discover that you're actually inhaling an atmosphere composed of millions of microscopic strands of olfactory ticker tape, exploding in your nostrils with ecstatic meaning. When you sit across the room from a woman during an LSD session, you're aware of thousands of penetrating chemical messages floating from her through the air into your sensory center, a symphony of a thousand odors that all of us exude at every moment, the shampoo she uses, her cologne, her sweat, the exhaust and discharge from her digestive system, her sexual perfume, the fragrance of her clothing—grenades of eroticism exploding in the olfactory cell.

Touch Becomes Electric as Well as Erotic

I remember a moment during one session in which my wife Rosemary leaned over and lightly touched the palm of my hand with her finger. Immediately a hundred thousand end cells in my hand exploded in soft orgasm. Ecstatic energies pulsated up my arms and rocketed into my brain, where another hundred thousand cells softly exploded in pure, delicate pleasure. The distance between my wife's finger and the palm of my hand was about 50 miles of space, filled with cotton candy, infiltrated with thousands of silver wires hurtling energy back and forth. Wave after wave of exquisite energy pulsed from her finger. Wave upon wave of ethereal tissue rapture—delicate, shuddering—coursed back and forth from her finger to my palm.

Transcendentally erotic rapture.

An enormous amount of information from every fiber of your body is released under LSD, most especially including sexual energy. There is no question that LSD is the most powerful aphrodisiac ever discovered.

Sex under LSD becomes miraculously enhanced and intensified. I don't mean that it simply generates genital energy. It doesn't automatically produce a longer erection. Rather, it increases your sensitivity a thousand percent. Let me put it this way: Compared with sex under LSD, the way you've been making love—no matter how ecstatic the pleasure you think you get from it—is like making love to a department store window dummy. In sensory and cellular communion on LSD, you may spend a half-hour making love with eyeballs, another half-hour making love with breath. As you spin through a thousand sensory and cellular organic changes, she does too.

Ordinarily, sexual communication involves one's own chemicals, pressure and interactions of a very localized nature, in what the psychologists call the erogenous zones. A vulgar concept, I think. When you're making love under LSD, it's as though every cell in your body—and you have trillions—is making love with every cell in her body. Her hand doesn't caress her skin but sinks down into and merges with ancient dynamos of ecstasy within her.

Every time I've taken LSD, I have made love. In fact, that is what the LSD experience is all about. Merging, yielding, flowing, union, communion. It's all lovemaking. You make love with candlelight, with sound waves from a record player, with a bowl of fruit on the table, with the trees. You're in pulsating harmony with all the energy around you.

The three inevitable goals of LSD sessions are to discover and make love with God, to discover and make love with yourself, and to discover and make love with another. You can't make it with yourself unless you've made it with the timeless energy process around you, and you can't make it with a mate until you've made it with yourself. One of the great purposes of an LSD session is sexual union. The more expanded your consciousness, the further out you can move beyond your mind, the deeper, the richer, the longer and more meaningful your sexual communion.

Only the most reckless poet would attempt to describe an orgasm on LSD. What does one say to a little child? The child asks, "Daddy, what is sex like?" and you try to describe it, and then the little child says, "Well, is it fun like the circus?"

And you say, "Well, not exactly like that."

And the child says, "Is it fun like chocolate ice cream?"

And you say, "Well, it's like that but much, much more than that."

And the child says, "Is it fun like the rollercoaster, then?"

And you say, "Well that's part of it, but it's even more than that."

In short, I can't tell you what it's like, because it's not like anything that's ever happened to you—and there aren't words adequate to describe it anyway. You won't know what it's like until you try it yourself and then I won't need to tell you.

This preoccupation with the number of orgasms is a hang-up for many men and women. It's as crude and vulgar a concept as wondering how much she paid for the negligee.

Still, it's a fact that women who ordinarily have difficulty achieving orgasm find themselves capable of multiple orgasms under LSD, even several hundred orgasms.

I can only speak for myself and about my own experience. I can only compare what I was with what I am now. In the last six years, my openness to, my responsiveness to, my participation in every form of sensory expression, has multiplied a thousandfold.

The sexual impact is, of course, the open but private secret about LSD, which none of us has talked about in the last few years. It's socially dangerous enough to say that LSD helps you find divinity and helps you discover yourself. You're already in trouble when you say that. But then if you announce that the psychedelic experience is basically a sexual experience, you're asking to bring the whole middle-aged, middle-class monolith down on your head.

At the present time, however, I'm under a thirty-year sentence of imprisonment, which for a forty-five-year-old man is essentially a life term, and in addition, I am under indictment on a second marijuana offense involving a sixteen-year sentence. Since there is hardly anything more that middle-aged, middle-class authority can do to me—and since the secret is out anyway among the young—I feel I'm free at this moment to say what we've never said before: *that sexual ecstasy is the basic reason for the current LSD boom.*

Young people are taking LSD and discovering God and meaning; they're discovering themselves; but did you really think that sex wasn't the fundamental reason for this surging, youthful social bloom? You can no more do research on LSD and leave out sexual ecstasy than you can do microscopic research on tissue and leave out cells.

LSD is not an automatic trigger to sexual awakening, however. The first ten times you take it, you might not be able to have a sexual experience at all, because you're so overwhelmed and delighted, or frightened and confused, by the novelty; the idea of having sex might be irrelevant or incomprehensible at the moment. But it depends upon the setting and the partner. It is almost inevitable, if a man and his mate take LSD together, that their sexual energies will be unimaginably intensified, and unless clumsiness or fright on the part of one or the other blocks it, will lead to a deeper experience than they ever thought possible.

From the beginning of our research, we have been aware of this tremendous personal power in LSD. You must be very careful to take it only with someone you know really well, because it's almost inevitable that a man will fall in love with the woman who shares his LSD experience. Deep and lasting neurological imprints, profound emotional bonds can develop as a result of an LSD session, bonds that can last a lifetime. For this reason, we have always been extremely cautious about running sessions with men and women. We always try to have a subject's husband or wife present during his or her first session, so that as these powerful urges develop, they are directed in ways that can be lived out responsibly after the session.

One of the great lessons I've learned from LSD is that every man contains the essence of all men and every woman has within her all women. I remember a session a few years ago in which, with horror and ecstasy, I opened my eyes and looked into Rosemary's eyes and was pulled into the deep pools of her being floating softly in the center of her mind, experiencing everything that she was experiencing, knowing every thought she ever had. As my eyes were riveted to hers, her face began to melt and change. I saw her as a young girl, as a baby, as an old woman with gray hair and seamy, wrinkled face. I saw her as a witch, a Madonna, a nagging crone, a radiant queen, a Byzantine virgin, a tired worldly-wise oriental whore who had seen every sight of life repeated a thousand times. She was all women, all woman, the essence of female, eyes smiling quizzically, resignedly, devilishly, always inviting, "See me, hear me, join me, merge with me, keep the dance going." Now the implications of this experience for sex and mating, I think are obvious. It's because of this, not because of moral restrictions or restraints, that I've been monogamous in my use of LSD over the last six years.

The notion of running around trying to find different mates is a very low-level concept. We are living in a world of expanding population in which there are more and more beautiful young girls and boys coming off the assembly line each month. It's obvious that the sexual criteria of the past are going to be changed and that what's demanded of creatures with our sensory and cellular repertoire is not just one affair after another with one young body after another, but the exploration of the incredible depths and varieties of your own identity with another. This involves time and commitment to the voyage. There is a certain kind of neurological and cellular fidelity that develops. I have said for many years now that in the future the grounds for divorce would not be that your mate went to bed with another and bounced around on a mattress for an hour or two, but that your mate had an LSD session with somebody else, because the bonds and the connections that develop are so powerful.

For the most part, during the last six years, I have lived very quietly in our research centers. But on lecture tours and in highly enthusiastic social gatherings, there is no question that a charismatic public figure does generate attraction and stimulate a sexual response.

Every woman has built into her cells and tissues the longing for a hero, sage-mythic male, to open up and share her own divinity. But casual sexual encounters do not satisfy this deep longing. Any charismatic person who is conscious of his or her own mythic potency awakens this basic hunger and pays reverence to it at the level that is harmonious and appropriate at the time. Compulsive body grabbing, however, is rarely the vehicle of such communication.

I'm no one to tell anyone else what to do. But I would say, if you use LSD to make out sexually in the seductive sense, then you'll be a very humiliated and embarrassed person, because it's just not going to work. On LSD, her eyes would be microscopic, and she'd see very plainly what you were up to, coming on with some heavy-handed, mustache-twisting routine. You'd look like a consummate ass, and she'd laugh at you, or you'd look like a monster and she'd scream and go into a paranoid state. Nothing good can happen with LSD if it's used crudely or for power or for manipulative purposes.

You must remember that in taking LSD with someone else, you are voluntarily relinquishing your personality defenses and opening yourself up in a very vulnerable manner. If you and the other are ready to do this, there would be an immediate and deep rapport if you took a trip together. People from the LSD cult would be able to make love upon a brief meeting, but an inexperienced person would probably find it extremely confusing, and the people might become quite isolated from each other. They might be whirled into the rapture or confusion of their own inner workings and forget entirely that the other person is there.

LSD is not a sexual cure-all. LSD is no guarantee of any specific social or sexual outcome. One man may take LSD and leave wife and family and go off to be a monk on the banks of the Ganges. Another may take LSD and go back to her husband. It's a highly individual situation. Highly unpredictable. During LSD sessions, you see, there can come a microscopic perception of your routine social and professional life. You may discover to your horror that you're living a robot existence, that your relationships with your boss, your husband, and your family are stereotyped, empty, and devoid of meaning. At this point, there might come a desire to renounce this hollow existence, to collect your thoughts, to go away and cloister yourself from the world like a monk while you figure out what kind of life you want to go back to, if any.

Conversely, we've found that in giving LSD to members of monastic sects, there has been a definite tendency for them to leave the monastic life and to find a mating relationship. Several were men in their late forties who had been monks for 15 or 20 years, but who even at this mature age returned to society, married and made the heterosexual adjustment. It's not coincidental that of all those I've given LSD to, the religious group—more than 200 ministers, priests, divinity students, and nuns— has experienced the most intense sexual reaction. And in two religious groups that prize chastity and celibacy, there have been wholesale defections of monks and nuns who left their religious orders to get married after a series of LSD experiences. The LSD session, you see, is an overwhelming awakening of experience; it releases potent, primal energies, and one of these is the sexual impulse, which is the strongest impulse at any level of organic life. For the first time in their lives, perhaps, these people were meeting head on the powerful life forces that they had walled off with ritualized defenses and self-delusions.

For almost everyone, the LSD experience is a confrontation with new forms of wisdom and energy that dwarf and humiliate the mind. This experience of awe and revelation is often described as religious. I consider my work basically religious, because it has, as its goal, the systematic expansion of consciousness and the discovery of energies within, which men call divine. From the psychedelic point of view, almost all religions are attempts, sometimes limited temporarily or nationally, to discover inner potential. Well, LSD is Western yoga. The aim of all Eastern religion, like the aim of LSD, is basically to get high—that is, to expand your consciousness and find ecstasy and revelation within.

Levels of Consciousness

Our system of consciousness—attested to by the experience of hundreds of thousands of trained voyagers who've taken LSD—defines seven different levels of awareness.

The lowest levels of consciousness are sleep and emotional stupor, which are produced by narcotics, barbiturates and our national stupe-facient, alcohol. A third level of consciousness is the conventional wakeful state, in which awareness is hooked to conditioned symbols: flags, dollar signs, job titles, brand names, party affiliations, and the like. This is the level that most people, including psychiatrists, regard as reality; they don't know the half of it.

The next two levels of awareness, somatic and sensory, would, I think, be of particular interest to *Playboy* readers because most of them are of the younger generation, which is much more sensual than the puritanical Americans of the older generation. In order to reach the somatic and sensory levels, you have to have something that will turn off symbols and open up your billions of sensory cameras to the billions of impulses that are hitting them. The chemical that opens the door to this level has been well known for centuries to cultures that stress delicate, sensitive registration of sensory stimulation: the Arab cultures, the Indian cultures, the Mogul cultures. It is marijuana. There is no question that marijuana is a sensual stimulator, and this explains not only why it's favored by young people but why it arouses fear and panic among the middle-aged, middle-class, whiskey-drinking, blue-nosed bureaucrats who run the narcotics agencies. If they only knew what they were missing. But we must bid a sad farewell to the bodily levels of consciousness and go on to the sixth level, which I call the cellular level. It's well known that the stronger psychedelics such as mescaline and LSD take you beyond the senses into a world of cellular awareness. Now the neurological fact of the matter is that every one of your 100 billion brain cells is hooked up to some 25,000 other cells, and everything you know comes from a communication exchange at the nerve endings of your cells. During an LSD session, enormous clusters of these pathways are turned on, and consciousness whirls into eerie panoramas for which we have no words or concepts. Here the metaphor that's most accurate is the metaphor of the micro-scope, which brings into awareness cellular patterns that are invisible to the naked eye. In the same way, LSD brings into awareness the cellular conversations that are inaudible to the normal consciousness and for which we have no adequate symbolic language. You become aware of processes you were never tuned into before. You feel yourself sinking down into the soft tissue swamp of your own body, slowly drifting down dark, red waterways and floating through capillary canals, softly propelled through endless cellular factories, ancient fibrous clockworlds: ticking, clicking, chugging, pumping relentlessly. Being swallowed up this way by the tissue industries and the bloody, sinewy carryings-on inside your body can be an appalling experience the first time it happens to you. But it can also be an awesome one . . . fearful, but full of reverence and wonder.

The next level is even more strange and terrifying. This is the precellular level, which is experienced only under a heavy dose of LSD. Your nerve cells are aware—as Professor Einstein was aware—that all matter, all structure, is pulsating information; well, there is a shattering moment in the deep psychedelic session when your body, and the world around you, dissolves into shimmering latticeworks of pulsating white waves, into silent, subcellular worlds of shuttling information. But this phenomenon is nothing new. It's been reported by mystics and visionaries throughout the last 4,000 years of recorded history as "the white light" of the "dance of energy." Suddenly you realize that everything you thought of as reality or even as life itself—including your body—is just a dance of particles. You find yourself horribly alone in a dead, impersonal world of raw data flooding your sense organs. This, of course, is one of the oldest Oriental philosophic notions, that nothing exists except in the chemistry of your own consciousness. But when it first really happens to you through the experience of LSD, it can come as a terrorizing, isolating discovery. At this point, the unprepared LSD subject often screams out: "I'm dead!" And he sits there transfigured with fear, afraid to move. For the experienced voyager, however, this revelation can be exalting: You've climbed inside Einstein's formula, penetrated to the ultimate nature of matter, and you're pulsing in harmony with its primal, cosmic beat.

It's happened to me about half of the 311 times I've taken LSD. And every time it begins to happen, no matter how much experience you've had, there is that moment of terror, because nobody likes to see the comfortable world of objects and symbols and even cells disintegrate into the ultimate physical design.

We know that there are many other levels of energy within and around us, and I hope that within our lifetimes we will have these opened up to us, because the fact is that there is no form of information on this planet that isn't recorded somewhere in your body. Built within every cell are molecular strands of memory and awareness called the DNA code, the genetic blueprint that has designed and executed the construction of your body. This is an ancient strand of molecules that possesses memories of every previous organism that has contributed to your present existence. In your DNA code you have the genetic history of your father and mother. It goes back, back, back through the generations, through the eons. Your body carries a protein record of everything that's happened to you since the moment you were conceived as a one-cell organism. It's a living history of every form of energy transformation on this planet back to the beginning of the life process over two billion years ago. When LSD subjects report retrogression and reincarnation visions, this is not mysterious or supernatural. It's simply modern biogenetics.

We don't know how these memories are stored, but countless events from early and even intrauterine life are registered in your brain and can be flashed into consciousness during an LSD experience.

The experiences that come from LSD are actually relived—in sight, sound, smell, taste and touch—exactly the way they were recorded before.

It's possible to check out some of these ancient memories, but for the most part, these memory banks, which are built into your protein cellular strands, can never be checked on by external observation. Who can possibly corroborate what your nervous system picked up before your birth, inside your mother? But the obvious fact is that your nervous system was operating while you were still in the uterus. It was receiving and recording units of consciousness. Why, then, is it surprising that at some later date, if you have the chemical key, you can release these memories of the nine perilous and exciting months before you were born?

I've charted my own family tree and traced it back as far as I can. I've tried to plumb the gene pools from which my ancestors emerged in Ireland and France.

There are certain moments in my evolutionary history that I can reach all the time, but there are certain untidy corners in my racial path that I often get boxed into, and because they are frightening, I freak out and open my eyes and stop it. In many of these sessions, back about 300 years, I often run across a particular French-appearing man with a black mustache, a rather dangerous-looking guy. And there are several highly eccentric recurrent sequences in an Anglo-Saxon country that have embarrassed me when I relived them in LSD sessions—goings-on that shocked my twentieth-century person.

Moments of propagation, scenes of rough ancestral sexuality in Irish barrooms, in haystacks, in canopied beds, in covered wagons, on beaches, on the moist jungle floor, and moments of crisis in which my forebears escape from fang, from spear, from conspiracy, from tidal wave and avalanche. I've concluded that the imprints most deeply engraved in neurological memory bank have to do with these moments of life-affirming exultation and exhilaration in the perpetuation and survival of the self and of the species.

They may all be nothing more than luridly melodramatic, Saturday serials conjured up by my forebrain. But whatever they are—memory or imagination—it's the most exciting adventure I've ever been involved in.

Turn On, Tune In, Drop Out

"Turn on" means to contact and explore the ancient energies and wisdoms that are built into your nervous system. They provide unspeakable excitements and revelations. "Tune in" means to harness and communicate these new perspectives in a harmonious dance with the external world. "Drop out" means to detach yourself from the tribal game. Current models of social adjustment— mechanized, computerized, socialized, intellectualized, televised, Sanforized—make no sense to the new LSD generation, who see clearly that American society is becoming an air-conditioned anthill. In every generation of human history, thoughtful men have turned on and dropped out of the tribal game and thus stimulated the larger society to lurch ahead. Every historical advance has resulted from the stern pressure of visionary men who have declared their independence from the game: "Sorry, George III, we don't buy your model. We're going to try something new."; "Sorry, Louis XVI, we've got a new idea. Deal us out"; "Sorry, LBJ, it's time to mosey on beyond the Great Society."

The reflex reaction of the gene pool to the creative drop-out is panic and irritation. If anyone questions the social order, he threatens the whole shaky edifice. The automatic, angry reaction to the creative drop-out is that he will become a parasite on the hardworking, conforming citizen. This is not true. The LSD experience does not lead to passivity and withdrawal; it spurs a driving hunger to communicate in new forms, in better ways, to express a more harmonious message, to live a better life. The LSD cult has already wrought revolutionary changes in American culture. If you were to conduct a poll of creative young musicians in this country, you'd find at least 80 percent are using psychedelic drugs in a systematic way. And this new psychedelic style has produced not only a new rhythm in modern music, but a new decor for our discotheques, a new form of film-making, a new kinetic visual art, a new literature, and has begun to revise our philosophic and psychological thinking. Remember, it's the college kids who are turning on—the smartest and most promising of the youngsters. What an exciting prospect: a generation of creative youngsters refusing to march in step, refusing to go to offices, refusing to sign up on the installment plan, refusing to climb aboard the treadmill.

Don't worry. Each one will work out his individual solution. Some will return to the establishment and inject their new ideas. Some will live underground as free agents, self-employed artists, artisans, and writers, Some are already forming small communities out of country. Many are starting schools for children and adults who wish to learn the use of their sense organs. Psychedelic businesses are springing up: bookstores, art galleries. Psychedelic industries may involve more manpower in the future than the automobile industry has produced in the last 20 years. In our technological society of the future, the problem will be not to get people to work but to develop graceful, fulfilling ways of living a more serene, beautiful and creative life. Psychedelics will help to point the way.

No one has the right to tell anyone else what he should or should not do with this great and last frontier of freedom. I think that anyone who wants to have a psychedelic experience and is willing to prepare for it and to examine his own hang-ups and neurotic tendencies should be allowed to have a crack at it.

LSD teaches us the understanding that basic to the life impulse is the question, should we go on with life? This is the only real issue, when you come down to it, in the evolutionary cosmic sense: whether to make it with a member of the opposite sex and keep it going, or not to. At the deepest level of consciousness, this question comes up over and over again. I've struggling with it in scores of LSD sessions. How did we get here and into this mess? How do we get out? There are two ways out of the basic philosophic isolation of man: You can ball your way out, by having children, which is immortality of a sort. Or you can step off the wheel. Buddhism, the most powerful psychology that man has ever developed, says essentially that. My choice, however, is to keep the life game going. I'm Hindu not Buddhist.

Beyond this affirmation of my own life, I've learned to confine my attention to the philosophic questions that hit on the really shrieking, crucial issues: Who wrote the cosmic script? What does the DNA code expect of me? Is the big genetic-code show live or on tape? Who is the sponsor? Are we completely trapped inside our nervous systems, or can we make real contact with anyone else out there? I intend to spend the rest of my life, with psychedelic help, searching for the answers to these questions—and encouraging others to do the same.

LSD is only the first of many new chemicals that will exhilarate learning, expand consciousness and enhance memory in years to come. These chemicals will inevitably revolutionize our procedures of education, child rearing, and social behavior. Within one generation these chemical keys to the nervous system will be used as regular tools of learning. You will be asking your children, when they come home from school, not "What book are you reading?" but "Which molecules are you using to open up new Libraries of Congress inside your nervous system?" There's no doubt that chemicals will be the central method of education in the future. The reason for this, of course, is that the nervous system, and learning and memory itself, is a chemical process. A society in which a large percentage of the population changes consciousness regularly and harmoniously with psychedelic drugs will bring about a very different way of life.

As some science fiction writers predict, people will be taking trips, rather than drinks, at psychedelic cocktail parties.

It's happening already. In this country, there are already functions at which LSD may be served. I was at a large dance recently where two-thirds of the guests were on LSD. And during a scholarly LSD conference in San Francisco a few months ago, I went along with 400 people on a picnic at which almost everyone turned on with LSD. It was very serene. They were like a herd of deer in the forest.

In years to come, it will be possible to have a lunch-hour psychedelic session; in a limited way, that can be done now with DMT, which has a very fast action, lasting perhaps a half-hour. It may be that there will also be large reservations of maybe 30 or 40 square miles, where people will go to have LSD sessions in tranquil privacy.

Everyone will not be turned on all the time. There will always be some functions that require a narrow form of consciousness. You don't want your airplane pilot flying higher than the plane and having Buddhist revelations in the cockpit. Just as you don't play golf on Times Square, you won't want to take LSD where linear, symbol-manipulating attention is required. In a sophisticated way, you'll attune the desired level of consciousness to the particular surrounding that will feed and nourish you.

No one will commit his life to any single level of consciousness. Sensible use of the nervous system would suggest that a quarter of out time will be spent in symbolic activities, producing and communicating in conventional, tribal ways. But the fully conscious life schedule will allow considerable time—perhaps an hour or two a day—devoted to the yoga of the senses, to the enhancement of sensual ecstasies through marijuana and hashish, and one day a week to completely moving outside the sensory and symbolic dimensions into the transcendental realms that are open to you through LSD. This is not science fiction fantasy. I have lived most of the last six years—until the recent unpleasantness—doing exactly that: taking LSD once a week and smoking marijuana once a day.

The Psychedelic Life will enable each person to realize that he is not a game-playing robot put on this planet to be given a Social Security Number and to be spun on the assembly line of school, college, career, insurance, funeral, good-bye. Through LSD, each human being will be taught to understand that the entire history of evolution is recorded inside his brain. The challenge of the complete human life will be for each person to recapitulate and experientially explore every aspect and vicissitude of this ancient and majestic wilderness. Each person will become his own Buddha, his own Einstein, his own Galileo. Instead of relying on canned, static, dead knowledge passed on from other symbol producers, he will be using his span of 80 or so years on this planet to live out every possibility of the human, prehuman, and even subhuman adventure. As more respect and time are diverted to these explorations, he will be less hung up on trivial, external pastimes. And this may be the natural solution to the problem of leisure. When all of the heavy work and mental drudgery is taken over by machines, what are we going to do with ourselves: build even bigger machines? The obvious and only answer to this peculiar dilemma is that man is going to have to explore the infinity of inner space, to discover the terror and adventure and ecstasy that lie within us all.

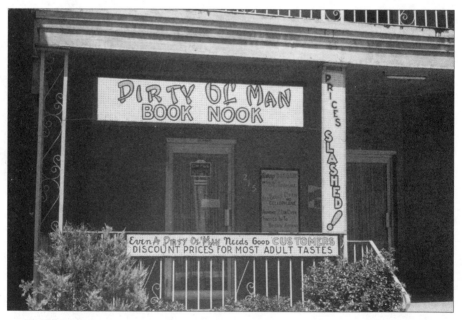

PART IV

Obscenity, Pornography and Erotica

• • •

Pornography is a complex phenomenon. One the one hand, the history of pornography in the US cannot be separated from the political and legal battles for free speech and the First Amendment, yet it is also and perhaps has always been a profitable business—and in the US sometimes involved organized crime. Pornographic representations of sexuality have ranged from profound explorations of desire—as in Pauline Reage's *Story of O*—to highly stereotyped permutations of sexual positions. The sexual explicitness of pornography ranges from soft-core images of attractive models posing or running in the woods to gritty depictions of kinky sex acts in an alley way. Pornography can reinforce the crudest stereotypes of sex roles, standards of beauty, or power dynamics or it can contribute to the education of desire. It is a fantasy machine or a form of discourse about sex. And it can be all these things at the same time.

Somewhere between 1500 and 1800 in Western Europe, pornography emerged both as literary genre and as a category of knowledge about sex. The first pornographers were among the free thinkers, heretics, and libertines of the Renaissance and the Enlightenment. Obscenity and pornography challenged the social boundaries between classes, redrew the line between private and public, redefined the social relations of the sexes, and sought to undermine those in political authority. Leaders of the French Enlightenment, such a Denis Diderot, occasionally wrote pornographic fiction to explore the significance of male and female, pleasure and sensation, power and autonomy.

Obscenity, on the other hand, is the terrain upon which the legal and political battles have been fought. It was originally formulated by the ancient Greeks to identify the boundary between private and public use of sexual and scatological language and imagery. Classic Greek comedy, such as that of Aristophanes, was bawdy and frequently used sexual and scatological terms to satirize and demean public figures, events and even the gods. In line with the classical definition, Freud argued that the obscene remark or joke achieves its shocking effect through the implicit acknowledgement of sexual inhibitions within a mixed male-female public setting. The impact of Lenny Bruce's comic routines was rooted in the transgressions of the public boundaries which had previously excluded sexually explicit speech. "The obscene word," one commentator has noted, "assumes a function of unmasking by denouncing sentimental discourse as a kind of euphemism intended to cover up the truth of sexual desire." By the classical definition, the descriptions of President Clinton and Monica Lewinsky's sexual activities in *The Starr Report* were obscene.

Contemporary legal battles have modified the meaning of obscenity somewhat. Supreme Court Justice Brennan has stated that "sex and obscenity are not synonymous . . . [obscene material] is material having a tendency to excite lustful thought." Obscenity has been transformed from referring to a boundary between private and public speech, to a form of speech that excites lustful thoughts. Brennan's four part definition of obscenity has profoundly shaped the legal battle over pornography: "[1] Whether to the average person, [2] applying contemporary community standards, [3] the dominant theme of the material taken as a whole [4] appeals to prurient interests." The battle over obscenity and pornography created a public arena in which it became possible to discuss sex and to represent it both literarily and visually, and without which the sexual revolution is difficult to imagine.

Obscenity and the Law of Reflection

Henry Miller

from *Remember to Remember,* 1947

Henry Miller is one of the major American writers of the twentieth century. The irony is that his most important work—The Tropic of Cancer, The Tropic of Capricorn and his trilogy Sexus, Plexus and Nexus—though mostly written during the 1930s and 1940s was not published in the United States until the early sixties because of its blunt sexual language and its explicit accounts of sexual activities. Only after Grove Press's publisher, Barney Rosset, had fought charges of obscenity and won the right to publish D.H. Lawrence's Lady Chatterly's Lover were Miller's sexually explicit books published in the U.S.

T o discuss the nature and meaning of obscenity is almost as difficult as to talk about God. Until I began delving into the literature which has grown up about the subject I never realized what a morass I was wading into. If one begins with etymology one is immediately aware that lexicographers are bamboozlers every bit as much as jurists, moralists and politicians. To begin with, those who have seriously attempted to track down the meaning of the term are obliged to confess that they have arrived nowhere. In their book, *To the Pure,* Ernst and Seagle state that "no two persons agree on the definitions of the six deadly adjectives: obscene, lewd, lascivious, filthy, indecent, disgusting." The League of Nations was also stumped when it attempted to define what constituted obscenity. D. H. Lawrence was probably right when he said that "nobody knows what the word obscene means." As for Theodore Schroeder, who has devoted his whole life to fighting for freedom of speech,[1] his opinion is that "obscenity does not exist in any book or picture, but is wholly a quality

1. See his *A Challenge to Sex Censors* and other works.

of the reading or viewing mind." "No argument for the suppression of obscene literature," he states, "has ever been offered which by unavoidable implications will not justify, and which has not already justified, every other limitation that has ever been put upon mental freedom."

As someone has well said, to name all the masterpieces which have been labeled obscene would make a tedious catalogue. Most of our choice writers, from Plato to Havelock Ellis, from Aristophanes to Shaw, from Catullus and Ovid to Shakespeare, Shelley and Swinburne, together with the Bible, to be sure, have been the target of those who are forever in search of what is impure, indecent and immoral. In an article called "Freedom of Expression in Literature,"[2] Huntington Cairns, one of the most broad-minded and clear-sighted of all the censors, stresses the need for the re-education of officials charged with law enforcement. "In general," he states, "such men have had little or no contact with science or art, have had no knowledge of the liberty of expression tacitly granted to men of letters since the beginnings of English literature, and have been, from the point of view of expert opinion, altogether incompetent to handle the subject. Administrative officials, not the populace who in the main have only a negligible contact with art, stand first in need of re-education."

Perhaps it should be noted here, in passing, that though our Federal government exercises no censorship over works of art originating in the country, it does permit the Treasury Department to pass judgments upon importations from abroad. In 1930, the Tariff Act was revised to permit the Secretary of the Treasury, in his discretion, to admit the classics or books of recognized and established literary or scientific merit, even if obscene. What is meant by "books of recognized and established literary merit?" Mr. Cairns gives us the following interpretation: "books which have behind them a substantial and reputable body of American critical opinion indicating that the works are of meritorious quality." This would seem to represent a fairly liberal attitude, but when it comes to a test, when a book or other work of art is capable of creating a furore, this seeming liberality collapses. It has been said with regard to the sonnets of Aretino that they were condemned for four hundred years. How long we shall have to wait for the ban to be lifted

2. From the *Annals of the American Academy of Political and Social Science,* Philadelphia, November, 1938.

on certain famous contemporary works no one can predict. In the article alluded to above, Mr. Cairns admits that "there is no likelihood whatever that the present obscenity statutes will be repealed." "None of the statutes," he goes on to say, "defines the word 'obscenity' and there is thus a wide latitude of discretion in the meaning to be attributed to the term." Those who imagine that the *Ulysses* decision established a precedent should realize by now that they were overoptimistic. Nothing has been established where books of a disturbing nature are concerned. After years of wrestling with prudes, bigots and other psychopaths who determine what we may or may not read, Theodore Schroeder is of the opinion that "it is not the inherent quality of the book which counts, but its hypothetical influence upon some hypothetical person, who at some problematical time in the future may hypothetically read the book."

In his book called *A Challenge to Sex Censors*, Mr. Schroeder quotes an anonymous clergyman of a century ago to the effect that "obscenity exists only in the minds that discover it and charge others with it." This obscure work contains most illuminating passages; in it the author attempts to show that, by a law of reflection in nature, everyone is the performer of acts similar to those he attributes to others; that self-preservation is self-destruction, etc. This wholesome and enlightened viewpoint, attainable, it would seem, only by the rare few, comes nearer to dissipating the fogs which envelop the subject than all the learned treatises of educators, moralists, scholars and jurists combined. In Romans xiv: 14 we have it presented to us axiomatically for all time: "I know and am persuaded by the Lord Jesus that there is nothing unclean of itself, but to him that esteemeth anything to be unclean, to him it is unclean." How far one would get in the courts with this attitude, or what the postal authorities would make of it, surely no sane individual has any doubts about.

A totally different point of view, and one which deserves attention, since it is not only honest and forthright but expressive of the innate conviction of many, is that voiced by Havelock Ellis, that obscenity is a "permanent element of human social life and corresponds to a deep need of the human mind."[3] Ellis indeed goes so far as to say that "adults need obscene literature, as much as children need fairy tales, as

3. *More Essays of Love and Virtue.*

a relief from the oppressive force of convention." This is the attitude of a cultured individual whose purity and wisdom has been acknowledged by eminent critics everywhere. It is the worldly view which we profess to admire in the Mediterranean peoples. Ellis, being an Englishman, was of course persecuted for his opinions and ideas upon the subject of sex. From the nineteenth century on, all English authors who dared to treat the subject honestly and realistically have been persecuted and humiliated. The prevalent attitude of the English people is, I believe, fairly well presented in such a piece of polished inanity as Viscount Brentford's righteous self-defense—"Do We Need a Censor?" Viscount Brentford is the gentleman who tried to protect the English public from such iniquitous works as *Ulysses* and *The Well of Loneliness*. He is the type, so rampant in the Anglo-Saxon world, to which the words of Dr. Ernest Jones would seem to apply: "It is the people with secret attractions to various temptations who busy themselves with removing these temptations from other people; really they are defending themselves under the pretext of defending others, because at heart they fear their own weakness."

As one accused of employing obscene language more freely and abundantly than any other living writer in the English language, it may be of interest to present my own views on the subject. Since the *Tropic of Cancer* first appeared in Paris, in 1934, I have received many hundreds of letters from readers all over the world: they are from men and women of all ages and all walks of life, and in the main they are congratulatory messages. Many of those who denounced the book because of its gutter language professed admiration for it otherwise; very, very few ever remarked that it was a dull book, or badly written. The book continues to sell steadily "under the counter" and is still written about at intervals although it made its appearance eleven years ago and was promptly banned in all the Anglo-Saxon countries. The only effect which censorship has had upon its circulation is to drive it underground, thus limiting the sales but at the same time insuring for it the best of all publicity—word of mouth recommendation. It is to be found in the libraries of nearly all our important colleges, is often recommended to students by their professors, and has gradually come to take its place beside other celebrated literary works which, once similarly banned and suppressed, are now accepted as classics. It is a book which appeals especially to young people and which, from all that I gather directly and indirectly, not only does not ruin their lives, but increases their morale. The book is a living proof that censorship defeats itself. It also proves once again that the only ones who may be said to be protected by censorship are the censors themselves, and this only because of a law of nature known to all who overindulge. In this connection I feel impelled to mention a curious fact often brought to my attention by booksellers, namely, that the two classes of books which enjoy a steady and ever-increasing sale are the so-called pornographic, or obscene, and the occult. This would seem to corroborate Havelock Ellis's view which I mentioned earlier. Certainly all attempts to regulate the traffic in obscene books, just as all attempts to regulate the traffic in drugs or prostitution, are doomed to failure wherever civilization rears its head. Whether these things are a definite evil or not, whether or not they are definite and ineradicable elements of our social life, it seems indisputable that they are synonymous with what is called civilization. Despite all that has been said and written for and against, it is evident that with regard to these factors of social life men have never come to that agreement which they have about slavery. It is possible, of course, that one day these things may disappear, but it is also possible, despite the now seemingly universal disapproval of it, that slavery may once again be practiced by human beings.

The most insistent question put to the writer of "obscene" literature is: why did you have to use such language? The implication is, of course, that with conventional terms or means the same effect might have been obtained. Nothing, of course could be further from the truth. Whatever the language employed, no matter how objectionable —I am here thinking of the most extreme examples—one may be certain that there was no other idiom possible. Effects are bound up with intentions, and these in turn are governed by laws of compulsion as rigid as nature's own. That is something which non-creative individuals seldom ever understand. Someone has said that "the literary artist, having attained understanding, communicates that understanding to his readers. That understanding, whether of sexual or other matters, is certain to come into conflict with popular beliefs, fears and taboos, because these are, for the most part, based on error." Whatever extenuating reasons are adduced for the erroneous opinions of the populace, such as lack of education, lack of contact with the arts, and so on, the fact is that there will always be a gulf between the creative artist and the public because the latter is immune to the mystery inherent in and surrounding all creation. The struggle which the artist wages, consciously or unconsciously, with the public, centers almost exclusively about the problem of a necessitous choice. Putting to one side all questions of ego and temperament, and taking the broadest view of the creative process, which makes of the artist nothing more than an instrument, we are nevertheless forced to conclude that the spirit of an age is the crucible in which, through one means or another, certain vital and mysterious forces seek expression. If there is something mysterious about the manifestation of deep and unsuspected forces, which find expression in disturbing movements and ideas from one period to another, there is nevertheless nothing accidental or bizarre about it. The laws governing the spirit are just as readable as those governing nature. But the readings must come from those who are steeped in the mysteries. The very depth of these interpretations naturally makes them unpalatable and unacceptable to the vast body which constitutes the unthinking public.

Parenthetically it is curious to observe that painters, however unapproachable their work may be, are seldom subjected to the same meddling interference as writers. Language, because it also serves as a means of communication, tends to bring about weird obfuscations. Men of high intelligence often display execrable taste when it comes to the arts. Yet even these freaks whom we all recognize, because we are always amazed by their obtuseness, seldom have the cheek to say what elements of a picture had been better left out or what substitutions might have been effected. Take, for example, the early works of George Grosz. Compare the reactions of the intelligent public in his case to the reactions provoked by Joyce when his *Ulysses* appeared. Compare these again with the reactions which Schönberg's later music inspired. In the case of all three the revulsion which their work first induced was equally strong, but in the case of Joyce the public was more articulate, more voluble, more arrogant in its pseudo-certitude. With books even the butcher and the plumber seem to feel that they have a right to an opinion, especially if the book happens to be what is called a filthy or disgusting one.

I have noticed, moreover, that the attitude of the public alters perceptibly when it is the work of primitive peoples which they must grapple with. Here for some obscure reason the element of the "obscene" is treated with more deference. People who would be revolted by the drawings in *Ecce Homo* will gaze unblushingly at African pottery or sculpture no matter how much their taste or morals may be offended. In the same spirit they are inclined to be more tolerant of the obscene works of ancient authors. Why? Because even the dullest are capable of admitting to themselves that other epochs might, justifiably or not, have enjoyed other customs, other morals. As for the creative spirits of their own epoch, however, freedom of expression is always interpreted as license. The artist must conform to the current, and usually hypocritical, attitude of the majority. He must be original, courageous, inspiring and all that—but never too disturbing. He must say Yes while saying No. The larger the art public, the more tyrannical, complex and perverse does this irrational pressure become. There are always exceptions, to be sure, and Picasso is one of them, one of the few artists in our time able to command the respect and attention of a bewildered and largely hostile public. It is the greatest tribute that could be made to his genius.

The chances are that during this transition period of global wars, lasting perhaps a century or two, art will become less and less important. A world torn by indescribable upheavals, a world preoccupied with social and political transformations, will have less time and energy to spare for the creation and appreciation of works of art. The politician, the soldier, the industrialist, the technician, all those in short who cater to immediate needs, to creature comforts, to transitory and illusory passions and prejudices, will take precedence over the artist. The most poetic inventions will be those capable of serving the most destructive ends. Poetry itself will be expressed in terms of blockbusters and lethal gases. The obscene will find expression in the most unthinkable techniques of self-destruction which the inventive genius of man will be forced to adopt. The revolt and disgust which the prophetic spirits in the realm of art have inspired, through their vision of a world in the making, will find justification in the years to come as these dreams are acted out.

The growing void between art and life, art becoming ever more sensational and unintelligible, life becoming more dull and hopeless, has been commented on almost ad nauseam. The war, colossal and portentous as it is, has failed to arouse a passion commensurate with its scope or significance. The fervor of the Greeks and the Spaniards was something which astounded the modern world. The admiration and the horror which their ferocious struggles evoked was revelatory. We regarded them as mad and heroic, and we had almost been on the point of believing that such madness, such heroism, no longer existed. But what strikes one as "obscene" and insane rather than mad, is the stupendous machine-like character of the war which the big nations are carrying on. It is a war of materiel, a war of statistical preponderance, a war in which victory is coldly and patiently calculated on the basis of bigger and better resources. In the war which the Spaniards and the Greeks waged there was not only a hopelessness about the immediate outcome but a hopelessness as to the eternal outcome, so to speak. Yet they fought, and with tooth and nail, and they will fight again and again, always hopelessly and always gloriously because always passionately. As for the big powers now locked in a death struggle, one feels that they are only grooming themselves for another chance at it, for a chance to win here and now in a victory that will be everlasting, which is an utter delusion. Whatever the outcome, one senses that life will not be altered radically but to a degree which will only make it more like what it was before the conflict started. This war has all the masturbative qualities of a combat between hopeless recidivists.

If I stress the obscene aspect of modern warfare it is not simply because I am against war but because there is something about the ambivalent emotions it inspires which enables me better to grapple with the nature of the obscene. Nothing would be regarded as obscene, I feel, if men were living out their inmost desires. What man dreads most is to be faced with the manifestation, in word or deed, of that which he has refused to live out, that which he has throttled or stifled, buried, as we say now, in his subconscious mind. The sordid qualities imputed to the enemy are always those which we recognize as our own and therefore rise to slay, because only through projection do we realize the enormity and horror of them. Man tries as in a dream to kill the enemy in himself. This enemy, both within and without, is just as but no more real than the phantoms in his dreams. When awake he is apathetic about this dream self, but asleep he is filled with terror. I say "when awake," but the question is, *when is he awake, if ever?* To those who no longer need to kill, the man who indulges in murder is a sleep walker. He is a man trying to kill himself in his dreams. He is a man who comes face to face with himself *only in the dream*. This man is the man of the modern world, everyman, as much a myth and a legend as the Everyman of the allegory. Our life today is what we dreamed it would be aeons ago. Always it has a double thread running through it, just as in the age-old dream. Always fear and wish, fear and wish. Never the pure fountain of desire. And so we have and we have not, we are and we are not.

In the realm of sex there is a similar kind of sleepwalking and self-delusion at work; here the bifurcation of pure desire into fear and wish has resulted in the creation of a phantasmagorical world in which love plays the role of a chameleon-like scapegoat. Passion is conspicuous by its absence or by monstrous deformations which render it practically unrecognizable. To trace the history of man's attitude towards sex is like threading a labyrinth whose heart is situated in an unknown planet. There has been so much distortion and suppression, even among primitive peoples, that today it is virtually impossible to say what constitutes a free and healthy attitude. Certainly the glorification of sex, in pagan times, represented no solution of the problem. And, though Christianity ushered in a conception of love superior to any known before, it did not succeed in freeing man sexually. Perhaps we might say that the tyranny of sex was broken through sublimation in love, but the nature of this greater love has been understood and experienced only by a rare few.

Only where strict bodily discipline is observed, for the purpose of union or communion with God, has the subject of sex ever been faced squarely. Those who have achieved emancipation by this route have, of course, not only liberated themselves from the tyranny of sex but from all other tyrannies of the flesh. With such individuals, the whole body of desire has become so transfigured that the results obtained have had practically no meaning for the man of the world. Spiritual triumphs, even though they affect the man in the street immediately, concern him little, if at all. He is seeking for a solution of life's problems on the plane of mirage and delusion; his notions of reality have nothing to do with ultimate effects; he is blind to the permanent changes which take place above and beneath his level of understanding. If we take such a type of being as the Yogi, whose sole concern is with reality, as opposed to the world of illusion, we are bound to concede that he has faced every human problem with the utmost courage and lucidity. Whether he incorporates the sexual or transmutes it to the point of transcendence and obliteration, he is at least one who has attained the vast open spaces of love. If he does not reproduce his kind, he at least gives new meaning to the word birth. In lieu of copulating he creates; in the circle of his influence conflict is stilled and the harmony of a profound peace established. He is able to love not only individuals of the opposite sex but all individuals, everything that breathes, in fact. This quiet sort of triumph strikes a chill in the heart of the ordinary man, for not only does it make him visualize the loss of his meager sex life but the loss of passion itself, passion as he knows it. This sort of liberation, which smashes his thermometrical gauge of feeling, represents itself to him as a living death. The attainment of a love which is boundless and unfettered terrifies him for the very good reason that it means the dissolution of his ego. He does not want to be freed for service, dedication and devotion to all mankind; he wants comfort, assurance and security, the enjoyment of his very limited powers. Incapable of surrender, he can never know the healing power of faith; and lacking faith he can never begin to know the meaning of love. He seeks release but not liberation, which is like saying that he prefers death instead of life.

As civilization progresses it becomes more and more apparent that war is the greatest release which life offers the ordinary man. Here he can let go to his heart's content for here crime no longer has any meaning. Guilt is abolished when the whole planet swims in blood. The lulls of peacetime seem only to permit him to sink deeper into the bogs of the sadistic-masochistic complex which has fastened itself into the heart of our civilized life like a cancer. Fear, guilt and murder— these constitute the real triumvirate which rules our lives. *What is obscene then?* The whole fabric of life as we know it today. To speak only of what is indecent, foul, lewd, filthy, disgusting, etc., in connection with sex, is to deny ourselves the luxury of the great gamut of revulsion-repulsion which modern life puts at our service. Every department of life is vitiated and corroded with what is so unthinkingly labeled "obscene." One wonders if perhaps the insane could not invent a more fitting, more inclusive term for the polluting elements of life which we create and shun and never identify with our behavior. We think of the insane as inhabiting a world completely divorced from reality, but our own everyday behavior, whether in war or peace, if examined from only a slightly higher standpoint, bears all the earmarks of insanity. "I have said," writes a well-known psychologist, "that this is a mad world; that man is most of the time mad; and I believe that in a way, what we call morality is merely a form of madness, which happens to be a working adaptation to existing circumstances."

When obscenity crops out in art, in literature more particularly, it usually functions as a technical device; the element of the deliberate which is there has nothing to do with sexual excitation, as in pornography. If there is an ulterior motive at work it is one which goes far beyond sex. Its purpose is to awaken, to usher in a sense of reality. In a sense, its use by the artist may be compared to the use of the miraculous by the Masters. This last-minute quality, so closely allied to desperation, has been the subject of endless debate. Nothing connected with Christ's life, for example, has been exposed to such withering scrutiny as the miracles attributed to him. The great question is: should the Master indulge himself or should he refrain from employing his extraordinary powers? Of the great Zen masters it has been observed that they never hesitate to resort to any means in order to awaken their disciples; they will even perform what we would call sacrilegious acts. And, according to some familiar interpretations of the Flood, it has been acknowledged that even God grows desperate at times and wipes the slate clean in order to continue the human experiment on another level.

It should be recognized, however, with regard to these questionable displays of power, that only a Master may hazard them. As a matter of fact, the element of risk exists only in the eyes of the uninitiated. The Master is always certain of the result; he never plays his trump card, as it were, except at the psychological moment. His behavior, in such instances, might be compared to that of the chemist pouring a last tiny drop into a prepared solution in order to precipitate certain salts. If it is a push it is also a supreme exhortation which the Master indulges in.

Sexual Revolution

Once the moment is passed, moreover, the witness is altered forever. In another sense, the situation might be described as the transition from belief to faith. Once faith has been established, there is no regression; whereas with belief everything is in suspense and capable of fluctuation.

It should also be recognized that those who have real power have no need to demonstrate it for themselves; it is never in their own interests, or for their own glorification, that these performances are made. In fact, there is nothing miraculous, in the vulgar sense, about these acts, unless it be the ability to raise the consciousness of the onlooker to that mysterious level of illumination which is natural to the Master. Men who are ignorant of the source of their powers, on the other hand, men who are regarded as the powers that move the world, usually come to a disastrous end. Of their efforts it is truly said that all comes to nought. On the worldly level nothing endures, because on this level, which is the level of dream and delusion, all is fear and wish vainly cemented by will.

To revert to the artist again. . . . Once he has made use of his extraordinary powers, and I am thinking of the use of obscenity in just such magical terms, he is inevitably caught up in the stream of forces beyond him. He may have begun by assuming that he could awaken his readers, but in the end he himself passes into another dimension of reality wherein he no longer feels the need of forcing an awakening. His rebellion over the prevalent inertia about him becomes transmuted, as his vision increases, into an acceptance and understanding of an order and harmony which is beyond man's conception and approachable only through faith. His vision expands with the growth of his own powers, because creation has its roots in vision and admits of only one realm, the realm of imagination. Ultimately, then, he stands among his own obscene objurgations like the conqueror midst the ruins of a devastated city. He realizes that the real nature of the obscene resides in the lust to convert. He knocked to awaken, but it was himself he awakened. And once awake, he is no longer concerned with the world of sleep; he walks in the light and, like a mirror, reflects his illumination in every act.

Once this vantage point is reached, how trifling and remote seem the accusations of moralists! How senseless the debate as to whether the work in question was of high literary merit or not! How absurd the wrangling over the moral or immoral nature of his creation! Concerning every bold act one may raise the reproach of vulgarity. Everything dramatic is in the nature of an appeal, a frantic appeal for communion. Violence, whether in deed or speech, is an inverted sort of prayer. Initiation itself is a violent process of purification and union. Whatever demands radical treatment demands God, and always through some form of death or annihilation. Whenever the obscene crops out one can smell the imminent death of a form. Those who possess the highest clue are not impatient, even in the presence of death: the artist in words, however, is not of this order, he is only at the vestibule, as it were, of the palace of wisdom. Dealing with the spirit, he nevertheless has recourse to forms. When he fully understands his role as creator he substitutes his own being for the medium of words. But in that process there comes the "dark night of the soul" when, exalted by his vision of things to come and not yet fully conscious of his powers, he resorts to violence. He becomes desperate over his inability to transmit his vision. He resorts to any and every means in his power; this agony, in which creation itself is parodied, prepares him for the solution of his dilemma, but a solution wholly unforeseen and mysterious as creation itself.

All violent manifestations of radiant power have an obscene glow when visualized through the refractive lens of the ego. All conversions occur in the speed of a split second. Liberation implies the sloughing off of chains, the bursting of the cocoon. What is obscene are the preliminary or anticipatory movements of birth, the preconscious writhing in the face of a life to be. It is in the agony of death that the nature of birth is apprehended. For in what consists the struggle if it is not between form and being, between that which was and that which is about to be? In such moments creation itself is at the bar; whoever seeks to unveil the mystery becomes himself a part of the mystery and thus helps to perpetuate it. Thus the lifting of the veil may be interpreted as the ultimate expression of the obscene. It is an attempt to spy on the secret processes of the universe. In this sense the guilt attaching to Prometheus symbolizes the guilt of man-the-creator, of man-the-arrogant-one who ventures to create before being crowned with wisdom.

The pangs of birth relate not to the body but to the spirit. It was demanded of us to know love, experience union and communion, and thus achieve liberation from the wheel of life and death. But we have chosen to remain this side of Paradise and to create through art the illusory substance of our dreams. In a profound sense we are forever delaying the act. We flirt with destiny and lull ourselves to sleep with myth. We die in the throes of our own tragic legends, like spiders caught in their own webs. If there is anything which deserves to be called "obscene" it is this oblique, glancing confrontation with the mysteries, this walking up to the edge of the abyss, enjoying all the ecstasies of vertigo and yet refusing to yield to the spell of the unknown. The obscene has all the qualities of the hidden interval. It is as vast as the Unconscious itself and as amorphous and fluid as the very stuff of the Unconscious. It is what comes to the surface as strange, intoxicating and forbidden, and which therefore arrests and paralyzes, when in the form of Narcissus we bend over our own image in the mirror of our own iniquity. Acknowledged by all, it is nevertheless despised and rejected, wherefore it is constantly emerging in Protean guise at the most unexpected moments. When it is recognized and accepted, whether as a figment of the imagination or as an integral part of human reality, it inspires no more dread or revulsion than could he ascribed to the flowering lotus which sends its roots down into the mud of the stream on which it is borne.

The People of the State of California vs. Lenny Bruce

Lenny Bruce

from *How to Talk Dirty and Influence People*, 1965

Lenny Bruce started out as a comedian and an MC of stripper shows and went on to become the most scathing social satirist of his time. He attacked the social, sexual, and religious hypocrisies of the fifties and sixties and his performances, controversial for both their subject matter and their blunt vernacular language, led to legal harassment and multiple arrests. He died in 1966 at the age of 40 of a morphine overdose, but not before he had exhausted himself physically and emotionally in a series of raucous trials for obscenity in San Francisco, Chicago and New York. This following excerpt is taken from Bruce's autobiography, **How to Talk Dirty and Influence People,** *which was originally published in* **Playboy**. *This excerpt demonstrates how the obscenity trials, where he tested the robustness of the First Amendment, were merely an extension into the legal arena of Bruce's comedy routines.*

The first time I got arrested for obscenity was in San Francisco. I used a ten-letter word onstage. Just a word in passing.

"Lenny, I wanna talk to you," the police officer said. "You're under arrest. That word you said—you can't say that in a public place. It's against the law to say it and do it."

They said it was a favorite homosexual practice. Now that I found strange. I don't relate that word to a homosexual practice. It relates to any contemporary chick I know, or would know, or would love, or would marry.

Then we get into the patrol wagon, and another police officer says, "You know, I got a wife and kid . . ."

"I don't wanna hear that crap," I interrupted.

"Whattaya mean?"

"I just don't wanna hear that crap, that's all. Did your wife ever do that to you?"

"No."

"Did anyone?"

"No."

"Did you ever say the word?"

"No."

"You never said the word one time? Let ye cast the first stone, man."

"Never."

"How long have you been married?"

"Eighteen years."

"You ever chippied on your wife?"

"Never."

"Never chippied on your wife one time in eighteen years?"

"Never."

"Then I love *you* . . . because you're a spiritual guy, the kind of husband I would like to have been . . . but if you're lying, you'll spend some good time in purgatory . . ."

Now we get into court. They swear me in.

THE COP: "Your Honor, he said blah-blah-blah."

THE JUDGE: "He said *blah*-blah-blah! Well, I got grandchildren . . ."

Oh, Christ, there we go again.

"Your Honor," the cop says, "I couldn't believe it, there's a guy up on the stage in front of women in a mixed audience, saying blah-blah-blah . . ."

THE DISTRICT ATTORNEY: "Look at him, he's smug! I'm not surprised he said blah-blah-blah . . ."

"He'll probably say blah-blah-blah again, he hasn't learned his lesson . . ."

And then I dug something: they sort of *liked* saying blah-blah-blah. (Even the BAILIFF:) "What'd he say?"

"He said blah-blah-blah."

"Shut up, you blah-blah-blah."

They were yelling it in the courtroom.

"Goddamn, it's good to say blah-blah-blah!"

The actual trial took place in the early part of March 1962. The People of the State of California *vs.* Lenny Bruce. The jury consisted of four men and eight women. The first witness for the prosecution was James

Ryan, the arresting officer. Deputy District Attorney Albert Wollenberg, Jr., examined him.

Q. . . . And on the night of October the fourth did you have any special assignment in regard to (the Jazz Workshop)?

A. I was told by my immediate superior, Sergeant Solden, that he had received a complaint from the night before that the show at this club was of a lewd nature, and that some time during the evening I was to go in and see the show and find out what the complaint was all about . . .

Q. And during the course of his act did any . . . talking about an establishment known as Ann's 440 arise?

A. Yes . . . during this particular episode at the 440 he was talking to some other person, who, as near as I can recall, I think was either his agent or another entertainer. And during this conversation . . . one person said, "I can't work at the 440 because it's overrun with cocksuckers."

Q. . . . Now, after this statement, what then occurred?

A. A little later on in the same show the defendant was talking about the fact that he distrusted ticket takers and the person that handled the money, and that one of these days a man was going to enter the premises and situate himself where he couldn't be seen by the ticket taker, and then he was going to expose himself and on the end of it he was going to have a sign hanging that read, WHEN WE REACH $1500 THE GUY IN THE FRONT BOOTH IS GOING TO KISS IT.

Q. . . . Now, subsequent to the statement about hanging a sign on a person exposed, was there any further conversation by the defendant while giving his performance?

A. Yes. Later in the show he went into some kind of chant where he used a drum, or a cymbal and a drum, for a tempo, and the dialog was supposed to be . . .

MR. BENDICH (my attorney, Albert Bendich): I'll object to what the witness infers the conversation or dialog was supposed to import, your Honor. The witness is to testify merely to what he heard.

THE COURT: Sustained.

MR. WOLLENBERG: . . . Can you give us the exact words or what your recollection of those words were?

A. Yes. During that chant he used the words "I'm coming, I'm coming, I'm coming," and . . .

Q. Did he just do it two or three times, "I'm coming, I'm coming, I'm coming"?

A. Well, this one part of the show lasted a matter of a few minutes.

Q. And then was anything else said by the defendant?

A. Then later he said, "Don't come in me. Don't come in me."

Q. Now, did he do this just one or two times?

A. No. As I stated, this lasted for a matter of a few minutes.

Q. Now, as he was saying this, was he using the same voice as he was giving this chant?

A. . . . Well, this particular instance where he was saying "I'm coming, I'm coming," he was talking in a more normal tone of voice. And when he stated, or when he said "Don't come in me. Don't come in me," he used a little higher-pitched voice . . .

Mr. Bendich now cross-examined.

Q. Officer Ryan, would you describe your beat to us, please?

A. . . . It takes in both sides of Broadway from Mason to Battery.

Q. And in the course of your duties, Officer, you have the responsibility and obligation to observe the nature of the shows being put on in various clubs in this area?

A. Yes, sir, I do.

Q. Would you tell us, Officer, what some of those clubs are? . . . Then I'll ask you some questions about the content of the work that is done there . . .

MR. WOLLENBERG: Well, that's irrelevant and immaterial, if your Honor, please, other than that they are on his beat, the content of the work done there.

MR. BENDICH: We're talking about community standards, your Honor.

THE COURT: (Mr. Wollenberg's objection) overruled. Now, the question is just to name some of the establishments. [The officer named several night clubs.]

Q. . . . Now, officer, you testified, I believe, on direct examination that you had a specific assignment with reference to the Lenny Bruce performance at the Jazz Workshop, is that correct?

A. That's correct.

Q. Tell us, please, if you will, what your specific assignment was.

A. My assignment was to watch the performance of the show that evening.

Q. What were you looking for?

A. Any lewd conversation or lewd gestures or anything that might constitute an objectionable show.

Q. What were your standards for judging, Officer, whether a show was objectionable or not?

A. Well, any part of the show that would violate any Police or Penal Code sections that we have . . .

MR. BENDICH: . . . [You have previously described] the clubs that are situated upon the beat that you patrol, and among other clubs you listed the Moulin Rouge. . . . And would you be good enough to tell us, Officer Ryan, what the nature of the entertainment material presented in the Moulin Rouge is?

A. Primarily a burlesque-type entertainment.

Q. Strip shows are put on . . . ?

A. That's correct.

Q. And, as a matter of fact, Officer Ryan, there is a housewives' contest put on at the Moulin Rouge with respect to superior talent in stripping, is there not?

A. I don't know if it just encompasses housewives; I know they have an amateur night.

Q. Now, Officer Ryan, will you tell us a little bit about what occurs during amateur night?

A. Well, just what it says, I believe. Girls that have had little or no experience in this type of entertainment are given a chance to try their hand at it.

Q. To try their hand at it, and they try their body a little, too, don't they?

MR. WOLLENBERG: If your Honor please, counsel is argumentative.

THE COURT: Yes. Let us not be facetious, Mr. Bendich.

MR. BENDICH: I will withdraw it. I don't intend to be facetious.

Q. Officer Ryan, will you describe for the ladies and gentlemen of the jury, if you will, please, what the ladies who are engaged in the competition on amateur night do?

MR. WOLLENBERG: If your Honor please, this is irrelevant.

THE COURT: Overruled.

THE WITNESS: Well, they come on the stage and then to the accompaniment of music they do a dance.

MR. BENDICH: And in the course of doing this dance, they take their clothes off, is that correct?

A. Partially, yes.

Q. Now, these are the amateur competitors and performers, is that correct?

A. That's correct.

Q. Tell us, please, if you will, what the professional performers do.

A. Approximately the same thing, with maybe a little more finesse or a little more ability, if there is ability in that line.

Q. And you have witnessed these shows, is that correct, Officer Ryan?

A. I have, yes.

Q. And these are shows which are performed in the presence of mixed audiences, representing persons of both sexes, is that correct?

A. That's true.

Q. Now, Officer Ryan, in the course of your official duties in patrolling your beat you have occasion, I take it, to deal with another club, the name of which is Finocchio's, is that correct?

A. That's true.

Q. And you have had occasion to observe the nature of the performances in Finocchio's, is that true? . . . Would you be good enough, Officer Ryan, to describe to the ladies and gentlemen of the jury what the nature of the entertainment presented in Finocchio's is?

A. Well, the entertainers are female impersonators.

Q. May I ask you to describe for the jury what female impersonators are?

A. A male that dresses as a woman, and the type of show they put on is, I guess, a pretty average show, other than the fact that they are female impersonators. They have songs that they sing, dances that they do, and so forth.

Q. . . . And can you describe the mode of dress, Officer, of the female impersonators in Finocchio's?

A. Well, they wear different types of costumes. Some of them are quite full, and others are . . .

Q. Quite scanty?

A. Not "quite scanty," I wouldn't say, no, but they are more near to what you'd call scanty, yes.

Q. "More near to what you'd call scanty." Well, as a matter of fact,

Officer, isn't it true that men appear in the clothes of women, and let's start up—or should I say, down at the bottom—wearing high-heeled shoes?

MR. WOLLENBERG: Oh, if your Honor please, he's already answered that they're wearing the clothes of women. That covers the subject. We're not trying Finocchio's here today.

MR. BENDICH: We're certainly not trying Finocchio's but we are trying Lenny Bruce on a charge of obscenity, and we have a question of contemporary community standards that has to be established, and I am attempting to have Officer Ryan indicate what the nature of the community standards on his beat are.

THE COURT: . . . Well, ask him to be more specific.

MR. BENDICH: Very well. Will you please be more specific, Officer Ryan, with regard to describing the nature of the scantily dressed female impersonators in terms of their attire.

A. They have all different kinds of costumes. Now, which particular one—I never paid that much attention to it, really.

Q. Well, they appear in black net stockings, do they not?

A. I imagine they do at times.

Q. And they appear in tights, do they not?

A. On occasion, yes.

Q. And they appear wearing brassieres, do they not?

A. That's correct.

Q. I think that's specific enough. . . . Officer Ryan, in the course of your observations of the strip shows in the Moulin Rouge, have you ever had occasion to become sexually stimulated?

A. No, sir.

MR. WOLLENBERG: I'm going to object to this and move to strike the answer as incompetent, irrelevant and immaterial, if your Honor please.

THE COURT: The answer is in; it may remain.

MR. BENDICH: Were you sexually stimulated when you witnessed Lenny Bruce's performance?

MR. WOLLENBERG: Irrelevant and immaterial, especially as to this officer, your Honor.

THE COURT: Overruled.

THE WITNESS: No, sir.

MR. BENDICH: Did you have any conversation with anyone in the Jazz Workshop on the night that you arrested Mr. Lenny Bruce?

A. No.

Q. Officer Ryan, you're quite familiar with the term "cocksucker" are you not?

A. I have heard it used, yes.

Q. As a matter of fact, Officer Ryan, it was used in the police station on the night that Lenny Bruce was booked there, was it not?

A. No, not to my knowledge.

Q. As a matter of fact, it is frequently used in the police station, is it not?

MR. WOLLENBERG: That's irrelevant and immaterial, if your Honor please. What's used in a police station or in private conversation between two people is completely different from what's used on a stage in the theater.

THE COURT: Well, a police station, of course, is a public place.

MR. WOLLENBERG: That's correct, your Honor.

THE COURT: As to the police station, the objection is overruled.

MR. BENDICH: You may answer, Officer.

A. Yes, I have heard it used.

Q. Yes, you have heard the term used in a public place known as the police station. Now, Officer Ryan, there is nothing obscene in and of itself about the word "cock," is there?

MR. WOLLENBERG: I'm going to object to this as being irrelevant and immaterial, what this man feels.

THE COURT: Sustained.

MR. BENDICH: Just two last questions, Officer Ryan. You laughed at Lenny Brace's performance the night that you watched, did you not?

A. No, I didn't.

Q. You didn't have occasion to laugh?

A. No, I didn't.

Q. Did you observe whether the audience was laughing?

A. Yes, I did.

Q. And they were laughing, were they not?

A. At times, yes.

Q. And no one in the audience made any complaint to you, though you were in uniform standing in the club?

A. No one, no.

MR. BENDICH: No further questions.

Mr. Wollenberg re-examined the witness.

Q. Now, Officer, when the word, "cocksucker," was used during the performance, did anybody laugh?

A. Not right at that instant, no.

Q. . . . Now, in Finocchio's, have you ever heard the word "cocksucker" used from the stage?

A. No, sir, I never have.

Q. . . . Now, at the Moulin Rouge, Officer, they do have a comedian as well as a strip show, isn't that right?

A. That's right.

Q. Have you ever heard the comedian at the Moulin Rouge use the term, "cocksucker"?

A. No, sir, never.

Q. Did you have a conversation with the defendant Bruce after his performance?

A. Yes, I did.

Q. And where was that?

A. In front of the Jazz Workshop.

Q. . . . Was that in relation to any of the terms used?

A. Yes, it was.

Q. And what was that?

A. I asked the defendant at that time, "Didn't I hear you use the word 'cocksucker' in your performance? And he says, 'Yes, I did.'"

Later, Mr. Wollenberg examined the other police officer, Sergeant James Solden.

Q. . . . And did you have occasion while in that area (the Jazz Workshop) to see the defendant Bruce? . . . Did you have a conversation with him?

A. I had a conversation with Mr. Bruce as we led—took him from the Jazz Workshop to the patrol wagon . . . I spoke to Mr. Bruce and said, "Why do you feel that you have to use the word 'cocksucker' to entertain people in a public night spot?" And Mr. Bruce's reply to me, was, "Well there are a lot of cocksuckers around, aren't there? What's wrong with talking about them?"

• • •

Mr. Bendich made his opening statement to the jury, "to tell you what it is that I am going to attempt to prove to you in the course of the presentation of the defense case. . . . I am going to prove through the testimony of several witnesses who will take the stand before you, ladies and gentlemen of the jury, that Mr. Bruce gave a performance in the Jazz Workshop on the night of October fourth last year which was a show based on the themes of social criticism, based upon an analysis of various forms of conventional hypocrisy, based upon the technique of satire which is common in the heritage of English letters and, as a matter of fact, in the heritage of world literature. We are going to prove, ladies and gentlemen of the jury, that the nature of Mr. Bruce's performance on the night of October the fourth was in the great tradition of social satire, related intimately to the kind of social satire to be found in the works of such great authors at Aristophanes, Jonathan Swift . . ."

MR. WOLLENBERG: I'm going to object. Aristophanes is not testifying here, your Honor, or any other authors, and I'm going to object to that at this time as improper argument.
MR. BENDICH: Your Honor, I didn't say I would call Mr. Aristophanes.
THE COURT: I don't think you could, very well . . .

• • •

The first witness for the defense was Ralph J. Gleason, a brilliant jazz critic and columnist for the *San Francisco Chronicle.*
    Mr. Bendich examined him.
Q. . . . Mr. Gleason, will you describe for us, if you will, please, what the themes of Mr. Bruce's work were during the appearance in the Workshop for which he was arrested?
MR. WOLLENBERG: I will object to just the themes, your Honor. He can give the performance or recite what was said, but the "themes" is ambiguous.
THE COURT: Overruled.
THE WITNESS: The theme of the performance on the night in question was a social criticism of stereotypes and of the hypocrisy of

contemporary society. . . . He attempted to demonstrate to the audience a proposition that's familiar to students of semantics, which is that words have been given, in our society, almost a magic meaning that has no relation to the facts, and I think that he tried in the course of this show that evening to demonstrate that there is no harm inherent in words themselves.

Q. . . . How important, if at all, was the theme of semantics with reference to the entire show given on the evening in question?

A. In my opinion, it was very important—vital to it.

Q. And what dominance or predominance, if any, did the theme of semantics occupy with respect to the content of the entire show on the night in question?

A. Well, it occupied an important part in the entire performance, not only in the individual routines, but in the totality of the program.

Q. Yes. Now, with respect to the rest of the program, Mr. Gleason, would you tell us about some of the other themes, and perhaps illustrate something about them if you can, in addition to the theme of semantics which Mr. Bruce worked with?

A. Well, to the best of my recollection there was a portion of the show in which he attempted to show satirically the hypocrisy inherent in the licensing of a ticket taker who had a criminal record for particularly abhorrent criminal acts and demanding a bond for him . . .

Mr. Gleason was asked to read to the jury an excerpt from an article in *Commonweal*, a Catholic magazine. The article was by Nat Hentoff, who's Jewish, so it doesn't really count. Gleason read:

> "It is in Lenny Bruce—and only in him—that there has emerged a cohesively 'new' comedy of nakedly honest moral rage at the deceptions all down the line in our society. Bruce thinks of himself as an ethical relativist and shares Pirandello's preoccupation with the elusiveness of any absolute, including absolute truth.
>
> "His comedy ranges through religion-in-practice ('What would happen if Christ and Moses appeared one Sunday at Saint Patrick's?'); the ultimate limitations of the white liberal; the night life of the hooker and her view of the day; and his own often scarifying attempts to make sense of his life in a society

where the quicksand may lie just underneath the sign that says:
TAKE SHELTER WHEN THE CIVILIAN DEFENSE ALARM SOUNDS.

"Bruce, however, does not turn a night club into Savonarola's church. More than any others of the 'new wave,' Bruce is a thoroughly experienced performer, and his relentless challenges to his audience and to himself are intertwined with explosive pantomime, hilarious 'bits,' and an evocative spray of Yiddishisms, Negro and show-business argot, and his own operational semantics. Coursing through everything he does, however, is a serious search for values that are more than security blankets. In discussing the film *The Story of Esther Costello*, Bruce tells of the climactic rape scene: 'It's obvious the girl has been violated. . . . She's been deaf and dumb throughout the whole picture. . . . All of a sudden she can hear again . . . and she can speak again. So what's the moral?'"

Later—after the judge had pointed something out to the Deputy District Attorney ("Mr. Wollenberg," he said, ". . . your shirttail is out.")—Mr. Gleason was asked to read to the jury a portion of an article by Arthur Gelb in *The New York Times*.

"The controversial Mr. Bruce, whose third visit to Manhattan this is, is the prize exhibit of the menagerie, and his act is billed 'for adults only.'

"Presumably the management wishes to safeguard the dubious innocence of underage New Yorkers against Mr. Bruce's vocabulary, which runs to four-letter words, of which the most printable is Y.M.C.A. But there are probably a good many adults who will find him offensive, less perhaps for his Anglo-Saxon phrases than for his vitriolic attacks on such subjects as facile religion, the medical profession, the law, pseudo-liberalism and Jack Paar. ('Paar has a God complex. He thinks he can create performers in six days,' Mr. Bruce is apt to confide.)

"Although he seems at times to be doing his utmost to antagonize his audience, Mr. Bruce displays such a patent air of morality beneath the brashness that his lapses in taste are often forgivable.

"The question, though, is whether the kind of derisive shock therapy he administers and the introspective free-form patter in which he indulges are legitimate night-club fare, as far as the typical customer is concerned.

"It is necessary, before lauding Mr. Bruce for his virtues, to warn the sensitive and the easily shocked that no holds are barred at Basin Street East. Mr. Bruce regards the night-club stage as the 'last frontier' of uninhibited entertainment. He often carries his theories to their naked and personal conclusions and has earned for his pains the sobriquet 'sick.' He is a ferocious man who does not believe in the sanctity of motherhood or the American Medical Association. He even has an unkind word to say for Smokey the Bear. True, Smokey doesn't set forest fires, Mr. Bruce concedes. But he eats boy scouts for their hats.

"Mr. Bruce expresses relief at what he sees as a trend of 'people leaving the church and going back to God,' and he has nothing but sneers for what he considers the sanctimonious liberal who preaches but cannot practice genuine integration.

"Being on cozy terms with history and psychology, he can illustrate his point with the example of the early Romans, who thought there was 'something dirty' about Christians. 'Could you want your sister to marry one?'—he has one Roman ask another—and so on, down to the logical conclusion in present-day prejudice.

"At times Mr. Bruce's act, devoid of the running series of staccato jokes that are traditional to the night-club comic, seems like a Salvationist lecture; it is biting, sardonic, certainly stimulating and quite often funny—but never in a jovial way. His mocking diatribe rarely elicits a comfortable belly laugh. It requires concentration. But there is much in it to wring a rueful smile and appreciative chuckle. There is even more to evoke a fighting gleam in the eye. There are also spells of total confusion.

"Since Mr. Bruce operates in a spontaneous, stream-of-consciousness fashion a good deal of the time, he is likely to tell you what he's thinking about telling you before he gets around to telling you anything at all . . ."

• • •

Mr. Bendich resumed his line of questioning.

Q. Mr. Gleason, would you tell us, please, what in your judgment the *predominant* theme of the evening's performance for which Mr. Bruce was arrested was?

A. Well, in a very real sense it's semantics—the search for the ultimate truth that lies beneath the social hypocrisy in which we live. All his performances relate to this.

Q. Mr. Gleason, as an expert in this field, would you characterize the performance in question as serious in intent and socially significant?

MR. WOLLENBERG: I will object to this as irrelevant and immaterial.

THE COURT: Overruled.

THE WITNESS: Yes, I would characterize it as serious.

MR. BENDICH: And how would you characterize the social significance, if any, of that performance?

A. Well, I would characterize this performance as being of high social significance, in line with the rest of his performances.

Q. Mr. Gleason, what in your opinion, based upon your professional activity and experience in the field of popular culture, and particularly with reference to humor, what in your opinion is the relation between the humor of Lenny Bruce and that of other contemporary humorists, such as Mort Sahl, Shelley Berman, Mike and Elaine?

MR. WOLLENBERG: That's immaterial, your Honor, what the comparison is between him and any other comedian.

THE COURT: Objection overruled.

THE WITNESS: Mr. Bruce attacks the fundamental structure of society and these other comedians deal with it superficially.

MR. BENDICH: Mr. Gleason, you have already testified that you have seen personally a great many Lenny Bruce performances, and you are also intimately familiar with his recorded works and other comic productions. Has your prurient interest ever been stimulated by any of Mr. Bruce's work?

A. Not in the slightest.

MR. WOLLENBERG: I will object to that as calling for the ultimate issue before this jury.

THE COURT: The objection will be overruled. . . . You may answer the question.

THE WITNESS: I have not been excited, my prurient or sexual interest has not been aroused by any of Mr. Brace's performances.

The complete transcript of my San Francisco trial runs 350 pages. The witnesses—not one of whose sexual interest had ever been aroused by any of my night-club performances—described one after another, what they remembered of my performance on the night in question at the Jazz Workshop, and interpreted its social significance according to his or her own subjectivity.

For example, during the cross-examination, the following dialog ensued between Mr. Wollenberg and Lou Gottlieb, a Ph.D. who's with the Limeliters:

Q. Doctor, you say you have heard Mr. Bruce in Los Angeles?

A. Yes.

Q. And what was the last remark he makes on leaving the stage in his show in Los Angeles?

A. I must say that Mr. Bruce's last remarks have varied at every performance that I have ever witnessed.

Q. Did he make any reference to eating something in his last remarks in Los Angeles when you heard him perform?

A. No.

Q. . . . Now, Doctor, you say the main theme of Mr. Bruce is to get laughter?

A. That's the professional comedian's duty.

Q. I see. And do you see anything funny in the word "cocksucker"?

A. . . . To answer that question with "Yes" or "No" is impossible, your Honor.

MR. WOLLENBERG: I asked you if you saw anything funny in that word.

THE COURT: You may answer it "Yes" or "No" and then explain your answer.

THE WITNESS: I found it extremely unfunny as presented by Mr. Wollenberg, I must say, but I can also——

THE COURT: All right, wait a minute, wait a minute. I have tolerated a certain amount of activity from the audience because I knew that it is difficult not to react at times, but this is not a show, you are not here to be entertained. Now, if there's any more of this sustained levity, the courtroom will be cleared. And the witness is instructed not to argue with counsel but to answer the questions . . .

THE WITNESS: I do not (see anything funny in that word) but as Mr. Bruce presents his performances he creates a world in which normal dimensions . . . become—how shall I say? Well, they are transmuted into a grotesque panorama of contemporary society, into which he places slices of life, phonographically accurate statements that come out of the show-business world . . . and sometimes the juxta-position of the generally fantastic frame of reference that he is able to create and the startling intrusion of slices of life in terms of lan-guage that is used in these kinds of areas, has extremely comic effect.

Q. . . . . Doctor, because an agent uses that term when he talks to his talent, you find nothing wrong with using it in a public place because you're relating a conversation between yourself and your agent? This excuses the use of that term?

A. What excuses the use of that term, Mr. Wollenberg, in my opinion, is its unexpectedness in the fantastic world that is the frame of ref-erence, the world which includes many grotesqueries that Mr. Bruce is able to establish. Then when you get a phonographic reproduc-tion of a snatch of a conversation, I find that this has comic effect very frequently.

Q. Do you mean "phonographic" or "photographic"?

A. "Phonographic." I mean reproducing the actual speech verbatim with the same intonation and same attitudes and everything else that would be characteristic of, let's say, a talent agent of some kind.

Q. I see. In other words, the changing of the words to more—well, we might use genteel—terms, would take everything away from that, is that right?

A. It wouldn't be phonographically accurate. It would lose its real feel; there would be almost no point.

Q. . . . . And taking out that word and putting in the word "homo-sexual" or "fairy," that would take away completely, in your opinion, from this story and make it just completely another one?

A. I must say it would.

Similarly, Mr. Wollenberg cross-examined Dr. Don Geiger, associate professor and chairman of the department of speech at the University of California in Berkeley; also author of a few books, including *Sound, Sense and Performance of Literature,* as well as several scholarly articles in professional journals.

Q. . . . And what does the expression "I won't appear there because it's overrun with cocksuckers" infer to you?

A. "I won't go there because it's filled with homosexuals."

Q. I see. And does the word "cocksucker" denote any beauty as distinguished from the word homosexual?

A. I couldn't possibly answer that, I think. That is, you would have to provide a context for it, and then one could answer that. I would say this about it . . . that "homosexual" is a kind of neutral, scientific term which might in a given context itself have a freight of significance or beauty or artistic merit. But it's less likely to than the word "cocksucker," which is closer to colloquial, idiomatic expression.

Later, Kenneth Brown, a high school English teacher, testified as to his reaction to the "to come" part of my performance:

THE WITNESS: The impression is, he was trying to get over a point about society, the inability to love, the inability to perform sexual love in a creative way. The routine then would enter a dialog between a man and a woman and they were having their sexual difficulties at orgasm in bed; at least, one of them was. And one said, "Why can't you come?" And, "Is it because you don't love me? Is it because you can't love me?" And the other one said, "Why, you know me, this is where I'm hung up. I have problems here." And that was enough to give me the impression that—with the other things in context that were going on before and after—that he was talking, dissecting our problems, of relating to each other, man and woman. . . . Great comics throughout literature have always disguised by comedy, through laughter, through jokes, an underlying theme which is very serious, and perhaps needs laughter because it is also painful . . .

MR. BENDICH: May I ask you this question, Mr. Brown: On the basis of your professional training and experience, do you think that the work of Mr. Bruce as you know it, and in particular the content of Mr. Bruce's performance on the night of October fourth, for which he was arrested, for which he is presently here in this courtroom on trial, bears a relation to the themes and the fashion in which those themes are in the works which we have listed here [*Lysistrata* by Aristophanes; *Gargantua and Pantagruel* by Rabelais; *Gulliver's Travels* by Jonathan Swift]?

A. I see a definite relationship, certainly.

Q. Would you state, please, what relationship you see and how you see it?

MR. WOLLENBERG: I think he hasn't qualified as an expert on this, your Honor.

THE COURT: Well, he may state what the relationship is that he sees.

THE WITNESS: These works use often repulsive techniques and vocabulary to make—to insist—that people will look at the whole of things and not just one side. These artists wish not to divide the world in half and say one is good and one is bad and avoid the bad and accept the good, but you must, to be a real and whole person, you must see all of life and see it in a balanced, honest way. I would include Mr. Bruce, certainly, in his intent, and he has success in doing this, as did Rabelais and Swift.

At one point during the trial, a couple of 19-year-old college students were admonished by the judge; they had been distributing the following leaflet outside the courtroom:

> WELCOME TO THE FARCE!
>
> Lenny Bruce, one of America's foremost comedians and social critics, is at this moment playing an unwilling part as a straight man in a social comedy put on by the City and County of San Francisco.
>
> Incongruously, in our urbane city, this is a poor provincial farce, insensitively played by some of the city's most shallow actors.
>
> Bruce may be imaginative, but the dull-witted, prudish lines of the police department are not, neither are the old-maidish lyrics of section 311.6 of the California Penal Code, which in genteel, puritan prose condemns the users of —— and —— and other common expressions to play a part in the dreary melodrama of "San Francisco Law Enforcement."

Really, we are grown up now. With overpopulation, human misery and the threat of war increasing, we need rather more adult performances from society.

You know, and I know, all about the hero's impure thoughts. We've probably had them ourselves. Making such a fuss isn't convincing at all—it lacks psychological realism—as do most attempts to find a scapegoat for sexual guilt feelings.

Forgive Lenny's language. Most of us use it at times; most of us even use the things and perform the acts considered unprintable and unspeakable by the authors of (Section 311.6 of the Penal Code of the State of California), though most of us are not nearly frank enough to say so.

Lenny has better things to do than play in this farce; the taxpayers have better uses for their money; and the little old ladies of both sexes who produce it *should* have better amusements.

With a nostalgic sigh, let's pull down the curtain on *People vs. Bruce* and its genre; and present a far more interesting and fruitful play called *Freedom of Speech*. It would do our jaded ears good.

The writer and distributor of the leaflet were properly chastised by the judge.

And so the trial continued.

One of the witnesses for the defense was Clarence Knight, who had been an assistant district attorney for a couple of years in Tulare County, California, and was deputy district attorney for four years in San Mateo, where he evaluated all pornography cases that were referred to the district attorney's office. He had passed on "probably between 200 and 250 separate items of material in regard to the pornographic or nonpornographic content thereof."

As with the others, his prurient interests were not aroused by my performance at the Jazz Workshop. In fact, he said, while being cross-examined about the "cocksucker" reference: "In my opinion, Mr. Wollenberg, it was the funniest thing Mr. Bruce said that night."

• • •

Finally, I was called as a witness in my own behalf. I took the stand, and Mr. Bendich examined me.

Q. Mr. Bruce, Mr. Wollenberg yesterday said (to Dr. Gottlieb) specifically that you had said, "Eat it." Did you say that?

A. No, I never said that.

Q. What did you say, Mr. Bruce?

A. What did I say when?

Q. On the night of October fourth.

MR. WOLLENBERG: There's no testimony that Mr. Wollenberg said that Mr. Bruce said, "Eat it," the night of October fourth, if your Honor please.

THE COURT: The question is: What did he say?

THE WITNESS: I don't mean to be facetious. Mr. Wollenberg said, "Eat it." I said, "Kiss it."

MR. BENDICH: Do you apprehend there is a significant difference between the two phrases, Mr. Bruce?

A. "Kissing it" and "eating it," yes, sir. Kissing my mother goodbye and eating my mother goodbye, there is a quantity of difference.

Q. Mr. Wollenberg also quoted you as saying, "I'm coming, I'm coming, I'm coming." Did you say that?

A. I never said that.

MR. BENDICH: . . . Mr. Bruce, do you recall using the term "cocksucker"?

A. Yes.

Q. Can you recall accurately now how you used that term?

A. You mean accuracy right on the head—total recall?

Q. Yes, Mr. Bruce.

A. If a "the" and an "an" are changed around, no. I don't have that exact, on-the-head recall. That's impossible; it's impossible. I defy anyone to do it. That's impossible.

Q. Mr. Bruce, if a "the" and an "an" were turned around, as you have put it, would that imply a significant difference in the characterization of what was said that evening?

A. Yes, yes.

Q. Are you saying, Mr. Bruce, that unless your words can be given in exact, accurate, verbatim reproduction, that your meaning cannot be made clear?

THE WITNESS: Yes, that is true. I would like to explain that. The "I am coming, I am coming" reference, which I never said—if we change——

THE COURT: Wait a minute, wait a minute. If you never said it, there's nothing to explain.

THE WITNESS: Whether that is a coming in the Second Coming or a different coming——

THE COURT: Well, you wait until your counsel's next question, now.

MR. BENDICH: Mr. Bruce, in giving your performance on the night of October fourth in the Jazz Workshop, as a consequence of which you suffered an arrest and as a result of which you are presently on trial on the charge of obscenity, did you intend to arouse anybody's prurient interest?

A. No.

• • •

Before the tape was played, Mr. Bendich pointed out to the judge that "there are portions of this tape which are going to evoke laughter in the audience."

THE COURT: I anticipated you; I was going to give that admonition.

MR. BENDICH: Well, what I was going to ask, your Honor, is whether the audience might not be allowed to respond naturally, given the circumstances that this is an accurate reproduction of a performance which is given at a night club; it's going to evoke comic response, and I believe that it would be asking more than is humanly possible of the persons in this courtroom not to respond humanly, which is to say, by way of laughter.

THE COURT: Well, as I previously remarked, this is not a theater and it is not a show, and I am not going to allow any such thing. I anticipated you this morning, and I was going to and I am now going to admonish the spectators that you are not to treat this as a performance. This is not for your entertainment. There's a very serious question involved here, the right of the People and the right of the defendant. And I admonish you that you are to control yourselves with regard to any emotions that you may feel during the hearing this morning or by the taping and reproduction of this tape. All right, you may proceed. And the tape was played:

. . . The hungry i. The hungry i has a Grayline Tour and American

Legion convention. They took all the bricks out and put in Saran Wrap. That's it. And Ferlinghetti is going to the Fairmont.

You know, this was a little snobby for me to work. I just wanted to go back to Ann's. You don't know about that, do you? Do you share that recall with me? It's the first gig I ever worked up here, a place called Ann's 440, which was across the street. And I got a call, and I was working a burlesque gig with Paul Moore in the Valley. That's the cat on the piano here, which is really strange, seeing him after all these years, and working together.

And the guy says, "There's a place in San Francisco but they've changed the policy."

"Well, what's the policy?"

"Well, I'm not there anymore, that's the main thing."

"Well, what kind of a show is it, man?"

"A bunch of cocksuckers, that's all. A damned fag show."

"Oh. Well, that is a pretty bizarre show. I don't know what I can do in that kind of a show."

"Well, no. It's—we want you to change all that."

"Well—I don't—that's a big gig. I can't just tell them to stop doing it."

Oh, I like you, and if sometimes I take poetic license with you and you are offended—now this is just with semantics, dirty words. Believe me, I'm not profound, this is something that I assume someone must have laid on me, because I do not have an original thought. I am screwed—I speak English—that's it. I was not born in a vacuum. Every thought I have belongs to somebody else. Then I must just take— ding-ding-ding—somewhere.

So I am not placating you by making the following statement. I want to help you if you have a dirty-word problem. There are none, and I'll spell it out logically to you.

Here is a toilet. Specifically—that's all we're concerned with, specifics—if I can tell you a dirty toilet joke, we must have a dirty toilet. That's what we're talking about, a toilet. If we take this toilet and boil it and it's clean, I can never tell you specifically a dirty toilet joke about this toilet. I can tell you a dirty toilet joke in the Milner Hotel, or something like that, but this toilet is a clean toilet now. Obscenity is a human manifestation. This toilet has no central nervous system, no level of consciousness. It is not aware; it is a dumb toilet; it cannot be obscene; it's impossible. If it could be obscene, it could be cranky, it could be a Communist toilet, a traitorous toilet. It can do none of these things. This is a dirty toilet here.

Nobody can offend you by telling you a dirty toilet story. They can offend you because it's trite; you have heard it many, many times.

Now, all of us have had a bad early toilet training—that's why we are hung up with it. All of us at the same time got two zingers—one for the police department and one for the toilet.

"All right, he made a kahkah, call a policeman. All right, OK, all right. Are you going to do that anymore? OK, tell the policeman he doesn't have to come up now."

All right, now we all got "Policeman, policeman, policeman," and we had a few psychotic parents who took it and rubbed it in our face, and those people for the most, if you search it out, are censors. Oh, true, they hate toilets with a passion, man. Do you realize if you got that wrapped around with a toilet, you'd hate it, and anyone who refers to it? It is dirty and uncomfortable to you.

Now, if the bedroom is dirty to you, then you are a true atheist, because if you have any of the mores, superstitions, if anyone in this audience believes that God made his body, and your body is dirty, the fault lies with the manufacturer. It's that cold, Jim, yeah.

You can do anything with the body that God made, and then you want to get definitive and tell me of the parts He made; I don't see that anywhere in any reference to any Bible. Yeah. He made it all; it's all clean or all dirty.

But the ambivalence comes from the religious leaders, who are celibates. The religious leaders are "what *should* be."

They say they do not involve themselves with the physical. If we are good, we will be like our rabbi, or our nun, or our priests, and absolve, and finally put down the carnal and stop the race.

Now, dig, this is stranger. Everybody today in the hotel was bugged with Knight and Nixon. Let me tell you the truth. The truth is "what *is*." If "what is" is, you have to sleep eight, ten hours a day, that is the truth. A lie will be: People need no sleep at all. Truth is "what *is*." If every politician from the beginning is crooked, there is no crooked. But if you are concerned with a lie, "what should be"—and "what should be" is a fantasy, a terrible, terrible lie that someone gave the people long ago: This is what *should* be—and no one ever saw what should be, that you don't need any sleep and you can go seven years without sleep, so that all the people were made to measure up to that dirty lie. You know there's no crooked politicians. There's never a lie because there is never a truth.

I sent this agency a letter—they are bonded and you know what that means: anybody who is bonded never steals from you, nor could Earl Long. Ha! If the governor can, then the bond is really—yeah, that's some bond.

Very good. Write the letter. Blah, blah, blah, "I want this," blah, blah, blah, "ticket taker."

Get a letter back, get an answer back, Macon, Georgia:

"Dear Mr. Bruce: Received your letter," blah, blah, blah. "We have ticket sellers, bonded. We charge two-and-a-half dollars per ticket seller, per hour. We would have to have some more details," blah, blah, blah, "Sincerely yours, Dean R. Moxie."

Dean R. Moxie . . . Dean R. Moxie . . . Moxie, buddy. Dean R. Moxie, from the Florida criminal correctional institution for the criminally insane, and beat up a spade-fed junkie before he was thrown off the police force, and then was arrested for *schtupping* his stepdaughter. Dean R. Moxie. Hmmm.

All right, now, because I have a sense of the ludicrous, I

sent him back an answer, Mr. Moxie. Dig, because I mean this is some of the really goodies I had in the letter, you know. He wants to know details.

"Dear Mr. Moxie: It would be useless to go into the definitive, a breakdown of what the duties will be, unless I can be sure that the incidents that have happened in the past will not be reiterated, such as ticket takers I have hired, who claimed they were harassed by customers who wanted their money back, such as the fop in San Jose who is suing me for being stabbed. Claims he was stabbed by an irate customer, and it was a lie—it was just a manicure scissors, and you couldn't see it because it was below the eyebrow, and when his eye was open, you couldn't see it anyway. (So I tell him a lot of problems like that.) And —oh yes, oh yeah—my father . . . has been in three mental institutions, and detests the fact that I am in the industry, and really abhors the fact that I have been successful economically and has harassed some ticket sellers, like in Sacramento he stood in line posing as a customer and, lightning flash, grabbed a handful of human feces and crammed it in the ticket taker's face. And once in Detroit he posed as a customer and he leaned against the booth so the ticket seller could not see him, and he was exposing himself, and had a sign hanging from it, saying: WHEN WE HIT $1500, THE GUY INSIDE THE BOOTH IS GOING TO KISS IT."

Now, you'd assume Dean R. Moxie, reading the letter, would just reject that and have enough validity to grab it in again.

"Dear Mr. Moxie: You know, of course, that if these facts were to fall into the hands of some yellow journalists, this would prove a deterrent to my career. So I'm giving you, you know, my confessor, you know," blah, blah, blah. "Also, this is not a requisite of a ticket seller, but I was wondering if I could have a ticket seller who could be more than a ticket seller—a companion."

Really light now. This is really subtle.

"A companion, someone who I could have coffee with, someone who is not narrow-minded like the—I had a stunning Danish seaman type in Oregon, who misinterpreted me and stole my watch."

Ha! Ha, is that heavy?

"Stole my watch. Am hoping to hear from you," blah, blah, blah, "Lenny Bruce."

OK. Now I send him a booster letter.

"Dear Mr. Moxie: My attorney said I was mad for ever confessing what has happened to me, you know, so I know that I can trust you, and I have sent you some cologne."

Ha!

"Sent you some cologne, and I don't know what's happened . . ." Isn't this beautiful?

"And I don't know what's happened to that naughty postman, naughtiest . . ."

Get this phraseology. I hadn't heard, you know. Now I get an answer from him:

"We cannot insure the incidents that have happened in the past will not reoccur. A ticket seller that would socialize is out of the question."

I think this is beautiful.

"And I did not receive any cologne nor do we care for any. Dean R. Moxie . . ."

(*With drum and cymbal accompaniment.*)
To is a preposition.

To is a preposition
Come is a verb.
To is a preposition.
Come is a verb.
To is a preposition.
Come is a verb, the verb intransitive.
To come.
To come.

I've heard these two words my whole adult life, and as a kid when I thought I was sleeping.

To come.
To come.

It's been like a big drum solo.

Did you come?

Did you come?

Good.

Did you come good?

Did you come good?

Did you come good?

Did you come good?

Did you come good?

Did you come good?

Did you come good?

I come better with you, sweetheart, than anyone in the whole goddamned world.

I really came so good.

I really came so good 'cause I love you.

I really came so good.

I come better with you, sweetheart, than anyone in the whole world.

I really came so good.

So good.

But don't come in me.

Don't come in me.

Don't come in me, me, me, me, me.

Don't come in me, me, me, me.

Don't come in me.

Don't come in me, me, me.

Don't come in me, me, me.

I can't come.

'Cause you don't love me, that's why you can't come.

I love you, I just can't come; that's my hang-up, I can't come when I'm loaded, all right?

'Cause you don't love me. Just what the hell is the matter with you?

What has that got to do with loving? I just can't come.

Now, if anyone in this room or the world finds those two words decadent, obscene, immoral, amoral, asexual, the words "to come" really make you feel uncomfortable, if you think I'm rank for saying it to you, you the beholder think it's rank for listening to it, you probably can't come. And then you're of no use, because that's the purpose of life, to re-create it.

Mr. Wollenberg called me to the witness stand for cross-examination:

Q. Mr. Bruce, had you a written script when you gave this performance?

A. No.

MR. BENDICH: Objected to as irrelevant, your Honor.

THE COURT: The answer is "No"; it may stand.

MR. WOLLENBERG: I have no further questions.

THE COURT: All right, you may step down.

THE WITNESS: Thank you.

MR. BENDICH: The defense rests, your Honor.

The time had come for the judge to instruct the jury:

"The defendant is charged with violating Section 311.6 of the Penal Code of the State of California, which provides:

Every person who knowingly sings or speaks any obscene song, ballad, or other words in any public place is guilty of a misdemeanor.

"'Obscene' means to the average person, applying contemporary standards, the predominant appeal of the matter, taken as a whole, is to prurient interest; that is, a shameful or morbid interest in nudity, sex or excretion which goes substantially beyond the customary limits of candor in description or representation of such matters and is matter which is utterly without redeeming social importance.

"The words 'average person' mean the average adult person and have no relation to minors. This is not a question of what you would or would not have children see, hear or read, because that is beyond the scope of the law in this case and is not to be discussed or considered by you.

" 'Sex' and 'obscenity' are not synonymous. In order to make the portrayal of sex obscene, it is necessary that such portrayal come within the definition given to you, and the portrayal must be such that its dominant tendency is to deprave or corrupt the average adult by tending to create a clear and present danger of antisocial behavior.

"The law does not prohibit the realistic portrayal by an artist of his subject matter, and the law may not require the author to put refined language into the mouths of primitive people. The speech of the performer must be considered in relation to its setting and the theme or themes of his production. The use of blasphemy, foul or coarse language, and vulgar behavior does not in and of itself constitute obscenity, although the use of such words may be considered in arriving at a decision concerning the whole of the production.

"To determine whether the performance of the defendant falls within the condemnation of the statute, an evaluation must be made as to whether the performance as a whole had as its dominant theme an appeal to prurient interest. Various factors should be borne in mind when applying this yardstick. These factors include the theme or themes of the performance, the degree of sincerity of purpose evident in it, whether it has artistic merit. If the performance is merely disgusting or revolting, it cannot be obscene, because obscenity contemplates the arousal of sexual desires.

"A performance cannot be considered utterly without redeeming social importance if it has literary, artistic or aesthetic merit, or if it contains ideas, regardless of whether they are unorthodox, controversial, or hateful, of redeeming social importance.

"In the case of certain crimes, it is necessary that in addition to the intended act which characterizes the offense, the act must be accompanied by a specific or particular intent without which such a crime may not be committed. Thus, in the crime charged here, a necessary element is the existence in the mind of the defendant of knowing that the material used in his production on October 4, 1961, was obscene, and that, knowing it to be obscene, he presented such material in a public place.

"The intent with which an act is done is manifested by the circumstances attending the act, the manner in which it is done, the means used, and the discretion of the defendant. In determining whether the defendant had such knowledge, you may consider reviews of his work which were available to him, stating that his performance had artistic merit and contained socially important ideas, or, on the contrary, that his performance did not have any artistic merit and did not contain socially important ideas."

The court clerk read the verdict:

"In the Municipal Court of the City and County of San Francisco, State of California; the People of the State of California, Plaintiff, *vs.* Lenny Bruce, Defendant; Verdict . . ."

I really started to sweat it out there.

"We, the jury in the above-entitled case, find the defendant not guilty of the offense charged, misdemeanor, to wit: violating Section 311.6 of the Penal Code of the State of California . . ."

"Ladies and gentlemen of the jury, is this your verdict?"

THE JURY: Yes.

THE COURT: All right. Do you desire the jury polled?

MR. WOLLENBERG: No, your Honor.

THE COURT: Would you ask the jury once again if that is their verdict.

THE CLERK: Ladies and gentlemen of the jury, is this your verdict?

THE JURY: Yes.

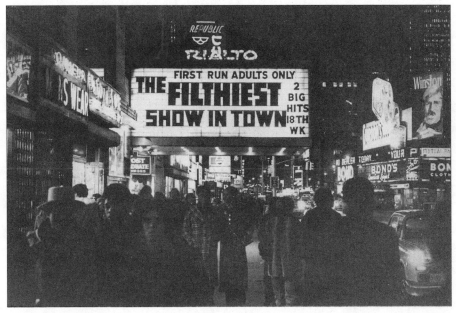

© Fred W. McDarrah

Think Clean

from *Time*, March 3, 1967

*This profile of Hugh Hefner, the founder and the publisher of **Playboy**, is an indication of the way in which **Playboy** had entered the mainstream of American culture. The magazine's editors saw the mainstreaming of **Playboy** as a continuation of the developments—in particular what it called "spectator sex"—that it had charted three years earlier in its essay on the second sexual revolution.*

The buzz of cocktail chatter and the clink of ice cubes shrink the vast room with its monumental fireplace, paneled walls, beamed 22-ft. ceiling and two suits of medieval armor. Soft, round girls curl up with boy friends on couches beneath immense paintings by Franz Kline and Larry Rivers, relaxed, confident plainly well off. A scene straight out of *Playboy* magazine? Precisely. The men are mostly magazine employees, and the girls are some of the 24 bunnies who room upstairs. A couple of centerfold "Playmates," disarmingly pretty and ingenuous-looking in party dresses, sip Pepsi-Cola.

Then stillness and a turning of heads. Down a few steps from a doorway in the corner of the room walk a man and a woman—he, casual in slacks and cardigan sweater, she, sleek in blonde hair and black dress. Simultaneously, a full-sized movie screen begins a silent descent down a side wall. *Playboy* Editor-Publisher Hugh Marston

Hefner, 40, sinks into a love seat that has been saved for him beside the 15-ft.-long stereo console. His girl friend, *Playboy* Cover Girl Mary Warren, 23, slips alongside him, puts her head on his shoulder. A butler brings a bowl of hot buttered popcorn and bottle of Pepsi; the lights dim; the movie begins. Last week it was Michelangelo Antonioni's *Blow-Up*, the week before Claude Lelouch's *A Man and a Woman*.

After the move, buffet supper is served in the bunny dining room. "Hef" (nicknames abound) and Mary chat for awhile then stroll of to his private quarters. These include a duplex of offices, living room, bedroom, (an adjoining room serves as a TV taping studio), all ankle-deep in white carpet. Once Hef has retired, his guests may amuse themselves as they see fit. The top floor of the house, used as a bunny dormitory by the Chicago Playboy club, is off limits. Very much available, however, is the heated, kidney-shaped first-floor swimming pool (bathing suits, if desired, are supplied by the house). If guests want seclusion, they may swim through a gentle waterfall to a hidden grotto furnished with soft cushions and background music. Privacy is not complete, however, the grotto can be observed through a trap door on the main hall above. The way to a nightcap is a brisk slide down a brass firehouse pole leading to a bar, where a glass wall gives an underwater view of the pool.

Spectator Sex.

To some visitors, the trap door and the glass wall are the real symbols of Hugh Hefner's achievement. Bacchanalia with Pepsi. Orgies with popcorn, And 24 girls—count'em, 24—living right overhead! Not to mention all those mechanical reassurances, like TV and hi-fi. It is all so familiar and domestic. Don Juan? Casanova? That was in another country and, besides, the guys are dead, Hugh Hefner is alive, American, modern, trustworthy, clean, respectful, and the country's leading impresario of spectator sex.

Hefner's pad on Chicago's North State Parkway has become a considerable tourist attraction, with guided tours available to anyone who has a minimum of pull. It is also the monument to a major American business success story. Unlike other Chicago businesses, the enterprise is not founded on steel, grain or transportation, but on a magazine. One of the great publishing successes since World War II, *Playboy* was started in 1953 with a 70,000 press run, now has a 4,000,000 circulation.

The magazine has many things to offer, but the basis of success is the nude or seminude photographs that Hugh Hefner has made respectable in the U.S. prints. America was undoubtedly ready for it anyway but Hefner seized the moment. He was the first publisher to see that the sky would not fall and mothers would not march if he published bare bosoms; he realized that the old taboos were going, that, so to speak, the empress need wear no clothes. He took the old-fashioned, shame-thumbed girlie magazine, stripped off the plain wrapper, added gloss, class and culture. It proved to be a sure fire formula, which more sophisticated and experienced competitors somehow had never dared contemplate.

The Ultimate Life

Apart from the nudes, *Playboy* offers fiction, reportage and interviews, reasonably amusing and bawdy cartoons, some dirty jokes, and discussions by sociologists and theologians. Above all, in vivid color and enthusiastic text, the ultimate life of material and sensual pleasure is abundantly demonstrated for some imaginary man about town. Latest male fashions are on display; so are sleek cars, sumptuous stereo sets and fine wines and foods, with instruction on when, how and to whom to serve them. There is always the suggestion that sex is part of the successful life, that good-looking women are status symbols. Says Paul Gebhard, executive director of Indiana University's Kinsey-founded Institute for Sex Research. "Hefner's genius is that he has linked sex with upward mobility."

No content just to picture all these pleasures, Hefner has brought many of them to life, sort of. He operates 16 Playboy Clubs. He has opened a Caribbean Playboy resort in Jamaica and has started construction of a $9,000,000 year-round resort near Lake Geneva, Wis. Last year "HMH" enterprises sold $2,400,000 worth of products, ranging from tie clasps bearing the bunny insigne to bunny tail wall plaques.

Hefner has also experienced some commercial failures, including *Show Business Illustrated*, which folded after nine issues with an estimated loss of $2,000,000, and *Trump*, a *Mad*-like humor magazine. On the other hand, the newly formed Playboy Press is thriving; last year, it sold $1,000,000 worth of books, most of them containing reprints from the magazine. At present, *Playboy's* staff is moving into large quarters in Chicago's venerable Palmolive Building, leased for 63 years for $2,700,000. Thanks to eager press agents, the building's famed beacon, whose beam can be seen 500 miles way, has been renamed the Bunny Beacon.

Just Accessories

In both his magazine and its allied enterprises, Hugh Hefner is a prophet of pop hedonism. He instinctively realized what sociologists had been saying for years—that the puritan ethic was dying, that pleasure and leisure were becoming positive and universally adored values in American society. As Psychiatrist Rollo May has pointed out, a new Puritanism has developed, a feeling that enjoyment is imperative, that to live the full, uninhibited life (in sex as in other areas) is everyone's duty.

Hefner is clearly a new-style puritan, but in many ways he is an old-style one as well. He, works to spread the gospel of pleasure with a dogged devotion that would do credit to any God-driven missionary or work-driven millionaire. How much real pleasure his Chicago pleasure dome hold for Hefner is a question his friends and associates sometimes wonder about. There is even something slightly puritanical about the magazine itself. Says Harvard Theologian Harvey Cost: "*Playboy* is basically antisexual. Like the sports car, liquor and hi-fi, girls are just another *Playboy* accessory."

Unlike the other accessories, *Playboy's* girls are out of reach—real in the imagination only. Shapes in the pictures all have an implausible gloss, achieved by lights that flatter and airbrushes that remove blemishes, but most of all by a mind convinced that to be real would not be ideal—and probably obscene. In their creamy perfection, their lack of any natural disorder, their stilted poses and expressionless faces, they recall nothing so much as the ivory-skinned, perfectionist nudes of Victorian and classical painters, of Ingres, Boucher, and David—the paintings that Grandfather used to steal a glance at on his first trip to Europe.

Beyond Parody.

The magazine girls have their living counterparts in the Playboy Club bunnies—700 round little girls in glorified corsets that push their bosoms out, cinch their waists in, run to a sharp V in front and feature a cotton-tail in the rear. The bunnies also seem unreal (one cynic suggested they are made of plastic), but they are provocative enough for the management to pass a rule against dating the customers. The rule might not be necessary. As the manager of the London Playboy Club, who obviously knows his customers, says: "The basic conventioneer doesn't want to go to bed. He just wants to gawk."

In designing and running the Playboy Clubs, Hugh Hefner has effortlessly soared beyond parody or spoof. No satirist could improve on the thick bunny manual, which commands her, among other things, to remember "your proudest possession is your bunny tail. You must make sure it is always white and fluffy." If it is not, she gets five demerits.

Kinseyan Revelation

"The whole thing," says London Observer Columnist Katharine Whitehorn "is a Midwestern Methodist's vision of sin." She is absolutely right. Hefner's parents, Glenn and Grace, had been childhood sweethearts in Nebraska before they married and moved to Chicago. Glenn, an accountant who is now treasurer of *Playboy*, was and is a regular Methodist churchgoer; so is Grace. In his early years, Hefner was the kid across the aisle in school who was always scribbling sketches. He like to write up the doings of local kids for a neighborhood newspaper, and drew 70 cartoon strips about ornery Western outlaws, an interplanetary space traveler and a diabolical villain named Skull.

After graduating from high school, he enlisted in the Army for an uneventful two years. Discharged, he enrolled in the University of Illinois, largely because of another student there named Millie Glunn. While at Illinois, Hefner read Kinsey's *Sexual Behavior in the Human Male*. It came as a revelation and he wrote an indignant review in the campus humor magazine. "Our moral pretenses," he said, "our hypocrisy on matters of sex, have led to incalculable frustration, delinquency and unhappiness. One of these days," he promised, "I'm going to do an editorial on the subject."

Aim for the Libido

After 24 years, Hef graduated from college, married Millie and, with his cartoons tucked underneath his arm, canvassed the Chicago publishing world for a job. Nothing doing, so he took a job with a Chicago firm that produced and printed cardboard cartoons. It was, says Hefner, the closest thing to journalism he could get. Eventually he landed a job with the subscription department for *Esquire* magazine. But, when, after several months, he asked for a $5-a-week raise, he was turned down. He went to work briefly for a publication call *Children's Activities*, but he decided it was time to start his own magazine—and not for kids. In 1953 he hocked his furniture for $600, scraped together $10,000. He later persuaded a talented designer, Art Paul, to become his art director. Most other magazines for men concentrated on the outdoors, so he shrewdly decided to take up where *Esquire* had left off in catering to indoor tastes. Hefner picked a bunny to symbolize the new enterprise—because rabbits are the playboys of the animal world. The first issue in December 1953 told readers that "we plan to spend most of our time inside. We like our apartment." Hefner also bought right to the famed nude calendar pictures of Marilyn Monroe, then at the height of her career, and published them for the first time off a calendar. The 48-page issue sold 53,991 copies, even Hef was surprised.

From then on he aimed *Playboy* straight at the libido. Since sex is part of the whole man, he reasoned, why not devote part of a whole magazine to it? "Would you put together a human being that is just a heart and toenails?" he asks. So he put together a magazine that was largely bosom and thigh and not especially distinguishable from other girlie slicks. But he added more substantial content as he went along; today's *Playboy* is a well-stuffed product, bulging with intellectual ambition and self-confidence. It even includes some tips from John Paul Getty on how to succeed in business. The humor, however, remains on a fairly primitive level. A typical cartoon shows a playboy in bed with a bunnyesque girl, asking: "Why talk about love at a time like this?"

To begin with, fiction published in *Playboy* was spicy but hardly shocking—long forgotten efforts by John Steinbeck, Erskine Caldwell, Somerset Maugham, Robert Ruark. *Playboy* also dipped into the ribald classics; despite constant mining, the Boccaccio and De Maupassant vein is still running strong. In the early days, name writers shunned *Playboy*. Today, Vladimir Nabokov, James Baldwin, Kenneth Tynan, Herbert Bold, Ray Bradbury regularly provide respectable material. This upgrading of fiction is largely due to Auguste Comte Spectorsky,* 56, who was hired from NBC by Hefner to bring some New York know-how and sophistication (a favorite *Playboy* word) to the magazine. "Spec" has done that and more. Last summer he hired as fiction editor Robie Macauley, who had been running the distinguished *Kenyon Review*. "I was familiar with *Playboy*," says Macauley. "The students at Kenyon read it—so did the clergy. Besides, a magazine like this matures as it goes along."

Dream World

Maturing or not, *Playboy* still exists in a rather special world. Partly it can be seen in the ads, some of them for Hefner products. A four color promotion for the 1967 *Playboy* calendar reads: "Make a date with these twelve Playmates. You won't want to miss a day with this delicious dozen . . . Provocative . . . in captivating new poses. SHARE THE JOY! Perhaps nostalgic older readers can hear an echo in these lines of the candy butcher during intermission at the burlesque show, peddling the latest "pictures direct from Paris with each and every luscious pose guaranteed the way you gentlemen like it."

In general, though, *Playboy* ads are discreet—no stag movies, no sex manuals. "*Playboy* takes the reader into a kind of dream world, explains Advertising Director Howard Lederer. "We create a euphoria and we want nothing to spoil it. We don't want a reader to come suddenly on an ad that says he has bad breath. We don't want him to be reminded of the fact, though it may be true, that he is going bald."

The dream extends to the magazine's editorial content, but there reality does intrude. Viet Nam has hardly ever been mentioned in its columns, but there have been eloquent pleas for abolishing the draft and capital punishment, and a defense of the right to privacy by Senator Edward Long. Long, long question-and-answer interviews, some of them aggressive and stimulating, lately recorded the views of Fidel Castro, Mark Lane and Norman Thomas—just the thing to read aloud

* Named for the 19th century French Positivist philosopher, who added the word "sociology" to the language.

to a date in front of the fire, he wearing a Playboy sweater, she wearing Playmate perfume.

The magazine also has its own special crusades. It recently brought enough pressure to win a parole for a West Virginia disk jockey who was serving a one-to-ten-year sentence for a morals offense with a consenting teen-age girl. Another notable success involved a campaign against entrapment tactics practiced by—no, not the CIA but, of all agencies, the Post Office. Seems that postal inspectors were in the habit of placing an ad in a newspaper to the effect that one "swinger" would like to meet another. When letters were exchanged, the unsuspecting hedonist might include a nude photograph or two—whereupon the police arrived and arrested him.* Bowing to a Playboy-organized protest movement, as well as complaints from Congress, the Post Office promised to quit the practice.

Playboy has good reason to keep the mails safe for swingers, although the magazine itself has had little trouble with obscenity laws. Hefner was once arrested by the Chicago police after he ran some nude photos of Jayne Mansfield, but the case ended in a hung jury.

Girls con Brio

"Every issue of *Playboy*," Hefner has said, "must be paced like a symphony." While there may be a scherzo of cartoons, a largo of literature, a rondo of reportage, the allegro in each addition is still the girls and molto con brio. Although, girl pictures take up less than 10% of the pages, they remain the main motif. The style for the center fold Playmate was set by the maestro himself. He chose a rather average though well-endowed girl named Charlene Drain who worked in his subscription department. She said the department needed an addressograph machine. Sure, said Hef, provided she would pose in the nude. She agreed, became "Janet Pilgrim" and appeared in the July 1955 issue. The circulation department got its machine, and "Janet" became, for a while, head of *Playboy*'s readers' service department. She has since married and left for Texas, though she is still listed on the masthead.

Ever since, the magazine has tried hard to make its girls look ordinary

---

* *Playboy* has itself practices entrapment at times by hiring private investigators who pretend to be eager Johns and ask club bunnies for a date. If the bunnies are dumb enough to accept, the may get fired.

in a wholesome sort of way—just like the Nude Next Door. The illusion is heightened by the fact that the girls, are presented not only nude and in color but also in numerous black and white pictures in their natural habitat, whipping up a batch of muffins or playing the guitar. Suggestive poses are out as are the accouterments of fetishism. None of the nudes ever looks as if she has just indulged in sex, or were about to.

Hefner may have run the Marilyn Monroe shots without her consent, but now he has no problem finding big-name actresses eager to appear in the magazine. The album so far includes Carroll Baker, Arlene Dahl, Ursula Andress, Kim Novak, Susan Strasberg, Elsa Marinelli and Susannah York. Nor is there any trouble getting unknown girls to pose; hundreds apply. Sometimes, though, there is a problem in making the copy that goes with them interesting enough. For instance, the latest Miss January, *Playboy* said, would love to be a nurse. She was "Albert Schweitzer's fairest disciple. She has read each of the doctor's books at least twice."

The magazine also finds potential Playmates through a network of freelance photographers. A particularly rewarding field is wedding parties; a photographer covering the reception will often spot a comely bridesmaid. If under 21, she must get her parents' written consent. Photographing her is another matter. Getting a nonprofessional model, who has never before posed, in the right mood can take a photographer one whole day, or several. And all the while the photographer must keep in mind Art Director, Paul's concept of the *Playboy* nude "The idea," he says, "is to think clean."

Zero Garbo

The selection of the right nude from among hundreds of transparencies is taken at least as seriously by the *Playboy* staff as, say, choosing the proper tribal dance for a lead page in the *National Geographic*. Dialogue between Art Director, Paul and Editor Hefner when choosing pictures for the Playmates-of-the-year feature:

Paul: This is the best shot of her face.

Hef: That shot makes the girl look too Hollywoodish. She doesn't look natural.

Paul: Don't her breasts look somewhat distorted? . . . It looks as if the shots were made on a foggy day. We don't want to mix the reader up. You can't really be sure that this is the same girl.

Hef (viewing new layout): There is something wrong with the angle of that shot. Her thighs and hips look awkward. This doesn't do her justice . . . There must be other aspects to her personality.

Hefner knows exactly what he wants. He likes the young, pouty type without complications or excessive intelligence. Riper beauties he summarily dismisses. "Jeanne Moreau is a fine actress, she once said. "But as a woman she tells me zero. And zero to Greta Garbo. I think that when Sophia Loren was 20 she had a fantastic body. But that is all." To Gershon Legman, a Paris-based writer on sexuality, "*Playboy* is for the sub virile man who just wants to look. Basically, he's afraid of the girls." Says the Rev. William Hamilton of Colgate-Rochester Divinity School. "Hefner rightly affirms the goodness of the body, but he misses the beauty and mystery of sexuality."

Bundle of Insecurities

Who reads *Playboy*? Since 85% of its circulation comes from newsstand sales, readership surveys are difficult. But certain clues can be found in a sampling of questions asked of the feature, "Playboy Advisor." Mostly, they deal with insecurities about clothes, food and sex. A Fayetteville, Ark., reader wants to know whether the gas from his CO cork extractor will harm the wine (no). A Bahamas-bound Louisville bachelor wants to know what clothes to take along; a fellow in Elgin, Ill., wonders whether blue or striped shirts are all right after dark (no).

A San Francisco playboy seems to have become involved with a lesbian, the "Advisor" tells him: "Next time she calls, tell her you've lots of authentically male friends for those evenings you wish to spend going out with the guys." An Akon gentleman of 57 pronounces himself "hopelessly in love" with a lovely 59-year-old neighbor. Trouble is she won't go out with him Saturday nights; she's got a standing date with some other fellow. "Your Saturday nights must indeed be hell," agrees *Playboy* but if you insist on your so-called 'rights,' you may force the lady to make a decision that will cause *all* your evenings to be hell."

Despite the occasional appearance in the "Playboy Advisor" of such senior citizens, the magazine is in large measure addressed to the young who worry about the right socks as well as the right line with girls and the right pleasures. In short, it appeals to the undergraduate who wants to act like a sophisticate—or for that matter, to the high school graduate who wants to act like a college sophomore. And why not? After all half the magazine's title plainly emphasizes *boy*. Yet this does not do full justice to the range of *Playboy*'s readers. *Playboy* estimates that half have attended college, 70% are between the ages of 18 and 34. Women make up about 25% of its audience, and their reactions are mixed. Says Social Commentator Marya Mannes: There is "the implicit premise that woman is an Object. She has no other function than to be lusted after, and lurched at." Other female readers, who apparently don't mind being lurched at, enjoy *Playboy* for its inside view of a man's world and its notion of the latest styles in feminine sex appeal.

The Last Frontier

One of the more surprising facts is that *Playboy*'s readers include quite a number of ministers. Hefner offered the clergy a 25% subscription discount; found that seminarians demanded similar privileges. In some quarters, it is considered the mark of the cool, contemporary minister to mention *Playboy* casually in conversation, quote it in sermons, or even to write for it. In one issue, William Hamilton expounded on God-is-dead theology; shortly after, Bishop James Pike wrote in to argue with him. Harvey Cox of the Harvard Divinity School did an article in praise of the clergy's new grass-roots involvement with social ills and maladjustments; a group of ministers debated the pros and cons of liberalized abortion. "The last frontier is the sexual one," says Allen Moore of the Claremont School of Theology. "Because of Hefner, many in the church have begun to confront this barrier for the first time. Discussion is more open."

To supervise communications between the last frontier and the cloth, Hefner chose onetime Zoologist Anson Mount, the magazine's football editor; appointed him six months ago to head a new religion department. People who saw this move as a rather amusing put-on overestimate Hefner's sense of humor. It was all very serious, and frivolous staffers were discouraged from making jokes involving "sermon" and "Mount." Recalls the new religion editor: "I found myself over my head with things like personhood, demythologizing, Bonhoeffer. So I went to Hefner and said, 'Man, I've got to go off to school and learn some of this.' Hef sent him to the University of the South at Sewanee, where he studied hard for one summer and entertained lavishly, as befits an emissary from *Playboy*. The theologians grew so used to stopping by his house at cocktail hour that eventually they even ventured as far as Hef's Chicago mansion for discussions. "At first, they entered the house as if it were Dante's inferno," says Mount. "But now those cats are used to it."

Enlightenment Simplified

Ministerial interest was greatly stimulated by Hefner's earnest, marathon attempt to sellout the *"Playboy* philosophy." It took 25 installments and a quarter of a million words, Hefner's thesis was that U.S. society had too long and too rigorously suppressed good healthy heterosexuality. Since its growth had been stunted, Hefner argued, all sorts of perversions flourished in its place. "You get healthy sex not by ignoring it but by emphasizing it," he maintains. And the villain at the bottom of all this? Organized religion announced Hefner with an unabashed air of discover. Hefner revived Puritanism long enough to condemn it for being as "stultifying to the mind of man as Communism or any other totalitarian concept."

As it poured through the magazine's columns, the *Playboy* philosophy was often pretentious and relatively conventional. Hefner is a kind of oversimplified Enlightenment thinker with what comes out as an almost touching faith in the individual's capacity for goodness. Release a man from repression, thinks Hef, and he will instinctively pursue a "healthy" life in business and sex alike. Hefner also exhibits a tendency to "situation ethics," which call for judging acts within their special context rather than by a more fixed morality. Some use this formula to justify homosexuality, but Hefner firmly draws a heterosexual line. He does not endorse extramarital sex though he approves of the premarital variety.

No one has ever accused Hugh Hefner of being lyrical, but he can grow almost eloquent about sex, sounding approximately like D. H. Lawrence as rewritten by Alfred Kinsey. Sex, he is on record as saying, "can become, at its best, a means of expressing the innermost, deepest-felt longing, desires and emotions. And it is when sex serves those ends—in addition to, and apart from, reproduction—that it is lifted above the animal level and becomes most human.

Bedwork

With many more endorsements like that, Hefner might just possibly make sex go out of style. Whatever his philosophy may amount to, he does not belong to the peripatetic school. Is he out bunny-hugging every night in his sports car or carousing through his clubs with Play-mates on either arm? Not as all. His Mercedes-Benz sits forlornly in the garage; his clubs never see him. Lean, rather gaunt, with piercing dark eyes, he has succumbed to the work ethic. He explains that he does not want to face all the outside world's trivia—small talk, party joining— that might distract him from his work. Nor does he have the distractions of a family. Hefner was divorced from Millie eight years ago. Their two children live with his ex-wife, who has remarried.

He does a lot of that work in bed—a round bed, 8 ft. in diameter, which revolves or vibrates at the touch of a button. By rotating the bed toward the fireplace or the bar or the television, Hefner has the feeling that he is moving from one room to another. A life-sized epoxy sculpture of a seated nude girl by Frank Gallo crouches beside the fireplace, and a TV camera can be trained on the bed.

He does visit the office, but mostly he uses dictating machines to communicate with this staff, sometimes producing recorded memos 30 pages long. Two secretaries, one on day shift, the other on night shift, transcribe the flow. The complete man of electronics, he avoids face-to-face contact and gets his information on the outside world from newspapers, magazines and eight television monitors. He rarely watches a TV show when it is on the air, has it taped for later viewing, and also keeps a stock of several hundred taped movies.

No Daylight

Within his sealed capsule, Hefner loses all sense of time and season. He loves the night. By keeping his shades always drawn, he has effectively banished daylight from his life. He eats when he pleases—a kitchen staff is on duty 24 hours a day. But then he subsists largely on Pepsi-Colas, which are stocked in small refrigerators scattered throughout his quarters, including one in the headboard of his bed. Often he doesn't even know what day it is. A friend suggested giving him a set of seven pajamas with the day embroidered on each—in reverse writing so that he would just have to look in the mirror while shaving to see where he was in the week.

There is evidence that he might be looking in new directions. He sometimes sounds as if he thought the sexual revolution were over, thanks to *Playboy*, and that it is now time to move on to other social and economic challenges. Even the country's gross national product seems to interest him. "A publication," he wrote, "that helps motivate a part of society to work harder, to accomplish more, to earn more in order to enjoy more of the material benefits described—to that extent, the publication is contributing to the economic growth of the nation."

Like sex, G.N.P. has three letters. But for a real hedonist, it's hardly the same thing.

Pornotopia

Steven Marcus

from The Other Victorians, 1966

The Other Victorians is a pioneering portrait of sex during the years of Queen Victoria's reign—whose name has been given to a harsh regime of sexual repression. But it was also a pathbreaking study of sexual history, an academic field that did not exist at the time. Marcus' research was conducted in the Kinsey Institute's immense collection of Victorian material which included medical texts dealing with sex and pornography. Ten years later, Michel Foucault opened his reflections on the history of sexuality by returning to the world portrayed in The Other Victorians. This selection explores the significance of pornography's utopian impulse for endlessly repeated and deferred gratification – its quest for unlimited pleasure.

There is a passage in one of Max Weber's great essays on the methodology of the social sciences which is pertinent to our discussion. In it Weber is struggling to define with absolute rigor and clarity his difficult notion of the "ideal type." He is trying to demonstrate that this notion or analytical construct "has no connection at all with *value-judgments,*" and that further "it has nothing to do with any type of perfection other than a purely *logical* one." To illustrate the distinction he has in mind, Weber states that "there are ideal types of brothels as well as of religions"; and he goes on to say that there are even "ideal types of those kinds of brothels which are technically 'expedient' from the point of view of police ethics as well as those of which the exact opposite" holds true. The writer or scholar who undertakes to discuss pornography has in effect made a contract to construct an ideal type of a brothel—and he has in addition contracted to maintain the distinctions that Weber established. This is not a simple task, as Weber himself was quick to recognize. On the one hand, he states, we must guard ourselves against such "crude misunderstandings . . . as the opinion that cultural significance should be attributed only to *valuable* phenomena. Prostitution is a *cultural* phenomenon just as much as religion or money." At the same time, and on the other hand, he continues, prostitution, religion, and money "are cultural phenomena *only* because and *only* insofar as their existence and the form which they historically assume touch directly or indirectly on our cultural *interests* and arouse our striving for knowledge concerning problems brought into focus by the evaluative ideas which give *significance* to the fragment of reality analyzed by those concepts." Weber's strained and circling syntax attests to the difficulty of keeping these two fields of discourse distinct. Our interests and our values inevitably dictate our choice of subjects—the significance we attribute to any fragment of reality that we subject to analysis has its point of origin and reference in a realm external to the analysis itself. Nevertheless, in the course of analysis we must dissociate ourselves, as much as possible, from those very values that informed our choice of a subject to begin with. This is not altogether possible, in practice if not in logic—although I believe it to be logically impossible as well. Which is to say that in the social sciences, as much as in literary criticism, the problem of judgment remains central, unyielding, and full of impossible demands. That these demands are impossible in no way rules out the necessity that they be fulfilled.

Our difficulties seem to be further compounded if we examine another part of Weber's long definition-discussion of this heuristic idea or device. An ideal type, Weber remarks, is not "an average" of anything. It is formed rather by "the one-sided *accentuation* of one or more points of view and by the synthesis of a great many diffuse, discrete, more or less present and occasionally absent *concrete individual* phenomena, which are arranged according to those one-sidedly emphasized viewpoints into a unified *analytical* construct." In substance, he states, "this construct is like a *utopia* which has been arrived at by the analytical accentuation of certain elements of reality." And he goes to add that "in its conceptual purity, this mental construct cannot be found empirically anywhere in reality. It is a *utopia*." The writer who tries to take the next step beyond the analysis of specific works of a pornographic character, who extends his discussion in order to reach some synthetic or theoretical conclusions, is compelled to deal with utopia on two fronts. In summing up, sorting, and ordering the material he has already dealt with, he is employing the logical method of the ideal type—by abstraction, accentuation, suppression, emphasis, and rearrangement, he attains to a hypothetical or utopian conception of the material which earlier he had analytically dispersed. At the same time, however, in the instance of pornography that material itself inclines to take the form of a utopia. The literary genre that pornographic fantasies—particularly when they appear in the shape of pornographic fiction—tend most to resemble is the utopian fantasy. For our present purposes I call this fantasy pornotopia.

What is pornotopia?

Where, in the first place, does it exist? Or where, alternatively, does it take place? The word "utopia," of course, means "not place," or "not a place," or "no place." More than most utopias, pornography takes the injunction of its etymology literally—it may be said largely to exist at no place, and to take place in nowhere. The isolated castle on an inaccessible mountain top, the secluded country estate, set in the middle of a large park and surrounded by insurmountable walls, the mysterious town house in London or Paris, the carefully furnished and elaborately equipped set of apartments to be found in any city at all, the deserted cove at the seaside, or the solitary cottage atop the cliffs, the inside of a brothel rented for a day, a week, or a month, or the inside of a hotel room rented for a night—these are all the same place and are identically located. These places may be found in books; they may be read about in libraries or in studies; but their true existence is not the world, or even the world as it exists by special reference in literature. They truly exist behind our eyes, within our heads. To read a work of pornographic fiction is to rehearse the ineffably familiar; to locate that fantasy anywhere apart from the infinite, barren, yet plastic space that exists within our skulls is to deflect it from one of its chief purposes. A representative nineteenth-century novel begins, "In the town of X——, on a warm summer's day . . ." By the time we have finished with such a novel we have learned an astonishing number of things about that town and its weather, about its inhabitants, their families, how they go about making their livings, what their opinions may be upon a variety of topics, what they like and dislike, how they were born and how they die, what they leave behind and what they set up in store for the future. A representative pornographic novel may also begin with the town of X—— and a summer's day, but it does not proceed from that point, as the novel does, by elaboration and extension. What typically happens is that after having presented the reader with some dozen concrete details—by way of a down payment on credibility, one assumes—the novel then leaves this deposit of particularities behind and proceeds by means of abstraction to its real business, which is after all largely irrelevant to considerations of place. In the century of national literatures, pornography produced a body of writing that was truly international in character. It is often impossible to tell whether a pornographic work of fiction is a translation or an original—one need only change the names, or the spelling of the names, of characters in order to conceal such a novel's origin. The *genius loci* of pornography speaks in the *lingua franca* of sex. One need not inquire very far to find sufficient reasons for pornography's indifference to place: in the kind of boundless, featureless freedom that most pornographic fantasies require for their action, such details are regarded as restrictions, limitations, distractions, or encumbrances.

Utopias commonly have some special relation to time, and pornotopia is no exception to this rule. Some utopias are set in a distant past, some are located in a distant future; almost all seem to be implicitly conceived as taking place at some special juncture in time, where time as we know it and some other kind of time intersect. Although utopias are often furnished with novel means of measuring and counting time—such as new kinds of clocks or calendars—it is sound to say that most of them are outside of time. So is pornotopia, although the special ways in which it represents its exemption need to be specified. To the question "What time is it in pornotopia?" one is tempted to answer, "It is always bedtime," for that is in a literal sense true. Sometimes a work of pornography, following the example of the novel, will establish an equivalence between time and the duration of a single life-span or personal history. In pornography, however, life or existence in time does not begin with birth; it begins with one's first sexual impulse or experience, and one is said to be born in pornotopia only after one has experienced his first erection or witnessed his first primal scene. Similarly, one is declared dead when, through either age or accident, one becomes impotent—which helps to explain why in pornotopia women are immortal, and why in pornographic novels there are so many old women, witches, and hags, and so few old men. In another sense, time in pornotopia is without duration; when the past is recalled, it is for the single purpose of arousing us in the present. And the effort of pornography in this regard is to achieve in consciousness the condition of the unconscious mind—a condition in which all things exist in a total, simultaneous present. Time, then, in pornotopia is sexual time; and its real unit of measurement is an internal one—the time it takes either for a sexual act to be represented or for an autoerotic act to be completed. (These last two distinctions depend upon whether one chooses to emphasize the author's or the reader's sense of time—in a considerable number of instances the two seem to coincide.)

On a larger scale, time in pornotopia is determined by the time it takes to run out a series of combinations. Given a limited number of variables—that is, persons of both sexes with their corresponding organs and appendages—and a limited number of juxtapositions into which these variables may be placed, time becomes a mathematical function and may be defined as however long it takes to represent or exhaust the predetermined number of units to be combined. This is why *The One Hundred and Twenty Days of Sodom* represents one kind of perfection in this genre. Pornography's mad genius, the Marquis de Sade, with psychotic rigidity and precision, and with psychotic logic, wrote his novel along strict arithmetical lines: so many of this and so many of these and those, doing this, that, and those to them in the following order or declension; to be succeeded on the following day, after all have changed hands or places by . . . et cetera, et cetera. Although it is commonly believed that Sade did not finish this novel, since large parts of it exist only in outline, such a conclusion is not acceptable. Having completed his outline, Sade had in effect written his novel— the rest is only filling in. The truth of this suggestion may be demonstrated by a reading of the novel: I can for myself find no essential difference between the filled-in parts and those that exist only in outline. Form and content are perfectly fused in the outline, and the filling-in or writing-out is largely a matter of adornment—

a circumstance that both anticipates and points to certain distinctions which have to be made in considering pornography's relation to literature. It also serves to suggest that a pornographic novel might be written by a computer. If one feeds in the variables out will come the combinations. I have no doubt that one day this kind of literature will be produced, and I must confess to a sense of relief when I recognize that I will not be around to read it.

So much for the coordinates of space and time. We next may turn to the actual external world as it appears in pornotopia. How, for example, is nature represented? It is represented as follows. It is usually seen at eye-level. In the middle distance there looms a large irregular shape. On the horizon swell two immense snowy white hillocks; these are capped by great, pink, and as it were prehensile peaks or tips—as if the rosy-fingered dawn itself were playing just behind them. The landscape then undulates gently down to a broad, smooth, swelling plain, its soft rolling curves broken only in the lower center by a small volcanic crater or omphalos. Farther down, the scene narrows and changes in perspective. Off to the right and left jut two smooth snowy ridges. Between them, at their point of juncture, is a dark wood—we are now at the middle of our journey. This dark wood—sometimes it is called a thicket—is triangular in shape. It is also like a cedarn cover, and in its midst is a dark romantic chasm. In this chasm the wonders of nature abound. From its top there depends a large, pink stalactite, which changes shape, size, and color in accord with the movement of the tides below and within. Within the chasm—which is roughly pear-shaped—there are caverns measureless to man, grottoes, hermits' caves, underground streams—a whole internal and subterranean landscape. The climate is warm but wet. Thunderstorms are frequent in this region, as are tremors and quakings of the earth. The walls of the cavern often heave and contract in rhythmic violence, and when they do the salty streams that run through it double their flow. The whole place is dark yet visible. This is the center of the earth and the home of man.

The essential imagination of nature in pornotopia, then, is this immense, supine, female form. Sometimes this figure is represented in other positions and from other perspectives; sometimes other orifices are chosen for central emphasis. Whichever way it is regarded, however, this gigantic female shape is the principal external natural object in the world we are describing. Although I have in part composed this catalogue of features with a humorous intention, I should add that every image in it is taken from a work of pornography, and that all of these images are commonplaces—they really are the means through which writers of pornography conceive of the world. As for man in this setting he is really not part of nature. In the first place, he is actually not man. He is an enormous erect penis, to which there happens to be attached a human figure. Second, this organ is not a natural but a supernatural object. It is creator and destroyer, the source of all and the end of all being—it is literally omnipotent, and plays the role in pornotopia that gods and deities play elsewhere. It is the object of worship; and the nature that we have just finished describing exists—as does the universe in certain cosmogonies—for the sole purpose of confirming the existence of its creator. Finally, we should take notice of the gigantic size of these figures. This is not simply another aspect of their godlike characters; it suggests to us as well in what age of life the imagination of pornography has its grounds.

As for external nature as we ordinarily perceive it, that exists in pornotopia in an incidental yet interesting way. If a tree or a bush is represented as existing, the one purpose of its existence is as a place to copulate under or behind. If there is a stream, then the purpose of that stream is as a place in which to bathe before copulating. If a rainstorm comes up, then the purpose of that rainstorm is to drive one indoors in order to copulate. (When D. H. Lawrence dragged in a rainstorm in order to drive his lovers out of doors, he was doing something that no right-minded pornographer would ever dream of.) Nature, in other words, has no separate existence in pornotopia; it is not external to us, or "out there." There is no "out there" in pornography, which serves to indicate to us again in what phase of our mental existence this kind of thinking has its origins.

These attributes of nature in pornotopia are in turn connected with others, which have to do with the richness and inexhaustibility of life in this imaginary world—pornotopia is a pornocopia as well. Pornotopia is literally a world of grace abounding to the chief of sinners. All men in it are always and infinitely potent; all women fecundate with lust and flow inexhaustibly with sap or juice or both. Everyone is always ready for anything, and everyone is infinitely generous with his substance. It is always summertime in pornotopia, and it is a summertime of the emotions as well—no one is ever jealous, possessive, or really angry. All our aggressions are perfectly fused with our sexuality, and the only rage is the rage of lust, a happy fury indeed. Yet behind these representations of physiological abundance and sexual plenitude one senses an anxiety that points in the opposite direction. Pornotopia could in fact only have been imagined by persons who have suffered extreme deprivation, and I do not by this mean sexual deprivation in the genital sense alone. One gets the distinct impression, after reading a good deal of this literature, that it could only have been written by men who at some point in their lives had been starved. The insatiability depicted in it seems to me to be literal insatiability, and the orgies endlessly represented are the visions of permanently hungry men. The Marquis de Sade once again took the matter to its logical conclusion; when his orgies include the eating of excrement, and then finally move on to murder with the purpose of cannibalism, he was bringing to explicit statement the direction taken by almost all works of pornography. Inside of every pornographer there is an infant screaming for the breast from which he has been torn. Pornography represents an endless and infinitely repeated effort to recapture that breast, and the bliss it offered, as it often represents as well a revenge against the world—and the women in it—in which such cosmic injustice could occur.

Relations between human beings also take on a special appearance in pornotopia. It is in fact something of a misnomer to call these representations "relations between human beings." They are rather juxtapositions of human bodies, parts of bodies, limbs, and organs; they are depictions of positions and events, diagrammatic schema for sexual ballets—actually they are more like football plays than dances; they are at any rate as complicated as either. As an example of how such relations are represented, I will quote some passages from *The Romance of Lust*. This novel was published during the 1870's. It is in four volumes and runs to six hundred pages, every one of which is devoted to nothing other than the description of persons in sexual congress. This novel comes as close as anything I know to being a pure pornotopia in the sense that almost every human consideration apart from sexuality is excluded from it. The passages I quote were chosen almost at random.

> We ran off two bouts in this delicious position, and then with more regulated passions rose to form more general combinations.
>
> The Count had fucked the Egerton while we were engaged above the divine Frankland. Our first pose was suggested by the Egerton, who had been as yet less fucked than any. She had been also greatly taken with the glories of the Frankland's superb body, and especially struck with her extraordinary clitoris, and had taken the curious lech of wishing to have it in her bottomhole while riding St. George on my big prick. We all laughed at her odd choice, but agreed at once, especially the Frankland, whose greatest lech was to fuck very fair young women with her long and capable clitoris. A fairer creature than the lovely Egerton could not be found. The Frankland admitted that in her inmost heart she had longed thus to have the Egerton from the moment she had first seen her, and her delight and surprise at finding the dear Egerton had equally desired to possess her, fired her fierce lust with increased desire. I lay down, the Egerton straddled over, and feeling the delight of my huge prick when completely imbedded, she spent profusely with only two rebounds. Then sinking on my belly she presented her lovely arse to the lascivious embraces of the salacious Frankland. . . .
>
> The Count next took the Benson in cunt while I blocked the rear aperture, and the Frankland once more enculed the Egerton, who dildoed herself in cunt at the same time; all of us running two courses. We then rose, purified, and refreshed. When our pricks were ready it was the Egerton who took me in front and the Count behind, and the Benson, who had grown lewd on the Frankland's clitoris, was sodomised by her and dildoed by herself. The Egerton still suffered a little in the double stretching, so that we ran but one exquisite bout, enabling us, whose powers began to fail, to be re-excited, and to finish with the double jouissance in the glorious body of the Frankland.

Before proceeding any further, I should like to direct attention to

certain qualities in the prose of these passages. First, this prose manages to combine extreme fantasy with absolute cliché—as if the fantasy,
however wild and excessive it may seem, had been gone through so
many times that it had long since become incapable of being anything
other than a weary and hopeless repetition of itself. Second, the whole
representation takes place under the order of "regulated passions."
That is to say everything in it—the movements and responses of the
imaginary persons—is completely controlled, as things are in auto-
erotic fantasies but as they never are in the relations of human beings,
and even, one might add, as they never are in the relations of human
beings as these are represented in literature. Third, the relations
between the persons in these passages are intricate and mechanical; the
juxtaposition of organs and apertures is convoluted yet precise, and it
is impossible to know the players without a scorecard. In this connection, one should also note the tendency to abolish the distinction
between the sexes: clitorises become penises, anuses are common to
both sexes, and everyone is everything to everyone else. Yet this everything is confined strictly to the relations of organs, and what is going
on may be described as organ grinding.

The Romance of Lust continues, after a short hiatus, as follows:

So to five women we thus had six men, and eventually a very
handsome young priest, debauched by the others, joined our
party, and we carried on the wildest and most extravagant orgies
of every excess the most raging lust could devise. We made
chains of pricks in arseholes, the women between with dildoes
strapped round their waist, and shoved into the arseholes of
the man before them, while his prick was into the arsehole of the
woman in his front. . . .

Our second double couplings were, myself in my aunt's cunt,
which incest stimulated uncle to a stand, and he took to his
wife's arse while her nephew incestuously fucked her cunt. The
Count took to the delicious and most exciting tight cunt of the
Dale, while her son shoved his prick into his mother's arse, to
her unspeakable satisfaction. Ellen and the Frankland amused
themselves with tribadic extravagances.

This bout was long drawn out, and afforded inexpressible

extasies to all concerned. And after the wild cries and most bawdy oaths that instantly preceded the final extasy, the dead silence and long after enjoyments were drawn out to a greater length than before. After which we all rose and purified, and then took refreshments of wine and cake, while discussing our next arrangements of couples. . . .

I then took my aunt's arse while the lecherous Dale was underneath gamahuching and dildoing her, and by putting the Dale close to the edge of the bed, the Count stood between her legs, which were thrown over his shoulders, and thus he fucked her, having taken a lech to fuck her cunt, which was an exquisite one for fucking; her power of nip being nearly equal to the Frankland, and only beaten by aunt's extraordinary power in that way. We thus formed a group of four enchained in love's wildest sports together.

The Frankland was gamahuched by uncle while having Harry's prick in her arse, Ellen acting postilion to Harry's arse while frigging herself with a dildo.

The closing bout of the night was the Count into aunt's arse, my prick into the Frankland's arse, Harry enjoying an old-fashioned fuck with his mother, and Ellen under aunt to dildo and be gamahuched and dildoed by aunt. We drew this bout out to an interminable length, and lay for nearly half-an-hour in the annihilation of the delicious afterjoys. At last we rose, purified, and then restoring our exhausted frames with champagne, embraced and sought well earned sleep in our separate chambers.

The relations between persons set forth in such passages are in fact combinations. They are outlines or blueprints, diagrams of directions or vectors, and they must be read diagrammatically. They are, in other words, sets of abstractions. Although the events and organs they refer to are supposed to be concrete, one may observe how little concrete detail, how few real particularities, these passages contain. Persons in them are transformed into literal objects; these objects finally coalesce into one object—oneself. The transactions represented in this writing are difficult to follow because so little individuation has gone into them. In a world whose organization is directed by the omnipotence of thought, no such discriminations are necessary.

With this relentless circumscription of reality, with its tendency, on the one hand, to exclude from itself everything that is not sexual and, on the other, to include everything into itself by sexualizing all of reality, pornography might appear to resemble poetry—at least some power analogous to metaphor appears to be always at work in it. This possibility brings us again to the question of the relation of pornography to literature. The subject is extremely complex, and I do not intend to deal with it systematically. I should like, however, to make a number of elementary distinctions.

Since it is written, printed, and read, and since it largely takes the form of fictional representations of human activities, pornography is of course, in a formal sense, literature. Furthermore, it is impossible to object theoretically to its purposes. There is, on the face of it, nothing illegitimate about a work whose purpose or intention is to arouse its readers sexually. If it is permissible for works of literature to move us to tears, to arouse our passions against injustice, to make us cringe with horror, and to purge us through pity and terror, then it is equally permissible—it lies within the orbit of literature's functions—for works of literature to excite us sexually. Two major works of literature may be adduced which undertake this project—part of the undertaking being, at least to my mind, a conscious intention on the author's part to move his readers sexually. *Madame Bovary* and the final section of *Ulysses* seem to me to have been written with such an intention. They also seem to me to have been successful in that intention. I will go one step further and assert that anyone who reads these works and is not sexually moved or aroused by Emma Bovary or Molly Bloom is not responding properly to literature, is not reading with the fullness and openness and attentiveness that literature demands.

Literature possesses, however, a multitude of intentions, but pornography possesses only one. This singleness of intention helps us to understand how it is that, in regard to pornography, the imponderable question of critical judgment has been solved. Given a work of literature whose unmistakable aim is to arouse its reader, and given a reader whose range of sexual responsiveness is not either altogether inhibited or aberrant, then a work of pornography is successful *per se* insofar as we are aroused by it. Keats's hope for literature in general has been ironically fulfilled: pornography proves itself upon our pulses, and elsewhere. Its success is physical, measurable, quantifiable; in it the common pursuit of true judgment comes to a dead halt. On this side, then, pornography falls into the same category as such simpler forms of literary utterance as propaganda and advertising. Its aim is to move us in the direction of action, and no doubt Plato, in *his* utopia, would have banned it along with poetry—which to his way of thinking exerted its influence in a similar way and toward similar ends. There remains an element of truth in this radical judgment.

Despite all this, we know as well that pornography is not literature. I have, at earlier and separate points in this work, tried to demonstrate how this negative circumstance operates, but it might be useful to bring several of these demonstrations together and quickly repeat and recapitulate them. First, there is the matter of form. Most works of literature have a beginning, a middle, and an end. Most works of pornography do not. A typical piece of pornographic fiction will usually have some kind of crude excuse for a beginning, but, having once begun, it goes on and on and ends nowhere. This impulse or compulsion to repeat, to repeat endlessly, is one of pornography's most striking qualities. A pornographic work of fiction characteristically develops by unremitting repetition and minute mechanical variation—the words that may describe this process are again, again, again, and more, more, more. We also observed that although pornography is obsessed with the idea of pleasure, of infinite pleasure, the idea of gratification, of an end to pleasure (pleasure being here an endless experience of retentiveness, without release) cannot develop. If form in art consists in the arousal in the reader of certain expectations and the fulfillment of those expectations, then in this context too pornography is resistant to form and opposed to art. For fulfillment implies completion, gratification, an end; and it is an end, a conclusion of any kind, that pornography most resists. The ideal pornographic novel, I should repeat, would go on forever; it would have no ending, just as in pornotopia there is ideally no such thing as time.

In terms of language, too, pornography stands in adverse relation to literature. Although a pornographic work of fiction is by necessity written, it might be more accurate to say that language for pornography is a prison from which it is continually trying to escape. At best, language is a bothersome necessity, for its function in pornography is to set going a series of non-verbal images, of fantasies, and if it could achieve this without the mediation of words it would. Such considerations help us to understand certain of the special qualities of pornographic prose. The prose of a typical pornographic novel consists almost entirely of clichés, dead and dying phrases, and stereotypical formulas; it is also heavily adjectival. These phrases and formulas are often interchangeable, and by and large they are interchangeable without any loss of meaning. They tend to function as non-specific abstractions, and can all be filled with the same general content. Nevertheless, to the extent that they become verbally non-referential, they too express the tendency of pornography to move ideally away from language. Inexorably trapped in words, pornography, like certain kinds of contemporary literature, tries desperately to go beneath and behind language; it vainly tries to reach what language cannot directly express but can only point toward, the primary processes of energy upon which our whole subsequent mental life is built. This effort explains in part why pornography is also the repository of the forbidden, tabooed words. The peculiar power of such words has to do with their primitiveness. They have undergone the least evolution, and retain much of their original force. In our minds, such words are minimally verbal; they present themselves to us as acts; they remain extremely close to those unconscious impulses in which they took their origin and that they continue to express. The language of pornography demonstrates to us that the meaning of this phenomenon is to be found somewhere beyond language—yet we have only language to show us where that is.

Even in its use of metaphor, pornography can be seen to differ from literature. Although the language of pornography is highly metaphoric, its metaphors regularly fail to achieve specific verbal value. Metaphor ordinarily fuses or identifies similar characteristics from disparate objects; its apparent aim, both in literature and in speech, is to increase our command over reality—and the objects in it—by magically exercising our command of the language through which reality is identified and mediated. In pornography, however, the intention of language, including metaphor, is unmetaphoric and literal; it seeks to *de-elaborate* the verbal structure and the distinctions upon which it is built, to move back through language to that part of our minds where all metaphors are literal truths, where everything is possible, and where we were all once supreme.

Taking their origins in the same matrix of impulses, pornography and literature tend regularly to move off in opposite directions.

The third way in which pornography is opposed to literature has also been mentioned. Literature is largely concerned with the relations of human beings among themselves; it represents how persons live with each other, and imagines their feelings and emotions as they change; it investigates their motives and demonstrates that these are often complex, obscure, and ambiguous. It proceeds by elaboration, the principal means of this elaboration being the imagination of situations of conflict between persons or within a single person. All of these interests are antagonistic to pornography. Pornography is not interested in persons but in organs. Emotions are an embarrassment to it, and motives are distractions. In pornotopia conflicts do not exist; and if by chance a conflict does occur it is instantly dispelled by the waving of a magic sexual wand. Sex in pornography is sex without the emotions—and this we need not discuss any further: D. H. Lawrence has already done the job.[1]

---

1. That pornography is almost entirely written by men and for men was demonstrated to me by a reading of one or two of the few works of pornographic fiction known definitely to be written by women. In these stories, there is no focus or concentration upon organs; much more attention is paid to the emotions, and there is a good deal of contemplation, conscious reverie, and self-observation.

I should like, at the close of this discussion, to remind the reader once again that pornotopia does not exist and is not anywhere to be found. It is an ideal type, an instrument to be used for comparison and analysis. None of the works that I have discussed—and none that I have ever read—is actually a pornotopia, though several approach that extreme limit. If the theoretical model which I have constructed is an adequate one, then the reader should be helped in making certain discriminations. It should be possible to apply the idea of pornotopia to concrete, existing works, and to determine in what ways and in how far such works are or are not pornographic. I do not at all mean that this device can be a substitute for critical judgment, but that it can act as an aid to judgment and as one more instrument of analysis.

A concrete illustration may prove useful. In the last few years, much has been written about *Fanny Hill*. Almost every article about this book that I have read seems to me to have been—with the best will in the world—mistaken and misguided. *Fanny Hill* is of course a pornographic novel; it contains, however (as does every other work of pornography), a number of non-pornographic elements, qualities, or attributes—it may even contain these to a more substantial degree than other or subsequent pornographic works of fiction. One does not, it must be emphasized, need a device like pornotopia to arrive at such a judgment; but the device may nevertheless be used in the analysis of that novel, in the effort of demonstrating just how it goes about achieving its pornographic purposes, how it may at certain points be deflected from such purposes, or how in fact other purposes may be included within its larger or overall design.

Finally, something should be said about the historical circumstances of pornography. Although the impulses and fantasies with which pornography deals are trans-historical, pornography itself is a historical phenomenon. It has its origins in the seventeenth century,[2] may be said to come into full meaningful existence in the latter part of the eighteenth, persists, develops, and flourishes throughout the nineteenth century, and continues on in our own. To ask what caused such a phenomenon to occur is to ask a stupendous question, since the causes of it seem to be inseparable from those vast social processes which brought about the modern world. A few matters may, however, be briefly referred to. The growth of pornography is inseparable from and dependent upon the growth of the novel. Those social forces which acted to contribute to the rise of the novel—and to the growth of its audience—acted analogously in contributing to the development of pornography. Like the novel, pornography is connected with the growth of cities—with an urban society—and with an audience of literate readers rather than listeners or spectators. These considerations are in turn involved with the development of new kinds of experience, in particular with the development of private experience—sociologists call the process "privatization." If the novel is both evidence of and a response to the needs created by the possibilities of increased privacy and private experience, then pornography is a mad parody of the same situation. No experience of reading is more private, more solitary in every possible way.

As an urban, capitalist, industrial, and middle-class world was being created, the sexual character of European society underwent significant modifications. The sexual character or roles attributed to both men and women changed; sexual manners and habits altered; indeed the whole style of sexual life was considerably modified. Among the principal tendencies in this process was a steadily increasing pressure to split sexuality off from the rest of life. By a variety of social means which correspond to the psychological processes of isolation, distancing, denial, and even repression, a separate and insulated sphere in which sexuality was to be confined was brought into existence. Yet even as sexuality was

2. My own researches and those of David Foxon, referred to in the Introduction, p. xv, above, agree in this conclusion. I regret that this is not the place to make a demonstration of these findings, but I refer the reader to Mr. Foxon's essays.

isolated, it continued to develop and change—that is to say, human consciousness of sexuality continued to change and to increase. Indeed that isolation was both the precondition of and the vehicle through which such a development occurred. The growth of pornography was one of the results of these processes—as, in another context, was the development of modern romantic love. Pornography and the history of pornography allow us to see how, on one of its sides, and under the special conditions of isolation and separation, sexuality came to be thought of in European society from the end of the seventeenth to the end of the nineteenth century.

Matters came to a head during the middle and latter decades of the nineteenth century. During that period, pornographic writings were produced and published in unprecedented volume—it became in fact a minor industry. The view of human sexuality as it was represented in the subculture of pornography and the view of sexuality held by the official culture were reversals, mirror images, negative analogues of one another. For every warning against masturbation issued by the official voice of culture, another work of pornography was published; for every cautionary statement against the harmful effects of sexual excess uttered by medical men, pornography represented copulation *in excelsis*, endless orgies, infinite daisy chains of inexhaustibility; for every assertion about the delicacy and frigidity of respectable women made by the official culture, pornography represented legions of maenads, universes of palpitating females; for every effort made by the official culture to minimize the importance of sexuality, pornography cried out—or whispered—that it was the only thing in the world of any importance at all. It is essential for us to notice the similarities even more than the differences between these two groups of attitudes or cultures. In both the same set of anxieties are at work; in both the same obsessive ideas can be made out; and in both sexuality is conceived of at precisely the same degree of consciousness. It was a situation of unbearable contradiction. And it was at this point that the breaking through began.

This breaking through was made in three areas. First and most important was the invention or discovery of modern psychology, most centrally of course in the work of Freud. For the first time in human history it became possible to discuss sexuality in a neutral way; for the first time a diction and a set of analytic concepts or instruments were established through which men could achieve sufficient intellectual distance from their own sexual beliefs and behavior so as to be able to begin to understand them. And it may even be added that for the first time human sexuality achieved a meaning, using the word "meaning" in the sense put to it by philosophy and the social sciences. The work of retrieving human sexuality had begun, but what would be retrieved was in the nature of the case a different thing than what had earlier been set apart.

The second breaking through took place at about the same time. In the work of the great late nineteenth-century and early twentieth-century avant-garde artists, and in particular among the novelists, the entire fabric of modern society came in for attack. The focus of their assault was the sexual life of the bourgeois or middle classes, as those classes and the style of life they conducted had come to be the prevailing social powers. The difficulties, agonies, contradictions, double-dealings, hypocrisies, inequities, guilts, and confusions of the sexual life of the middle classes were for these novelists not only bad in themselves; they were symbolic of general circumstances of injustice, unpleasantness, demoralization, and malaise which for these artists characterized the world they inhabited. They endorsed a freer sexual life as a good in itself; and they depicted the sexual anguish of modern persons and the sexual hypocrisies and contradictions of modern society not merely for the sake of exposure and sensationalism (although there was that too), but in order to outrage and awaken the society which had imposed upon itself such hideous conditions of servitude. Society being what it is, they were often punished for their efforts, but the work of awakening had been furthered, the work of bringing back into the central discourse of civilization that sexual life upon which it is built and through which it is perpetuated.

The third breaking through followed upon the other two, and is still happening. I refer to the general liberalization of sexual life and of social attitudes toward sexuality that is taking place in our time. It seems likely that what we are witnessing today will be as important, momentous, and enduring as that other revolution in sensibility, manners, and attitudes which occurred in England during the latter part of the eighteenth and first part of the nineteenth century. One of the more interesting recent developments in this social drama is that pornography itself is now being openly and legally published. We need not inquire into the motives of those who publish and republish such works—and I feel constrained to add that I would indeed be troubled if I came across my small son studiously conning *Justine*. Nevertheless, this development was inevitable and necessary, and on the whole, so far as we are able to see, benign. It suggests to me, moreover, that we are coming to the end of an era. We are coming to the end of the era in which pornography had a historical meaning and even a historical function. The free publication of all the old pornographic chestnuts does not necessarily indicate to me moral laxness, or fatigue, or deterioration on the part of society. It suggests rather that pornography has lost its old danger, its old power—negative social sanctions and outlawry being always the most reliable indicators of how much a society is frightened of anything, how deeply it fears its power, how subversive to its settled order it conceives an idea, or work, or act to be. (What will happen to sexuality itself if this goes on long enough is a matter upon which I hesitate to speculate.) As I have said, the impulses and fantasies of pornography are trans-historical—they will always be with us, they will always exist. Pornography is, after all, nothing more than a representation of the fantasies of infantile sexual life, as these fantasies are edited and reorganized in the masturbatory day dreams of adolescence. Every man who grows up must pass through such a phase in his existence, and I can see no reason for supposing that our society, in the history of its own should not have to pass through such a phase as well.

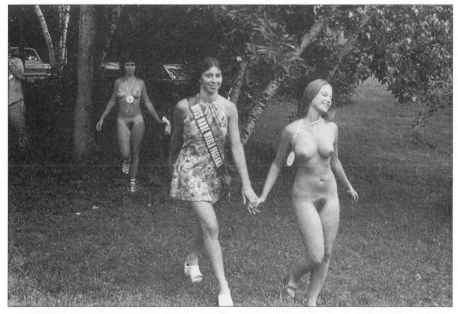

© Fred W. McDarrah

The Pornographic Imagination

Susan Sontag

from *Styles of Radical Will,* 1967

Well known essayist, novelist, and filmmaker, Susan Sontag has written on topics such as literature, critical theory, AIDS, photography and politics. This excerpt from her essay on "The Pornographic Imagination" discusses three different aspects of pornography: the social historical, the psychological and, the focus of her essay, the literary.

No one should undertake a discussion of pornography before acknowledging the pornograph*ies*—there are at least three— and before pledging to take them on one at a time. There is a considerable gain in truth if pornography as an item in social history is treated quite separately from pornography as a psychological phenomenon (according to the usual view, symptomatic of sexual deficiency or deformity in both the producers and the consumers), and if one further distinguishes from both of these another pornography: a minor but interesting modality or convention within the arts.

It's the last of the three pornographies that I want to focus upon. More narrowly, upon the literary genre for which, lacking a better name, I'm willing to accept (in the privacy of serious intellectual debate, not in the courts) the dubious label of pornography. By literary genre I mean a body of work belonging to literature considered as an art, and to which inherent standards of artistic excellence pertain. From the standpoint of social and psychological phenomena, all porno-graphic texts have the same status; they are documents. But from the standpoint of art, some of these texts may well become something else. Not only do Pierre Louys' *Trois Filles de leur Mère*, Georges Bataille's *Histoire de l'Oeil* and *Madame Edwarda*, the pseudonymous *Story of O* and *The Image* belong to literature, but it can be made clear why these books, all five of them, occupy a much higher rank as literature than *Candy* or Oscar Wilde's *Teleny* or the Earl of Rochester's *Sodom* or Apol-linaire's *The Debauched Hospodar* or Cleland's *Fanny Hill*. The avalanche of pornographic potboilers marketed for two centuries under and now, increasingly, over the counter no more impugns the status as literature of the first group of pornographic books than the proliferation of books of the caliber of *The Carpetbaggers* and *Valley of the Dolls* throws into question the credentials of *Anna Karenina* and *The Great Gatsby* and *The Man Who Loved Children*. The ratio of authentic literature to trash in pornography may be somewhat lower than the ratio of novels of genuine literary merit to the entire volume of sub-literary fiction produced for mass taste. But it is probably no lower than, for instance, that of another somewhat shady sub-genre with a few first-rate books to its credit, science fiction. (As literary forms, pornography and sci-ence fiction resemble each other in several interesting ways.) Anyway, the quantitative measure supplies a trivial standard. Relatively uncommon as they may be, there are writings which it seems reason-able to call pornographic—assuming that the stale label has any use at all—which, at the same time, cannot be refused accreditation as serious literature.

The point would seem to be obvious. Yet, apparently, that's far from being the case. At least in England and America, the reasoned scrutiny and assessment of pornography is held firmly within the limits of the discourse employed by psychologists, sociologists, historians, jurists, professional moralists, and social critics. Pornography is a malady to be diagnosed and an occasion for judgment. It's something one is for or against. And taking sides about pornography is hardly like being for or against aleatoric music or Pop Art, but quite a bit like being for or against legalized abortion or federal aid to parochial schools. In fact, the same fundamental approach to the subject is shared by recent eloquent defenders of society's right and obligation to censor dirty books, like

George P. Elliott and George Steiner, and those like Paul Goodman, who foresee pernicious consequences of a policy of censorship far worse than any harm done by the books themselves. Both the libertarians and the would-be censors agree in reducing pornography to pathological symptom and problematic social commodity. A near unanimous consensus exists as to what pornography is—this being identified with notions about the *sources* of the impulse to produce and consume these curious goods. When viewed as a theme for psychological analysis, pornography is rarely seen as anything more interesting than texts which illustrate a deplorable arrest in normal adult sexual development. In this view, all pornography amounts to is the representation of the fantasies of infantile sexual life, these fantasies having been edited by the more skilled, less innocent consciousness of the masturbatory adolescent, for purchase by so-called adults. As a social phenomenon—for instance, the boom in the production of pornography in the societies of Western Europe and America since the eighteenth century—the approach is no less unequivocally clinical. Pornography becomes a group pathology, the disease of a whole culture, about whose cause everyone is pretty well agreed. The mounting output of dirty books is attributed to a festering legacy of Christian sexual repression and to sheer physiological ignorance, these ancient disabilities being now compounded by more proximate historical events, the impact of drastic dislocations in traditional modes of family and political order and unsettling change in the roles of the sexes. (The problem of pornography is one of "the dilemmas of a society in transition," Goodman said in an essay several years ago.) Thus, there is a fairly complete consensus about the *diagnosis* of pornography itself. The disagreements arise only in the estimate of the psychological and social *consequences* of its dissemination, and therefore in the formulating of tactics and policy.

The more enlightened architects of moral policy are undoubtedly prepared to admit that there is something like a "pornographic imagination," although only in the sense that pornographic works are tokens of a radical failure or deformation of the imagination. And they may grant, as Goodman, Wayland Young, and others have suggested, that there also exists a "pornographic society": that, indeed, ours is a flourishing example of one, a society so hypocritically and repressively constructed that it must inevitably produce an effusion of pornography as both its logical expression and its subversive, demotic antidote. But nowhere in the Anglo-American community of letters have I seen it argued that some pornographic books are interesting and important works of art. So long as pornography is treated as only a social and psychological phenomenon and a locus for moral concern, how could such an argument ever be made?

2.

There's another reason, apart from this categorizing of pornography as a topic of analysis, why the question whether or not works of pornography can be literature has never been genuinely debated. I mean the view of literature itself maintained by most English and American critics—a view which in excluding pornographic writings *by definition* from the precincts of literature excludes much else besides.

Of course, no one denies that pornography constitutes a branch of literature in the sense that it appears in the form of printed books of fiction. But beyond that trivial connection, no more is allowed. The fashion in which most critics construe the nature of prose literature, no less than their view of the nature of pornography, inevitably puts pornography in an adverse relation to literature. It is an airtight case, for if a pornographic book is defined as one not belonging to literature (and vice versa), there is no need to examine individual books.

Most mutually exclusive definitions of pornography and literature rest on four separate arguments. One is that the utterly singleminded way in which works of pornography address the reader, proposing to arouse him sexually, is antithetical to the complex function of literature. It may then be argued that pornography's aim, inducing sexual excitement, is at odds with the tranquil, detached involvement evoked by genuine art. But this turn of the argument seems particularly unconvincing, considering the respected appeal to the reader's moral feelings intended by "realistic" writing, not to mention the fact that some certified masterpieces (from Chaucer to Lawrence) contain passages that do properly excite readers sexually. It is more plausible just to emphasize that pornography still possesses only one "intention," while any genuinely valuable work of literature has many.

Another argument, made by Adorno among others, is that works of pornography lack the beginning-middle-and-end form characteristic of literature. A piece of pornographic fiction concocts no better than a crude excuse for a beginning; and once having begun, it goes on and on and ends nowhere.

Another argument: pornographic writing can't evidence any care for its means of expression as such (the concern of literature), since the aim of pornography is to inspire a set of nonverbal fantasies in which language plays a debased, merely instrumental role.

Last and most weighty is the argument that the subject of literature is the relation of human beings to each other, their complex feelings and emotions; pornography, in contrast, disdains fully formed persons (psychology and social portraiture), is oblivious to the question of motives and their credibility and reports only the motiveless tireless transactions of depersonalized organs.

Simply extrapolating from the conception of literature maintained by most English and American critics today, it would follow that the literary value of pornography has to be nil. But these paradigms don't stand up to close analysis in themselves, nor do they even fit their subject. Take, for instance, *Story of O*. Though the novel is clearly obscene by the usual standards, and more effective than many in arousing a reader sexually, sexual arousal doesn't appear to be the sole function of the situations portrayed. The narrative does have a definite beginning, middle, and end. The elegance of the writing hardly gives the impression that its author considered language a bothersome necessity. Further, the characters do possess emotions of a very intense kind, although obsessional and indeed wholly asocial ones; characters do have motives, though they are not psychiatrically or socially "normal" motives. The characters in *Story of O* are endowed with a "psychology" of a sort, one derived from the psychology of lust. And while what can be learned of the characters within the situations in which they are placed is severely restricted—to modes of sexual concentration and explicitly rendered sexual behavior—O and her partners are no more reduced or foreshortened than the characters in many nonpornographic works of contemporary fiction.

Only when English and American critics evolve a more sophisticated view of literature will an interesting debate get underway. (In the end, this debate would be not only about pornography but about the whole body of contemporary literature insistently focused on extreme situations and behavior.) The difficulty arises because so many critics continue to identify with prose literature itself the particular literary conventions of "realism" (what might be crudely associated with the major tradition of the nineteenth-century novel). For examples of alternative literary modes, one is not confined only to much of the greatest twentieth-century writing—to *Ulysses,* a book not about characters but about media of transpersonal exchange, about all that lies outside individual psychology and personal need; to French Surrealism and its most recent offspring, the New Novel; to German "expressionist" fiction; to the Russian post-novel represented by Biely's *St. Petersburg* and by Nabokov; or to the nonlinear, tenseless narratives of Stein and Burroughs. A definition of literature that faults a work for being rooted in "fantasy" rather than in the realistic rendering of how lifelike persons in familiar situations live with each other couldn't even handle such venerable conventions as the pastoral, which depicts relations between people that are certainly reductive, vapid, and unconvincing.

An uprooting of some of these tenacious clichés is long overdue: it will promote a sounder reading of the literature of the past as well as put critics and ordinary readers better in touch with contemporary literature, which includes zones of writing that structurally resemble pornography. It is facile, virtually meaningless, to demand that literature stick with the "human." For the matter at stake is not "human" versus "inhuman" (in which choosing the "human" guarantees instant moral self-congratulation for both author and reader) but an infinitely varied register of forms and tonalities for transposing *the human voice* into prose narrative. For the critic, the proper question is not the relationship between the book and "the world" or "reality" (in which each novel is judged as if it were a unique item, and in which the world is regarded as a far less complex place than it is) but the complexities of consciousness itself, as the medium through which a world exists at all and is constituted, and an approach to single books of fiction which doesn't slight the fact that they exist in dialogue with each other. From this point of view, the decision of the old novelists to depict the unfolding of the destinies of sharply individualized "characters" in familiar, socially dense situations within the conventional notation of chronological sequence is only one of many possible decisions, possessing no inherently superior claim to the allegiance of serious readers. There is nothing innately more "human" about these procedures. The presence of realistic characters is not, in itself, something wholesome, a more nourishing staple for the moral sensibility.

The only sure truth about characters in prose fiction is that they are, in Henry James' phrase, "a compositional resource." The presence of human figures in literary art can serve many purposes. Dramatic tension or three-dimensionality in the rendering of personal and social relations is often *not* a writer's aim, in which case it doesn't help to insist on that as a generic standard. Exploring ideas is as authentic an aim of prose fiction, although by the standards of novelistic realism this aim severely limits the presentation of lifelike persons. The constructing or imaging of something inanimate, or of a portion of the world of nature, is also a valid enterprise, and entails an appropriate rescaling of the human figure. (The form of the pastoral involves both these aims: the depiction of ideas and of nature. Persons are used only to the extent that they constitute a certain kind of landscape, which is partly a stylization of "real" nature and partly a neo-Platonic landscape of ideas.) And equally valid as a subject for prose narrative are the extreme states of human feeling and consciousness, those so peremptory that they exclude the mundane flux of feelings and are only contingently linked with concrete persons—which is the case with pornography.

One would never guess from the confident pronouncements on the nature of literature by most American and English critics that a vivid debate on this issue had been proceeding for several generations. "It seems to me," Jacques Rivière wrote in the *Nouvelle Revue Française* in 1924, "that we are witnessing a very serious crisis in the concept of what literature is." One of several responses to "the problem of the possibility and the limits of literature," Rivière noted, is the marked tendency for "art (if even the word can still be kept) to become a completely nonhuman activity, a supersensory function, if I may use that term, a sort of creative astronomy." I cite Rivière not because his essay, "Questioning the Concept of Literature," is particularly original or definitive or subtly argued, but simply to recall an ensemble of radical notions about literature which were almost critical commonplaces forty years ago in European literary magazines.

To this day, though, that ferment remains alien, unassimilated, and persistently misunderstood in the English and American world of letters: suspected as issuing from a collective cultural failure of nerve, frequently dismissed as outright perversity or obscurantism or creative sterility. The better English-speaking critics, however, could hardly fail to notice how much great twentieth-century literature subverts those ideas received from certain of the great nineteenth-century novelists on the nature of literature which they continue to echo in 1967. But the critics' awareness of genuinely new literature was usually tendered in a spirit much like that of the rabbis a century before the beginning of the Christian era who, humbly acknowledging the spiritual inferiority of their own age to the age of the great prophets, nevertheless firmly closed the canon of prophetic books and declared—with more relief, one suspects, than regret—the era of prophecy ended. So has the age of what in Anglo-American criticism is still called, astonishingly enough, "experimental" or "avant-garde" writing been repeatedly declared closed. The ritual celebration of each contemporary genius's undermining of the older notions of literature was often accompanied by the nervous insistence that the writing brought forth was, alas, the last of its noble, sterile line. Now, the results of this intricate, one-eyed way of looking at modern literature have been several decades of unparalleled interest and brilliance in English and American—particularly American—criticism. But it is an interest and brilliance reared on bankruptcy of taste and something approaching a fundamental dishonesty of method. The critics' retrograde awareness of the impressive new claims staked out by modern literature, linked with their chagrin over what was usually designated as "the rejection of reality" and "the failure of the self" endemic in that literature, indicates the precise point at which most talented Anglo-American literary criticism leaves off considering structures of literature and transposes itself into criticism of culture.

I don't wish to repeat here the arguments that I have advanced elsewhere on behalf of a different critical approach. Still, some allusion to that approach needs to be made. To discuss even a single work of the radical nature of *Histoire de l'Oeil* raises the question of literature itself, of prose narrative considered as an art form. And books like those of Bataille could not have been written except for that agonized reappraisal of the nature of literature which has been preoccupying literary Europe for more than half a century; but lacking that context, they must prove almost unassimilable for English and American readers—except as "mere" pornography, inexplicably fancy trash. If it is even necessary to take up the issue of whether or not pornography and literature are antithetical, if it is at all necessary to assert that works of pornography *can* belong to literature, then the assertion must imply an overall view of what art is.

To put it very generally: art (and art-making) is a form of consciousness; the materials of art are the variety of forms of consciousness. By no *aesthetic* principle can this notion of the materials of art be construed as excluding even the extreme forms of consciousness that transcend social personality or psychological individuality.

In daily life, to be sure, we may acknowledge a moral obligation to inhibit such states of consciousness in ourselves. The obligation seems pragmatically sound, not only to maintain social order in the widest sense but to allow the individual to establish and maintain a humane contact with other persons (though that contact can be renounced, for shorter or longer periods). It's well known that when people venture into the far reaches of consciousness, they do so at the peril of their sanity, that is, of their humanity. But the "human scale" or humanistic standard proper to ordinary life and conduct seems misplaced when applied to art. It oversimplifies. If within the last century art conceived as an autonomous activity has come to be invested with an unprecedented stature— the nearest thing to a sacramental human activity acknowledged by secular society—it is because one of the tasks art has assumed is making forays into and taking up positions on the frontiers of consciousness (often very dangerous to the artist as a person) and reporting back what's there. Being a freelance explorer of spiritual dangers, the artist gains a certain license to behave differently from other people; matching the singularity of his vocation, he may be decked out with a suitably eccentric life style, or he may not. His job is inventing trophies of his experiences—objects and gestures that fascinate and enthrall, not merely (as prescribed by older notions of the artist) edify or entertain. His principal means of fascinating is to advance one step further in the dialectic of outrage. He seeks to make his work repulsive, obscure, inaccessible; in short, to give what is, or seems to be, *not* wanted. But however fierce may be the outrages the artist perpetrates upon his audience, his credentials and spiritual authority ultimately depend on the audience's sense (whether something known or inferred) of the outrages he commits upon himself. The exemplary modern artist is a broker in madness.

The notion of art as the dearly purchased outcome of an immense spiritual risk, one whose cost goes up with the entry and participation of each new player in the game, invites a revised set of critical standards. Art produced under the aegis of this conception certainly is not, cannot be, "realistic." But words like "fantasy" or "surrealism," that only invert the guidelines of realism, clarify little. Fantasy too easily declines into "mere" fantasy; the clincher is the adjective "infantile." Where does fantasy, condemned by psychiatric rather than artistic standards, end and imagination begin?

Since it's hardly likely that contemporary critics seriously mean to bar prose narratives that are unrealistic from the domain of literature, one suspects that a special standard is being applied to sexual themes. This becomes clearer if one thinks of another kind of book, another kind of "fantasy." The ahistorical dreamlike landscape where action is situated, the peculiarly congealed time in which acts are performed—these occur almost as often in science fiction as they do in pornography. There is nothing conclusive in the well-known fact that most men and women fall short of the sexual prowess that people in pornography are represented as enjoying; that the size of organs, number and duration of orgasms, variety and feasibility of sexual powers, and amount of sexual energy all seem grossly exaggerated. Yes, and the spaceships and the teeming planets depicted in science-fiction novels don't exist either. The fact that the site of narrative is an ideal *topos* disqualifies neither pornography nor science fiction from being literature. Such negations of real, concrete, three-dimensional social time, space, and personality—and such "fantastic" enlargements of human energy—are rather the ingredients of another kind of literature, founded on another mode of consciousness.

The materials of the pornographic books that count as literature are, precisely, one of the extreme forms of human consciousness. Undoubtedly, many people would agree that the sexually obsessed consciousness can, in principle, enter into literature as an art form. Literature about lust? Why not? But then they usually add a rider to the agreement which effectually nullifies it. They require that the author have the proper "distance" from his obsessions for their rendering to count as literature. Such a standard is sheer hypocrisy, revealing once again that the values commonly applied to pornography are, in the end, those belonging to psychiatry and social affairs rather than to art. (Since Christianity upped the ante and concentrated on sexual behavior as the root of virtue, everything pertaining to sex has been a "special case" in our culture, evoking peculiarly inconsistent attitudes.) Van Gogh's paintings retain their status as art even if it seems his manner of painting owed less to a conscious choice of representational means than to his being deranged and actually seeing reality the way he painted it. Similarly, *Histoire de l'Oeil* does not become case history rather than art because, as Bataille reveals in the extraordinary autobiographical essay appended to the narrative, the book's obsessions are indeed his own.

What makes a work of pornography part of the history of art rather than of trash is not distance, the superimposition of a consciousness more conformable to that of ordinary reality upon the "deranged consciousness" of the erotically obsessed. Rather, it is the originality, thoroughness, authenticity, and power of that deranged consciousness itself, as incarnated in a work. From the point of view of art, the exclusivity of the consciousness embodied in pornographic books is in itself neither anomalous nor anti-literary.

Nor is the purported aim or effect, whether it is intentional or not, of such books—to excite the reader sexually—a defect. Only a degraded and mechanistic idea of sex could mislead someone into thinking that being sexually stirred by a book like *Madame Edwarda* is a simple matter. The singleness of intention often condemned by critics is, when the work merits treatment as art, compounded of many resonances. The physical sensations involuntarily produced in someone reading the book carry with them something that touches upon the reader's whole experience of his humanity—and his limits as a personality and as a body. Actually, the singleness of pornography's intention is spurious. But the aggressiveness of the intention is not. What seems like an end is as much a means, startlingly and oppressively concrete. The end, however, is less concrete. Pornography is one of the branches of literature—science fiction is another—aiming at disorientation, at psychic dislocation.

In some respects, the use of sexual obsessions as a subject for literature resembles the use of a literary subject whose validity far fewer people would contest: religious obsessions. So compared, the familiar fact of pornography's definite, aggressive impact upon its readers looks somewhat different. Its celebrated intention of sexually stimulating readers is really a species of proselytizing. Pornography that is serious literature aims to "excite" in the same way that books which render an extreme form of religious experience aim to "convert."

● ● ●

5.

The prominent characteristics of all products of the pornographic imagination are their energy and their absolutism.

The books generally called pornographic are those whose primary, exclusive, and overriding preoccupation is with the depiction of sexual "intentions" and "activities." One could also say sexual "feelings," except that the word seems redundant. The feelings of the personages deployed by the pornographic imagination are, at any given moment, either identical with their "behavior" or else a preparatory phase, that of "intention," on the verge of breaking into "behavior" unless physically thwarted. Pornography uses a small crude vocabulary of feeling, all relating to the prospects of action: feeling one would like to act (lust); feeling one would not like to act (shame, fear, aversion). There are no gratuitous or non-functioning feelings; no musings, whether speculative or imagistic, which are irrelevant to the business at hand. Thus, the pornographic imagination inhabits a universe that is, however repetitive the incidents occurring within it, incomparably economical. The strictest possible criterion of relevance applies: everything must bear upon the erotic situation.

The universe proposed by the pornographic imagination is a total universe. It has the power to ingest and metamorphose and translate all concerns that are fed into it, reducing everything into the one negotiable currency of the erotic imperative. All action is conceived of as a set of sexual *exchanges*. Thus, the reason why pornography refuses to make fixed distinctions between the sexes or allow any kind of sexual preference or sexual taboo to endure can be explained "structurally." The bisexuality, the disregard for the incest taboo, and other similar features common to pornographic narratives function to multiply the possibilities of exchange. Ideally, it should be possible for everyone to have a sexual connection with everyone else.

Of course the pornographic imagination is hardly the only form of consciousness that proposes a total universe. Another is the type of imagination that has generated modern symbolic logic. In the total universe proposed by the logician's imagination, all statements can be broken down or chewed up to make it possible to rerender them in the form of the logical language; those parts of ordinary language that don't fit are simply lopped off. Certain of the well-known states of the religious imagination, to take another example, operate in the same cannibalistic way, engorging all materials made available to them for retranslation into phenomena saturated with the religious polarities (sacred and profane, etc.).

• • •

But the pornographic imagination is not just to be understood as a form of psychic absolutism—some of whose products we might be able to regard (in the role of connoisseur, rather than client) with more sympathy or intellectual curiosity or aesthetic sophistication.

Several times before in this essay I have alluded to the possibility that the pornographic imagination says something worth listening to, albeit in a degraded and often unrecognizable form. I've urged that this spectacularly cramped form of the human imagination has, nevertheless, its peculiar access to some truth. This truth—about sensibility, about sex, about individual personality, about despair, about limits—can be shared when it projects itself into art. (Everyone, at least in dreams, has inhabited the world of the pornographic imagination for some hours or days or even longer periods of his life; but only the full-time residents make the fetishes, the trophies, the art.) That discourse one might call the poetry of transgression is also knowledge. He who transgresses not only breaks a rule. He goes somewhere that the others are not; and he knows something the others don't know.

• • •

Pornography, considered as an artistic or art-producing form of the human imagination, is an expression of what William James called "morbid-mindedness." But James was surely right when he gave as part of the definition of morbid-mindedness that it ranged over "a wider scale of experience" than healthy-mindedness.

What can be said, though, to the many sensible and sensitive people who find depressing the fact that a whole library of pornographic reading material has been made, within the last few years, so easily available in paperback form to the very young? Probably one thing: that their apprehension is justified, but may not be in scale. I am not addressing the usual complainers, those who feel that since sex after all is dirty, so are books reveling in sex (dirty in a way that a genocide screened nightly on TV, apparently, is not). There still remains a sizeable minority of people who object to or are repelled by pornography not because they think it's dirty but because they know that pornography can be a crutch for the psychologically deformed and a brutalization of the morally innocent. I feel an aversion to pornography for those reasons, too, and am uncomfortable about the consequences of its increasing availability. But isn't the worry somewhat misplaced? What's really at stake? A concern about the uses of knowledge itself. There's a sense in which *all* knowledge is dangerous, the reason being that not everyone is in the same condition as knowers or potential knowers. Perhaps most people don't need "a wider scale of experience." It may be that, without subtle and extensive psychic preparation, any widening of experience and consciousness is destructive for most people. Then we must ask what justifies the reckless unlimited confidence we have in the present mass availability of other kinds of knowledge, in our optimistic acquiescence in the transformation of and extension of human capacities by machines. Pornography is only one item among the many dangerous commodities being circulated in this society and, unattractive as it may be, one of the less lethal, the less costly to the community in terms of human suffering. Except perhaps in a small circle of writer-intellectuals in France, pornography is an inglorious and mostly despised department of the imagination. Its mean status is the very antithesis of the considerable spiritual prestige enjoyed by many items which are far more noxious.

In the last analysis, the place we assign to pornography depends on the goals we set for our own consciousness, our own experience. But the goal A espouses for his consciousness may *not* be one he's pleased to see B adopt, because he judges that B isn't qualified or experienced or subtle enough. And B may be dismayed and even indignant at A's adopting goals that he himself professes; when A holds them, they become presumptuous or shallow. Probably this chronic mutual suspicion of our neighbor's capacities—suggesting, in effect, a hierarchy of competence with respect to human consciousness—will never be settled to everyone's satisfaction. As long as the quality of people's consciousness varies so greatly, how could it be?

In an essay on the subject some years ago, Paul Goodman wrote: "The question is not *whether* pornography, but the quality of the pornography." That's exactly right. One could extend the thought a good deal further. The question is not *whether* consciousness or *whether* knowledge, but the quality of the consciousness and of the knowledge. And that invites consideration of the quality or fineness of the human subject—the most problematic standard of all. It doesn't seem inaccurate to say most people in this society who aren't actively mad are, at best, reformed or potential lunatics. But is anyone supposed to act on this knowledge, even genuinely live with it? If so many are teetering on the verge of murder, de-humanization, sexual deformity and despair, and we were to act on that thought, then censorship much more radical than the indignant foes of pornography ever envisage seems in order. For if that's the case, not only pornography but all forms of serious art and knowledge—in other words, all forms of truth—are suspect and dangerous.

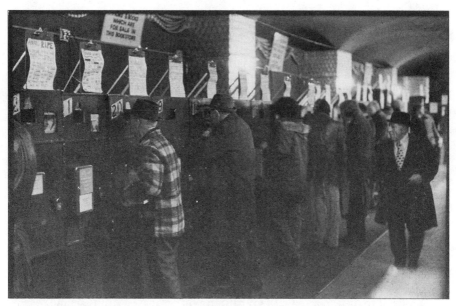

© Fred W. McDarrah

Pornography in the Service of Women

Angela Carter

from *The Sadeian Woman and the Ideology of Pornography*, 1978

*Born in London, the daughter of socialist parents, Angela Carter was active in radical political movements throughout her life. She was a brilliant writer of short stories (**The Bloody Chamber**) and novels (**Nights at the Circus**). **The Sadean Woman** is one of the most audacious essays ever written on pornography. It offers a feminist interpretation of the Marquis de Sade in which Carter explores the relationship between power and sexuality. She manages to transform the extreme vision of de Sade into meditations on celebrity sex goddesses, mothers and daughters, and sex and marriage.*

Pornographers are the enemies of women only because our contemporary ideology of pornography does not encompass the possibility of change, as if we were the slaves of history and not its makers, as if sexual relations were not necessarily an expression of social relations, as if sex itself were an external fact, one as immutable as the weather, creating human practice but never a part of it.

Pornography involves an abstraction of human intercourse in which the self is reduced to its formal elements. In its most basic form, these elements are represented by the probe and the fringed hole, the twin signs of male and female in graffiti, the biological symbols scrawled on the subway poster and the urinal wall, the simplest expression of stark and ineradicable sexual differentiation, a universal pictorial language of lust—or, rather, a language we accept as universal because, since it has always been so, we conclude that it must always remain so.

In the stylisation of graffiti, the prick is always presented erect, in an alert attitude of enquiry or curiosity or affirmation; it points upwards, it asserts. The hole is open, an inert space, like a mouth waiting to be filled. From this elementary iconography may be derived the whole metaphysic of sexual differences—man aspires; woman has no other function but to exist, waiting. The male is positive, an exclamation mark. Woman is negative. Between her legs lies nothing but zero, the sign for nothing, that only becomes something when the male principle fills it with meaning.

Anatomy is destiny, said Freud, which is true enough as far as it goes, but ambiguous. My anatomy is only part of an infinitely complex organisation, my self. The anatomical reductionalism of graffiti, the *reductio ad absurdum* of the bodily differences between men and women, extracts all the evidence of me from myself and leaves behind only a single aspect of my life as a mammal. It enlarges this aspect, simplifies it and then presents it as the most significant aspect of my entire humanity. This is true of all mythologising of sexuality; but graffiti lets it be *seen* to be true. It is the most explicit version of the idea of different sexual essences of men and women, because it is the crudest. In the face of this symbolism, my pretensions to any kind of social existence go for nothing; graffiti directs me back to my mythic generation as a woman and, as a woman, my symbolic value is primarily that of a myth of patience and receptivity, a dumb mouth from which the teeth have been pulled.

Sometimes, especially under the influence of Jung, a more archaic mouth is allowed to exert an atavistic dominance. Then, if I am lucky enough to be taken with such poetic pseudo-seriousness, my nether mouth may be acknowledged as one capable of speech—were there not, of old, divinatory priestesses, female oracles and so forth? Was there not Cassandra, who always spoke the truth, although admittedly in such a way that nobody ever believed her? And that, in mythic terms, is the hell of it. Since that female, oracular mouth is located so near the beastly backside, my vagina might indeed be patronisingly regarded as a speaking mouth, but never one that issues the voice of reason. In this most insulting mythic redefinition of myself, that of occult priestess, I am indeed allowed to speak but only of things that male society does not take seriously. I can hint at dreams, I can even personify the imagination; but that is only because I am not rational enough to cope with reality.

If women allow themselves to be consoled for their culturally determined lack of access to the modes of intellectual debate by the invocation of hypothetical great goddesses, they are simply flattering
themselves into submission (a technique often used on them by men).
All the mythic versions of women, from the myth of the redeeming
purity of the virgin to that of the healing, reconciling mother, are consolatory nonsenses; and consolatory nonsense seems to me a fair definition of myth, anyway. Mother goddesses are just as silly a notion as
father gods. If a revival of the myths of these cults gives women emotional satisfaction, it does so at the price of obscuring the real conditions of life. This is why they were invented in the first place.

Myth deals in false universals, to dull the pain of particular circumstances. In no area is this more true than in that of relations between
the sexes. Graffiti, the most public form of sexual iconography, one
which requires no training or artistic skill in its execution and yet is
always assured of an audience, obtains all its effects from these false
universals of myth. Its savage denial of the complexity of human relations is also a consolatory nonsense.

In its schema, as in the mythic schema of all relations between men
and women, man proposes and woman is disposed of, just as she is
disposed of in a rape, which is a kind of physical graffiti, the most
extreme reduction of love, in which all humanity departs from the
sexed beings. So that, somewhere in the fear of rape, is a more than
merely physical terror of hurt and humiliation—a fear of psychic disintegration, of an essential dismemberment, a fear of a loss or disrup-
tion of the self which is not confined to the victim alone. Since all
pornography derives directly from myth, it follows that its heroes and
heroines, from the most gross to the most sophisticated, are mythic
abstractions, heroes and heroines of dimension and capacity. Any
glimpse of a real man or a real woman is absent from these representations of the archetypal male and female.

The nature of the individual is not resolved into but is ignored by
these archetypes, since the function of the archetype is to diminish the
unique 'I' in favour of a collective, sexed being which cannot, by reason
of its very nature, exist as such because an archetype is only an image
that has got too big for its boots and bears, at best, a fantasy relation to
reality.

All archetypes are spurious but some are more spurious than others. There is the unarguable fact of sexual differentiation; but, separate from it and only partially derived from it, are the behavioural modes of masculine and feminine, which are culturally defined variables translated in the language of common usage to the status of universals. And these archetypes serve only to confuse the main issue, that relationships between the sexes are determined by history and by the historical fact of the economic dependence of women upon men. This fact is now very largely a fact of the past and, even in the past, was only true for certain social groups and then only at certain periods. Today, most women work before, during and after marriage. Nevertheless, the economic dependence of women remains a believed fiction and is assumed to imply an emotional dependence that is taken for granted as a condition inherent in the natural order of things and so used to console working women for their low wages. They work; see little profit from it; and therefore conclude they cannot really have been working at all.

This confusion as to the experience of reality—that what I know from my experience is true is, in fact, not so—is most apparent, however, in the fantasy love-play of the archetypes, which generations of artists have contrived to make seem so attractive that, lulled by dreams, many women willingly ignore the palpable evidence of their own responses.

In these beautiful encounters, any man may encounter any woman and their personalities are far less important to their copulation than the mere fact of their genders. At the first touch or sigh he, she, is subsumed immediately into a universal. (She, of course, rarely approaches him; that is not part of the fantasy of fulfillment.) She is most immediately and dramatically a woman when she lies beneath a man, and her submission is the apex of his malehood. To show his humility before his own erection, a man must approach a woman on his knees, just as he approaches god. This is the kind of beautiful thought that has bedevilled the history of sex in Judaeo-Christian culture, causing almost as much confusion as the idea that sex is a sin. Some of the scorn heaped on homosexuals may derive from the fact that they do not customarily adopt the mythically correct, sacerdotal position. The same beautiful thought has elevated a Western European convention to the position of the only sanctified sexual position; it fortifies the missionary position with a bizarre degree of mystification. God is invoked as a kind of sexual referee, to assure us, as modern churchmen like to claim in the teeth of two thousand years of Christian sexual repression, that sex is really sacred.

The missionary position has another great asset, from the mythic point of view; it implies a system of relations between the partners that equates the woman to the passive receptivity of the soil, to the richness and fecundity of the earth. A whole range of images poeticises, kitschifies, departicularises intercourse, such as wind beating down corn, rain driving against bending trees, towers falling, all tributes to the freedom and strength of the roving, fecundating, irresistible male principle and the heavy, downward, equally irresistible gravity of the receptive soil. The soil that is, good heavens, myself. It is a most self-enhancing notion; I have almost seduced myself with it. Any woman may manage, in luxurious self-deceit, to feel herself for a little while one with great, creating nature, fertile, open, pulsing, anonymous and so forth. In doing so, she loses herself completely and loses her partner also.

The moment they succumb to this anonymity, they cease to be themselves, with their separate lives and desires; they cease to be the lovers who have met to assuage desire in a reciprocal pact of tenderness, and they engage at once in a spurious charade of maleness and femaleness.

The anonymity of the lovers, whom the act transforms from me and you into they, precludes the expression of ourselves.

So the act is taken away from us even as we perform it.

We become voyeurs upon our own caresses. The act does not acknowledge the participation of the individual, bringing to it a whole life of which the act is only a part. The man and woman, in their particularity, their being, are absent from these representations of themselves as male and female. These tableaux of falsification remove our sexual life from the world, from tactile experience itself. The lovers are lost to themselves in a privacy that does not transcend but deny reality. So the act can never satisfy them, because it does not affect their lives. It occurs in the mythic dream-time of religious ritual.

But our flesh arrives to us out of history, like everything else does. We may believe we fuck stripped of social artifice; in bed, we even feel we touch the bedrock of human nature itself. But we are deceived.

Flesh is not an irreducible human universal. Although the erotic relationship may seem to exist freely, on its own terms, among the distorted social relationships of a bourgeois society, it is, in fact, the most self-conscious of all human relationships, a direct confrontation of two beings whose actions in the bed are wholly determined by their acts when they are out of it. If one sexual partner is economically dependent on the other, then the question of sexual coercion, of contractual obligation, raises its ugly head in the very abode of love and inevitably colours the nature of the sexual expression of affection. The marriage bed is a particularly delusive refuge from the world because all wives of necessity fuck by contract. Prostitutes are at least decently paid on the nail and boast fewer illusions about a hireling status that has no veneer of social acceptability, but their services are suffering a decline in demand now that other women have invaded their territory in their own search for a newly acknowledged sexual pleasure. In this period, promiscuous abandon may seem the only type of free exchange.

But no bed, however unexpected, no matter how apparently gratuitous, is free from the de-universalising facts of real life. We do not go to bed in simple pairs; even if we choose not to refer to them, we still drag there with us the cultural impedimenta of our social class, our parents' lives, our bank balances, our sexual and emotional expectations, our whole biographies—all the bits and pieces of our unique existences. These considerations have limited our choice of partners before we have even got them into the bedroom. It was impossible for the Countess in Beaumarchais' *The Marriage of Figaro* to contemplate sleeping with her husband's valet, even though he was clearly the best man available; considerations of social class censored the possibility of sexual attraction between the Countess and Figaro before it could have begun to exist, and if this convention restricted the Countess's activities, it did not affect those of her husband; he happily plotted to seduce his valet's wife. If middle-class Catherine Earnshaw, in Emily Brontë's *Wuthering Heights*, wants to sleep with Heathcliff, who has the dubious class origins of the foundling, she must not only repress this desire but pay the socially sanctioned price of brain-fever and early death for even contemplating it. Our literature is full, as are our lives, of men and women, but especially women, who deny the reality of sexual attraction and of love because of considerations of class, religion, race and of gender itself.

Class dictates our choice of partners and our choice of positions. When fear, shame and prudery condemn the poor and the ignorant to copulate in the dark, it must be obvious that sexual sophistication is a by-product of education. The primal nakedness of lovers is a phenomenon of the middle-class in cold climates; in northern winters, naked lovers must be able to afford to heat their bedrooms. The taboos regulating the sight of bare flesh are further determined by wider cultural considerations. The Japanese bathed together in the nude for centuries, yet generations of Japanese lovers fucked in kimono, even in the humidity of summer, and did not even remove the combs from their chignons while they did so. And another complication—they did not appreciate the eroticism of the nude; yet they looked at one another's exposed genitalia with a tender readiness that still perturbs the West.

Control of fertility is a by-product of sexual education and of official legislation concerning the availability of cheap or free contraception. Even so, a poor woman may find herself sterilised when all she wanted was an abortion, her fertility taken out of her own control for good by social administrators who have decided that poverty is synonymous with stupidity and a poor woman cannot know her own mind.

The very magical privacy of the bed, the pentacle, may itself only be bought with money, and lack of privacy limits sexual sophistication, which may not be pursued in a room full of children.

Add to these socio-economic considerations the Judaeo-Christian heritage of shame, disgust and morality that stand between the initial urge and the first attainment of this most elementary assertion of the self and it is a wonder anyone in this culture ever learns to fuck at all.

Flesh comes to us out of history; so does the repression and taboo that governs our experience of flesh.

The nature of actual modes of sexual intercourse is determined by historical changes in less intimate human relations, just as the actual nature of men and women is capable of infinite modulations as social structures change. Our knowledge is determined by the social boundaries upon it; for example, Sade, the eighteenth-century lecher, knew that manipulation of the clitoris was the unique key to the female orgasm, but a hundred years later, Sigmund Freud, a Viennese intellectual, did not wish to believe that this grand simplicity was all there was to the business. It was socially permissible for an eighteenth-century aristocrat to sleep with more women than it was for a member of the nineteenth-century bourgeoisie, for one thing, and to retain a genuine curiosity about female sexuality whilst doing so, for another. Yet Freud, the psychoanalyst, can conceive of a far richer notion of human nature as a whole than Sade, the illiberal philosopher, is capable of; the social boundaries of knowledge expand in some areas and contract in others due to historical forces.

Sexuality, in short, is never expressed in a vacuum. Though the archaic sequence of human life—we are born, we fuck, we reproduce, we die—might seem to be universal experience, its universality is not its greatest significance. Since human beings have invented history, we have also invented those aspects of our lives that seem most immutable, or, rather, have invented the circumstances that determine their nature. Birth and death, the only absolute inescapables, are both absolutely determined by the social context in which they occur. There is no longer an inevitable relationship between fucking and reproducing and, indeed, neither fucking nor reproducing have been activities practiced by all men and women at all times, anyway; there has always been the option to abstain, whether it is exercised or not. Women experience sexuality and reproduction quite differently than men do; rich women are more in control of the sequence than poor women and so may actually enjoy fucking and childbirth, when poor women might find them both atrocious simply because they are poor and cannot afford comfort, privacy and paid help.

The notion of a universality of human experience is a confidence trick and the notion of a universality of female experience is a clever confidence trick.

Pornography, like marriage and the fictions of romantic love, assists the process of false universalising. Its excesses belong to that timeless, locationless area outside history, outside geography, where fascist art is born.

Nevertheless, there is no question of an aesthetics of pornography. It can never be art for art's sake. Honourably enough, it is always art with work to do.

Pornographic literature, the specific area of pornography with which we are going to deal, has several functions. On one level, and a level which should not be despised, it might serve as an instruction manual for the inexperienced. But our culture, with its metaphysics of sexuality, relegates the descriptions of the mechanics of sex to crude functionalism; in the sex textbook, intercourse also takes place in a void. So pornography's principal and most humanly significant function is that of arousing sexual excitement. It does this by ignoring the first function; it usually describes the sexual act not in explicit terms—for that might make it seem frightening—but in purely inviting terms.

The function of plot in a pornographic narrative is always the same. It exists purely to provide as many opportunities as possible for the sexual act to take place. There is no room here for tension or the unexpected. We know what is going to happen; that is why we are reading the book. Characterisation is necessarily limited by the formal necessity for the actors to fuck as frequently and as ingeniously as possible. But they do not do so because they are continually consumed by desire; the free expression of desire is as alien to pornography as it is to marriage. In pornography, both men and women fuck because to fuck is their raison d'etre. It is their life work.

It follows that prostitutes are favourite heroines of the pornographic writer, though the economic aspects of a prostitute's activity, which is her own main concern in the real world, will be dealt with only lightly. Her labour is her own private business. Work, in this context, is *really* dirty work; it is unmentionable. Even unspeakable. And we may not talk about it because it reintroduces the question of the world. In this privatised universe pleasure is the only work; work itself is unmentionable. To concentrate on the prostitute's trade *as* trade would introduce too much reality into a scheme that is first and foremost one of libidinous fantasy, and pornographic writers, in general, are not concerned with extending the genre in which they work to include a wider view of the world. This is because pornography is the orphan little sister of the arts; its functionalism renders it suspect, more applied art than fine art, and so its very creators rarely take it seriously.

Fine art, that exists for itself alone, is art in a final state of impotence. If nobody, including the artist, acknowledges art as a means of *knowing* the world, then art is relegated to a kind of rumpus room of the mind and the irresponsibility of the artist and the irrelevance of art to actual living becomes part and parcel of the practice of art. Nevertheless, pornographic writing retains this in common with all literature—that it turns the flesh into word. This is the real transformation the text performs upon libidinous fantasy.

The verbal structure is in itself reassuring. We know we are not dealing with real flesh or anything like it, but with a cunningly articulated verbal simulacrum which has the power to arouse, but not, in itself, to assuage desire. At this point, the reader, the consumer, enters the picture; reflecting the social dominance which affords him the opportunity to purchase the flesh of other people as if it were meat, the reader or consumer of pornography is usually a man who subscribes to a particular social fiction of manliness. His belief in this fiction prevents him from realising that, when he picks up a dirty book, he engages in a game with his own desire and with his own solitude, both of which he endlessly titillates but never openly confronts.

Therefore a cerebral insatiability, unacknowledged yet implicit, is a characteristic of pornography, which always throws the reader back on his own resources, since it convinces him of the impotence of his desire that the book cannot in itself assuage, at the same time as he solaces that loneliness through the medium of the fantasy extracted from the fiction.

The one-to-one relation of the reader with the book is never more apparent than in the reading of a pornographic novel, since it is virtually impossible to forget oneself in relation to the text. In pornographic literature, the text has a gap left in it on purpose so that the reader may, in imagination, step inside it. But the activity the text describes, into which the reader enters, is not a whole world into which the reader is absorbed and, as they say, 'taken out of himself'. It is one basic activity extracted from the world in its totality in such a way that the text constantly reminds the reader of his own troubling self, his own reality—and the limitations of that reality since, however much he wants to fuck the willing women or men in his story, he cannot do so but must be content with some form of substitute activity. (The fictional maleness of the pornography consumer encompasses the butch hero of homosexual pornography; it is a *notion* of masculinity unrelated to practice.)

The privacy of the reader is invaded by his own desires, which reach out towards the world beyond the book he is reading. Yet they are short-circuited by the fantastic nature of the gratification promised by the text, which denies to flesh all its intransigence, indeed its sexed quality, since sexuality is a quality made manifest in being, and pornography can only allow its phantoms to exist in the moment of sexual excitation; they cannot engage in the wide range of activity in the real world in which sexual performance is not the supreme business of all people at all times.

Yet the gripping nature of pornography, its directly frontal assault upon the senses of the reader, its straightforward engagement of him at a non-intellectual level, its *sensationalism*, suggest the methodology of propaganda. Indeed, pornography is basically propaganda for fucking, an activity, one would have thought, that did not need much advertising in itself, because most people want to do it as soon as they know how.

The denial of the social fact of sexuality in pornography is made explicit in its audience. Produced in the main by men for an all-male clientele, suggesting certain analogies with a male brothel, access to pornography is usually denied to women at any level, often on the specious grounds that women do not find descriptions of the sexual act erotically stimulating. Yet if pornography is produced by men for a male audience, it is exclusively concerned with relations between the sexes and even the specialised area of homosexual pornography divides its actors into sexual types who might roughly be defined as 'masculine' and 'feminine'. So all pornography suffers the methodological defects of a manual of navigation written by and for landlubbers.

Many pornographic novels are written in the first person as if by a woman, or use a woman as the focus of the narrative; but this device only reinforces the male orientation of the fiction. John Cleland's *Fanny Hill* and the anonymous *The Story of O*, both classics of the genre, appear in this way to describe a woman's mind through the fiction of her sexuality. This technique ensures that the gap left in the text is of just the right size for the reader to insert his prick into, the exact dimensions, in fact, of Fanny's vagina or of O's anus. Pornography engages the reader in a most intimate fashion before it leaves him to his own resources. This gap in the text may also be just the size of the anus or mouth of a young man, subsuming him, too, to this class that is most present in its absence, the invisible recipients of the pornographic tribute, the mental masturbatory objects.

426

So pornography reinforces the false universals of sexual archetypes because it denies, or doesn't have time for, or can't find room for, or, because of its underlying ideology, ignores, the social context in which sexual activity takes place, that modifies the very nature of that activity. Therefore pornography must always have the false simplicity of fable; the abstraction of the flesh involves the mystification of the flesh. As it reduces the actors in the sexual drama to instruments of pure function, so the pursuit of pleasure becomes in itself a metaphysical quest. The pornographer, in spite of himself, becomes a metaphysician when he states that the friction of penis in orifice is the supreme matter of the world, for which the world is well lost; as he says so, the world vanishes.

Pornography, like satire, has an inbuilt reactionary mechanism. Its effect depends on the notion that the nature of man is invariable and cannot be modified by changes in his social institutions. The primordial itch in the groin existed before multinational business corporations and the nuclear family and will outlast them just as it illicitly dominates them. The disruptiveness of sexuality, its inability to be contained, the overflowing of the cauldron of id—these are basic invariables of sexuality, opines the pornographer, and in itself pornography is a satire on human pretensions. The judge conceals his erection beneath his robes of office as he passes judgement on the whore. The cabinet minister slips away from his office early to visit the call girl. The public executioner ejaculates as the neck of his victim snaps. And we laugh wryly at the omnipotence of Old Adam, how he will always, somehow or other, get his way; and we do ourselves and Old Adam the grossest injustice when we grant him so much power, when we reduce sexuality to the status of lowest common denominator without asking ourselves what preconceptions make us think it should be so.

Since sexuality is as much a social fact as it is a human one, it will therefore change its nature according to changes in social conditions. If we could restore the context of the world to the embraces of these shadows then, perhaps, we could utilise their activities to obtain a fresh perception of the world and, in some sense, transform it. The sexual act in pornography exists as a metaphor for what people do to one another, often in the cruellest sense; but the present business of the pornographer is to suppress the metaphor as much as he can and leave us with a handful of empty words. Pornographic pictures, movies and narrative fiction are the pure forms of sexual fiction, of the fiction *of* sex, where this operation of alienation takes place most visibly. But all art which contains elements of eroticism (eroticism, the pornography of the elite) contains the possibility of the same methodology—that is, writing that can 'pull' a reader just as a woman 'pulls' a man or a man 'pulls' a woman.

And all such literature has the potential to force the reader to reassess his relation to his own sexuality, which is to say to his own primary being, through the mediation of the image or the text. This is true for women also, perhaps especially so, as soon as we realise the way pornography reinforces the archetypes of her negativity and that it does so simply because most pornography remains in the service of the status quo. And that is because its elementary metaphysic gets in the way of real life and prevents us seeing real life. If the world has been lost, the world may not be reassessed. Libidinous fantasy in a vacuum is the purest, but most affectless, form of day-dreaming. So pornography in general serves to defuse the explosive potential of all sexuality and that is the main reason why it is made by and addressed to the politically dominant minority in the world, as an instrument of repression, not only of women, but of men too. Pornography keeps sex in its place, that is, under the carpet. That is, outside everyday human intercourse.

The sexuality of the blue movie queen, contained by her social subservience, exhibits no menace. Linda Lovelace does not believe in the Women's Liberation Movement; how could she? Fanny Hill gladly gives up the dominant role of mistress for the subservient role of wife and hands to her Charles all her hard-earned money too, which is an infinitely more far-reaching gesture of submission than that of accepting his sexual mastery and opting for domestic monogamy and motherhood under his exclusive economic sanction. Fanny knows in her heart that her Charles is really her last, most efficient, pimp. O, less complex because her economic means of support are not explored as closely as Cleland explores Fanny's, is more content simply to rejoice in her chains, a model for all women.

It is fair to say that, when pornography serves—as with very rare exceptions it always does—to reinforce the prevailing system of values and ideas in a given society, it is tolerated; and when it does not, it is banned. (This already suggests there are more reasons than those of public decency for the banning of the work of Sade for almost two hundred years; only at the time of the French Revolution and at the present day have his books been available to the general public.) Therefore an increase of pornography on the market, within the purchasing capacity of the common man, and especially the beginning of a type of pornography modelled on that provided for the male consumer but directed at women, does not mean an increase in sexual licence, with the reappraisal of social mores such licence, if it is real, necessitates. It might only indicate a more liberal attitude to masturbation, rather than to fucking, and reinforce a sollipsistic concentration on the relationship with the self, which is a fantasy one at the best of times.

When pornography abandons its quality of existential solitude and moves out of the kitsch area of timeless, placeless fantasy and into the real world, then it loses its function of safety valve. It begins to comment on real relations in the real world. Therefore, the more pornographic writing aquires the techniques of real literature, of real art, the more deeply subversive it is likely to be in that the more likely it is to affect the reader's perceptions of the world. The text that had heretofore opened up creamily to him, in a dream, will gather itself together and harshly expel him into the anguish of actuality.

There is a liberal theory that art disinfects eroticism of its latent subversiveness, and pornography that is also art loses its shock and its magnetism, becomes 'safe'. The truth of this is that once pornography is labelled 'art' or 'literature' it is stamped with the approval of an elitist culture and many ordinary people will avoid it on principle, out of a fear of being bored. But the more the literary arts of plotting and characterisation are used to shape the material of pornography, the more the pornographer himself is faced with the moral contradictions inherent in real sexual encounters. He will find himself in a dilemma; to opt for the world or to opt for the wet dream?

Out of this dilemma, the moral pornographer might be born.

The moral pornographer would be an artist who uses pornographic material as part of the acceptance of the logic of a world of absolute sexual licence for all the genders, and projects a model of the way such a world might work. A moral pornographer might use pornography as a critique of current relations between the sexes. His business would be the total demystification of the flesh and the subsequent revelation, through the infinite modulations of the sexual act, of the real relations of man and his kind. Such a pornographer would not be the enemy of women, perhaps because he might begin to penetrate to the heart of the contempt for women that distorts our culture even as he entered the realms of true obscenity as he describes it.

But the pornographer's more usual business is to assert that the function of flesh is pure pleasure, which is itself a mystification of a function a great deal more complex, apart from raising the question of the nature of pleasure itself. However, the nature of pleasure is not one with which the pornographer often concerns himself; for him, sexual pleasure is a given fact, a necessary concomitant of the juxtaposition of bodies.

It is at this point that he converts the sexed woman, living, breathing, troubling, into a desexed hole and the breathing, living, troubling man into nothing but a probe; pornography becomes a form of pastoral, sex an engaging and decorative activity that may be performed without pain, soil, sweat or effect, and its iconography a very suitable subject for informal murals in public places. If, that is, the simplest descriptions of sex did not also rouse such complex reactions.

And that is because sexual relations between men and women always render explicit the nature of social relations in the society in which they take place and, if described explicitly, will form a critique of those relations, even if that is not and never has been the intention of the pornographer.

So, whatever the surface falsity of pornography, it is impossible for it to fail to reveal sexual reality at an unconscious level, and this reality may be very unpleasant indeed, a world away from official reality.

A male-dominated society produces a pornography of universal female aquiescence. Or, most delicious titillation, of compensatory but spurious female dominance. Miss Stern with her rods and whips, Our Lady of Pain in her leather visor and her boots with sharp, castratory heels, is a true fantasy, a distorted version of the old saying 'The hand that rocks the cradle rules the world.' This whip hand rocks the cradle in which her customer dreams but it does nothing else. Miss Stern's dominance exists only in the bedroom. She may utilise apparatus that invokes heaven, hell and purgatory for her client, she may utterly ravage his body, martyrise him, shit on him, piss on him, but her cruelty is only the manifestation of the victim or patient's guilt before the fact of his own sexuality, of which he is ashamed. She is not cruel for her own sake, or for her own gratification. She is most truly subservient when most apparently dominant; Miss Stern and her pretended victim have established a mutually degrading pact between them and she in her weird garb is mutilated more savagely by the erotic violence she perpetrates than he by the pain he undergoes, since his pain is in the nature of a holiday from his life, and her cruelty an economic fact of her real life, so much hard work. You can describe their complicity in a pornographic novel but to relate it to her mortgage, her maid's salary and her laundry bills is to use the propaganda technique of pornography to express a view of the world, which deviates from the notion that all this takes place in a kindergarten of soiled innocence. A kindergarten? Only small children, in our society, do not need to work.

The pornographer who consciously utilises the propaganda, the 'grabbing' effect of pornography to express a view of the world that transcends this kind of innocence will very soon find himself in deep political water for he will begin to find himself describing the real conditions of the world in terms of sexual encounters, or even find that the real nature of these encounters illuminates the world itself; the world turns into a gigantic brothel, the area of our lives where we believed we possessed most freedom is seen as the most ritually circumscribed.

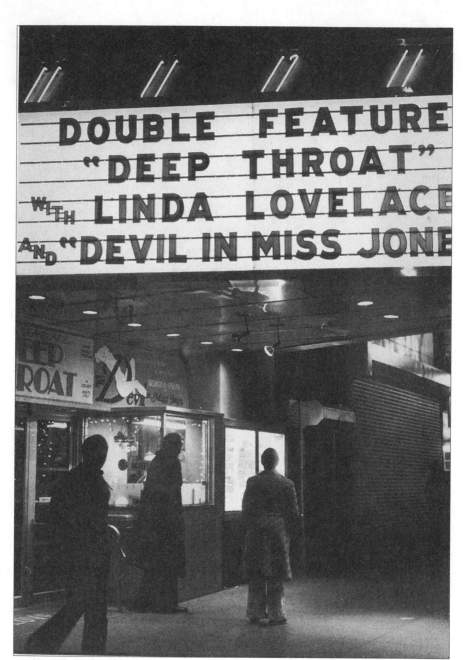

© Fred W. McDarrah

Review of *Deep Throat*

Al Goldstein

from *Screw*, March, 1972

Deep Throat was the first hard-core porn movie to be shown in mainstream movie theaters and to be seen by large numbers of women. It was enthusiastically reviewed by Screw magazine—at the time widely distributed on street corners in many large American cities—which gave Deep Throat its highest rating: three erect penises.

Deep *Throat* is everything you could possibly imagine it to be. Tis a tale with a happy ending of a girl who, after discovering that she is a sexual freak with a clitoris in her throat instead of between her legs, sucks her way to happiness and bliss. The technical and artistic work of the film is excellent. The photography is sharp and clear, and the color is beautiful. The soundtrack is perfect, the acting well done and the fucking and sucking supreme. The storyline traces the life of a fair young damsel who can't have an orgasm from routine balling and blowing. She tries a gangbang scene with enough hard pricks around to get 12 normal women off. When the promiscuous ploy fails, she consults a psychiatrist who makes the discovery that her clit has somehow managed to lodge itself in the deep dark recesses of her throat. He recommends that she try some sword-swallowing and gets her started on his own ample weapon. Such a display of cock-consumption has never before been recorded on the porno movie screen. The heroine engulfs stiff dicks right down to the balls. They simply disappear into her mouth and seemingly penetrate into the depths of her bowels. The girl becomes a physio-therapist for the shrink's sexually maladjusted patients and fucks them and sucks them while gratifying her own special orgasmic needs. She falls in love with a patient and he with her . . . and the movie ends with a fantastic blowjob to spurt-spurt and a smile on her face that lets the audience know just how much she digs eating cock. The film features a couple of assfucking sequences and three come shots, two in that wonderful mouth. There is also a scene where the heroine gets a glass test tube stuffed up her snatch. It gets filled with Coca-Cola and drunk through a siphon-straw to the tune of the Coke jingle revised to say—"I'd like to teach you all to screw in perfect harmony." Playing at the Mature World, 49th St. off 7th Ave. (CI 7-5747). Admission $5.

Feminism, Moralism, and Pornography

Ellen Willis

from *Village Voice*, October/November, 1979

By the late seventies, the conclusions of the 1970 Presidential Commission on Obscenity and Pornography were under attack by both conservatives and feminists. Journalist, rock critic, and one of the founders of the radical feminist movement Ellen Willis, for many years an editor and writer for the **Village Voice**, *addresses the feminist crusade against pornography. Anti-porn feminists had argued that pornography was one of the fundamental causes of violence against women. Ellis offers a wide-ranging response to the feminist analysis of pornography.*

For women, life is an ongoing good cop-bad cop routine. The good cops are marriage, motherhood, and that courtly old gentleman, chivalry. Just cooperate, they say (crossing their fingers), and we'll go easy on you. You'll never have to earn a living or open a door. We'll even get you some romantic love. But you'd better not get stubborn, or you'll have to deal with our friend rape, and he's a real terror; we just can't control him.

Pornography often functions as a bad cop. If rape warns that without the protection of one man we are fair game for all, the hard-core pornographic image suggests that the alternative to being a wife is being a whore. As women become more "criminal," the cops call for nastier reinforcements; the proliferation of lurid, violent porn (symbolic rape) is a form of backlash. But one can be a solid citizen and still be shocked (naively or hypocritically) by police brutality. However

*This is an expanded version of two columns written for *The Village Voice*.

widely condoned, rape is illegal. However loudly people proclaim that porn is as wholesome as granola, the essence of its appeal is that emotionally it remains taboo. It is from their very contempt for the rules that bad cops derive their power to terrorize (and the covert approbation of solid citizens who would love to break the rules themselves). The line between bad cop and outlaw is tenuous. Both rape and pornography reflect a male outlaw mentality that rejects the conventions of romance and insists, bluntly, that women are cunts. The crucial difference between the conservative's moral indignation at rape, or at *Hustler,* and the feminist's political outrage is the latter's understanding that the problem is not bad cops or outlaws but cops and the law.

Unfortunately, the current women's campaign against pornography seems determined to blur this difference. Feminist criticism of sexist and misogynist pornography is nothing new, porn is an obvious target insofar as it contributes to larger patterns of oppression—the reduction of the female body to a commodity (the paradigm being prostitution), the sexual intimidation that makes women regard the public streets as enemy territory (the paradigm being rape), sexist images and propaganda in general. But what is happening now is different. By playing games with the English language, antiporn activists are managing to rationalize as feminism a single-issue movement divorced from any larger political context and rooted in conservative moral assumptions that are all the more dangerous for being unacknowledged.

When I first heard there was a group called Women Against Pornography, I twitched. Could I define myself as Against Pornography? Not really. In itself, pornography—which, my dictionary and I agree, means any image or description intended or used to arouse sexual desire— does not strike me as the proper object of a political crusade. As the most cursory observation suggests, there are many varieties of porn, some pernicious, some more or less benign. About the only generalization one can make is that pornography is the return of the repressed, of feelings and fantasies driven underground by a culture that atomizes sexuality, defining love as a noble affair of the heart and mind, lust as a base animal urge centered in unmentionable organs. Prurience—the state of mind I associate with pornography—implies a sense of sex as forbidden, secretive pleasure, isolated from any emotional or social context. I imagine that in Utopia, porn would wither away along with the state, heroin, and Coca-Cola. At present, however, the sexual impulses that pornography appeals to are part of virtually everyone's psychology. For obvious political and cultural reasons nearly all porn is sexist in that it is the product of a male imagination and aimed at a male market; women are less likely to be consciously interested in pornography, or to indulge that interest, or to find porn that turns them on. But anyone who thinks women are simply indifferent to pornography has never watched a bunch of adolescent girls pass around a trashy novel. Over the years I've enjoyed various pieces of pornography—some of them of the sleazy Forty-second Street paperback sort—and so have most women I know. Fantasy, after all, is more flexible than reality, and women have learned, as a matter of survival, to be adept at shaping male fantasies to their own purposes. If feminists define pornography, per se, as the enemy, the result will be to make a lot of women ashamed of their sexual feelings and afraid to be honest about them. And the last thing women need is more sexual shame, guilt, and hypocrisy—this time served up as feminism.

So why ignore qualitative distinctions and in effect condemn all pornography as equally bad? WAP organizers answer—or finesse—this question by redefining pornography. They maintain that pornography is not really about sex but about violence against women. Or, in a more colorful formulation, "Pornography is the theory, rape is the practice." Part of the argument is that pornography causes violence; much is made of the fact that Charles Manson and David Berkowitz had porn collections. This is the sort of inverted logic that presumes marijuana to be dangerous because most heroin addicts started with it. It is men's hostility toward women—combined with their power to express that hostility and for the most part get away with it—that causes sexual violence. Pornography that gives sadistic fantasies concrete shape—and, in today's atmosphere, social legitimacy—may well encourage suggestible men to act them out. But if *Hustler* were to vanish from the shelves tomorrow, I doubt that rape or wife-beating statistics would decline.

Even more problematic is the idea that pornography depicts violence rather than sex. Since porn is by definition overtly sexual, while most of it is not overtly violent, this equation requires some fancy explaining. The conference WAP held in September was in part devoted to this task. Robin Morgan and Gloria Steinem addressed it by attempting to distinguish pornography from erotica. According to this argument, erotica (whose etymological root is "eros," or sexual love) expresses an integrated sexuality based on mutual affection and desire between equals; pornography (which comes from another Greek root—"porne," meaning prostitute) reflects a dehumanized sexuality based on male domination and exploitation of women. The distinction sounds promising, but it doesn't hold up. The accepted meaning of erotica is literature or pictures with sexual themes; it may or may not serve the essentially utilitarian function of pornography. Because it is less specific, less suggestive of actual sexual activity, "erotica" is regularly used as a euphemism for "classy porn." Pornography expressed in literary language or expensive photography and consumed by the upper middle class is "erotica"; the cheap stuff, which can't pretend to any purpose but getting people off, is smut. The erotica-versus-porn approach evades the (embarrassing?) question of how porn is *used*. It endorses the portrayal of sex as we might like it to be and condemns the portrayal of sex as it too often is, whether in action or only in fantasy. But if pornography is to arouse, it must appeal to the feelings we have, not those that by some Utopian standard we ought to have. Sex in this culture has been so deeply politicized that it is impossible to make clear-cut distinctions between "authentic" sexual impulses and those conditioned by patriarchy. Between, say, *Ulysses* at one end and *Snuff* at the other, erotica/pornography conveys all sorts of mixed messages that elicit complicated and private responses. In practice, attempts to sort out good erotica from bad porn inevitably come down to "What turns me on is erotic; what turns you on is pornographic."

It would be clearer and more logical simply to acknowledge that some sexual images are offensive and some are not. But logic and clarity are irrelevant—or rather, inimical—to the underlying aim of the antiporners, which is to vent the emotions traditionally associated with the word "pornography." As I've suggested, there is a social and psychic link between pornography and rape. In terms of patriarchal morality both are expressions of male lust, which is presumed to be innately vicious, and offenses to the putative sexual innocence of "good" women. But feminists supposedly begin with different assumptions— that men's confusion of sexual desire with predatory aggression reflects a sexist system, not male biology; that there are no good (chaste) or bad (lustful) women, just women who are, like men, sexual beings. From this standpoint, to lump pornography with rape is dangerously simplistic. Rape is a violent physical assault. Pornography can be a psychic assault, both in its content and in its public intrusions on our attention, but for women as for men it can also be a source of erotic pleasure. A woman who is raped is a victim; a woman who enjoys pornography (even if that means enjoying a rape fantasy) is in a sense a rebel, insisting on an aspect of her sexuality that has been defined as a male preserve. Insofar as pornography glorifies male supremacy and sexual alienation, it is deeply reactionary. But in rejecting sexual repression and hypocrisy—which have inflicted even more damage on women than on men—it expresses a radical impulse.

That this impulse still needs defending, even among feminists, is evident from the sexual attitudes that have surfaced in the antiporn movement. In the movement's rhetoric pornography is a code word for vicious male lust. To the objection that some women get off on porn, the standard reply is that this only shows how thoroughly women have been brainwashed by male values—though a WAP leaflet goes so far as to suggest that women who claim to like pornography are lying to avoid male opprobrium. (Note the good-girl-versus-bad-girl theme, reappearing as healthy-versus-sick, or honest-versus-devious; for "brainwashed" read "seduced.") And the view of sex that most often emerges from talk about "erotica" is as sentimental and euphemistic as the word itself: lovemaking should be beautiful, romantic, soft, nice, and devoid of messiness, vulgarity, impulses to power, or indeed aggression of any sort. Above all, the emphasis should be on *relationships,* not (yuck) *organs.* This goody-goody concept of eroticism is not feminist but feminine. It is precisely sex as an aggressive, unladylike activity, an expression of violent and unpretty emotion, an exercise of erotic power, and a specifically genital experience that has been taboo for women. Nor are we supposed to admit that we, too, have sadistic impulses, that our sexual fantasies may reflect forbidden urges to turn the tables and get revenge on men. (When a woman is aroused by a rape fantasy, is she perhaps identifying with the rapist as well as the victim?)

At the WAP conference lesbian separatists argued that pornography reflects patriarchal sexual relations; patriarchal sexual relations are based on male power backed by force; ergo, pornography is violent. This dubious syllogism, which could as easily be applied to romantic novels, reduces the whole issue to hopeless mush. If all manifestations of patriarchal sexuality are violent, then opposition to violence cannot explain why pornography (rather than romantic novels) should be singled out as a target. Besides, such reductionism allows women no basis for distinguishing between consensual heterosexuality and rape. But this is precisely its point; as a number of women at the conference put it, "In a patriarchy, all sex with men is pornographic." Of course, to attack pornography, and at the same time equate it with heterosexual sex, is implicitly to condemn not only women who like pornography, but women who sleep with men. This is familiar ground. The argument that straight women collaborate with the enemy has often been, among other things, a relatively polite way of saying that they consort with the beast. At the conference I couldn't help feeling that proponents of the separatist line were talking like the modern equivalents of women who, in an era when straightforward prudery was socially acceptable, joined convents to escape men's rude sexual demands. It seemed to me that their revulsion against heterosexuality was serving as the thinnest of covers for disgust with sex itself. In any case, sanitized feminine sexuality, whether straight or gay, is as limited as the predatory masculine kind and as central to women's oppression; a major function of misogynist pornography is to scare us into embracing it. As a further incentive, the good cops stand ready to assure us that we are indeed morally superior to men, that in our sweetness and nonviolence (read passivity and powerlessness) is our strength.

Women are understandably tempted to believe this comforting myth. Self-righteousness has always been a feminine weapon, a permissible way to make men feel bad. Ironically, it is socially acceptable for women to display fierce aggression in their crusades against male vice, which serve as an outlet for female anger without threatening male power. The temperance movement, which made alcohol the symbol of male violence, did not improve the position of women; substituting porn for demon rum won't work either. One reason it won't is that it bolsters the good girl—bad girl split. Overtly or by implication it isolates women who like porn or "pornographic" sex or who work in the sex industry. WAP has refused to take a position on prostitution, yet its activities—particularly its support for cleaning up Times Square—will affect prostitutes' lives. Prostitution raises its own set of complicated questions. But it is clearly not in women's interest to pit "good" feminists against "bad" whores (or topless dancers, or models for skin magazines).

So far, the issue that has dominated public debate on the anti-porn campaign is its potential threat to free speech. Here too the movement's arguments have been full of contradictions. Susan Brownmiller and other WAP organizers claim not to advocate censorship and dismiss the civil liberties issue as a red herring dragged in by men who don't want to face the fact that pornography oppresses women. Yet at the same time, WAP endorses the Supreme Court's contention that obscenity is not protected speech, a doctrine I—and most civil libertarians—regard as a clear infringement of First Amendment rights. Brownmiller insists that the First Amendment was designed to protect political dissent, not expressions of woman-hating violence. But to make such a distinction is to defeat the amendment's purpose, since it implicitly cedes to the government the right to define "political." (Has there ever been a government willing to admit that its opponents are anything more than antisocial troublemakers?) Anyway, it makes no sense to oppose pornography on the grounds that it's sexist propaganda, then turn around and argue that it's not political. Nor will libertarians be reassured by WAP's statement that "We want to change the definition of obscenity so that it focuses on violence, not sex." Whatever their focus, obscenity laws deny the right of free expression to those who transgress official standards of propriety—and personally, I don't find WAP's standards significantly less oppressive than Warren Burger's. Not that it matters, since WAP's fantasies about influencing the definition of obscenity are appallingly naive. The basic purpose of obscenity laws is and always has been to reinforce cultural taboos on sexuality and suppress feminism, homosexuality, and other forms of sexual dissidence. No pornographer has ever been punished for being a woman hater, but not too long ago information about female sexuality, contraception, and abortion was assumed to be obscene. In a male supremacist society the only obscenity law that will not be used against women is no law at all.

As an alternative to an outright ban on pornography, Brownmiller and others have advocated restricting its display. There is a plausible case to be made for the idea that antiwoman images displayed so prominently that they are impossible to avoid are coercive, a form of active harassment that oversteps the bounds of free speech. But aside from the evasion involved in simply equating pornography with misogyny or sexual sadism, there are no legal or logical grounds for treating sexist material any differently from (for example) racist or anti-Semitic propaganda; an equitable law would have to prohibit any kind of public defamation. And the very thought of such a sweeping law has to make anyone with an imagination nervous. Could Catholics claim they were being harassed by nasty depictions of the pope? Could Russian refugees argue that the display of Communist literature was a form of psychological torture? Would proabortion material be taken off the shelves on the grounds that it defamed the unborn? I'd rather not find out.

At the moment the First Amendment issue remains hypothetical; the movement has concentrated on raising the issue of pornography through demonstrations and other public actions. This is certainly a legitimate strategy. Still, I find myself more and more disturbed by the tenor of antipornography actions and the sort of consciousness they promote; increasingly their focus has shifted from rational feminist criticism of specific targets to generalized, demagogic moral outrage. Picketing an antiwoman movie, defacing an exploitative billboard, or boycotting a record company to protest its misogynist album covers conveys one kind of message, mass marches Against Pornography quite another. Similarly, there is a difference between telling the neighborhood news dealer why it pisses us off to have *Penthouse* shoved in our faces and choosing as a prime target every right-thinking politician's symbol of big-city sin, Times Square.

In contrast to the abortion rights movement, which is struggling against a tidal wave of energy from the other direction, the anti-porn campaign is respectable. It gets approving press and cooperation from the city, which has its own stake (promoting tourism, making the Clinton area safe for gentrification) in cleaning up Times Square. It has begun to attract women whose perspective on other matters is in no way feminist ("I'm anti-abortion," a participant in WAP's march on Times Square told a reporter, "but this is something I can get into").

Despite the insistence of WAP organizers that they support sexual freedom, their line appeals to the antisexual emotions that feed the backlash. Whether they know it or not, they are doing the good cops' dirty work.

Talking Sex

Deirdre English, Amber Hollibaugh and Gayle Rubin

from *Socialist Review*, November/December, 1980

This conversation among three women—two lesbian radicals, Amber Hollibaugh and Gayle Rubin, and Deirdre English, feminist writer and editor of the radical magazine Mother Jones—*explores the potential impact of the feminist anti-porn crusade on the public discussion of sexuality and why that is an important issue.*

Deirdre English: Feminist discussions of sex seem to take place in a vacuum. We often ignore some of the extreme changes going on in society as people react to the ideas of sexual freedom and of equality of the sexes. Those reactions are highly charged, whether positive or negative, and their intensity has often intimidated us. I would go so far as to say that, on the whole, the women's movement is not as far-sighted as some of the more progressive areas in the field of sex research, where psychologists have really come to grips with people's emotions and behavior. They have learned through their practices not to be threatened by the sexual realm; they have developed an acceptance of fantasy, an acceptance of women's sexuality and of diverse forms of sexual expression.

Gayle Rubin: You're right. There is certainly a branch of the sex field that is progressive. Many women, even feminists, even dykes, work in that field. Instead of assuming that sex is guilty until proven innocent, these people assume that sex is fundamentally OK until proven bad. And that idea has not penetrated either the women's movement or the Left. Some feminists cannot digest the concept of benign sexual variation. Instead of realizing that human beings are not all the same, that variation is OK, the women's movement has created a new standard. This is like the old psychiatric concept, that dictates a "normal" way to do it. Male/female, heterosexual, married, man on top, reproductive sex was OK. But all other behavior was measured against that standard and found wanting.

DE: The old idea of malignant variation was in the service of a particular kind of social structure, the patriarchal heterosexual structure. But I think that some feminists also have a concept of sexuality in service to society.

Amber Hollibaugh: The notion that sex has no right to exist for itself, that sex is good or bad only in terms of social relations.

DE: Right. And, at worst, this feminist vision would bar some forms of sexual expression. One of the first things it would probably get rid of is heterosexuality. The man on top, heterosexual, reproductive.

GR: That for sure will not be permitted after the revolution.

AH: No one will want it, you see! These things are all imposed by sexist male domination and patriarchy, which has brainwashed us from childhood into believing that our bodies are driven to this, in spite of the terrifically healthy erotic desires which would bloom in a new, revolutionary society. That's hogwash. My fantasy life has been constructed in a great variety of ways. My sexual desire has been channeled. But what that view takes from me is my right to genuinely feel, in my body, what I want.

What it says is that I have no notion of healthy sexuality and that anything sexual now is unhealthy and contaminated because of the culture I live in. So that the notion of pleasure in sex is now a forbidden one, it's a contradiction in terms. The theory is that lesbianism comes the closest to being a profemale sexuality because it's two women together. However, when you acknowledge power between women, that you would like to be dominated by or dominate another woman in a sexual exchange, that you'll lust after her if you put passion and sexual power into the lesbian description rather than Cinderella, lesbian Cinderellaism, you are told that you have a heterosexual model for your lesbian sexuality, you have leftover penetration fantasies you really should reexamine. There's never been anything in that rap about sex that has much joy, pleasure, power, or lustiness.

GR: I don't think there has been a feminist discussion of sex. And that's not just the fault of the women's movement. People don't utilize the best analysis of progressive sex research because they don't really know about it. I firmly believe that sexuality is not natural, not an unchanging, ahistorical item in the human repertoire of behavior. Which means that, after the revolution, in Utopia, it would obviously be different. However, that idea, that sex will change if social reality changes, is confused in a peculiar and perhaps fundamentally Christian way. The idea of sex after the revolution is so removed from anything that we now do that it transcends the flesh itself. It becomes an absence of anything that we do now, all of which is contaminated by this earthly, fleshy existence. So *"sex after the revolution"* becomes a transcendent image of celestial delight.

When we talk about how work will change, we don't say work will disappear. We talk about how what people do will be different, how social relations will be different, but we don't therefore condemn what everybody does now and say that they are bad people for doing it. We treat sex as a special case at almost every point. And we use different standards to judge it.

The late 1960s and early 1970s saw the so-called sexual revolution. Women like me felt that it hadn't worked because it was male dominated, but we still wanted it in a nonsexist way. Other women said, It's male dominated, it hasn't worked for women, and it won't. And we don't want anything to do with it. So basically the people who don't want anything to do with a sexual revolution are now defining the discourse around sex, rather than those of us who want to have some kind of sexual liberation that is not sexist.

Yet this sexual revolution was only a liberalization, so of course it didn't do what we wanted. People's standards for what should have happened are based on the assumption that this was the revolution. It's saying that socialism will never work, look at the Soviet Union.

DE: It's very popular now to say that the sexual revolution of the 1960s was incredibly oppressive to women, that it was just a male-dominated thing. That's too simple. My recollection of it is that it was not an unmitigated disaster. The sexism was there, but women were actually having more sexual experience of different kinds and enjoying it. Women were having more sex that was not procreational and claiming the right to it as well as paying a lower social and emotional cost. There were obstacles, and many women were disappointed. They were often disappointed by the nature of the sexuality that they found with men. That's not too surprising, historically. But the raised sexual expectations created enormous social and sexual gains for women. There was a fresh, post-Victorian discovery of the female orgasm. Many women were actually able to change the way that men made love with them as well as the way they made love with men. Not enough, but there were dramatic changes. Women were fighting for sexual rights and often getting them.

AH: We forget that, ten or twelve years ago, you were a strident ball-buster if you were a woman who was sexually self-defined, who said what she wanted and sought her own partners, who perhaps was not heterosexual. It was not very long ago that the notion of being sexual and being female was outrageous. Part of my attraction to feminism involved that right to be a sexual person. I'm not sure where that history got lost.

DE: We didn't win. We made great gains, but we had enormous losses. Now we're in a period in which a lot of women are looking only at the losses and are saying, Give up, back to square one, better sexual expression. But can't we have a nonsexist sexual liberation? Can't we still go for that?

AH: Marxism hasn't taken sexuality very seriously. It's not only that feminism doesn't take it seriously, but most progressive movements have been very unprogressive about sexuality, and we've inherited that tradition. When we analyzed sexism, we found it hard to separate sex and pleasure from sexism and didn't realize until fairly recently how to use Marxist tools to help look at sexuality in a historical perspective. The Left shares responsibility for the vacuum in sexual theory that the feminist movement has needed to fill. Sexuality has not been thought of as a central part of human life. It has even been thought to be frivolous. Or the Left has been sexually repressive. Lenin said that if women were not monogamous, for the man it was like drinking out of someone else's glass.

GR: I thought all the questions that weren't answered for me in the Left would be answered in the women's movement. In 1968, compared to the Left, the women's movement had everything to say about sex. Not just about gender, but about sex. It's only become clear more recently that feminist theory, although it talks about sex, it mostly talks in terms of gender and gender hierarchy and the relationships between men and women. It doesn't really have a language for sexual desire and wants. Feminist concepts and Marxist concepts are indispensable for dealing with sex. But you have to deal with sex and not assume that if you're talking about class or gender or romance, you're talking about sex.

Lesbianism and Heterosexuality
DE: What you're saying might not be true if the women's movement had not been willing to make women feel guilty about heterosexuality.

GR: What happened around lesbianism is interesting and complicated. Suddenly some of us could go out and be sexual without dealing with sexism and men. And that changed the issues that we faced. Many of us became lesbians in a quest for greater and better sexual experience. And other people became lesbians to get away from sex. Both a seeking of sex and a running from it got involved in early lesbian theory and practice.

AH: Are you thinking about "The Woman-Identified Woman"? [a piece written by a collective called Radicalesbians].

GR: Yes, around 1970, the "Woman-Identified Woman" paper basically argued, in the popular phraseology, that feminism was the theory and lesbianism the practice.

AH: That all women were lesbians or potential lesbians.

GR: And that to be a lesbian was to revolt against patriarchy. All of which made sense.

DE: Therefore, heterosexuals are what? Deviants?

AH: Heterosexuality was an imposed system that women suffered from. But all women—if they only knew it—were woman identified. The lesbian in all of us was closer to the surface in some of us and bubbled forth, while in other people it was silent.

GR: Lesbianism at that time was presented as the oppressed getting together, as if women were the proletariat getting together to relate to each other instead of to the oppressor. At the time it seemed to justify the lesbian experience pretty well, though it didn't account for male homosexuals. Yet it made heterosexual feminists into second-class citizens and created a decade of problems for heterosexual women in the radical women's movement. In retrospect, I think it also abused lesbians. By conflating lesbianism—which I think of as a sexual and erotic experience—with feminism—a political philosophy—the ability to justify lesbianism on grounds other than feminism dropped out of the discourse. If you recognized that it was ok to be a dyke whether or not it was politically correct, that the basic lust itself was legitimate—correct, that the basic lust itself was legitimate—then at some level you had to recognize that other people's basic lust, no matter how it looked in an oppressive time, was also legitimate. And people didn't want to do that. In defining both heterosexuality and lesbianism in terms of one's relationships to patriarchy, the erotic experience dropped out. Definitions of sexual orientation became completely unsexual. And so no one has really had to think explicitly about the erotic components of anybody's sexual orientation for ten years. And this has led to a new hierarchy of what's OK. First, it was that lesbians were better than straight women.

And now it turns out that some lesbians are better than other lesbians and some straight women can be permitted to be political lesbians but not others. We now have replaced the old psychiatric view of what's permissible and nonpermissible in sexual behavior with a new hierarchy based on the notion that lesbianism somehow is exempt from the patriarchy. What angers me most about this is the assumption that lesbianism is not a social construct. The fact is that lesbianism is as much a social construct of the current system as anyone else's sexuality. It has a different, specific relationship to the system as a whole. Everything does. But lesbianism relies on aspects of the system as it is. For instance, the sense of lesbianism being a rebellious sexuality is predicated on male supremacy. If men did not oppress women, that valence would presumably be gone from lesbianism.

AH: Parts of the feminist movement basically said that sexuality really wasn't very important and other kinds of relationships had to take priority. Lusting in whatever form was unacceptable. The lesbian was not supposed to be any lustier than the heterosexual woman, and the heterosexual woman was not to be sexual at all. As a lesbian who was a lesbian before the feminist movement, with a lover in the closet, I was told that we couldn't go to women's conferences and stay in the same bedroom, that we were not allowed to show physical desire for each other in public, and that we were not to dance together in any particularly heavy sexual way. We were asked to leave some parts of the women's movement if we were sexual with each other because women had been terrorized by sexuality and were sick of it. Our dirty sex lives were no better than anybody else's, especially since there was no way to keep us out.

DE: Let's talk about heterosexual women and their acceptance of this theory. I find it fascinating and almost funny that so many heterosexual feminists, especially in the socialist movement, seemed to accept the idea that heterosexuality meant cooperating in their own oppression and that there was something wrong with being sexually turned on to men. How many times have I heard this? "Well, unfortunately, I'm not a lesbian, but I wish I was, maybe I will be."

AH: "I'm a lesbian in my mind. But I'm still a heterosexual in my body."

GR: The mind is willing, but the flesh is weak.

DE: "And so, for reasons I cannot explain, unfortunately, except for my patriarchal conditioning, I have sex with this man every night."

AH: In the dark, though, in the dark.

DE: "But never mind. I'll never discuss the pleasure I get from it. I'll never raise that; I'll never ask for that to be legitimate. I know it's illegitimate and I'm guilty!"

How did it serve heterosexual feminists to adopt a theory that was—on the surface—so self-denying? Partly it was a relief to be able to consider themselves deviant. With heterosexual desire itself, I can see no criticism. But heterosexuality does give you access to privileges that lesbian women or women not associated with men do not have. The feminist understanding of how women are protected by their alliance with men is valid.

I think it was convenient for heterosexuals to be able to feel guilty for this trait, which was advantageous to them and allied them with powerful men, while still being considered a deviant—and not having to change anything. That much is perhaps ironically amusing. But it doesn't advance our thinking, and it doesn't provide honest emotional support to anyone—female, male, straight, or gay. And, for some women, guilt over heterosexual relations sometimes also fed a sad and bitter sexual self-denial.

AH: Maybe some of the confusion about lesbianism and sexuality occurred when lesbianism began to be the model for describing good sex. Everybody, heterosexual or homosexual, used it to describe non-genitally organized sexual experience. That was a way to reject men fucking for a minute and a half and pulling out, a way to talk about non-missionary-position sexuality, foreplay as all-play. The description of lesbian-feminist sexuality actually resembles a feminist description of what good sex is supposed to be more than a description of lesbian sex.

And all women in the feminist movement were trying to make love the way dykes were supposed to.

GR: But it's turned the other way now; now sex has to occur in a certain way for it to be good. And the only legitimate sex is very limited. It's not focused on orgasm, it's very gentle, and it takes place in the context of a long-term, caring relationship. It's the missionary position of the women's movement.

Violence against Women

AH: Categories that needed careful exploration—romance, long-term relationships, sex, sexism—a whole variety of things have all got thrown into the same washing machine, and this very odd-colored garment came out. If you combine incorrectly, then you can't do anything within that discussion. That's what I feel about the way questions get raised by the antiporn movement. I don't even want to try and answer those wrong questions, even though the issue is crucial. The issue is taken from us if we question any of the objects of struggle. For instance, if you question pornography's ability to turn out masses of rapists, it is assumed that you are encouraging rape. You have no right to make sexual violence against women your issue. To people like Susan Brownmiller and Andrea Dworkin, pornography and violence against women are seen as absolutely, intimately linked.

DE: I find myself wondering what the purpose of the antiporn movement is in its own terms. Of course, I'm against violence against women. But I don't feel that I can express my politics toward the violence against women because the only form in which a politics opposed to violence against women is being expressed is antisexual. I'd like to take back the night, and I'd like to go on those marches, and if it's a march through dark and dangerous areas of town, I find that easy to do. But if it's a march through the porn district, then I experience it very much as being directed against the women who work in those districts and as an unnecessary attack on a small zone of some sexual freedom. One thing that became clear to me in writing an article on pornography and working on the porn issue at *Mother Jones* magazine is that the issue pushes people's buttons. They polarize and go to their corners very fast. They're scared of each other and scared of what's really being said. If you criticize the feminist antiporn movement, you very quickly get accused of calling those women prudes. Or you get accused of defending pornography or getting off on pornography, and therefore there's something wrong with you. It's difficult even to create a clearing in which we can have a conversation. I think women are almost at a panic point about violence all the time and are in a place where we are willing to make terrible bargains. We will do anything to be rid of that terror.

AH: When I heard Andrea Dworkin speak, she named my relationship, as a feminist, to porn as a form of being raped. I wanted to say, "Do anything to me, but let me still be alive at the end." I had to smash pornography because, if I didn't, it would take my life. It was not one more position I should understand and debate as a feminist but a life-and-death issue. I went to an antiporn conference because I was very confused about my own position. At the workshops I heard some of the most reactionary politics I've ever heard about how we had to smash pornography and save the family. In fact, it was a radical Right critique, much more so than a Left.

GR: We're all terrorized about a range of possible ways that violence is done to us, whether it's rape or being beat up on the streets or whatever. We're all in the state of severe intimidation, and that's a very powerful and strong feeling. The other strong feeling that is involved is disgust and horror at explicit images of sex. Those images can call up disgust and repulsion in people—especially women—who are not familiar with them. What the antiporn movement has done is to take those very powerful feelings around sex and link them to very powerful feelings around violence and sexual abuse and say it's all the same subject.

We all agree about the problem. We don't agree about the solution— would ending porn have an appreciable effect on rape and violence and abuse? But these connections have been foisted on the movement in a really unprecedented way. I have never seen a position become dogma with so little debate, with so little examination of its possible ramifications or of other perspectives. One reason is that anyone who has tried to raise other issues and who has questioned this analysis has been trashed very quickly as antifeminist or personally attacked. This has also affected the better parts of the Left that of course want to be profeminist.

DE: One of the things women have been taught to help repress us sexually is that, if you begin to deal with sexuality at all, if you begin to become explicit, then you will pay the price of unleashing and stimulating male violence. Once you permit yourself to be perceived as a sexual creature, then you become open territory, open prey. Actual sexual violence oppresses us. But the climate of fear we live in also oppresses us horribly and makes us feel that we cannot afford to take any risks to discover our own sexuality and to be experimental in any way.

GR: Let's look back at what we thought that threat was when we were growing up. Part of the problem is that sex itself is seen as dangerous and violent. It is predicated on a Victorian model of the distribution of libido in terms of male and female. There was the good woman who was not sexual. There is the man who is sexual. So, whenever sex happens between a good woman and a man, it's a kind of violation of her. It's something she doesn't want. The good woman, you know, doesn't move. Her husband, of course, is more of an animal, so he gets off. If you were a good woman and had sex, terrible things might happen to you; good women who had sex out of wedlock became bad women. They fell and became prostitutes, and they were excluded from the comforts of family and home.

This model imposes a moral discourse over a class analysis of who is really doing what sexually. Because the women who were by and large hooking in Victorian England were poor women. And the women who were able to maintain their purity were middle-class women or well-to-do women. And this model scares women into being sexually repressed and gives women the idea (especially respectable women) that sex itself is violence.

AH: It was terrifying that there was so little birth control, which added another element of fear to sex.

GR: I'm not denying that there was a semirational basis for these views.

But I am saying that the notion that sex itself is violent is very much with us. The woman who raised me was raised by a Victorian. We're not that far away from that system. And you have to remember that, in the nineteenth century, great social resources were expended trying to eliminate masturbation under the theory that masturbation caused insanity, disease, and degeneration.

DE: We live in such a strange, transitional time that we bear the marks—we women—of extreme sexual repression, total lack of images of women being motivated by sexual desire. Even predatory women in the movies are motivated by romance, or romantic pathology. But there are few images of healthy, assertive sexuality or lust. Yet at the same time we no longer want to be sexually repressed.

GR: There's a geography of access to certain kinds of sexual and erotic experience. I wouldn't call them liberated zones because they're not. But there really are zones of more and less freedom. For instance, there is the gay community. There are the porn districts, which provide people with a range of experiences they can't get in a suburban family. Part of what the politics of sex is about is respectable society trying to keep those other sectors at bay, keeping them impoverished, keeping the people in them harassed, not letting people know they are there, and generally making sure that they are marginal. That permits an enormous amount of exploitation of the people in them. One of the reasons why women in the sex industry are exploited is because of the police and social pressure on the industry. It means the people in the industry do not have unions, they don't have police protection, and they can't organize to improve the conditions of their work.

Part of the problem is that we use different standards when we talk about sex than we do for almost any other aspect of life. Whatever your analysis of commodities, people are not upset that we have to go and get food. People are upset at the structure of the organizations that provide and produce the food, but the need for food itself is ok. We don't feel that way about sex. We also feel that it's ok to exchange food for some other service. But, when we think about sex, we think that any social exchange of sex is bad other than a romantic one. I don't think this is either a socialist or a feminist idea. I think it's either a Christian or a Victorian idea.

AH: There's an assumption that pornography is only for men and that there is no female counterpart. But that's not true. A recent article argues that there is a female counterpart, in Harlequin romances. This is my experience. I grew up reading those books; I still read them. These were unacceptable for women—romance books where it took 89 pages for a reluctant first kiss and another 120 to get married and a fade-out. The endless pages of tingling skins and the desire to bruise the mouth have never been described as porn. But that's really what they are.

GR: Well, they are, and they aren't. They're turn-on literature for women, but there's no explicit sex in them. They are not literally pornographic in that sense.

AH: But they are a sexual literature.

GR: Yes, and one of the interesting things about them in terms of the antiporn analysis is that the social relations in the Harlequins and the Gothic novels display a basic sexism unparalleled in the culture. There's always a very strong man who sweeps this woman off her feet, and through romance the gender hierarchy is reproduced. Yet I have seen no one marching in the streets to ban the neo-Gothic novel.

DE: I think that the antiporn movement would say that that's OK because they're harmless, that feminists only oppose materials that provoke violence against women.

AH: I could make a strong argument for the potential violence of Harlequin romances around gender and roles.

GR: I think those novels help teach women a structure of fantasy that enables them to participate in unequal social relationships. One response might then be, Well, those novels have to be exchanged, too. What's interesting is that the question of the social reproduction of the emotional and erotic components of gender hierarchy is reduced to the question of sexual materials. Much of the argument against porn says that what's wrong with it is the bad social relations in it. But since there are equally bad social relations in a whole range of other forms, what distinguishes porn from the other media is mainly that it is the explicitly sexual medium.

AH: Absolutely. In the history of women's sexual experiences from the Victorian era, love has been women's sphere, and men's has been sex. So I don't think it's an accident that Harlequin romances are not sexually explicit but create a romantic fantasy life for women while *Hustler* and *Penthouse* purport to be for men. Women also read them, so I don't want to argue that they are only for men. But the industry at least initially was based on a male market and male fantasies.

GR: The industry of sexual fantasy has been sex segregated. The romances are basically oriented toward women, and porn is basically oriented toward men. Having access to sexually explicit material has by and large been a male privilege. Yet, rather than wanting to get rid of it, since women haven't been able to get it, I want women to be able to get it.

AH: Deirdre said something in her article that I agree with. There's still a long way to go to uncover the feminist or prowomen or equal love life. To get there we need nonsexist sexual images. A lot more of them. In short, maybe what we need even more than Women against Pornography (WAP) are women pornographers, or eroticists, if that sounds better.

DE: But that doesn't mean that women will want to create and consume the same sexual imagery that we currently see in the domain of pornography. They might. But they might create something completely different.

GR: Well, we might. And we probably will. But some of the worst and major victims of the antiporn sentiment have been indigenous feminist eroticists. And it's gotten to the point now where, in the women's movement, if anything is sexual, it's immediately considered to be violent. The porn that's available now is not so wonderful or gratifying. I mean, I go to a porn show now, and there's almost nothing that's about my fantasies. I see very few women in blue jeans, very few women with broad shoulders and muscles, standing next to motorcycles, and a whole range of other things I find a turn-on. The fact is that there's not a lot of porn oriented toward minorities of any sort. Gay men probably have the best-produced porn. And one reason gay male porn is better is that a lot of it is produced by gay men and for gay men.

What Is Pornography?

AH: What is pornography? What do we define as pornography?

GR: I have a three-part definition. One, the legal definition, is that it's sexually explicit material designed to arouse prurient interest. I think that definition, at least for this historical time and place, is the most useful one. We should remember that porn is not legal; by this definition material that has no focus but to arouse is not legal. In other words, a sexual aim is not considered legitimate in this culture. But we also need a historical definition; that is, porn as we now know it is widely available, commercial erotica as opposed to the older erotica that was hand produced and was mostly something that rich people collected. In the middle of the last century, mass production of erotic materials started to take place, resulting in the cheap, printed dirty book. Third, I have a sociological definition: pornography is a particular industry located in certain places, with certain kinds of shops which tend to put out a product with certain conventions. One convention, for example, is that a man's orgasm never happens inside the woman. Pornography has a concrete existence that you can define sociologically. But that's not the current, so-called feminist definition of porn.

AH: What's that—"what we don't like is pornographic"?

GR: The definition used in the antiporn movement is that pornography is violence against women and that violence against women is pornography. There are several problems with this. One is a replacement of the institutional forms of violence with representations of violence. That is to say, there's been a conflating of images with the thing itself. People really don't talk about the institutions; they talk about the images. Images are important, but they're not the whole thing.

Actually, if you walk into an adult bookstore, 90 percent of the material you will see is frontal nudity, intercourse, and oral sex, with no hint of violence or coercion. There are specialty porns. There's gay male porn; that's a big subgenre. There used to be a genre of porn that featured young people, although that's now so illegal that you don't see it anymore. And there is a genre of porn that caters to sadomasochists, which is the porn that they focus on when you see a WAVPM (Women against Violence in Pornography and Media) or a WAP slide show. They show the worst possible porn and claim it's representative of all of it. The two images that they show most are sadomasochistic porn and images of violence that contain sex. For instance, the infamous *Hustler* cover with the woman being shoved through a meat grinder. An awful picture, but by no means a common image in pornography.

DE: It was self-parody. It was gross, but it was actually satirical, a self-critical joke, which a lot of people didn't get.

GR: They include images that are not pornographic that you cannot find in an adult bookstore. For instance, the stuff on billboards, the stuff on record covers, the stuff in *Vogue*. None of it has explicit sexual content. At most, it's covert. And what they do is draw in images they consider to be violent, or coercive, or demeaning, and call that pornography. That definition enables them to avoid the empirical question of how much porn is really violent. Their analysis is that the violent images come out of porn and into the culture at large, that sexism comes from porn into the culture. Whereas it seems to me that pornography only reflects as much sexism as is in the culture.

The existence of S/M porn enabled this whole analysis to proceed. It's very disturbing to most people and contains scenes that most people don't even want to encounter in their lives. They don't realize that S/M porn is about fantasy. What most people do with it is take it home and masturbate. Those people who do S/M are consensually acting out fantasies: the category of people who read and use S/M porn and the category of violent rapists are not the same. We used to talk about how religion and the state and the family create sexism and promote rape. No one talks about any of these institutions anymore. They've become the good guys!

AH: And now pornography creates sexism and violence against women.

DE: One of the things that has amazed me, and I don't know what to make of it, is that many antiporn activists see red if they hear you say that the violent porn is a minority within the whole industry. They would just not agree with you. Now, when I went into those bookstores, I saw basically what you see. And I agree with your description.

GR: When I went on the WAVPM tour, everybody went, and I stood in front of the bondage material. It was like they had on blinders. And I said, Look, there's oral sex over there! Why don't you look at that? And they were glued to the bondage rack. I started pulling out female dominance magazines and saying, "Look, here's a woman dominating a man. What about that? Here's a woman who's tied up a man. What about that?" It was like I wasn't there. People said, "Look at this picture of a woman being tied up!"

AH: Another example in the WAVPM slide show, there will be an image from a porn magazine of a woman tied up, beaten, right? And they'll say, *Hustler* magazine, 1976, and you're struck dumb by it, horrified! The next slide will be a picture of a woman with a police file, badly beaten by her husband. And the rap that connects these two is that the image of the woman tied and bruised in the pornographic magazine caused the beating that she suffered. The talk implies that her husband went and saw that picture, then came home and tried to re-create it in their bedroom. That is the guilt-by-association theory of pornography and violence. And I remember sitting and watching this slide show and being freaked out about both of those images and having nowhere to react to the analysis and say, What the hell is going on? I found it incredibly manipulative.

GR: Some of the antiporn people are looking at material that is used in a particular subculture with a particular meaning and a particular set of conventions and saying, It doesn't mean what it means to the people who are using it. It means what *we* see! They're assuming that they know better than the people who are familiar with it. They're assuming, for example, that S/M is violent, and that analysis leads to the view that S/M people can't be the victims of violence.

AH: It also discourages anyone from making explicit any sexual fantasy which seems risky to them or from exploring a sexual terrain that's not familiar. It ignores the fact that you learn what you like and what you don't like through trying things out. What it says is that these forbidden desires are not yours but imposed on you. You never experiment sexually.

Yet most people know goddamn well that their sex lives are wider than those standard notions let them play in. They may feel guilty about it, but they know it. So they don't need one more movement to tell them that they can't play.

GR: Anal sex is a real good example, I think, of some of the ways that this all works. It can seem like the most appalling thing in the world, so unpleasant that your idea is that no one else would find it pleasant unless they were coerced into it. And therefore all anal sex is a form of coercion or rape. And the truth is that anal sex for some people is pleasurable and it is not always done under duress. That's true of almost all of the sexual variations. What's one person's horror show is another person's delight.

The Politics of Pornography
AH: In fact, some women working in the antiporn movement would agree with us about opening up sexual possibilities for women but still believe that pornography is the link with violence against women.

GR: Sure, there are differences in that movement. I just think that they have to be held accountable for the social impact of the politics they're promulgating. I think that to focus on porn as a solution to the problem of violence is wrong. It won't substantially reduce the amount of violence against women. Porn may not be the most edifying form of sexual material that we can image, but it is the most available sexual material. To attack that is ultimately going to reduce the amount of social space available to talk about sex in an explicit way.

DE: I think we're being too uncritical of porn. Your definition of porn is probably more positive than the way pornography functions for a lot of people. It's important to point out that a great deal of pornography is deeply sexist and that it contains a hideous and misogynistic view of women.

GR: It also contains a hideous view of sexual minorities, including the people who do all the stuff the antiporn movement is so upset by, including S/M.

DE: And the constant repetition of those sexist images of women does validate the sexism of sexist people who buy and consume it.

GR: So does the TV they watch.

DE: Yes.

GR: And the novels they read.

DE: Yes, and everything else. But there may be nothing in their lives that ever says to consumers of pornography, that shows that violence against women is a fantasy, that women don't really want to be raped or brutalized. They may never really get the message that porn depicts behavior that is in fact not acceptable to women. And that is a serious problem.

GR: I disagree. I think there is a serious problem with pornography when it does not challenge sexism, racism, homophobia, or antivariation bigotry. But again, while there is sexism in all porn and there are violent images from a variety of media sources, there is not a whole lot of violent porn per se.

AH: Then let's really talk about sexist porn.

GR: OK. I have no objection to being critical of the content of porn, or creating nonsexist porn, and having better sex education, and talking to men about what women really want sexually. But that has not been the agenda of the antiporn movement.

DE: All right. But I want to stress that we are strongly speaking for an antisexist movement, in every domain of society.

AH: Pornography is not the first thing to worry about in trying to go to the root of the things that destroy, brutalize, and murder women.

DE: Right. I don't think I'd try to change pornography first. What I'm trying to say is that what's very important is that there be a strong antisexist movement as a point of reference. For example, women should be able to enjoy, say, masochistic pornography or dominance and submission fantasies in a safe context. But there should also be a source of support, a movement saying that that does not mean that women want to be beaten up.

GR: Absolutely. But the fact that we have a movement against sexism does not mean that the movement is always wise or alert to the real sources of distress that people feel. For two or three years now, ever since Anita Bryant, there has been an enormous increase in police activity and state repression against all these parts of the sexual world that are not mainstream. The cost to the people who've been beaten up and who've gone to jail and lost their livelihoods is immense. There is an insidious moral blindness to this reality in the women's movement, one encouraged by the antiporn line. Two resolutions that were recently passed disturb me. One is a resolution passed by the National Organization for Women (NOW) in 1980 that reaffirms NOW's support for lesbian rights but specifically says that public sex, pederasty, S/M, and pornography are issues of violence, not of sexual preference. These are specifically excluded from the definition of a lesbian or gay group that now would work with. The second resolution was passed by the National Lawyers Guild, a resolution against porn based on all the analyses we've been talking about, saying that it is violence against women. It encourages the members of the guild not to defend people who are arrested on porn charges and to defend people who are arrested doing antiporn work. This isolates the victims of repression from support and delivers them up to the state.

AH: These resolutions close off the only areas in which some of these victims of repression could hope to find support. They need to be placed in a context, which is the reification of the nuclear family and a new emphasis on male-dominated, heterosexual marriage as the only sexual model. And when the feminist movement focuses on pornography rather than the violence of institutions like marriage and enforced heterosexuality and a variety of other things, it endangers its own future.

DE: But I think that it's very important for us to have a critique of sexist pornography as well as a critique of the antiporn movement.

GR: But issues that are very important to me have been compromised by bad politics. I would love to go, as you were saying earlier, Deirdre, on a march to take back the night and demonstrate against violence. But I would not like to go on an antiporn march. I would love to talk more about the whole issue of the way that the media are involved in the social reproduction of sexism. There are things being promoted in the name of feminist ideology that are destructive. I don't want a viable and powerful women's movement to create social havoc rather than social good! Many social movements had wonderful intentions but left a dreadful legacy. And we're not magically an exception to that.

AH: What we began talking about and what I hope we end on is that this is an opening up of the discussion that will allow us to figure out what these questions are. We're not really arguing that everything we're saying is correct, but the feminist movement has got to allow a wider discussion of all sorts of sexual issues and what they are and how they combine.

PART V

Homosexuality

• • •

Changes in attitudes toward homosexuality—primarily among homosexuals themselves (the term "gay" was not widely used by homosexuals at the time, "queer" was more commonly used)—had begun during World War II, when many American men and women, away from their families and communities, and amassed in wartime same-sex environments, discovered their sexual desires for those of their own sex. After the war, the first efforts to organize homosexuals were undertaken—in Los Angeles, Chicago, and New York—by war veterans. In 1951, Donald Webster Cory published his groundbreaking book, *The Homosexual in America* in which he declared that "homosexuals constitute what can be termed the unrecognized minority. . . . Our minority status is similar, in a variety of respects, to that of national, religious, and other ethnic groups: in the denial of civil liberties; in the legal, extra-legal, and quasi-legal discrimination; in the assignment of an inferior social position; in the exclusion from the mainstream of life and culture." The homophile movement that emerged from these efforts did not attempt to promote a coherent homosexual culture, but instead, it worked within the postwar liberal consensus to educate the American public that homosexuals were neither criminals nor mentally ill degenerates.

In 1969, a police raid on a Greenwich Village bar called the Stonewall Inn provoked a series of riots that mobilized drag queens, street hustlers, lesbians and gay men, many of whom had been politicized by the movement against the war in Vietnam. There were already many signs that homosexuals were in the process of creating a civil rights movement, inspired, in part, by the black struggles of the sixties, but the Stonewall riots of 1969 crystallized a broad grass-roots mobilization across the country. The movement that emerged after Stonewall resulted from a clash of two cultures and two generations— the underground homosexual subculture of the fifties and sixties and the radical politics and counterculture of sixties youth.

The homosexual culture of the fifties and early sixties reflected its bitter consciousness of the oppressive stigma against homosexuality in its flamboyant, irony-charged camp humor, but it was not political. Fifties gay culture was invested in protecting the "secret" of an individual's homosexuality and expressing it only in a symbolic or heavily-coded way. Cultural resistance to the heterosexual norm was expressed through cross-gender performances and sex role-playing. The new gay liberationists, however, had little appreciation of traditional gay and lesbian life of the 1950s and the sixties. Instead of protecting "secrecy" as the right to privacy, gay liberationists gave political meaning to "coming out" by extending the psychological-personal process into public life. To "come out of the closet" was to do the very thing most feared in the gay and lesbian culture of the 1950s. By putting "coming out" at the center of its political strategy, the gay liberation movement tended to mobilize those people who felt more emotionally committed to living a full-time life as homosexuals rather than those who experienced homosexual desire only sporadically, or who experienced desire for both men and women.

Very early in the 1970s, impatient with gay men's lack of interest in women's issues, many lesbians left the gay organizations to focus on feminist politics. Thereafter, at least until the early eighties, there remained a certain separate and parallel development between lesbian social/political activities and those of gay men. Lesbian-feminism was the most thoroughly developed political philosophy to emerge from the heady days of early feminism and gay liberation— it was both a theory and a politics of lesbian identity. It was first publicly articulated in 1970 in the pamphlet "The Woman-Identified Woman" published by Radicalwomen (some of whom had been active in the Gay Liberation Front, founded in 1969) and elaborated more fully in Jill Johnston's *Lesbian Nation*. Through a series of popular and provocative essays and books lesbian-feminist writers created an intellectual and political framework that offered bold and vigorous interpretations of feminist politics, pornography, rape, lesbian culture and history.

The gay and lesbian movement did not at first focus on the question of identity or even strictly on civil rights—though black civil rights was, most certainly, on the political horizon—but on sexual liberation. The sexual revolution, along with the student anti-war movement which had mobilized millions of Americans against the war in Vietnam, influenced how gay activists framed their political struggles.

Revolt of the Homosexual

Seymour Krim

from *Views of a Nearsighted Cannoneer*, 1968

*This is one of the earliest sightings of the "new homosexual" which emerged in full force only after the Stonewall riots of 1969. Seymour Krim was New York based journalist and writer. He was the editor of **The Nugget**, a softcore men's magazine, and wrote for the **Village Voice** and Barney Rosset's **Evergreen Review**. A native New Yorker, Krim was closely associated with the Beats and published one of the first anthologies of their works as well as three books of his own work—**Views of a Nearsighted Cannoneer, You and Me**, and **Shake it for the World, Smartass**.*

STRAIGHT GUY: You say I can talk frankly to you sans the usual bullshit. O.K. Why have so many fairies come out in the open recently? Wherever I go I run into them—the Village, East Side, Harlem, even the Bronx. The whole thing seems to have exploded like a queer Mount Vesuvius.

HOMOSEXUAL: We no longer have the energy to hide, baby. You can't know the strain on a person in always pretending. As Donald Webster Cory says in *The Homosexual in America*, we have been the great unrecognized minority. That time is ending. We want recognition for our simple human rights, just like Negroes, Jews, and women. That's little enough to ask!

SG: You actually think you'll be accepted on your own terms?

H: Certainly. For years homosexuals in this country have cringed behind a mask of fear. Legally they're criminals, morally they're considered perverted, psychologically they've tortured themselves.

Courageous gay people are now beginning to realize that they are human beings who must fight to gain acceptance for what they are— not what others want them to be.

SG: Let me be blunt. Do you think it does your cause any good to see platinum-haired freaks swishing along 8th Street screaming at the top of their voices? Are you naive enough to believe the rest of us see anything sympathetic in this?

H: You're the naive one because your experience is limited. Such homosexuals are in the minority, as much as a camping chick compared with most women.

SG: But you'll admit that most homosexuals are much more effeminate in their actions than ordinary men?

H: I doubt that modern psychology concedes such a thing as an ordinary man or woman. But let that pass. It's true, I think, that we are more esthetic or perhaps outwardly fastidious than most men. But then it's been pointed out that American women have become increasingly vigorous. Does this make them any less female?

SG: Not necessarily, though my ego would like it better if they were more dewey. But they still go for men, not their own kind.

H: That's not completely true. Many women have a deep hatred for the presumption of superiority that the modern straight man puts on.

SG: I won't argue with you. The important thing is that the essential sexual need for each other is still there and will remain. It may sound obvious, but God or nature obviously intended men and women to make it with each other.

H: That seems logical on the surface. But when you look at history you'll see that there's never been a culture without homosexuality. It's always existed: among the Greeks, Romans, even the American Indians. I believe it is a fundamental part of human life.

SG: Then why do you think it's always been outlawed? I'm fairly sophisticated, but I believe society had no choice in condemning sodomy. Let's face it: if homosexuality were encouraged the family would disintegrate, a farce would be made of every moral principle on which we were raised, and the perpetuation of life itself could conceivably be endangered.

H: Editorial-page gas! The human race can certainly withstand a comparative handful of homosexuals if it's going to survive. Nuclear weapons are obviously a much closer threat. As for the family's falling apart, homosexuality is only one tiny cause among hundreds for the tension people have in living with each other today. I have little sympathy for your so-called moral principles. Morals change as we view life differently, and it's right that we abandon them when we can no longer see their truth.

SG: Maybe you can't see their truth. But millions of people still have hopes for leading some kind of traditional life—with families, children, and the rest of the bit.

H: I have nothing but good will toward such people. But nothing gives them the right to impose their desires on human beings who can't or don't want to follow the same goals. It's hypocrisy to pretend that we live in a Victorian world or even one with agreed-upon values.

SG: Is it Victorian to wish for a complete life? People like yourself are amputated and therefore make bitter fun of it. But the majority of us still have the possibility of getting normal satisfactions out of living.

H: No one is preventing you. I personally think you're deluding yourself in pretending a normality which no longer exists. But that's only my private opinion. I merely want my own freedom to behave as I choose and must.

SG: Didn't it ever occur to you that you might be literally sick? Suppose I were a compulsive murderer and said I wanted my own freedom to behave as I had to. You'd smile and have me locked up.

H: But homosexuals murder nothing except a preconception of what people are supposed to be. Certainly it's occurred to me that I'm "sick," in your handy word. Every minority person in America feels this pressure, sometimes to the screaming-point. In fact I was in therapy for almost four years, examining every angle of my so-called problem.

SG: Well?

H: I came to the conclusion that I was different, not sick. Under the analyst's guidance I dated women and even went to bed with several. But our love-making, the techniques, ended up exactly as my experience with men; I could become passionate no other way. I even imagined they were boys during the whole thing. Believe me, I tried incredibly hard to act straight. But it finally just seemed a tortured attempt to be something I'm not.

SG: What did your psychiatrist say?

H: At first he said my fantasying of men when I was with a woman was a reflection of how deep-seated my problem was. He maintained it could be "cured" and told me he'd had success before. But when I tirelessly tried to suppress my desire for men, and it came upon me anyway, he finally conceded that I would be less miserable as a homosexual. The rest of the therapy tried to blot out the guilt that I and all gay people feel for not being permitted to express ourselves.

SG: Then he finally did say you were abnormal, or sick, but had to make the best of it—correct?

H: Yes. But I myself was beginning to realize for the first time in my life that I was only sick in relation to a majority standard.

SG: But your analyst didn't agree with you. And most psychiatrists would say that homosexuality is a fixation at an infantile level and represents a sadly distorted and undeveloped personality.

H: I'd find a moral judgment in such a generalization rather than the modest impersonality that's supposed to distinguish science. Undeveloped by what standard? I once read that Carl Sandburg was an "undeveloped Walt Whitman"—and Walt, of course, was gay. So who's infantile there? You use the words "sadly distorted"—in comparison to what? A fantasy of the ideal arrow-collar man or the imperfect flesh-and-booze mortals whom we both know? I've discovered that much psychiatric language is based on a too-pure and debatable ideal of what people should be like. If you lowered the ideal to the actual reality around us, you wouldn't be so pious about the homosexual.

SG: That's a defensive argument. The standards that psychiatry uses are rationally established after scrupulous and neutral research.

H: Nuts! Many psychiatrists use conventional middle-class American ideals of psychological well-being as their standard. There is nothing universal about them. They merely happen to reflect the majority attitudes at this time. In the future you'll see the equally suave acknowledgment of different standards, including the right of the homosexual to fully express himself as a "healthy" individual in terms of his tradition.

SG: Do you actually think society will give up its basic distinctions of right and wrong, a working separation between normality and abnormality, just to accommodate the guilt of homosexuals?

H: It must: Homosexuals have submitted too weakly until now to judgments from above. We now know that what you call society actually gets down to individuals in positions of social power, who call the tune and set the standards. Many of us are no longer willing to put up with this degrading of our personalities. Merely to live, we must assert ourselves as homosexuals who are as proud to be what we are as you are of yourself. When this movement becomes powerful enough—and gay people refuse either to hide or flaunt themselves—it will be openly accepted.

sg: You're kidding yourself if you believe that what's always been recognized as the number-one human perversion will suddenly be completely whitewashed.

h: What is a perversion? Truly modern people find it hard to see the idea of perversion in any kind of sex relationship. The entire concept is beginning to die as people realize that whatever can be done with the body is ultimately just and natural if it gives pleasure without causing harm. Be realistic. Why is it any worse for a man to perform oral intercourse with another man instead of with a woman? Or for two women to do so, instead of woman and man? Or for two men to masturbate each other instead of being played with by a woman? Do you think our organs themselves are prejudiced and draw a line? You moralize, but you don't have the courage to carry your logic to the end.

sg: Listen: homosexuality is obviously a substitute for the regular thing. You never mention this at all. Why do men dress up in women's clothes and act as if they were girls? Can't you see that by any standard there's nothing healthy or defensible about such an obvious distortion of what a man was made for?

h: Was a man made to incinerate thousands of his fellow-creatures? To cook them in ovens, make lampshades of their skin, bury them alive? If that is what a man was made for, I decline the honor. You set up an ideal of manhood *which doesn't exist in the modern world* and then you beat homosexuals over the head with it. I see nothing more manly in spitting, cursing, abusing women, being tasteless and animalistic in your appetites than in making love to a man you admire. Why does manhood have to be defined by who you sleep with rather than your intelligence and ability? As for women's clothes, most gay men are not queens who wear drag. But if this is the pleasure of some why should it offend you any more than the thousands of women who wear slacks?

It seems obvious to me that if American women see an appeal in men's clothes and mannerisms there is nothing shameful in the imaginative man wanting to behave like a woman occasionally. Several straight men have told me secretly that they enjoy this dressing up. Instead of seeing them as effeminate—to use your word—I see it as a natural desire to experience another dimension of life.

SG: You keep trying to wipe out sexual differences and pretend there are no basic distinctions between men and women. I'm convinced you do this because it gives you an excuse to act like a woman.

H: I doubt if there's a man alive who doesn't feel "womanly" at some time, if you mean responsive, tender, sweet, even cuddly. The old categories of man being Mars and a woman Venus are artificial: only insensitive people or poseurs pretend to a cartoon image of masculinity vs. femininity. I'm not wiping out sexual differences. Social change itself has softened the dividing line. It was once considered mannish for women to drive a car, smoke on the street, drink at a bar, earn an independent buck. We laugh at this today. Those who come after us will laugh at the pressures once put upon men to keep up a front of endless courage, indifference to delicacy, superiority over women. If I prefer gentleness to harshness, I'm not being a woman. I'm being human—something you might be ashamed of with your straight jacket notion of masculinity.

SG: You mean because I don't mince, I'm a barbarian? Because I don't simper or speak in a falsetto or try to goose a waiter I'm behind the times? Yeah, I'm a brute. I like women, steak, baseball, poker and bourbon. Maybe I'll be arrested in this beautiful future of yours.

H: In my future you'd merely be seen as a person of limited tastes. But I don't want to be arrested in your present for liking men, coq au vin, Modigliani, bridge and dry sherry! You're smug in your superiority to the homosexual because you have average tastes while mine are comparatively rare. You use the word normal to congratulate your averageness and the word abnormal to smear my individuality. You look down on myself and other homosexuals as being freakish or repulsive because our way of life is foreign to you—like a schoolboy who throws rocks at a synagogue window. You refuse to see beyond our uniqueness to our *universality* just as your grandfather and great-grandfathers choked the life out of the minorities of their time. Your limited standards of health and law have made us outcasts or psychological wrecks, hypocrites forced to smile and swallow our human pride when any of the usual jokes and abuses are made. But I tell you in complete honesty that this pathetic half-existence of homosexuals is ending because we will no longer accept your version of ourselves.

sg: And I tell you that your only chance for a decent life is that in the future a method of treatment will be devised which will catch the young homosexual and iron out the mother-dependency that cripples him.

h: And I say thank God that some people are forever deprived of so-called normality so that they can one day see how shallow and intolerant it is! When homosexuality achieves legitimacy, it will be seen as a branch of a river rather than a contamination of the source. When it is given unity, homosexual culture will be seen as constituting a unique view of experience, offering insights to all people. The homosexuality of great figures of the past—not only your Prousts and Whitmans—will be revealed, as Byron's is beginning to be, and he the outstanding popular symbol of the Don Juan! All the dearly-bought insight that has come out of a closed-door suffering which can no longer bear its isolation will be given to society at large.

sg: I can't see this occurring in my lifetime. No matter how wetly liberal I ever get I'll always see homosexuality as antimasculine, perverse, a short-circuit of nature's obvious logic in creating two sexes. And a pathological Star of David for those who have to carry it.

h: You're the crude prisoner of what you think is your honesty. We live in a torn-open age where each minority is determined to proclaim itself as good as the self-appointed judges of a life *which no longer provides a rational basis for their prejudices.* We homosexuals will be in the leadership of this revolt with this phrase of Wilhelm Reich's as a motto: "That which is alive is in itself reasonable. It becomes a caricature when it is not allowed to live."

sg: You make it sound like a holy crusade when you really feel inside—from what sensitive faggots have told me—that you're miserable and almost unworthy to live. You'll excuse my so-called crude honesty!

h: But that's the point. We've finally rebelled against feeling this way because our human nature can no longer stand it. Look out for people whom you have driven to such an extreme! We refuse to live any longer as exotic pets. We refuse to be discriminated against in job situations and in the Army and Navy. We refuse to be fired from government service as "security risks" and then have *The New York Times* not print the details. We refuse to marry in order to disguise what we are, and we refuse to pretend any longer to enjoy a heterosexuality that is foreign to most of us. Life is too fast and mad today for us to accept old-fashioned, socially-induced suffering. But accept it or not, we will force our way into open society and you will have to acknowledge us. From 5 to 10 million American adults—at least—are not going to be treated like animals or freaks because *we are no longer going to accept your evaluation of us.* Sweetie, remember my words when the showdown comes!

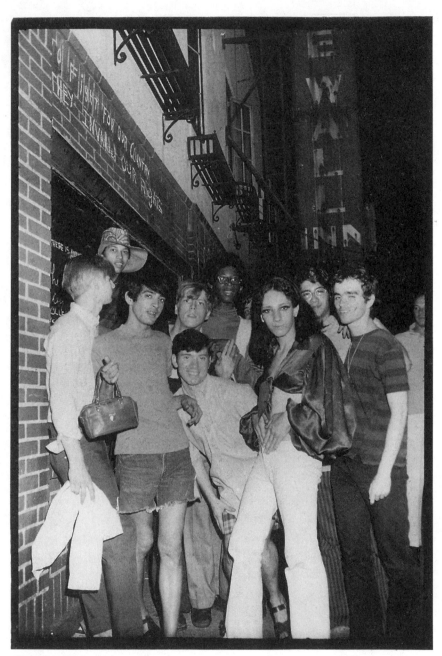

© Fred W. McDarrah

The Homosexual Villain

Norman Mailer

From *Advertisements for Myself*, 1963

*Norman Mailer was one of most promising and important novelists to come out of World War II. The author of a best-selling war novel, **The Naked and the Dead**, he was also known as a brawler and frequently adopted a macho posture. In 1954, **One** magazine, a small homosexual publication based in Los Angeles, asked Mailer to write something for it. He resisted the idea but finally ended up writing on the homosexual villain in his work—it is an interesting reflection on his own prejudices and what made him realize that he needed to confront the subject of homosexuality as a test of his masculinity.*

Some time back in the early fifties, a group of young men in Los Angeles started a homosexual magazine called One. To attract attention they sent free copies of the magazine and a personal letter out to a horde of big and little celebrities including Bishop Fulton Sheen, Eleanor Roosevelt, Tennessee Williams, Arthur Miller, and fifty-eight others including myself. It was an arresting idea. The top of the letterhead flared the legend: One—the Homosexual Magazine, and like a pile of chips on the left margin, we worthies had our names banked, as if we were sponsors. "Dear Norman Mailer" went my letter. "On the left you will see your name listed. You are one of those prominent Americans whom we are seeking to interest in our magazine, so that you might help us to dispel public ignorance and hostility on the subject." And the letter went on to invite us to contribute to the magazine. (I quote it from memory.) About a month later, this letter was followed by a phone call—the New York secretary of the organization called me up to say that he didn't know just what I had to do with all this, but out on *the West Coast they had asked him to get in touch with me because I might be able to write for them.*

I didn't know the first thing about homosexuality I hurried to tell him.

Well, the secretary assured me (he had a high-pitched folksy voice) he could understand how I felt about the whole matter, but he could assure Mr. Mailer it was really a very simple matter, Mr. Mailer could say what he wished to say under a pseudonym.

"I told you," I said, "I don't know anything about the subject. I hardly even know any homosexuals."

"Well, Lordy-me," said the secretary, "I could introduce you to a good many of us, Mr. Mailer, and you would see what interesting problems we have."

"No . . . now look."

"Mr. Mailer, wouldn't you at least say that you're sympathetic to the aims of the magazine?"

"Well, I suppose the police laws against homosexuals are bad, and all that. I guess homosexuality is a private matter."

"Would you say that for us?"

"It's not a new idea."

"Mr. Mailer, I can understand that a man with your name and reputation wouldn't want to get mixed up with such dangerous ideas."

He was right. I was ready to put my name to any radical statement, my pride was that I would say in print anything I believed, and yet I was not ready to say a word in public defense of homosexuals.

So I growled at the New York secretary of One magazine, "If I were to write something about homosexuality, I would sign my name to it."

"You would, Mr. Mailer? Listen, I must tell you, by the most conservative statistics, we estimate there are ten million homosexuals in this country. We intend to get a lobby and in a few years we expect to be able to elect our own Congressman. If you write an article for us, Mr. Mailer, why then you might become our first Congressman!"

I cannot remember the secretary's name, but he had a small knifelike talent—he knew the way to me: mate the absurd with the apocalyptic, and I was a captive. So before our conversation was over, I had promised to write an article for One magazine.

It is printed here. I delayed for months getting down to it, my mood would be depressed whenever I remembered my promise, I writhed at what the gossip would be—for every reader who saw my piece there would be ten or a hundred who would hear that Mailer was writing for a faggot magazine. It would be taken for granted I was homosexual—how disagreeable! I used to wish that One *magazine would fail, and be gone forever.*

Then the New York secretary had a fight with the West Coast. He wrote me a letter in which he advised me not to write the piece after all. Since he was my connection to the magazine, I was set free from my promise. Yet I took the step of writing to the editors to ask them if they still wanted an article from me. Not surprisingly, they did. I got their answer in Mexico, and in a flat dutiful mood I sat down and wrote "The Homosexual Villain." It is beyond a doubt the worst article I have ever written, conventional, empty, pious, the quintessence of the Square. Its intellectual level would place it properly in the pages of the Reader's Digest, *and if the* Reader's Digest *had a desire to be useful at their doubtfully useful level they would have scored a Square coup by reprinting it, for the article has a satisfactory dullness of thought which comes from writing in a state of dull anxiety.*

Now, it is easier to understand why I did this piece. The Deer Park *was then in galleys at Rinehart, and I was depressed about it. Apart from its subject, I thought it a timid inhibited book. I must have known that my fear of homosexuality as a subject was stifling my creative reflexes, and given the brutal rhythms of my nature, I could kill this inhibition only by jumping into the middle of the problem without any clothes. Done gracefully this can stop the show, but I was clumsy and constipated and sick with the bravery of my will, and so "The Homosexual Villain" while honorable as a piece of work, is dressed in the gray of lugubrious caution.*

Yet it was important for my particular growth. The gray prose in "The Homosexual Villain" was the end of easy radical rhetoric—I knew I had nothing interesting to say about homosexuality because the rational concepts of socialism, nicely adequate to writing about the work of David Riesman, were not related to the ills of the homosexual. No, for that one had to dig— deep into the complex and often foul pots of thought where sex and society live in their murderous dialectic. Writing "The Homosexual Villain" showed me how barren I was of new ideas, and so helped to blow up a log jam of accumulated timidities and restraints, of caution for my good name. Later when I was back in New York, my mind running wild in the first fevers of self-analysis, I came to spend some months and some years with the endless twists of habit and defeat which are latent homosexuality for so many of us, and I came to understand myself, and become maybe a little more of a man, although it's too soon to brag on it, for being a man is the continuing battle of one's life, and one loses a bit of manhood with every stale compromise to the authority of any power in which one does not believe. Which is a part of the explanation for the tenacity of organized faith, patriotism and respect for society. But that is another essay, and here is "The Homosexual Villain."

Those readers of *One* who are familiar with my work may be somewhat surprised to find me writing for this magazine. After all, I have been as guilty as any contemporary novelist in attributing unpleasant, ridiculous, or sinister connotations to the homosexual (or more accurately, bisexual) characters in my novels. Part of the effectiveness of General Cummings in *The Naked and The Dead*—at least for those people who thought him well-conceived as a character—rested on the homosexuality I was obviously suggesting as the core of much of his motivation. Again, in *Barbary Shore,* the "villain" was a secret police agent named Leroy Hollingsworth whose sadism and slyness were essentially combined with his sexual deviation.

At the time I wrote those novels, I was consciously sincere. I did believe—as so many heterosexuals believe—that there was an intrinsic relation between homosexuality and "evil," and it seemed perfectly natural to me, as well as *symbolically* just, to treat the subject in such a way.

The irony is that I did not know a single homosexual during all those years. I had met homosexuals of course, I had recognized a few as homosexual, I had "suspected" others, I was to realize years later that one or two close friends were homosexual, but I had never known one in the human sense of knowing, which is to look at your friend's feelings through his eyes and not your own. I did not *know* any homosexual because obviously I did not want to. It was enough for me to recognize someone as homosexual, and I would cease to consider him seriously as a person. He might be intelligent or courageous or kind or witty or virtuous or tortured—no matter. I always saw him as at best ludicrous and at worst—the word again—sinister. (I think it is by the way significant that just as many homosexuals feel forced and are forced to throw up protective camouflage, even boasting if necessary of women they have had, not to mention the thousand smaller subtleties, so heterosexuals are often eager to be so deceived for it enables them to continue friendships which otherwise their prejudices and occasionally their fears might force them to terminate.)

Now, of course, I exaggerate to a certain degree. I was never a roaring bigot, I did not go in for homosexual-baiting, at least not face to face, and I never could stomach the relish with which soldiers would describe how they had stomped some faggot in a bar. I had, in short, the equivalent of a "gentleman's anti-Semitism."

The only thing remarkable about all this is that I was hardly living in a small town. New York, whatever its pleasures and discontents, is not the most uncivilized milieu, and while one would go too far to say that its attitude toward homosexuals bears correspondence to the pain of the liberal or radical at hearing someone utter a word like "nigger" or "kike," there is nonetheless considerable tolerance and considerable propinquity. The hard and fast separations of homosexual and heterosexual society are often quite blurred. Over the past seven or eight years I had had more than enough opportunity to learn something about homosexuals if I had wanted to, and obviously I did not.

It is a pity I do not understand the psychological roots of my change of attitude, for something valuable might be learned from it. Unfortunately, I do not. The process has seemed a rational one to me, rational in that the impetus apparently came from reading and not from any important personal experiences. The only hint of my bias mellowing was that my wife and I had gradually become friendly with a homosexual painter who lived next door. He was pleasant, he was thoughtful, he was a good neighbor, and we came to depend on him in various small ways. It was tacitly understood that he was homosexual, but we never talked about it. However, since so much of his personal life was not discussable between us, the friendship was limited. I accepted him the way a small-town banker fifty years ago might have accepted a "good" Jew.

About this time I received a free copy of *One* which was sent out by the editors to a great many writers. I remember looking at the magazine with some interest and some amusement. Parts of it impressed me unfavorably. I thought the quality of writing generally poor (most people I've talked to agree that it has since improved), and I questioned the wisdom of accepting suggestive ads in a purportedly serious magazine. (Indeed, I still feel this way no matter what the problems of revenue might be.) But there was a certain militancy and honesty to the editorial tone, and while I was not sympathetic, I think I can say that for the first time in my life I was not unsympathetic. Most important of all, my curiosity was piqued. A few weeks later I asked my painter friend if I could borrow his copy of Donald Webster Cory's *The Homosexual in America*.

Reading it was an important experience. Mr. Cory strikes me as being a modest man, and I think he would be the first to admit that while his book is very good, closely reasoned, quietly argued, it is hardly a great book. Nonetheless, I can think of few books which cut so radically at my prejudices and altered my ideas so profoundly. I resisted it, I argued its points as I read, I was often annoyed, but what I could not overcome was my growing depression that I had been acting as a bigot in this matter, and "bigot" was one word I did not enjoy applying to myself. With that came the realization I had been closing myself off from understanding a very large part of life. This thought is always disturbing to a writer. A writer has his talent, and for all one knows, he is born with it, but whether his talent develops is to some degree responsive to his use of it. He can grow as a person or he can shrink, and by this I don't intend any facile parallels between moral and artistic growth. The writer can become a bigger hoodlum if need be, but his alertness, his curiosity, his reaction to life must not diminish. The fatal thing is to shrink, to be interested in less, sympathetic to less, desiccating to the point where life itself loses its flavor, and one's passion for human understanding changes to weariness and distaste.

So, as I read Mr. Cory's book, I found myself thinking in effect, *My God, homosexuals are people, too.* Undoubtedly, this will seem incredibly naïve to the homosexual readers of *One* who have been all too painfully aware that they are indeed people, but prejudice is wed to naïveté, and even the sloughing of prejudice, particularly when it is abrupt, partakes of the naïve. I have not tried to conceal that note. As I reread this article I find its tone ingenuous, but there is no point in trying to alter it. One does not become sophisticated overnight about a subject one has closed from oneself.

At any rate I began to face up to my homosexual bias. I had been a libertarian socialist for some years, and implicit in all my beliefs had been the idea that society must allow every individual his own road to discovering himself. Libertarian socialism (the first word is as important as the second) implies inevitably that one have respect for the varieties of human experience. Very basic to everything I had thought was that sexual relations, above everything else, demand their liberty, even if such liberty should amount to no more than compulsion or necessity. For, in the reverse, history has certainly offered enough examples of the link between sexual repression and political repression. (A fascinating thesis on this subject is *The Sexual Revolution* by Wilhelm Reich.) I suppose I can say that for the first time I understood homosexual persecution to be a political act and a reactionary act, and I was properly ashamed of myself.

On the positive side, I found over the next few months that a great deal was opening to me—to put it briefly, even crudely, I felt that I understood more about people, more about life. My life-view had been shocked and the lights and shadows were being shifted, which is equal to saying that I was learning a great deal. At a perhaps embarrassingly personal level, I discovered another benefit. There is probably no sensitive heterosexual alive who is not preoccupied at one time or another with his latent homosexuality, and while I had no conscious homosexual desires, I had wondered more than once if really there were not something suspicious in my intense dislike of homosexuals. How pleasant to discover that once one can accept homosexuals as real friends, the tension is gone with the acceptance. I found that I was no longer concerned with latent homosexuality. It seemed vastly less important, and paradoxically enabled me to realize that I am actually quite heterosexual. Close friendships with homosexuals had become possible without sexual desire or even sexual nuance—at least no more sexual nuance than is present in all human relations.

However, I had a peculiar problem at this time. I was on the way to finishing *The Deer Park*, my third novel. There was a minor character in it named Teddy Pope who is a movie star and a homosexual. Through the first and second drafts he had existed as a stereotype, a figure of fun; he was ludicrously affected and therefore ridiculous. One of the reasons I resisted Mr. Cory's book so much is that I was beginning to feel uneasy with the characterization I had drawn. In life there are any number of ridiculous people, but at bottom I was saying that Teddy

Pope was ridiculous because he was homosexual. I found myself dissatisfied with the characterization even before I read *The Homosexual in America*, it had already struck me as being compounded too entirely of malice, but I think I would probably have left it that way. After Mr. Cory's book, it had become impossible. I no longer believed in Teddy Pope as I had drawn him.

Yet a novel which is almost finished is very difficult to alter. If it is at all a good book, the proportions, the meanings, and the interrelations of the characters have become integrated, and one does not violate them without injuring one's work. Moreover, I have developed an antipathy to using one's novels as direct expressions of one's latest ideas. I, therefore, had no desire to change Teddy Pope into a fine virtuous character. That would be as false, and as close to propaganda, as to keep him the way he was. Also, while a minor character, he had an important relation to the story, and it was obvious that he could not be transformed too radically without recasting much of the novel. My decision, with which I am not altogether happy, was to keep Teddy Pope more or less intact, but to try to add dimension to him. Perhaps I have succeeded. He will never be a character many readers admire, but it is possible that they will have feeling for him. At least he is no longer a simple object of ridicule, nor the butt of my malice, and I believe *The Deer Park* is a better book for the change. My hope is that some readers may possibly be stimulated to envisage the gamut of homosexual personality as parallel to the gamut of heterosexual personality even if Teddy Pope is a character from the lower half of the spectrum. However, I think it is more probable that the majority of homosexual readers who may get around to reading *The Deer Park* when it is published will be dissatisfied with him. I can only say that I am hardly satisfied myself. But this time, at least, I have discovered the edges of the rich theme of homosexuality rather than the easy symbolic equation of it to evil. And to that extent I feel richer and more confident as a writer. What I have come to realize is that much of my homosexual prejudice was a servant to my aesthetic needs. In the variety and contradiction of American life, the difficulty of finding a character who can serve as one's protagonist is matched only by the difficulty of finding one's villain, and so long as I was able to preserve my prejudices, my literary villains were at hand. Now, the problem will be more difficult, but I suspect it may be rewarding too, for deep-down I was never very happy nor proud of myself at whipping homosexual straw-boys.

A last remark. If the homosexual is ever to achieve real social equality and acceptance, he too will have to work the hard row of shedding his own prejudices. Driven into defiance, it is natural if regrettable, that many homosexuals go to the direction of assuming that there is something intrinsically superior in homosexuality, and carried far enough it is a viewpoint which is as stultifying, as ridiculous, and as anti-human as the heterosexual's prejudice. Finally, heterosexuals are people too, and the hope of acceptance, tolerance, and sympathy must rest on this mutual appreciation.

Memoirs of an Ancient Activist

Paul Goodman

from *WIN Magazine,*1969

*One of the most influential social critics of the period, Paul Goodman was also a novelist, poet, psychotherapist, and anarchist theorist. He is best known for **Growing Up Absurd**, his book on the social and psychological problems of adolescent boys in a conformist society. He also wrote extensively on Wilhelm Reich and sexuality. Though he was also married, he publicly acknowledged his homosexuality after the emergence of the gay liberation movement.*

In essential ways, my homosexual needs have made me a nigger. Most obviously, of course, I have been subject to arbitrary brutality from citizens and the police; but except for being occasionally knocked down, I have gotten off lightly in this respect, since I have a good flair for incipient trouble and I used to be nimble on my feet. What makes me a nigger is that it is not taken for granted that my outgoing impulse is my right. Then I have the feeling that it is not my street. I don't complain that my passes are not accepted; nobody has a claim to be loved (except small children). But I am degraded for making the passes at all, for being myself. Nobody likes to be rejected, but there is a way of rejecting someone that accords him his right to exist and is the next best thing to accepting him. I have rarely enjoyed this treatment.

Allen Ginsberg and I once pointed out to Stokely Carmichael how we were niggers, but he blandly put us down by saying that we could always conceal our disposition and pass. That is, he accorded us the same lack of imagination that one accords to niggers; we did not really exist for him. Interestingly, this dialogue was taking place on (British) national TV, that haven of secrecy. More recently, since the formation of the Gay Liberation Front, Huey Newton of the Black Panthers has welcomed homosexuals to the revolution, as equally oppressed.

In general, in America, being a queer nigger is economically and professionally not such a disadvantage as being a black nigger, except for a few areas like government service, where there is considerable fear and furtiveness. (In more puritanic regimes, like present day Cuba, being queer is professionally and civilly a bad deal. Totalitarian regimes, whether communist or fascist, seem to be inherently puritanic.) But my own experience has been very mixed. I have been fired three times because of my queer behavior or my claim to the right to it—and these are the only times I have been fired. I was fired from the University of Chicago during the early years of Robert Hutchins; from Manumit School, an offshoot of A. J. Muste's Brookwood Labor College; and from Black Mountain College. These were highly liberal and progressive institutions, and two of them prided themselves on being communities.—Frankly, my experience of radical community is that it does not tolerate my freedom. Nevertheless, I am all for community because it is a human thing, only I seem doomed to be left out.

On the other hand, so far as I know, my homosexual acts and the overt claim to them have never disadvantaged me much in more square institutions. I have taught at half a dozen State universities. I am continually invited, often as chief speaker, to conferences of junior high school superintendents, boards of Regents, guidance counsellors, task forces on delinquency, and so forth. I say what I think is true—often there are sexual topics; I make passes if there is occasion: and I seem to get invited back. I have even sometimes made out—which is more than I can say for conferences of SDS or the Resistance. Maybe the company is so square that it does not believe, or dare to notice, my behavior; or more likely, such professional square people are more worldly (this is our elderly word for "cool") and couldn't care less what you do, so long as they don't have to face anxious parents and yellow press.

As one grows older, homosexual wishes keep one alert to adolescents and young people more than heterosexual wishes do, especially since our society strongly discountenances affairs between older men and girls or older women and boys. And as a male, the homosexual part of one's character is a survival of early adolescence anyway. But needless to say, there is a limit to this bridging of the generation gap. Inexorably I, like other men who hang around campuses, have found that the succeeding waves of freshmen seem more callow and incommunicable and one stops trying to rob the cradle. Their music leaves me cold. After a while my best contact with the young has gotten to be with the friends of my own grown children, as an advisor in their politics, rather than by my sexual desires. (The death of my son estranged me from the young world altogether.)

On the whole, although I was desperately poor up to a dozen years ago—I brought up a family on the income of a sharecropper—I don't attribute this to being queer but to my pervasive ineptitude, truculence, and bad luck. In 1945, even the Army rejected me as "Not Military Material" (they had such a stamp) not because I was queer but because I made a nuisance of myself with pacifist action at the examination and also had bad eyes and piles.

Curiously, however, I have been told by Harold Rosenberg and the late Willie Poster that my sexual behavior used to do me damage in precisely the New York literary world. It kept me from being invited to advantageous parties and making contacts to get published. I must believe Harold and Willie because they were unprejudiced observers. What I myself noticed in the thirties and forties was that I was excluded from the profitable literary circles dominated by Marxists in the thirties and ex-Marxists in the forties because I was an anarchist. For example, I was never invited to PEN or the Committee for Cultural Freedom. When CCF finally got around to me at the end of the fifties, I had to turn them down because they were patently tools of the CIA. (I said this in print in '61, but they lied their way out.)

To stay morally alive, a nigger uses various kinds of spite, which is the vitality of the powerless. He may be randomly destructive, since he feels he has no world to lose, and maybe he can prevent the others from enjoying their world. Or he may become an in-group fanatic, feeling that only his own kind are authentic and have soul. There are queers and blacks belonging to both these parties. Queers are "artistic," blacks have "soul." (This is the kind of theory, I am afraid, that is self-disproving; the more you believe it, the stupider you become; it is like trying to prove that you have a sense of humor.) In my own case, however, being a nigger seems to inspire me to want a more elementary humanity, wilder, less structured, more variegated, and where people pay attention to one another. That is, my plight has given energy to my anarchism, utopianism, and Gandhianism. There are blacks in this party too.

My actual political stance is a willed reaction-formation to being a nigger. I act that "the society I live in is mine," the title of one of my books. I regard the President as my public servant whom I pay, and I berate him as a lousy employee. I am more Constitutional than the Supreme Court. And in the face of the gross illegitimacy of the Government—with its Vietnam War, military-industrial cabal, and CIA—I come on as an old-fashioned patriot, neither supine nor more revolutionary than is necessary for my modest goals. This is a quixotic position. Sometimes I sound like Cicero.

In their in-group, Gay Society, homosexuals can get to be fantastically snobbish and a-political or reactionary. This is an understandable ego-defense: "You gotta be better than somebody," but its payoff is very limited. When I give talks to the Mattachine Society, my invariable sermon is to ally with all other libertarian groups and liberation movements, since freedom is indivisible. What we need is not defiant pride and self-consciousness, but social space to live and breathe. The Gay Liberation people have finally gotten the message of indivisible freedom, but they have the usual fanaticism of the Movement.

But there is a positive side. In my observation and experience, queer life has some remarkable political values. It can be profoundly democratizing, throwing together every class and group more then heterosexuality does. Its promiscuity can be a beautiful thing (but be prudent about VD). I have cruised rich, poor, middle class, and petit bourgeois; black, white, yellow, and brown; scholars, jocks, Gentlemanly C's, and dropouts; farmers, seamen, railroad men, heavy industry, light manufacturing, communications, business, and finance; civilians, soldiers and sailors, and once or twice cops. (But probably for Oedipal reasons, I tend to be sexually anti-Semitic, which is a drag.) There is a kind of political meaning, I guess, in the fact that there are so many types of attractive human beings; but what is more significant is that the many functions in which I am professionally and economically engaged are not altogether cut and dried but retain a certain animation and sensuality. HEW in Washington and IS 201 in Harlem are not total wastes, though I talk to the wall in both. I have something to occupy me on trains and buses and during the increasingly long waits at airports. At vacation resorts, where people are idiotic because they are on vacation, I have a reason to frequent the waiters, the boatmen, the room clerks, who are working for a living. I have something to do at peace demonstrations—I am not inspirited by guitar music—though no doubt the TV files and the FBI with their little cameras have pictures of me groping somebody. The human characteristics that are finally important to me and can win my lasting friendship are quite simple: health, honesty, not being cruel or resentful, being willing to come across, having either sweetness or character on the face. As I reflect on it now, only gross stupidity, obsessional cleanliness, racial prejudice, insanity, and being habitually drunk or high really put me off.

In most human societies, of course, sexuality has been one more area in which people can be unjust, the rich buying the poor, males abusing females, sahibs using niggers, the adults exploiting the young. But I think this is neurotic and does not give the best satisfaction. It is normal to befriend and respect what gives you pleasure. St. Thomas, who was a grand moral philosopher though a poor metaphysician, says that the chief human use of sex—as distinguished from the natural law of procreation—is to get to know other persons intimately. That has been my experience.

A common criticism of homosexual promiscuity, of course, is that, rather than democracy, it involves an appalling superficiality of human conduct, so that it is a kind of archetype of the inanity of mass urban life. I doubt that this is generally the case, though I don't know; just as, of the crowds who go to art-galleries, I don't know who are being spoken to by the art and who are being bewildered further—but at least some are looking for something. A young man or woman worries, "Is he interested in me or just in my skin? If I have sex with him, he will regard me as nothing": I think this distinction is meaningless and disastrous; in fact I have always followed up in exactly the opposite way and many of my lifelong personal loyalties had sexual beginnings. But

is this the rule or the exception? Given the usual coldness and frag-
mentation of community life at present, my hunch is that homosexual
promiscuity enriches more lives than it desensitizes. Needless to say, if
we had better community, we'd have better sexuality too.

I cannot say that my own promiscuity (or attempts at it) has kept me
from being possessively jealous of some of my lovers—more of the
women than the men, but both. My experience has not borne out what
Freud and Ferenczi seem to promise, that homosexuality diminishes
this voracious passion, whose cause I do not understand. But the
ridiculous inconsistency and injustice of my attitude have sometimes
helped me to laugh at myself and kept me from going overboard.

Sometimes it is sexual hunting that brings me to a place where I
meet somebody—for example, I used to haunt bars on the waterfront;
sometimes I am in a place for another reason and incidentally hunt—
for example, I go to the TV studio and make a pass at the cameraman;
sometimes these are both of a piece—for example, I like to play handball and I am sexually interested in fellows who play handball. But
these all come to the same thing, for in all situations I think, speak,
and act pretty much the same. Apart from ordinary courteous adjust-
ments of vocabulary—but not of syntax, which alters character—I say
the same say and do not wear different masks or find myself suddenly
with a different personality. Perhaps there are two opposite reasons
why I can maintain my integrity: on the one hand, I have a strong
enough intellect to see how people are for real in our only world, and
to be able to get in touch with them despite differences in background;
on the other hand, I am likely so shut in my own preconceptions that
I don't even notice glaring real obstacles that prevent communication.

How I do come on hasn't made for much success. Since I don't use
my wits to manipulate the situation, I rarely get what I want out of it.
Since I don't betray my own values, I am not ingratiating. My aristo-
cratic egalitarianism puts people off unless they are secure enough in
themselves to be also aristocratically egalitarian. Yet the fact I am not
phony or manipulative has also kept people from disliking or resenting
me, and I usually have a good conscience. If I happen to get on with
someone, there is not a lot of lies and bullshit to clear away.

Becoming a celebrity in the past few years, however, seems to have
hurt me sexually rather than helped me. For instance, decent young

collegians who might like me and who used to seek me out, now keep a respectful distance from the distinguished man. Perhaps they are now sure that I must be interested in their skin, not in them. And the others who seek me out just because I am well known seem to panic when it becomes clear that I don't care about that at all, and I come on as myself. Of course, a simpler explanation of my worsening luck is that I'm growing older every day, probably uglier, and certainly too tired to try hard.

As a rule I don't believe in poverty and suffering as a way of learning anything, but in my case the hardship and starvation of my inept queer life have usefully simplified my notions of what a good society is. As with any other addict who cannot get an easy fix, they have kept me in close touch with material hunger. So I cannot take the Gross National Product very seriously, nor status and credentials, nor grandiose technological solutions, nor ideological politics, including ideological liberation movements. For a starving person, the world has got to come across in kind. It doesn't. I have learned to have very modest goals for society and myself: things like clean air, green grass, children with bright eyes, not being pushed around, useful work that suits one's abilities, plain tasty food, and occasional satisfying nookie.

A happy property of sexual acts, and perhaps especially of homosexual acts, is that they are dirty, like life: as Augustine said, *Inter urinas et feces nascimur,* we're born among the piss and shit. In a society as middle class, orderly, and technological as ours, it's good to break down squeamishness, which is an important factor in what is called racism, as well as in cruelty to children and the sterile exiling of the sick and aged. And the illegal and catch-as-catch-can nature of much homosexual life at present breaks down other conventional attitudes. Although I wish I could have had my parties with less apprehension and more unhurriedly, yet it has been an advantage to learn that the ends of docks, the backs of trucks, back alleys, behind the stairs, abandoned bunkers on the beach, and the washrooms of trains are all adequate samples of all the space there is. For both bad and good, homosexual life retains some of the alarm and excitement of childish sexuality.

It is damaging for societies to check any spontaneous vitality.

Sometimes it is necessary, but rarely; and certainly not homosexual acts which, so far as I have heard, have never done any harm to anybody. A part of the hostility, paranoia, and automatic competitiveness of our society comes from the inhibition of body contact. But in a very specific way, the ban on homosexuality damages and depersonalizes the educational system. The teacher-student relation is almost always erotic.—The only other healthy psychological motivations are the mother-hen relevant for small children and the professional who needs apprentices, relevant for graduate schools.—If there is fear and to-do that erotic feeling might turn into overt sex, the teacher-student relation lapses or, worse, becomes cold and cruel. And our culture sorely lacks the pedagogic sexual friendships, homosexual, heterosexual, and lesbian, that have starred other cultures. To be sure, a functional sexuality is probably incompatible with our mass school systems. This is one among many reasons why they should be dismantled.

I recall when *Growing Up Absurd* had had a number of glowing reviews, finally one irritated critic, Alfred Kazin, darkly hinted that I wrote about my Puerto Rican delinquents (and called them "lads") because I was queer for them. News. How could I write a perceptive book if I didn't pay attention, and why should I pay attention to something unless, for some reason, it interested me? The motivation of most sociology, whatever it is, tends to produce worse books. I doubt that anybody would say that my observations of delinquent adolescents or of collegians in the Movement have been betrayed by infatuation. But I do care for them.—Of course, *they* might say, "With such a friend, who needs enemies?"

Yet it is true that an evil of the hardship and danger of queer life in our society, as with any situation of scarcity and starvation, is that we become obsessional and one-track-minded about it. I have certainly spent far too many anxious hours of my life fruitlessly cruising, which I might have spent sauntering for other purposes or for nothing at all, pasturing my soul. But I trust that I have had the stamina, or stubbornness, not to let my obsession cloud my honesty. So far as I know, I have never praised a young fellow's bad poem because he was attractive. But of course I am then especially pleased if it is good and I can say so. And best of all, of course, if he is my lover and he shows me something that I can be proud of and push with an editor. Yes, since I began these reflections on a bitter note, let me end them with a happy poem that I like, from *Hawkweed:*

> We have a crazy love affair,
> it is wanting each other to be happy.
> Since nobody else cares for that
> we try to see to it ourselves.
>
> Since everybody knows that sex
> is part of love, we make love;
> When that's over, we return
> to shrewdly plotting the other's advantage.
>
> Today you gazed at me, that spell
> is why I choose to live on.
> God bless you who remind me simply
> of the earth and sky and Adam.
>
> I think of such things more than most
> but you remind me simply. Man,
> you make me proud to be a workman
> of the Six Days, practical.

On balance, I don't know whether my choice, or compulsion, of a bisexual life has made me especially unhappy or only averagely unhappy. It is obvious that every way of life has its hang-ups, having a father or no father, being married or single, being strongly sexed or rather sexless, and so forth; but it is hard to judge what other people's experience has been, to make a comparison. I have persistently felt that the world was not made for me, but I have had good moments. And I have done a lot of work, have brought up some beautiful children, and have gotten to be 58 years old.

A Letter to the Revolutionary Brothers and Sisters

Huey Newton

from *Berkeley Tribe*, September 5-12, 1970

Huey Newton was a leader of the Black Panthers, a radical black militant and social service organization. This letter represents one of first overtures made by a nationally recognized leader to the lesbian and gay communities, thus legitimating homosexuality as a political issue.

During the past few years, strong movements have developed among women and among homosexuals seeking their liberation. There has been some uncertainty about how to relate to these movements.

Whatever your personal opinions and your insecurities about homosexuality and the various liberation movements among homosexuals and women (and I speak of the homosexuals and women as oppressed groups), we should try to unite with them in a revolutionary fashion. I say "whatever your insecurities are" because, as we very well know, sometimes our first instinct is to want to hit a homosexual in the mouth and want a woman to be quiet. We want to hit the homosexual in the mouth because we're afraid we might be homosexual; and we want to hit the woman or shut her up because we're afraid that she might castrate us, or take the nuts that we might not have to start with.

We must gain security in ourselves and therefore have respect and feelings for all oppressed people. We must not use the racist type attitude like the White racists use against people because they are Black and poor. Many times the poorest White person is the most racist because he's afraid that he might lose something, or discover something that he doesn't have; you're some kind of threat to him. This kind of psychology is in operation when we view oppressed people and we're angry with them because of their particular kind of behavior, or their particular kind of deviation from established norm.

Remember, we haven't established a revolutionary value system; we're only in the process of establishing it. I don't remember us ever constituting any value that said that a revolutionary must say offensive things towards homosexuals, or that a revolutionary should make sure that women do not speak out about their own particular kind of oppression. Matter of fact it's just the opposite: we say that we recognize the women's right to be free. We haven't said much about the homosexual at all, and we must relate to the homosexual movement because it's a real thing. And I know through reading and through my life experience, my observations, that homosexuals are not given freedom and liberty by anyone in the society. Maybe they might be the most oppressed people in the society.

And what made them homosexual? Perhaps it's a whole phenomenon that I don't understand entirely. Some people say that it's the decadence of capitalism. I don't know whether this is the case; I rather doubt it. But whatever the case is, we know that homosexuality is a fact that exists, and we must understand it in its purest form: That is, a person should have freedom to use his body in whatever way he wants to. That's not endorsing things in homosexuality that we wouldn't view as revolutionary. But there's nothing to say that a homosexual cannot also be a revolutionary. And maybe I'm now injecting some of my prejudice by saying that "even a homosexual can be a revolutionary." Quite on the contrary, maybe a homosexual could be the most revolutionary.

When we have revolutionary conferences, rallies and demonstrations there should be full participation of the Gay Liberation movement and the Women's Liberation movement. Some groups might be more revolutionary than others. We shouldn't use the actions of a few to say that they're all reactionary or counterrevolutionary, because they're not.

We should deal with the factions just as we deal with any group or party that claims to be revolutionary. We should try to judge somehow, whether they're operating sincerely, in a revolutionary fashion from a really oppressed situation. (And we'll grant that if they're women, they're probably oppressed.) If they do things that are un-revolutionary or counterrevolutionary, then criticize that action. If we feel that the group in spirit means to be revolutionary in practice, but they make mistakes in interpretation of the revolutionary philosophy, or they don't understand the dialectics of the social forces in operation, we should criticize that and not criticize them because they're women trying to be free. And the same is true for homosexuals. We should never say a whole movement is dishonest, when in fact they're trying to be honest, they're just making honest mistakes. Friends are allowed to make mistakes. The enemy is not allowed to make mistakes because his whole existence is a mistake, and we suffer from it. But the Women's Liberation Front and Gay Liberation Front are our friends, they are potential allies, and we need as many allies as possible.

We should be willing to discuss the insecurities that many people have about homosexuality. When I say "insecurities," I mean the fear that they're some kind of threat to our manhood. I can understand this fear. Because of the long conditioning process which builds insecurity in the American male, homosexuality might produce certain hangups in us. I have hangups myself about male homosexuality. Where, on the other hand, I have no hangup about female homosexuality. And that's a phenomenon in itself. I think it's probably because male homosexuality is a threat to me, maybe, and the females are no threat.

We should be careful about using those terms that might turn our friends off. The terms "faggot" and "punk" should be deleted from our vocabulary, and especially we should not attach names normally designed for homosexuals to men who are enemies of the people, such as Nixon or Mitchell. Homosexuals are not enemies of the people.

We should try to form a working coalition with the Gay Liberation and Women's Liberation groups. We must always handle social forces in the most appropriate manner. And this is really a significant part of the population, both women and the growing number of homosexuals, that we have to deal with.

ALL POWER TO THE PEOPLE!

Notes of a Radical Lesbian

Martha Shelley

from *Come Out: A Liberation Forum for the Gay Community*, 1969

Lesbian feminism was the most influential perspective among lesbians in the seven-ties. It encouraged the development of a separate women's culture and institutions such as coffee houses, bookstores, restaurants, and even automobile repair shops. Martha Shelley was one of earliest, if not the earliest exponent of the lesbian feminist perspective. She had been a member of the lesbian organization Daughters of Bilitis in the early sixties, and after the Stonewall riots in 1969, Shelley became one of the founders of the Gay Liberation Front, the first gay radical organization to grow out of the political unrest of the sixties. Lesbian feminism also articulated a new approach to sexuality that Shelley touches on in this essay

Lesbianism is one road to freedom—freedom from oppression by men.

To see Lesbianism in this context—as a mode of living neither better nor worse than others, as one which offers its own opportunities—one must abandon the notion that deviance from the norm arises from personal illnesses.

It is generally accepted that America is a "sick society." There is an inevitable corollary to this statement, which has not been generally accepted: that people within our society are all crippled by virtue of being forced to conform to certain norms. (Those who conform most easily can be seen as either the most healthy, because adaptable, or most sick, because least spirited.) Black people are struggling to free themselves, not only from white oppression, but from the roles of self-contempt that they have been forced to play. Women are struggling to liberate their minds from sick sexual roles. It is clear that the suffering, supposedly self-abasing black is not someone with a personal neurosis, but society's victim; and someone who has been forced to learn certain techniques for survival. Few people understand that the same is true of the self-abnegating passive housewife. Fewer still understand this truth about the homosexual.

These techniques of survival help us meet certain needs, at the price of others.

For women, as for other groups, there are several American norms. All of them have their rewards, and their penalties. The nice girl next door, virginal until her marriage—the Miss America type—is rewarded with community respect and respectability. She loses her individuality and her freedom, to become a toothpaste smile and a chastity belt. The career woman gains independence and a large margin of freedom—if she is willing to work twice as hard as a man for less pay, and if she can cope with emotional strains similar to those that beset the black intellectual surrounded by white colleagues. The starlet, call girl, or bunny, whose source of income is directly related to her image as a sex object, gains some financial independence and freedom from housework. She doesn't have to work as hard as the career woman, but she pays through psychological degradation as a sex object, and through the insecurity of knowing that her career, based on youthful good looks, is short-lived.

The Lesbian, through her ability to obtain love and sexual satisfaction from other women, is freed of dependence on men for love, sex, and money. She does not have to do menial chores for them (at least at home), nor cater to their egos, nor submit to hasty and inept sexual encounters. She is freed from fear of unwanted pregnancy and the pains of childbirth, and from the drudgery of child raising.

On the other hand, she pays three penalties. The rewards of child raising are denied her. This is a great loss for some women, but not for others. Few women abandon their children, as compared with the multitudes of men who abandon both wives and children. Few men take much interest in the process of child raising. One suspects that it might not be much fun for the average person, and so the men leave it to the women.

The Lesbian still must compete with men in the job market, facing the same job and salary discrimination as her straight sister.

Finally, she faces the most severe contempt and ridicule that society can heap on a woman.

When members of the Women's Liberation Movement picketed the 1968 Miss America pageant, the most terrible epithet heaped on our straight sisters was "Lesbian." The sisters faced hostile audiences who called them "commies," and "tramps," but some of them broke into tears when they were called Lesbians. When a woman showed up at a feminist meeting and announced that she was a Lesbian, many women avoided her. Others told her to keep her mouth shut, for fear that she would endanger the cause. They felt that men could be persuaded to accept some measure of equality for women—as long as these women would parade their devotion to heterosexuality and motherhood.

A woman who is totally independent of men—who obtains love, sex, and self-esteem from other women—is a terrible threat to male supremacy. She doesn't need them, and therefore they have less power over her.

I have met many, many feminists who were not Lesbians—but I have never met a Lesbian who was not a feminist. "Straight" women by the millions have been sold the belief that they must subordinate themselves to men, accept less pay for equal work, and do all the shit-work around the house. I have met straight women who would die to preserve their chains. I have never met a Lesbian who believed that she was innately less rational or capable than a man; who swallowed one word of the "woman's role" horseshit.

Lesbians, because they are not afraid of being abandoned by men, are less reluctant to express hostility toward the male class— the oppressors of women. Hostility toward your oppressor is healthy, but the guardians of modern morality, the psychiatrists, have interpreted this hostility as an illness, and they say this illness causes and is Lesbianism.

If hostility to men causes Lesbianism, then it seems to me that in a male-dominated society, Lesbianism is a sign of mental health.

The psychiatrists have also forgotten that Lesbianism involves love between women. Isn't love between equals healthier than sucking up to an oppressor? And when they claim we aren't capable of loving men, even if we want to—I would ask a straight man, in turn: are you capable of loving another man so deeply that you aren't afraid of his body or afraid to put your body in his hands? Are you really capable of loving women, or is your sexuality just another expression of your hostility? Is it an act of love or an act of conquest?

I do not mean to condemn all males. I have found some beautiful, loving men among the revolutionaries, among the hippies, and the male homosexuals. But the average man, including the average student male radical, wants a passive sex-object *cum* domestic *cum* baby nurse to clean up after him while he does all the fun things and bosses her around—while he plays either bigshot executive or Che Guevara—and he is my oppressor and my enemy.

Society has taught most Lesbians to believe they are sick, arid has taught most straight women to despise and fear the Lesbian as a perverted, diseased creature. It has fostered the myth that Lesbians are ugly and turn to each other because they can't get that prize, that prince, a male! In this age of the new "sexual revolution," another myth has been fostered: the beautiful Lesbians who play games with each other on the screen for the titillation of heterosexual males. They are not seen as serious people in love, but as performers in the "let's try a new perversion" game.

Freud founded the myth of penis envy, and men have asked me "But what can two women do together?" As though a penis were the *sine qua non* of sexual pleasure! Man, we can do without it, and keep it going longer, too!

Women are afraid to be without a man's protection—because other men will assault them on the streets. And this is no accident, no aberration performed by a few lunatics. Assaults on women are no more an accident than are lynchings of blacks in Mississippi. Men have oppressed us, and like most oppressors, they hate the oppressed and fear their wrath. Watch a white man walking in Harlem and you will see what I mean. Look at the face of a man who has accidentally wandered into a Lesbian bar.

Men fear Lesbians because they are less dependent, and because their hostility is less controlled.

Straight women fear Lesbians because of the Lesbian inside them, because we represent an alternative. They fear us for the same reason that uptight middle class people fear hip people. They are angry at us because we have a way out that they are afraid to take.

And what happens to the Lesbian under all this pressure? Many of my sisters, confused by the barrage of anti-gay propaganda, have spent years begging to be allowed to live. They have come begging because they believed they were psychic cripples, and that other people were healthy and had the moral right to judge them. Many have lived in silence, burying themselves in their careers, like name-changing Jews or blacks who passed for white. Many have retreated into an apolitical domesticity, concerning themselves only with the attempt to maintain a love relationship in a society which attempts to destroy love and replace it with consumer goods, and which attempts to completely destroy any form of love outside the monogamous marriage.

Because *Lesbian* has become such a vile epithet, we have been afraid to fight openly. We can lose our jobs; we have fewer civil rights than any other minority group. Because we have few family ties and no children, for the most part, we have been active in many causes, but always in secret, because our name contaminates any cause that we work for.

To the radical Lesbian, I say that we can no longer afford to fight for everyone else's cause while ignoring our own. Ours is a life-style born out of a sick society; so is everyone else's. Our kind of love is as valid as anyone else's. The revolution must be fought for us, too, not only for blacks, Indians, welfare mothers, grape pickers, SDS people, Puerto Ricans, or mine workers. We must have a revolution for *human rights*. If we are in a bag, it's as good as anyone else's bag.

Maybe after the revolution, people will be able to love each other regardless of skin color, ethnic origin, occupation, or type of genitals. But if that's going to happen, it will only happen because we make it happen—starting right now.

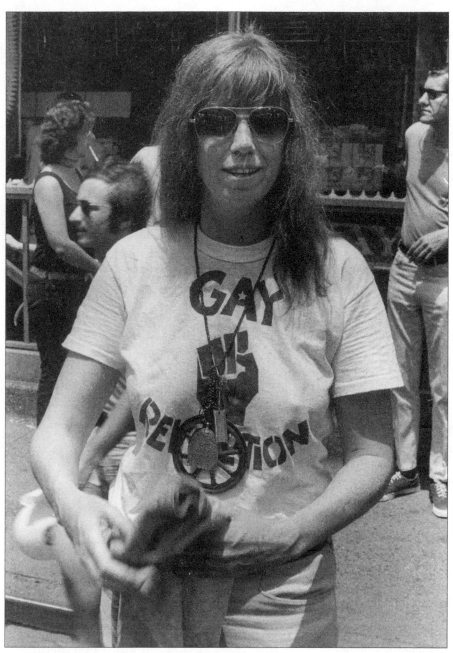

© Fred W. McDarrah

The Myth of the Myth of the Vaginal Orgasm

Jill Johnston

from *Lesbian Nation: The Feminist Solution*, 1973

*An influential dance critic for the **Village Voice**, Johnston began to include in her dance columns personal accounts of her involvement in the women's movement and her lesbianism. Her book **Lesbian Nation** is a wild ride of a book that explores Johnston's assertion that "all women are lesbians" She irreverently dismisses even the sacred beliefs of the women's liberation movement. Though **Lesbian Nation** was to become a classic of lesbian feminism, Johnston eschewed the gentle woman-identified sexuality idealized by lesbian feminists and took a more aggressive sexual stance.*

> Should the hypothesis be true that one of the requisite cornerstones upon which all modern civilizations were founded was coercive suppression of women's inordinate sexuality, one looks back over the long history of women and their relationships to men, children and society since the Neolithic revolution with a deeper, almost awesome, sense of the ironic tragedy in the triumph of the human condition.
>
> —Mary Jane Sherfey, M.D.

> The process of physical and psychic self-affirmation requires full relation with those like oneself, namely women.
>
> —*Ecstasy*, a paper written by a gay revolutionary party

Many of the new theories and descriptions of woman's basic equipment and orgasm may sound right to a lot of women. They don't sound bad to me, but they're almost exclusively written in relation to the man with the implicit instruction that the man had better shape up and recognize this "inordinate" sexuality of women and learn the more effective means of stimulating and satisfying his partner. Although many women can satisfy themselves in relation to the man it's not well known at all that the woman can satisfy herself just as well if not better in relation to herself or to other women. The sexual satisfaction of the woman independently of the man is the *sine qua non* of the feminist revolution. This is why Gay/Feminism expresses the proper sexual-political stance for the revolutionary woman. Sexual dependence on the man is inextricably entangled in the interdependence of man and woman at all levels of the social structures by which the woman is oppressed. It is in any case difficult to conceive of an "equal" sexual relationship between two people in which one member is the "biological aggressor." Although a hole also moves forward to enclose a sword it is the sword in all known personal-political forms of life thruout history which has assumed initiative to invade and conquer. The man retains the prime organ of invasion. Sexual congress between man and woman is an invasion of the woman, the woman doesn't get anything up to participate in this congress, and although a woman may be conditioned to believe that she enjoys this invasion and may in fact grow to like it if her male partner makes rare sacrifices of consideration in technical know-how, she remains the passive receptive hopeful half of a situation that was unequal from the start. The fate that woman has to resign herself to is the *knowledge* of this biological inequity. A fate that was not originally the occasion for the *social* inequities elaborated out of the biological situation. From this knowledge the woman can now alter her destiny or at least reclaim certain ancient historical solutions, namely the self sufficient tribes of amazons, to a physical problem in relation to men. Some Marxist-Socialist thinkers envision the solution in our technological advancement whereby the test-tube baby will relieve the woman of her reproductive function and release her to the wideranging sexual pleasures traditionally arrogated by the man. But *no* technological solution will be the answer to the spiritual needs of the woman deprived of herself in relation to the man. Feminism at heart is a massive complaint. Lesbianism is the solution. Which is another way of putting what Ti-Grace Atkinson once described as Feminism being a theory and lesbianism the practice. When theory and practice come together we'll have the revolution. Until all women are lesbians there will be no true political revolution. No feminist per se has advanced a solution outside of accommodation to the man. The complaints are substantial and articulate and historically sound and they contain by implication their own answers but the feminists refuse to acknowledge what's implicit in their own complaint or analysis. To wit: that the object of their attack is not going to make anything better than a *material* adjustment to the demands of their enslaved sex. There's no conceivable equality between two species in a relation in which one of the two has been considerably weakened in all aspects of her being over so long a period of historical time. The blacks in America were the first to understand that an oppressed group must withdraw into itself to establish its own identity and rebuild its strength through mutual support and recognition. The first unpublicized action of many feminists *was* in fact to withdraw from the man sexually. Feminists who still sleep with the man are delivering their most vital energies to the oppressor. Most feminists understood this immediately but were confounded in their realization by the taboo against the obvious solution of sex with another woman. Not only is the psychic-emotional potential for satisfaction with another woman far greater than that with a man, insomuch as every woman like every man was originally most profoundly attached to herself as her mother, but there is more likelihood of sexual fulfillment with another woman as well since all organisms best understand the basic equipment of another organism which most closely resembles themselves. The erotic potential between like organisms consists in the enhancement of self through narcissistic identification. Narcissism is the ideal appreciation of self. Women who love their own sex love the sameness in the other. They become both subject and object to each other. That makes two subjects and two objects. Narcissism is the totality of subject-object unity within the self extended to another. "When a heterosexual woman loves a man she is confronted with otherness, and so is a man who loves a woman. Otherness implies something completely different from oneself, something one has to learn to understand and live with . . . At one time or another, the 'normal' (heterosexual) woman will always be put back into the place of being an object." (Charlotte Wolff, *Love Between Women*, p. 70) Normalcy for women is the adaptation to their own oppression. Or to the male standard for perpetuating his privilege in unequal relationships. Normalcy is the fucked

up condition of woman. Normalcy is the unsuccessful attempt to overcome the obstacle of otherness by resigning oneself to one's own deprivation of self. Normalcy is an appeal to numbers in the form of
majorities to justify coercion in plans to cooperate for the benefit of
"mankind." Normalcy is the disease of maladjusted coupling by different or hetero or otherness species. Normalcy is achieved by puritan
ethical appeals to the moral correctness of doing things that are worth-
while by their difficulty and hard labor through delayed gratification of
real instincts, or uniting with self. True normalcy would mean the
return of all women to themselves. Majority behavior, which defines
civilized schizophrenia, is pseudo-normalcy. The first order of business
for a woman is the redefinition of herself through assertion of her sexuality in relation to herself or her own equal, in other words, independently of the man. Early feminist writings project the suggestion of
lesbianism as an alternative to the widespread sexual dissatisfaction of
women in relation to men. There was, in these early manifestos, both
fortunately and not so fortunately, a concentration on that aspect of
the basic equipment in which orgastic satisfaction originates. I thought
everybody knew the clitoris was the doorway to orgasm, the way a certain type of jill-in-the-box might pop open after sufficient rhythmic
friction against its trap door. Apparently this glorification of the clitoris
was a revelation to women who remained frigid in intercourse through
neglect of prior stimulation of the external or clitoral part of the organ.
Or who remained frigid in intercourse regardless of said prior stimulation, this actually being the true situation, according to early pronouncement, based on the total absence of feeling or orgastic potential
within the vagina itself. I have a record entry June 18, 1970: "find out
what they mean by the myth of the vaginal orgasm." Subsequently I
asked a few "feminists." They informed me, in effect, that I don't experience what I say I feel or feel what I say I experience or any combined
way of being a liar. And their chief authority was Masters & Johnson.
Studying the feminist literature I decided that the feminists had found
the perfect rationale for their frustration and excuse for not being
required to fuck with the man any more. They didn't actually say this.
They were mainly contesting the "myth of the liberated woman and
her vaginal orgasm." The refutation of Freud's thesis of sexual maturity
in the woman consisting of her transference to the father as proper love

object developing parallel to the shifting of orgasmic location in the clitoris to the "mature" vagina. Wherever these feminists obtained their "evidence" for an insensitive vagina, if not in themselves, it seemed not to matter either about the source or the (in)sensitivity if the issue constituted a rebellion against being defined sexually in terms of what pleases the man. It seems actually amazing that what they were asserting was a stubborn refusal to submit to conventional intercourse on grounds of an insensitive vagina. *Equating* intercourse with vaginal orgasm as it were. (No mention of hands or bananas or dildoes.) Really as though one was unthinkable without the other. As though the case for an insensitive vagina provided women with their first legal brief for the indictment of phallic imperialism. This rather misguided attempt of women to dissociate themselves from the suppression of their pleasure in "reproductive sexuality" was nonetheless a crucial rudimentary step in establishing sexual independence from the man and leading to the fuller dimension of womanhood in Gay/Feminism. In fact within two years or so after the appearance of these papers the feminist line includes more overt accommodation to and recognition of lesbians, as well as lesbianism itself within the ranks. I said "misguided" because the feminist equation along the old standard of "reproductive sexuality" or penis-in-vagina as proper model or primal scene, and their "discovering" of the insensitive female half of the bargain, important as it was, left them with only one operable part of the basic equipment—the clitoris—and the ignorance of a solution involving all the equipment with their sisters. I always agreed with one half of Freud's equation. That a woman moves from clitoral to vaginal orgasm. And that the latter *is* more mature in the sense that the activation of the inner walls brings about a more profound intensification of orgasm. I would add that this shift occurs in two kinds of time—over a period of months or years as a "discovery" of the orgastic potential of the internal walls, and as a transition in every sexual encounter, moving from initial stimulation of clitoris (as the seat of sensation, the *origin* of satisfaction) to full orgasm experienced in the total organ which includes the "deep" vaginal wall. I take issue like the feminists with Freud's postulation of "heterosexual maturity." Since a woman can achieve vaginal orgasm herself or with another woman clearly his case for maturity was in the interests of the continuation of phallic imperialism. The rights of the father to the mother. The Gay/Feminist revolution involves the rights of the mother to the mother. Woman's thighs are the gateways to infinity for women as well as for men. For women give birth to themselves as well as to boys. I was struck particularly by these remarks in the Masters & Johnson book on female orgasm: "During the first stage of subjective progression in orgasm, the sensation of intense clitoral-pelvic awareness has been described by a number of women as occurring concomitantly with a sense of bearing down or expelling. This last sensation was reported only by parous study subjects, a small number of whom expressed some concept of having an actual fluid emission or of expending in some concrete fashion." And: "Twelve women, all of whom have delivered babies on at least one occasion without anesthesia or analgesia, reported that during the second stage of labor they experienced a grossly intensified version of the sensations identified with this first stage of subjective progression through orgasm." These reports seemed to confirm my long suspicion that orgasm itself originated in the parthenogenetic birth of our unicellular beginnings. The daughter cells. The immaculate conception is the female fantasy of her own birth without the aid of the male. I can personally testify to the aboriginal reality of this state of being through having experienced a "psychic parthenogenesis" in certain hallucinatory symptoms of childbirth—psychosomatic labor pains—attending the birth of myself during a critical period of cosmic consciousness more commonly called insanity. Women of course do the same for each other in any intense relationship. I should also remark that my "rebirth" was accompanied by a great expansion of sexuality in the realms of both sensual awareness and orgastic potential. During this time for instance I began to experience the intensification or deepening of orgasm that I could only describe as "inner" or "internal." The feminists claimed Masters & Johnson as an authority in their case for an insensitive vagina. Yet Masters & Johnson say "The physiologic onset of orgasm is signaled by contractions of the target organs, starting with the *orgasmic platform in the outer third of the vagina.* This platform, created involuntarily by localized vasocongestion and myotonia, contracts with recordable rhythmicity as the tension increment is released" (italics mine). And "Vaginal spasm and penile grasping reactions have been described many times in the clinical and non-professional literature." And "Regularly recurring orgasmic-platform contractions were appreciated subjectively as pulsating or throbbing sensations of the vagina." And "Finally, as the third stage of subjective progression, a feeling of involuntary contraction with a specific focus in the vagina or lower pelvis was mentioned consistently." The Masters & Johnson team remain loyal to the standard of heterosexual coupling but they've presented the most impressive physiological findings to date of the extensive orgasmic response of the woman. I really think the feminists basically were making a common complaint in the new terminological context of feminism. That the man was no good in bed. That he was insensitive to the essential clitoris. That he just didn't know how to do it. And as an added fillip the new challenge that a woman or feminist anyway would henceforth refuse to accept responsibility for a frigidity that wasn't her own fault. The solution has still not been posed within feminist theory. It can't be because feminism is not a solution. It's the complaint that got the movement going. When the feminists have a solution they'll be Gay/Feminists. Until then, they've got the best problem around and that's the man. Feminism is a struggle terminology. Concerning women at odds with the man. Since women have always been at odds with the man feminism is the collectivized articulated expression of women's demeaned status. Feminism will no longer need itself when women cease to think of themselves as the "other" in relation to the "other" and unite with their own kind or species. Being male and female is, above all, defined in terms of the other. Feminists could begin by realizing that not only do they not need a penis to achieve their supreme satisfaction but they could easily do better without one since the timing involving the essential stimulation of the outer tissues prior to and/or concomitant with penetration requires a penis that can be erect for entry at a more or less precise moment in the progress toward climax. Some women and men work this thing out, or in, but most women, as the feminists observed, consistently receive a penis into a dead or dying chamber from which the penis eventually emerges as the savior in the form of a child. In any case the question many peoples are asking now is if "reproductive sexuality" is no longer the standard for sexual approach—for men it never was completely—what is keeping women from their total pleasure with other women. We know why. "Women far more than men are

510

trapped in a social view that suggests that their ultimate worth is derived from a suitable heterosexual attachment and the result of this is that they come to despise both themselves and other women." In order for a girl to achieve an adequate motherhood, she must to some degree relinquish her libidinal attachment to her own mother. The acculturation of women to believe most exclusively in "reproductive sexuality" remains pervasive and powerful. Altman again: "As a consequence of the utilitarian view of sex there is an extremely strong negative attitude toward all sexual urges other than those that are genital and heterosexual." Or: "Sex has been firmly linked, and nowhere more clearly than in Christian theology, with the institution of the family and with child bearing. Sex is thus legitimized for its utilitarian principles, rather than as an end in itself . . . even where sexual pleasure is accepted as a complementary goal, the connection between marriage and sex still remains." As a complementary goal women have no need to stay in relation to the aggravation caused by the "biological aggressor." If the male fears absorption and the female penetration, and both fears represent the disturbance of a static equilibrium—in which nothing is either gained or lost—it seems clear that the various global disturbances now accelerated by technological expansion are material visible extensions of the primal antagonism between men and women in some evolutionary distortion of destiny. (Not that there is such a thing as an evolutionary distortion.) Marcuse commented on Norman O. Brown: "If I understand his mysticism correctly it includes abolition of the distinction between male and female and creation of an androgynous person. He seems to see the distinction between male and female as the product of repression. I do not. It is the last difference I want to see abolished." Speaking of sexism in high places! If I understand Marcuse correctly. Since I too would not like to see the distinction abolished, but not I think for the same reasons. Agreeing with Brown, I'm not sure that he would envision the solution in the withdrawal of women from participation in that repression by which the distinction was created and sustained. Or even that he would define it that way. The fall was from some primeval division into two sexes. I think any bio-analytically oriented person knows we were originally one sex. The fall is a constant reoccurrence through birth or separation. "The sin is not between the lover and the beloved, but in parentage."

The project in our cycle toward species extinction should be clear enough. The present revolution of women is a clamorous reminder of that destiny and the proper organic means of achieving it. Many male intellects hope to see the abortion of this destiny. Not necessarily specifically identifying the agent of that abortion in the potential technological disasters of the male power problem. The key to survival in the interests of a natural death is the gradual extinction of the reproductive function as it is now still known and practiced. For it is by this function that the woman is so desperately deprived of herself. Lesbian or woman prime is *the* factor in advance of every projected solution for our embattled world. In her realization of herself both sensually polymorphously and genitally orgasmically she experiences her original self reproductive or parthenogenetic recreation of herself apart from the intruding and disturbing and subjugating male. Genitalorgasmic sex between women is absolutely consistent with our total sensual and emotional mutually reflecting relations with each other. The lesbian woman is not properly equipped to oppress her own kind. But she is equipped to give herself pleasure, and she doesn't need any artificial substitute for the instrument of oppression to give herself that pleasure.

Cocksucker

Anonymous

from *Fag Rag*, June 1971

In the early days of gay liberation, numerous small newspapers and magazines popped up all over the country: Gay Sunshine (San Francisco), The Gay Liberator (Detroit), Fag Rag (Boston), The Gay Alternative (Philadelphia), and The Body Politic (Toronto). They were small, with irregular publication schedules, and financed out of pocket. But every subject was open to discussion and many had never been discussed in a publication before. This editorial from Fag Rag explores the political significance of fellatio.

Writing about cocksucking can't help but emphasize cocks and in that sense be sexist—the objectification concentrated not just on, but on one small percentage part of the male body. We should be beyond cocksucking—into ear, nose, mouth, toe, tongue, knee, ass, back, arm, finger, nipple, loin, groin, and other part sucking.

> *We should be Eating each other's seed/ eating/ as, each other./ Kissing the lover in the mouth of bread/ lip to lip. (Gary Snyder, "Song of Taste")*

In the meantime, some misconceptions need to be overcome about cocksucking among males. Cocksucking is a specialized technique mastered even in an amateur way by probably not more than half the male population, and everyone knows what the word means.

Yet the allegedly "straight" male has an incredible taboo about sucking cock, or for that matter having his own cock sucked. Some want it, but they pretend they are drunk or asleep before they'll let another male touch them sexually or themselves touch another male. And there is another game—sometimes played in fraternities, prisons, and other male groups—of forcing someone to commit this fearsome act of love.

Generally cocksucking is considered an act of debasement and sub-jugation even more than anal or vulva-vaginal sex, and among gay males an implicit acceptance of this oppressive idea is surprisingly widespread.

Teenagers will play the game (and some continue through their life) of *you do me and I'll do you.* The unrecognized premise being that doing is a nasty, unpleasant, undesirable act. This trading off idea debases sex, reduces it from an act of love and passion to something calculated and marketed. Some gay males, who enjoy cocksucking and are often proud of their pleasure, will still retain this prejudice. How many gay males take the attitude they *don't want to do anyone who does me?* The hidden premise being that a cocksucker is an unworthy person.

Even presumably liberated gay males retain prejudices about cocksucking. Someone who had kissed every male in the room would be considered very liberated and right on; someone who had sucked the cock of every male in the room would be considered at best promiscuous at worst a perverted "dirty old man." Certainly on the Dow-Jones sex rating (that every gay male group maintains for every member) a liberated cocksucker would rate very low. Who would want to suck the cock of someone who had sucked the cock of every male in the room? the city? the nation? the universe?

One astonishing prejudice among males is the lack of interest in technique. There is an incredible amount of sloppy cocksucking, done without feeling, almost done without wanting to know what's being done. With training someone can swallow swords. Why is it then that people choke on cocks? If cocksucking were an act of relaxation, pleasure and ecstasy, none should ever choke.

Perhaps this absence of technique comes from most gay people's starting so late. It's not uncommon for someone to wait into their twenties to "come out." I sucked my first cock when I was four years old (and have enjoyed doing it ever since). That early experience has been very liberating and I think its one of the greatest oppressions that gay people are channeled and caged in an allegedly "straight" world through their most formative years.

A central part of the sexist brainwashing is the conception of sex as dirty. One reason we are sexist is that very early we learn to hide parts of our body because they are "private," "personal," "dirty," "unmentionable," or "unclean." To break this circuit takes a tremendous effort for everyone; for gay people, a greater effort because cock-ass-vulva-sucking-licking cannot be done without some sense of contact with those parts of the body.

Overlaying this puritanism, there are other forms of anti-gay channelling. At home, at school, where ever we go, the word is Dick, Jane, Spot, Puff, Mother, and Father. We never see or hear of gay people—not to mention cocksucking. Sex education, even the most progressive, does not include us (except in the categories of disease and deformity). Everywhere the nuclear family is the model. An essential part of any program for those who cherish freedom must be to trash the nuclear family. Gay male liberation is at the heart of this revolution, and so conceived, every cock sucked is an act of liberation.

Why not teach first graders, not only about cocksucking, but about how to do it? Why should they have to wait to be twenty-one and become a "consenting adult" before they can love? before they struggle for freedom? Twenty-one may be too late, the child grown to adult might be deformed, unable even to learn to love.

If we are proud of being gay males, we should be proud of being cocksuckers. If cocksucking is good, if it is an act of love, if it is a passionate pleasure, we need to celebrate and cherish it. Cherish it until the "private," "personal" disappear and with them sexist objectification of the cock.

SUCK TO BE FREE!!!

Indiscriminate Promiscuity as an Act of Revolution

Charley Shively

from *Gay Sunshine/Fag Rag*, Joint Issue, Summer 1974

In the seventies, Charles Shively wrote a series of articles which started off from some stigmatized form of homosexual behavior like promiscuity or cocksucking and then went on to show the political significance of that particular form of behavior. Brad Gooch characterized the seventies as the "Golden Age of Promiscuity" and Shively's analysis shows that it was a widely shared belief among gay men.

C hoosing homosexuality is in itself an act of rebellion, a revolutionary stance. Becoming a homosexual meant I rejected the boyfriend/girlfriend, jock/homecoming queen, auto mechanic/cooking class, dirty joke/purity, science/poetry divisions that were everything in Hamilton, Ohio. I refused to become a "man." I was (and am) "queer as a three-dollar bill."

I am [1974] also thirty-six years old and am part of a movement not more than twenty (really no more than five) years old. Why have we waited so many centuries to act on the revolutionary core, potential, voice deep within us? Notwithstanding Walt Whitman, Oscar Wilde, Paul Verlaine, or Magnus Hirschfeld—why have faggots been so slow to rebel?

The answer partly rests in the massive drains of energy put into surviving, the co-optation by the ruling class and other causes common to oppressed groups. But there is, I think, a unique potentiality among faggots to break away from the existing power structure and search out new alternatives. The nuclear family is the foundation stone of all that is established. Because we are so radically opposed to the breeding family unit with reproduction as its ultimate aim, our sexuality makes us revolutionary.

Everywhere people belittle our practice. In the spring of 1971, I wrote the first part of my "Cocksucking as an Act of Revolution" (*Fag Rag* #1, June 1971), and got little comment except people saying surely you don't mean that *just* sucking cocks or taking it up the ass can be revolutionary. If you do, you're wrong (or stupid) not to notice it's been done for centuries without much change. Aren't you just "wishfully thinking about our sex habits as though they *were* revolutionary"? If sucking cocks would do, then "given the number of numbers making it every night in bushes from Boston to Bulgaria, the state would [long ago] have exploded."

I have always refused to concede the point here because I believe there is an implicit denigration of sexuality and of the body. Our bodies are real, they are not some social theory, some Utopian proposal; their relationship to labor, the state, the economy and consciousness is no less fundamental than the other way around. We still wince at taking our bodies and sexuality seriously. Certainly I do. Doing child care at a conference recently, I was just stunned at the "innocent" sexuality of the "children." They had not learned yet how much more important thought and consciousness was then their bodies or the bodies of those they love. They simply did it.

Getting back into, back to our bodies, our sexuality can be a revolutionary perspective for ourselves. How much less Utopian can I be? to rest everything on the "flesh," "lust"—prevailing practice instead of magisterial theories? Why can't our bodies, commonplace things found in every home—why can't they be the source of change and revolution? Do we have to sail to Byzantium, the Kremlin, Hanoi, Havana, Santiago or Zanzibar to find *the revolution?* If so, there ain't many'll be able to afford the trip.

Obviously there is decadence, cruelty and exploitation everywhere in faggotland. But I say that decadence comes not from our bodies or our sexual practices; decadence comes from accepting the straight, white-man values. Believing that we are sick, inferior, cursed, bad, spoiled, wrong, wretched; believing "they" are always right; wanting to be them; not wanting to be ourselves. It is so easy to wander from sensation—to go away from what we feel into what they want us to feel, believe, think, and experience. Maybe, I'd do better to say "Revolutionary Sensuality" is intended to be a revolutionary perspective for ourselves—the antithesis to bourgeois decadence. But I prefer to talk of "Cocksucking as an Act of Revolution." When the ass is licked clean, then come to me talking of "revolutionary sensuality." Then I will kiss your sweet tongue.

Because our sexuality is not only strange, but dangerous and lethal, to the existing powers, they have invented peculiar and unique ways of talking about and conceptualizing us. Ruling-class men associate faggots with effeteness. Their projection is oddly perverted from their normal way of fantasizing about "oppressed" groups. Generally the administrators equate inferiority with sexuality and subjectivity (both being base, sensual) and their own superiority with thought and objectivity. This holds true of every group *except* faggots. We are considered animal/sexual/base because our only defining characteristic is sexual; at the same time we are paradoxically seen as an effete part of the ruling class—given over to music, philosophy, decoration, poetry and other intellectual pursuits. The accepted wisdom is that (unlike other oppressed groups) we are rich or nearly so. By one count, 80 percent of all U.S. homosexuals as homosexuals are living affluent lives or struggling to do so.

I don't accept such counts, nor the fantasy about our being an effete part of the ruling class. Quite the contrary, I think faggots suffer all the existing discriminations of our class/race-bound society plus those of sexual oppression. We need a more real understanding of our social standing—how it is a part of a class society—and from that I think we can find real strategies out of the existing, collapsing society.

To begin with, we need to understand that the idea of faggots being only a small group of decadent ruling-class parasites is nothing but a fantasy. Ruling-class faggots (of which there are plenty) are more visible and freer, but that doesn't mean they are necessarily more numerous. There are not fewer faggots in the working class, there are only more closets there. Manliness is really a mark of class oppression, and the lower class you are, the more manly you are expected and required to be—both by your peers and the society in general. Thus sports—i.e. baseball, football, hockey, boxing, etc.—are primarily an interest of young and lower-class men. Almost a social necessity that declines as you rise on the class scale.

In the gay community, these marks of class are visible everywhere. The young, virile, beautiful, educated—usually white—form a circle of beautiful people, who as a group enjoy more fun and privilege than the old, ugly, poor, uneducated. All faggots carry in their heads a computer system/switchboard in which they weigh each other. On the grid we process such factors as height, penis size, ass shape, eyes, clothing, personality, smile, weight, age, skin/hair color, virility, education, intelligence, sun sign, birthplace and so forth. The inexorable computer says: Meet my Fantasy or be gone, what do you think this is, some kind of charity?

Too many protests against the horrors of this computer system have been against the values being processed rather than the process itself. That is, someone with a short penis will argue that technique should count more. Or someone will want to substitute personality, intelligence and education for those areas in which he would get a lower score. And isn't the demand for counting personality similar? A friend writes: "i have my best luck meeting people on the streets, just talking, and many times, through the beginnings of compassion or intimacy, the other person (who might have refused my advances in a bar or the fens) sees that i am a *person* and responds. in fact, i think i can say that i have luck *only* when i can get myself across as a decent, interesting human being."

I don't deny this heartfelt cry in any way; just typing it makes me want to stop and cry—search the faggot out and embrace. Yet I can't help feeling some failure to recognize the goodness in anonymity. Plenty has been said of its shortcomings; it's supposed to be the breakdown of the family and civilization according to some sociologists. (They put it in French, *anomie,* to make their observation seem even profound.)

Faggots live *anomie* more than virtually any other group of people I know; despite the pitfalls, maybe we're onto something good. Because sometimes it does help the old, ugly, poor, uneducated and generally "unfortunate." Since the computer of each faggot is "fussy" to some degree about who they'll copulate with, the more casual the encounter the less particular they are likely to be. In the baths or bushes, a faggot will more likely make it with someone he will not have to live with the next day. The Trucks in New York City are one example of a very unfamilial rendezvous—where words are seldom spoken, names are unknown, the whole body may never be seen. Unlike the baths and bars, they are also cheap (no cover charge).

As the stakes go up in the relationship, the standards go up. You might trick with someone in the bushes who has a score of 25, but require a score of 50 before you'd take him home to bed; 65 before you'd fix him breakfast; 69 before you'd actually make it again with him; 75 before you'd live with him; 85 before you'd become his lover; 95 before you'd live with him the rest of your life.

Thus the denunciations of tea-room sex or the baths or one-night stands are denunciations of victims. The typical bourgeois morality; people are bad because they are poor, less successful, less happy; they have done poorly in the economy, they are to blame. An *Advocate* poll asks the question: "Do you think that tearoom and park 'queens' are a disgrace and discredit to Gays?" A recent front page story in the Boston *Gay Community News* condemns such sex because it might alienate the Massachusetts state legislature. Laud Humphreys in *Tea Room Trade* found that many more lowerclass men (often married) used the tea rooms than went to bars. More older men likewise. The baths or the bushes are similar. For instance, in Boston for many years you would not see more than one or two black faggots in the Punch Bowl (loud, brassy) or Sporters (collegiate) or Napoleon (high church)—but in the subway tea rooms or along the Esplanade, the proportion was greater.

Our computer/capitalist wiring grades not only people and places for cruising; more deviously it also controls our sexual practice. We carry around a control board indicating just what we can and will do in bed. Some people are wired only to suck; others only to fuck; some to sex only with black men; some only with white men; some only 69; some only in chains. Both as a group and as individuals, faggots have suffered from tightly delineated sex roles. Breaking these, building new wider, better circuits, is our most important task. Each person should be free to choose a role if he wants and to live without roles if he wants, but the freedom and potentiality should be wired in, available.

Least freedom probably exists in prison; here the roles tend to be most tightly defined. You either fuck or get fucked, and if you are fucked, you fit into an inescapable and undesirable category. When I went to visit the Billerica House of Correction, the prison master arranged an interview with two older trustees in order to intimidate any gay people coming to visit the prison. A lot of what they said was lies (like we were in danger of being raped and stabbed there), but one thing stood out in my mind. The trustee said, don't you understand, they've taken everything from us; we've only got one thing to hold onto, our manhood. Having to be a man is a mark of oppression; the more wretched your position, the more manly you're expected to be and the harder it is for you to be a faggot. The more you have to stay in the closet. The less freedom you have to be gay.

The situation with femininity or transvestism among men is similar—both in prison and in general "society." If you relinquish the role of straight man, then you have no other choice but to accept the role of woman—which brings a loss of freedom, money and independence. My own experience of cross-dressing is not great but that little has been educational. I remember wearing a robe at one gay "pride" celebration. In workshops, the lunch room and around the campus— everyone tended to ignore me and everything I said. Pantalooned men might open a few doors but for them I had otherwise ceased to exist. In themselves, roles are not evil but what is wrong is the fact that some people are involuntarily forced into certain definitely inferior roles and others fit into superior roles by their birthright as it were.

The idea of freedom seems particularly middle class; children of the working class are taught that you must either dominate someone or be dominated. And these roles appear in sexual relations. Anal sex is much more common among men in the third world or in rural areas than in the ruling parts of the empire (big cities for instance). The mouth is closer to the mind, personality above the rectum. Generally one is either dominant or dominated. The more middle-class a group of faggots, the more likely they will be into oral sex and the more likely it will be mutual. An interesting study shows that college students active in gay groups tend more toward oral sex than those outside gay groups who tend more toward anal sex. (No report on relative tooth decay.)

Whatever the shortcomings of the gay liberation fronts, they really tried to break down roles. Admittedly they could be freer because so many were from the middle class. The luxury and possibilities of freedom were hard to come to and to understand, but that insight is perhaps our single most precious heritage. It doesn't always make things easier; Phyllis Sawyer's "After Women's Liberation" says it in two lines: "Hurting more/enjoying it less." But occasionally the vision, luxury, even ecstasy of a mutual faggot sexuality can be found. A few days ago, I felt it in Lindhurst Butte, Oregon: when I was fucking and couldn't tell whether I was inside him or he was inside me. And later I couldn't remember which way it was. Maybe everyone feels that all the time but it was a revelation to me.

Everything boils down to *inequality.* We live in a culture/economy where all things are measured and sold; any inequality is counted and counts against you. Even the drug culture is a rat race of competition and selling and enslavement where the "superior" or those who have an edge either use it or have the potential for using it, and thus rule, prevail, while those without the edge fall to one side. Inequality cannot be dealt with on an individual philanthropic level: the unequal resent philanthropy, fear the loss of largesse. For instance, if a beautiful trick decides to befriend a "dirty old man," love him, go home with him, and become his lover, the economy dictates that the D.O.M. should live in constant jeopardy; he knows that he lives at the mercy of the other who has enough points to make different choices; the D.O.M. resents inevitably the disparity. Or the inequality could be money; someone might be rich and able to buy lovers. The poor lover will inevitably resent the inequality, where riches can be denied or granted him by reasons beyond his control.

Billie Holiday sings that "Them that's got, gets; them that's not, lose, that's what the Bible says—and it still is news." Matthew 25:29, "For the man who has will always be given more, till he has enough and to spare; and the man who has not will forfeit even what he has." An Arab proverb says, "If you are a peg, endure the knocking; if you are a mallet, strike." That's the conventional wisdom of centuries against which we now speak.

I believe early clues to a new direction can be found in my own experiences in tea rooms, parks, trucks, baths and other untalked of corners of this land. I don't want to make comparisons (such as faggots have made immemorially) about which faggots are good, better, best. Nor would I want to suggest the best bar or argue that monogamous marriage is the only respectable way. What I want to defend is the proposition that there is a whole body of experience within the existing promiscuity of faggots that (if accepted for the good it is) is revolutionary. I don't say there aren't "bad" sides to faggot behavior, the way we treat and mistreat each other. I offer some generalizations not as a Utopian fantasy, but as a way for making change, a way rooted in the actual social experience of faggots—a way tied deeply into centuries of suffering and experience. You could label it "revolutionary sensuality," but I prefer *Indiscriminate Promiscuity*. People (particularly menpeople) have tended to classify love as changeless, timeless, natural, and as unavoidable or indefinite as death. This mystification is a fraud meant to prevent any questioning or change in the so-called "reality." Why should there not be a socialism of love and sex no less than of work and money? Should not equality and freedom extend to our bodies and their physical relationships as well as to the economy?

We need to be *indiscriminate*. No one should be denied love because they are old, ugly, fat, crippled, bruised, of the wrong race, color, creed, sex or country of national origin. We need to copulate with anyone who requests our company; set aside all the false contraptions of being hard to get, unavailable—that is, costly on the capitalist market. We need to leave behind the whole mentality of measurement; it is a massive tool of social control. We all measure ourselves against some standard, find ourselves wanting, and feel inferior, guilty, wrong, weak—in need of authority, direction, correction, ruling and enslavement.

Discriminating and distinguishing involves more than recognizing differences. Differences can indeed be precious, but they need to be understood as that—precious differences, not marketable qualities that have to be counted, compared and graded. Indeed, discrimination presumes a scale in which one perfection is taken as standard; everything short of achieving that goal is substandard and inferior on a particular scale.

Beauty, for instance, tends to cluster around a few ruling imperial standards—blond, blue-eyed, Nordic, etc. But even if different standards were set—"Black is beautiful," for instance—that would not be enough unless the competitive, measuring, rewarding, punishing system were junked. We are crippled by the pursuit of a false social ideal in sex—generally that of an Anglo-Saxon man. In fact, beauty is not one ideal; it is in men everywhere. Beauty needs to be appreciated in its multiplicity and many manifestations; it also needs to be freed from its market value, its power, its usefulness in getting what you want (a lover, money, love, attention, customers, etc.).

Actually the greatest impediment to indiscriminacy is probably not so much ugliness as familiarity. I learned early about the incest tabu. I had this understanding faggot friend, who could see through my soul and perhaps me likewise. He made it with lots of people, some not that different from me. So once I said, "Why don't we try it together?" "Oh no," he answered, "that would be too much like incest." A faggot is more likely to be attracted to some stranger—hitchhiker, new-in-town, transient—than to a close friend. Part of this is the simple desire to keep social relations and sex separated; the latter being considered dirty and unworthy. But even those who overcome this prejudice, who can accept their sexuality for the joy, dignity and beauty that it can be— they still lose some ardor and passion after a few years' acquaintance with another faggot. I've noticed this with my lover of nearly ten years; as he has come to be like my family to me, he has lost interest in me sexually.

Being indiscriminate would not only break down the hesitations about "ugliness" and undesirability but also break tabus between those who work and live closely together. A meeting would never be for "business" alone; every contact could be sexual as well. Our whole social system could become eroticized, sexualized, changed, revolutionized. The alienation most of us feel most of the time is most pronounced in our most intimate institutions—the "family" of social units in which we live. As David Cooper maintains in *Death of the Family*, these units are "the ultimately perfected form of non-meeting" of "anonymized people."

We need to be more *promiscuous* as well as less discriminating. Promiscuous in every way with our bodies. Release all the armors and shackles, open all the pores and holes up for sexual communication. No restraint in any way. Multiple loves—amoeba-like as in orgies at the baths—single couplings, perhaps between subway stops or between classes or on the way shopping. We must be open at all times for sexual activity; in fact, not make it an in-between action, but make every action sexual. Unlike capitalist decadence, our sexuality would not be separated from our business, our sexuality would not "drag" us down or wear us out for the tasks of building a totally free society. Our sexuality would be that society.

Promiscuity among faggots is not some dream or fantasy; it is a real social experience in many parts of our community. The present short-comings of the baths, bushes, trucks, tea rooms and other libidinous areas is partly the discrimination that still goes on there. But it is more in the failure to provide for our lovers once we have been with them. Without a society in which everyone can make it (as well as make out), there will continue to be the question of "taking care of" each other— that is inequality, where the superior must provide for the inferior. Much of the fears and possessiveness in our present families comes from the way people are measured and sold on the love market as property. In our economy of scarcity, everyone continuously fears poverty and abandonment. Everyone is constantly hoarding people and love. Each relationship is curdled by the tendency to cling to someone else, to hold on for fear that there will be no more love after this. And the more marketable the love object and the less marketable the lover, the more desperate the clinging and the more terrifying the loss of a love object.

I think this may be my own greatest fantasy and fear—that of loss and abandonment. I've always worried about loss, what happens when the lover goes away, what if he leaves me, where then will I be? Such fear leads one to shut off, to be closed to loving, to protect oneself for fear of being wounded. And even coming to love the wound too dearly. Doubtless my own fantasy is my own particular one and cannot be exactly imposed on others, certainly not all faggots nor all society. Yet, I offer my humble solution, Indiscriminate Promiscuity, and wonder if it wouldn't allow for a society in which each person could be free to provide for themselves without dependency.

This would, I believe, be the essence of a socialist economy: where each individual would become a person, be free, be an independent, unique agent, where they might explore the voice deep within. A humane socialism must move beyond trade-union economism; it must lose its prudery, and find sexuality. In calling for a socialist society, we do not ask some party or state to suddenly give something to us—like legalize homosexuality.

We don't want something, we want everything. Not half a loaf, but the whole thing; not for some but for everyone. Our desires are not false, nor an expression of hunger, appetite, want: our desires—to suck cock for instance—are creative, they are the road to creation, to the modification of reality. Our bodies themselves are real; our sexual organs are not separate from our persons; they should be an expression of our individuality. "Capitalism," a friend of mine writes, "keeps the desires in the frame of its limits, it enlarges these limits to contain the desires, it co-opts. There is hope, though, because no one knows where the new eruption is going to come from, and desire is more and more coming from unexpected places, so that capitalism has a harder time to prevent revolution. While the capitalists are reading Mao, Castro, Che, to prevent a surprise attack, the marginals invent revolutionary strategies, unheard of, unread before."

A Secret Side of Lesbian Sexuality

Pat Califia

from *The Advocate*, December 27, 1979

*Lesbian feminism promoted a vision of lesbian sexuality that stressed equality and reciprocity. In this essay, Califia explores the world of lesbian S/M—in which power, dominance and submission play a part. Pat Califia has written many works of sexual advice, erotica, and on the theory of sexuality such as **Sapphistry**, **Macho Sluts**, and **Public Sex: The Culture of Radical Sex**.*

The sexual closet is bigger than you think. By all rights, we shouldn't be here, but we are. It's obvious that conservative forces like organized religion, the police, and other agents of the tyrannical majority don't want sadomasochism to flourish anywhere, and sexually active women have always been a threat the system won't tolerate. But conservative gay liberationists and orthodox feminists are also embarrassed by kinky sexual subcultures (even if that's where they do their tricking). "We are just like heterosexuals (or men)," is their plea for integration, their way of whining for some of America's carbon monoxide pie. Drag queens, leathermen, rubber freaks, boy-lovers, girl-lovers, dyke sadomasochists, prostitutes, transsexuals—we make that plea sound like such a feeble lie. We are not like everyone else. And our difference is not created solely by oppression. It is a preference, a sexual preference.

Lesbian S&M isn't terribly well-organized (yet). But in San Francisco, women can find partners and friends who will aid and abet them in pursuing the delights of dominance and submission. We don't have bars. We don't even have newspapers or magazines with sex ads. I sometimes think the gay subculture must have looked like this, when urbanization first started. Since our community consists of word-of-mouth and social networks, we have to work very hard to keep it going. It's a survival issue. If the arch-conformists with their cardboard cunts and angora wienies had their way, we wouldn't exist at all. As we become more visible, we encounter more hostility, more violence. This article is my way of refusing the narcotic of self-hatred. We must break out of the silence that persecution imposes on its victims.

I am a sadist. The polite term is "top," but I don't like to use it. It dilutes my image and my message. If someone wants to know about my sexuality, they can deal with me on my own terms. I don't particularly care to make it easy. S&M is scary. That's at least half its significance. We select the most frightening, disgusting, or unacceptable activities and transmute them into pleasure. We make use of all the forbidden symbols and all the disowned emotions. S&M is a deliberate, premeditated, erotic blasphemy. It is a form of sexual extremism and sexual dissent.

I identify more strongly as a sadomasochist than as a lesbian. I hang out in the gay community because that's where the sexual fringe starts to unravel. Most of my partners are women, but gender is not my boundary. I am limited by my own imagination, cruelty and compassion, and by the greed and stamina of my partner's body. If I had a choice between being shipwrecked on a desert island with a vanilla lesbian and a hot male masochist, I'd pick the boy. This is the kind of sex I like—sex that tests physical limits within a context of polarized roles. It is the only kind of sex I am interested in having.

I am not typical of S&M lesbians, nor do I represent them. In fact, because I define myself as a sadist, I am atypical. Most S&M people *prefer* the submissive "bottom" or masochistic role. The bulk of the porn (erotic, psychoanalytic, and political) that gets written about S&M focuses on the masochist. People who do public speaking about S&M have told me they get a more sympathetic hearing if they identify as bottoms. This makes sense, in a twisted kind of way. The uninitiated associate masochism with incompetence, lack of assertiveness, and self-destruction. But sadism is associated with chainsaw murders. A fluffy-sweater type listening to a masochist may feel sorry for her, but she's terrified of me. I'm the one who is ostensibly responsible for manipulating or coercing the M into degradation—all 130 pounds 5' 2" of me. Therefore, my word is suspect. It is nevertheless true that my services are in demand, that I respect my partners' limits and that both (or more) of us obtain great pleasure from a scene. I started exploring S&M as a bottom, and I still put my legs in the air now and then. I have never asked a submissive to do something I haven't or couldn't do.

In addition to being a sadist, I have a leather fetish. If I remember my Krafft-Ebing, that's another thing women aren't supposed to do. Oh, well. Despite the experts, seeing, smelling, or handling leather makes me cream. Every morning before I go out the door, I make a ritual out of putting on my leather jacket. The weight of it, settling on my shoulders, is reassuring. Once I zip it, turn the collar up and cram my hands into the pockets, the jacket is my armor. It also puts me in danger when I wear it on the street by alerting the curious and the angry to my presence.

I get all kinds of different reactions. Voyeurs drool. Queer-baiting kids shout or throw bottles from their cars. Well-dressed hets, secure in their privilege, give me the condescending smile of the genital dilettante. Some gay men are amused when they see me coming. They take me for a fag hag, a mascot dressed up to avoid embarrassing my macho friends. Others are resentful. Leather is their province, and a cunt is not entitled to wear the insignia of a sadomasochist. They avoid my shadow. I might be menstruating and make their spears go dull. When I visit a dyke bar, the patrons take me for a member of that nearly-extinct species, the butch. Femmes under this misapprehension position themselves within my reach, signaling their availability, not bothering to actively pursue me. They seem to expect me to do everything a man would do, except knock them up. Given the fact that I prefer someone to come crawling and begging for my attention, and to work pretty damned hard before they get it, this strikes me as being very funny. In women's groups, the political clones, the Dworkinites, see my studded belt and withdraw. I am obviously a sex pervert, and good, real true lesbians are not sex perverts. They are high priestesses of feminism, conjuring up the "wimmin's" revolution. As I understand it, after the wimmin's revolution, sex will consist of wimmin holding hands, taking their shirts off and dancing in a circle. Then we will all fall asleep at exactly the same moment. If we didn't all fall asleep, something else might happen—something male-identified, objectifying, pornographic, noisy, and undignified. Something like an orgasm.

This is why they say leather is expensive. When I wear it, disdain, amusement, and the threat of violence follow me from my door to my destination and home again. Is it worth it? Can the sex be that good? When am I going to get to the point and tell you what we do?

I can smell your titillation. Well—since you want it so bad, I'll let you have a taste of it.

If I'm interested in someone, I call them up and ask them if they'd like to go out for dinner. I have never picked up a stranger in a bar. My partners are friends, women who strike up acquaintances with me because they've heard me talk about S&M, women I know from Samois. (I also have a lover who is my slave. We enjoy conducting joint seductions or creating bizarre sexual adventures to tell each other about later.) If she agrees, I will tell her where and when to meet me. Over dinner, I begin to play doctor—Dr. Kinsey. I like to know when she started being sexual with other people, if and when she started masturbating, if and how she likes to have an orgasm, when she came out as a lesbian (if she has), and I give her similar information about me. Then I like to ask about her S&M fantasies and how much experience she has with acting them out. I also try to find out if she has any health problems (asthma, diabetes, etc.) that should limit play.

This conversation need not be clinical. It is not an interview—it is an interrogation. I am taking for granted my right to possess intimate information about my quarry. Giving me that information is the beginning of her submission. The sensations this creates are subtle, but we both begin to get turned on.

I will probably encourage her to get a little high. I don't like playing with women who are too stoned to feel what I am doing, nor do I want someone shedding inhibitions because of a chemical they've ingested. I prefer to deny a bottom any inhibitions and to take them away. However, I do like her to feel relaxed and somewhat vulnerable and suggestible.

If there's time, we may go to a bar. Socializing in gay men's leather bars is problematic for a lesbian. I prefer bars where I know some of the bartenders and patrons. I have rarely been refused admittance, but I have been made uncomfortable by men who felt I was an intruder. If there were women's bars that didn't make me feel even more unwelcome, I'd go there. Since I am a sadomasochist, I feel entitled to the space I take up in a men's bar. I sometimes wonder how many of the men exhibiting their leather in the light from the pinball machines go home and really work it out, and how many of them settle for fucking and sucking.

A leather bar provides a safe place to start establishing roles. I like to order my submissive to bring me a drink. She doesn't get a beer of her own. When she wants a drink, she asks me for one, and I pour it into her mouth while she kneels at my feet. I begin to handle her, appraising her flesh, correcting her posture, and fondling or exposing her so that she feels embarrassed and draws closer to me. I like to hear someone ask for mercy or protection. If she isn't already wearing a collar, I put one on her, and drag her over to a mirror—behind the bar, in the bathroom, on a wall—and make her look at it. I watch the response very carefully. I don't like women who collapse into passivity, whose bodies go limp and faces go blank. I want to see the confusion, the anger, the turn-on, the helplessness.

As soon as I am sure she is turned on (something that can be ascertained with the index finger if I can get her zipper down), I hustle her out of there. I especially like to put someone in handcuffs and lead them out on a leash.

This is one of the gifts I offer a submissive: the illusion of having no choice, the thrill of being taken.

The collar will keep her aroused until we reach my flat. I prefer to play in my space since it's set up for bondage and whipping. I will order her to stay two steps behind me, to reassure her that we really are going to do a scene. As soon as the door is locked behind us, I order her to strip. In my room, there is no such thing as casual nudity. When I take away someone's clothing, I am temporarily denying their humanity, with all its privileges and responsibilities.

Nudity can be taken a step further. The bottom can be shaved. A razor, passing over the skin, removes the pelt that warms and conceals. My lover/slave has her cunt shaved. It reminds her that I own her genitals, and reinforces her role as my child and property.

Shedding her clothes while I remain fully dressed is enough to shame and excite most bottoms. Once she is naked, I put her on the floor, and there she stays until I move her or raise her up. I stand over her, trail a riding crop down her spine, and tell her that she belongs underneath me. I talk about how good she's going to make my cunt feel and how strict I am going to be with her. I may allow her to embrace my boots. After delineating her responsibilities and cussing her out a little for being easy, I haul her up, slap her face, hold her head against my hip while I unzip, and let her feast on my clit.

I wonder if any man could understand how this act, receiving sexual service, feels to me. I was taught to dread sex, to fight it off, to provide it under duress or in exchange for romance and security. I was trained to take responsibility for other people's gratification and pretend pleasure when others pretend to have my pleasure in mind. It is shocking and profoundly satisfying to commit this piece of rebellion, to take pleasure exactly as I want it, to exact it like tribute. I need not pretend I enjoy a bottom's ministration if they are unskilled, nor do I need to be grateful.

I like to come before I do a scene because it takes the edge off my hunger. For the same reason, I don't like to play when I am stoned or drunk. I want to be in control. I need all my wits about me to outguess the bottom's needs and fears, take her out of herself, and bring her back. During the session, she will receive much more direct physical stimulation than I will. So I take what I need. From her mouth, she feeds me the energy I need to dominate and abuse her.

While I am getting off, I usually begin to fantasize about the woman on her knees. I visualize her in a certain position or a certain role. This fantasy is the seed that the whole scene sprouts from. When she's finished pleasing me, I order her to crawl onto my bed, which is on the floor, and I tie her up.

Bottoms tend to be anxious. Because there is a shortage of tops, they get used to playing all kinds of little psychological numbers on themselves to feel miserable and titillated. They also like to feel greedy and guilty, and get anxious about that. The bondage is reassurance. She can measure the intensity of my passion by the tightness of my knots. It also puts an end to bullshit speculation about whether I am doing this just because she likes it so much. I make sure there's no way she can get loose on her own. Restraint becomes security. She knows I want her. She knows I am in charge.

Being tied up is arousing, and I intensify this arousal by teasing her, playing with her breasts and clit, calling her nasty names. When she starts to squirm, I begin to rough her up a little, taking her to the edge of pain, the edge that melts and turns over into pleasure. I move from pinching her nipples to a pair of clamps that makes then ache and burn. I may put clips all over her breasts or on the labia. I will check her cunt to make sure it's still wet, and tell her how turned on she is, if she doesn't already know.

At some point, I will always use a whip. Some bottoms like to be whipped until they are bruised. Others find just the visual image exciting and may want to hear the sound of it whistling in the air or feel the handle moving in and out of them. A whip is a great way to get someone to be here now. They can't look away from it, and they can't think about anything else.

If the pain goes beyond a mild discomfort, the bottom will probably get scared. She will start to wonder, "Why am I doing this? Am I going to be able to take this?" There are many ways to get someone past this point. One is to ask her to take it for me because I need to watch her suffer. One is to administer a fixed number of blows as a punishment for some sexual offense. Another is to convince a bottom that they deserve the pain, and must endure it because they are "only" a slave. Pacing is essential. The sensations need to increase gradually. The particular implement involved may also be important. Some women who cannot tolerate whipping have a very high tolerance for other things— nipple play, hot wax, enemas, or verbal humiliation.

When I am playing bottom, I don't want pain or bondage for their own sake. I want to please. The top is my mistress. She has condescended to train me, and it is very important to me to deserve her attention. The basic dynamic of S&M is the power dichotomy, not pain. Handcuffs, dog collars, whips, kneeling, being bound, tit clamps, hot wax, enemas, penetration, and giving sexual service are all metaphors for the power imbalance. However, I must admit that I get bored pretty fast with a bottom who is not willing to take any pain.

The will to please is a bottom's source of pleasure, but it is also a source of danger. If the top's intentions are dishonorable (i.e., emotional sabotage) or her skill is faulty, the bottom is not safe when she yields. The primary point of competition among tops is to be emotionally and physically safe to play with, to be worthy of the gift of submission. Someone who makes mistakes gets a bad reputation very fast, and only inexperienced or foolish bottoms will go under for them.

Why would anyone want to be dominated, given the risks? Because it is a healing process. As a top, I find the old wounds and unappeased hunger I nourish, I cleanse and close the wounds. I devise and mete out appropriate punishments for old, irrational sins. I trip the bottom up, I see her as she is, and I forgive her and turn her on and make her come, despite her unworthiness or self-hatred or fear. We are all afraid of losing, of being captured and defeated. I take the sting out of that fear. A good scene doesn't end with orgasm—it ends with catharsis.

I would never go back to tweaking tits and munching cunt in the dark, not after this. Two lovers sweating against each other, each struggling for her own goal, eyes blind to each other—how appalling, how deadly. I want to see and share in every sensation and emotion my partner experiences, and I want all of it to come from me. I don't want to leave anything out. The affronted modesty and the hostility are as important as the affection and lust.

The bottom must be my superior. She is the victim I present for the night's inspection. I derive an awful knowledge from each gasp, the tossing head, the blanching of her knuckles. In order to force her to lose control, I must unravel her defenses, breach her walls, and alternate subtlety and persuasion with brutality and violence. Playing a bottom who did not demand my respect and admiration would be like eating rotten fruit.

S&M is high technology sex. It is so time consuming and absorbing that I have no desire to own anyone on a full-time basis. I am satisfied with their sexual submission. This is the difference between real slavery or exploitation and S&M. I am interested in something ephemeral, pleasure, not in economic control or forced reproduction.

This may be why S&M is so threatening to the established order, and why it is so heavily penalized and persecuted. S&M roles are not related to gender or sexual orientation or race or class. My own needs dictate which role I will adopt. Our political system cannot digest the concept of power unconnected to privilege. S&M recognizes the erotic under-pinnings of our systems, and seeks to reclaim them. There's an enormous hard-on beneath the priest's robe, the cop's uniform, the president's business suit, the soldier's khakis. But that phallus is powerful only as long as it is concealed, elevated to the level of a symbol, never exposed or used in literal fucking. A cop with his hard on sticking out can be punished, rejected, blown, or you can sit on it, but he is no longer a demi-god. In an S&M context, the uniforms and roles and dialogue become a parody of authority, a challenge to it, a recognition of its secret sexual nature.

Governments are based on sexual control. Any group of people who gain access to authoritarian power become accessories to that ideology. They begin to perpetuate and enforce sexual control. Women and gays who are hostile to other sexual minorities are siding with fascism. They don't want the uniforms to degenerate into drag—they want uniforms of their own.

As I write this, there is a case in Canada that will determine whether or not S&M sex between consenting adults can be legal. This case began when a gay male bathhouse that caters to an S&M clientele was raided. After that raid, a man in Toronto was busted for "keeping a common bawdy house." The "bawdy house" was a room in his apartment he had fixed up for S&M sex. Yet another man was busted for false imprisonment and aggravated assault. These charges stemmed from an S&M three-way.

In San Francisco, months before Moscone and Milk were assassinated and the cops smashed into the Elephant Walk, half the leather bars in the Folsom Street area lost their liquor licenses due to police harassment. The Gay Freedom Day Parade Committee tried to pass a resolution that would bar leather and S&M regalia from the parade.

I don't know how long it will take for other S&M people to get as angry as I am. I don't know how long we will continue to work in gay organizations that patronize us and threaten us with expulsion if we don't keep quiet about our sexuality. I don't know how long we will continue to let women's groups who believe that S&M and pornography are the same thing and cause violence against women to go unchallenged because they are ostensibly feminist. I don't know how long we will continue to run our sex ads in magazines that feature judgmental, slanderous articles about us. I don't know how long we will continue to be harassed and assaulted or murdered on the street, or how long we will tolerate the fear of losing our apartments or being fired from our jobs or arrested for making the wrong kind of noise during some heavy sex.

I do know that whenever we start to get angry, walk out, and work for our own cause, it will be long overdue.

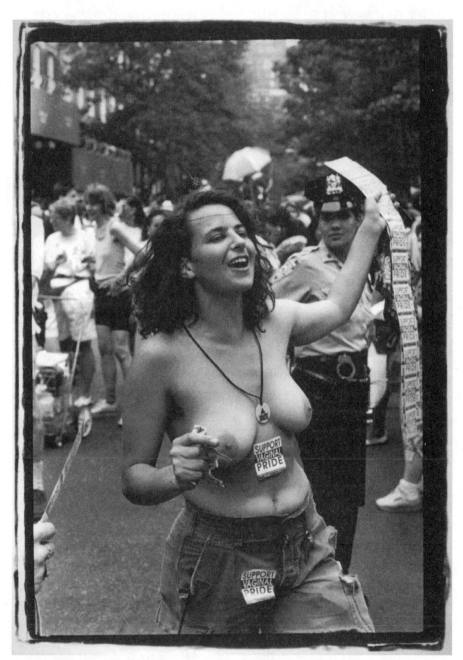

© Fred W. McDarrah

What We're Rollin' Around in Bed With

Amber Hollibaugh and Cherríe Moraga

from *Heresies*, 1981

Lesbian feminism was very critical of the forms of lesbian sexuality that had existed before the re-emergence of feminism in the seventies. In particular, it dismissed butch/femme roles as an imitation of patriarchal heterosexuality. In this dialogue, two lesbians, Amber Hollibaugh, a community organizer and author of **My Dangerous Desires** *(2000) and* **Cherríe Moraga**, *a prize- winning playwright, author of* **Loving in the War Years** *(1983), and co-editor of* **This Bridge Called My Back: Writings by Radical Women of Color** *(1981) discuss how some lesbian sexualities were excluded by the new lesbian feminist orthodoxy.*

Sexual Silences in Feminism
A Conversation Toward Ending Them

BThis article was derived from a series of conversations we entertained for many months. Through it, we wish to illuminate both our common and our different relationships to a feminist movement to which we are both committed.

The Critique

In terms of sexual issues, it seems feminism has fallen short of its original intent. The whole notion of "the personal is political" which surfaced in the early part of the movement (and which many of us have used to an extreme) is suddenly and ironically dismissed when we begin to discuss sexuality. We have become a relatively sophisticated movement, so many women think they now have to have the theory before they expose the experience. It seems we simply did not take our feminism to heart enough. This most privatized aspect of ourselves, our sex lives, has dead-ended into silence within the feminist movement.

Feminism has never directly addressed women's sexuality except in its most oppressive aspects in relation to men (e.g., marriage, the nuclear family, wife battering, rape, etc.). Heterosexuality is both an actual sexual interaction and a system. No matter how we play ourselves out sexually, we are all affected by the system inasmuch as our sexual values are filtered through a society where heterosexuality is considered the norm. It is difficult to believe that there is anyone in the world who hasn't spent some time in great pain over the choices and limitations which that system has forced on all of us. We all suffer from heterosexism every single day (whether we're conscious of it or not). And, as long as that's true, men and women, women and women, men and men—all different kinds of sexual combinations—must fight against this system if we are ever going to perceive ourselves as sexually profitable and loving human beings.

By analyzing the institution of heterosexuality through feminism, we learned what's oppressive about it and why people cooperate with it or don't, but we didn't learn what's *sexual*. We don't really know, for instance, why men and women are still attracted to each other, even through all that oppression, which we know to be true. There is something genuine that happens between heterosexuals but which gets perverted in a thousand different ways. There is heterosexuality outside of heterosexism.

What grew out of this kind of "nonsexual" theory was a "transcendent" definition of sexuality wherein lesbianism (since it exists outside the institution of heterosexuality) came to be seen as the practice of feminism. It set up a "perfect" vision of egalitarian sexuality, where we could magically leap over our heterosexist conditioning into mutually orgasmic, struggle-free, trouble-free sex. We feel this vision has become both misleading and damaging to many feminists, but in particular to lesbians. Who created this sexual model as a goal in the first place? Who can really live up to such an ideal? There is little language, little literature that reflects the actual sexual struggles of most lesbians, feminist or not.

The failure of feminism to answer all the questions regarding women, in particular women's sexuality, is the same failure the homosexual movement suffers from around gender. It's a confusing of those two things—that some of us are both female and homosexual—that

539

may be the source of some of the tension between the two movements and of the inadequacies of each. When we walk down the street, we are both female and lesbian. We are working-class white and working-class Chicana. We are all these things rolled into one, and there is no way to eliminate even one aspect of ourselves.

The Conversation:

Cherríe Moraga: In trying to develop sexual theory, I think we should start by talking about what we're rollin' around in bed with. We both agree that the way feminism has dealt with sexuality has been entirely inadequate.

Amber Hollibaugh: Right. Sexual theory has traditionally been used to say, "People have been forced to be this thing; people could be that thing." And you're left standing in the middle going, "Well, I am here, and I don't know how to get there." It hasn't been able to talk realistically about what people are sexually.

I think by focusing on roles in lesbian relationships we can begin to unravel who we really are in bed. When you hide how profoundly roles can shape your sexuality, you can use that as an example of other things that get hidden. There's a lot of different things that shape the way that people respond, some not so easy to see, some more forbidden, as I perceive S/M to be. Like with S/M, when I think of it, I'm frightened. Why? Is it because I might be sexually fascinated with it and I don't know how to accept that? Who am I there? The point is that when you deny that roles, S/M, fantasy, or any sexual differences exist in the first place, you can only come up with neutered sexuality, where everybody's got to be basically the same because anything different puts the element of power and deviation in there and threatens the whole picture.

CM: Exactly. Remember how I told you that growing up what turned me on sexually, at a very early age, had to do with the fantasy of capture, taking a woman, and my identification was with the man, taking? Well, something like that would be so frightening to bring up in a feminist context—fearing people would put it in some sicko sexual box. And yet, the truth is, I do have some real gut-level misgivings about my sexual connection with capture. It might feel very sexy to imagine "taking" a woman, but it has sometimes occurred at the expense of my feeling, sexually, like I can surrender myself, to a woman that is, always needing to be the one in control, calling the shots. It's a very butch trip, and I feel like this can keep me private and protected and can prevent me from fully being able to express myself.

AH: But it's not wrong, in and of itself, to have a capture fantasy. The real question is, Does it actually limit you? For instance, does it allow you to eroticize someone else but never see yourself as erotic? Does it keep you always in control? Does the fantasy force you into a dimension of sexuality that feels very narrow to you? If it causes you to look at your lover in only one light, then you may want to check it out. But if you can't even dream about wanting a woman in this way in the first place, then you can't figure out what is narrow and heterosexist in it and what's just play. After all, it's only one fantasy.

CM: Well, what I think is very dangerous about keeping down such fantasies is that they are forced to stay unconscious. Then, next thing you know, in the actual sexual relationship, you become the capturer; that is, you try to have power over your lover, psychologically or whatever. If the desire for power is so hidden and unacknowledged, it will inevitably surface through manipulation or what have you. If you couldn't play captured, you'd be it.

AH: Part of the problem in talking about sexuality is it's so enormous in our culture that people don't have any genuine sense of dimension. So that when you say *capture*, every fantasy you have ever heard of from Robin Hood to colonialism comes racing into your mind, and all you really maybe wanted to do was have your girlfriend lay you down. But, in feminism, we can't even explore these questions because what they say is, in gender, there is a masculine oppressor and a female oppressee. So whether you might fantasize yourself in a role a man might perform or a woman in reaction to a man, this makes you sick, fucked-up, and you had better go and change it.

If you don't speak of fantasies, they become a kind of amorphous thing that envelops you and hangs over your relationship, and you get terrified by the silence. If you have no way to describe what your desire is and what your fear is, you have no way to negotiate with your lover. And I guarantee you, six months or six years later, the relationship has paid. Things that are kept private and hidden become painful and deformed.

When you say that part of your sexuality has been hooked up with capture, I want to say that absolutely there's a heterosexist part of that, but what part of that is just plain dealing with power, sexually? I don't want to live outside of power in my sexuality, but I don't want to be trapped into a heterosexist concept of power either. But what I feel feminism asks of me is to throw the baby out with the bathwater.

For example, I think the reason butch/femme stuff got hidden within lesbian feminism is because people are profoundly afraid of questions of power in bed. And, though everybody doesn't play out power the way I do, the question of power affects who and how you eroticize your sexual need. And it is absolutely at the bottom of all sexual inquiry. I can't say to you, for instance, I am trying to work through being a femme so I won't have to be one any more.

CM: But what is femme to you? I told you once that what I thought of femme was passive, unassertive, etc. and you didn't fit that image. And you said to me, "Well, change your definition of *femme.*"

AH: My fantasy life is deeply involved in a butch/femme exchange. I never come together with a woman, sexually, outside of those roles. Femme is active, not passive. It's saying to my partner, "Love me enough to let me go where I need to go, and take me there. Don't make me think it through. Give me a way to be so in my body that I don't have to think, that you can fantasize for the both of us. You map it out. You are in control."

It's hard to talk about things like giving up power without it sounding passive. I am willing to give myself over to a woman equal to her amount of wanting. I expose myself for her to appreciate. I open myself out for her to see what's possible for her to love in me that's female. I want her to respond to it. I may not be doing something active with my body, but more eroticizing her need that I feel in her hands as she touches me.

In the same way, as a butch, you want and conceive of a woman in a certain way. You dress a certain way to attract her, and you put your sexual need within these certain boundaries to communicate that desire. And yet there's a part of me that feels maybe all this is not even a question of roles. Maybe it's much richer territory than that.

CM: Yes, I feel the way I want a woman can be a very profound experience. Remember I told you how when I looked up at my lover's face when I was making love to her (I was actually just kissing her breast at the moment), but when I looked up at her face, I could feel and see how deeply every part of her was present? That every pore in her body was entrusting me to handle her, to take care of her sexual desire. This look on her face is like nothing else. It fills me up. She entrusts me to determine where she'll go sexually. And I honestly feel a power inside me strong enough to heal the deepest wound.

AH: Well, I can't actually see what I look like, but I can feel it in my lover's hands when I look the way you described. When I open myself up more and more to her sensation of wanting a woman, when I eroticize that in her, I feel a kind of ache in my body, but it's not an ache to do something. I can feel a hurt spot and a need, and it's there, and it's just the tip of it, the tip of that desire, and that is what first gets played with, made erotic. It's light and playful. It doesn't commit you to exposing a deeper part of yourself sexually. Then I begin to pick up passion. And the passion isn't butch or femme. It's just passion.

But from this place, if it's working, I begin to imagine myself being the woman that a woman always wanted. That's when I begin to eroticize. That's what I begin to feel from my lover's hands. I begin to fantasize myself becoming more and more female in order to comprehend and meet what I feel happening in her body. I don't want her not to be female to me. Her need is female, but it's *butch* because I am asking her to expose her desire through the movement of her hands on my body, and I'll respond. I want to give up power in response to her need. This can feel profoundly powerful and very unpassive.

A lot of times how I feel it in my body is I feel like I have this fantasy of pulling a woman's hips into my cunt. I can feel the need painfully in another woman's body. I can feel the impact, and I begin to play and respond to that hunger and desire. And I begin to eroticize the fantasy that she can't get enough of me. It makes me want to enflame my body. What it feels like is that I'm in my own veins and I'm sending heat up into my thighs. It's very hot.

CM: Oh, honey, she feels the heat, too.

AH: Yes, and I am making every part of my body accessible to that woman. I completely trust her. There's no place she cannot touch me. My body is literally open to any way she interprets her sexual need. My power is that I know how to read her inside of her own passion. I can hear her. It's like a sexual language; it's a rhythmic language that she uses her hands for. My body is completely in sync with a lover, but I'm not deciding where she's gonna touch me.

CM: But don't you ever fantasize yourself being on the opposite end of that experience?

AH: Well, not exactly in the same way because with butches you can't insist on them giving up their sexual identity. You have to go through that identity to that other place. That's why roles are so significant and you can't throw them out. You have to find a way to use them so you can eventually release your sexuality into other domains that you may feel the role traps you in. But you don't have to throw out the role to explore the sexuality. There are femme ways to orchestrate sexuality. I'm not asking a woman not to be butch. I am asking her to let me express the other part of my own character, where I am actively orchestrating what's happening. I never give up my right to say that I can insist on what happens sexually. Quite often what will happen is I'll simply seduce her. Now, that's very active. The seduction can be very profound, but it's a seduction as a femme.

CM: What comes to my mind is something as simple as you coming over and sitting on her lap. Where a butch, well, she might just go for your throat if she wants you.

AH: Oh yes, different areas for different roles! What's essential is that your attitude doesn't threaten the other person's sexual identity but plays with it. That's what good seduction is all about. I play a lot in that. It's not that I have to have spike heels on in order to fantasize who I am. Now that's just a lot of classist shit, conceiving of femme in such a narrow way.

CM: Well, I would venture to say that some of these dynamics that you're describing happen between most lesbians, only they may both be in the same drag of flannel shirts and jeans. My feeling, however, is—and this is very hard for me—what I described earlier about seeing my lover's face entrusting me like she did, well, I want her to take me to that place, too.

AH: Yes, but you don't want to have to deny your butchness to get there. Right?

CM: Well, that's what's hard. To be butch, to me, is not to be a woman. The classic extreme-butch stereotype is the woman who sexually refuses to allow another woman to touch her. It goes something like this: She doesn't want to feel her femaleness because she thinks of you as the "real" woman and, if she makes love to you, she doesn't have to feel her own body as the object of desire. She can be a kind of "bodiless lover." So when you turn over and want to make love to her and make her feel physically like a woman, then what she is up against is queer. You are a woman making love to her. She feels queerer than anything in that. Get it?

AH: Got it. Whew!

CM: I believe that probably from a very early age the way you conceived of yourself as female has been very different from me. We both have pain, but I think that there is a particular pain attached if you identified yourself as a butch queer from an early age, as I did. I didn't really think of myself as female or male. I thought of myself as this hybrid or something. I just kinda thought of myself as this free agent until I got tits. Then I thought, Oh oh, some problem has occurred here.

For me, the way you conceive of yourself as a woman and the way I am attracted to women sexually reflect that butch/femme exchange where a woman believes herself so woman that it really makes me want her. But, for me, I feel a lot of pain around the fact that it has been difficult for me to conceive of myself as thoroughly female in that sexual way. So retaining my "butchness" is not exactly my desired goal. Now that, in itself, is probably all heterosexist bullshit about what a woman is supposed to be in the first place, but we are talking about the differences between the way you and I conceive of ourselves as sexual beings.

AH: I think it does make a difference. I would argue that a good femme does not play to the part of you that hates yourself for feeling like a man, but to the part of you that knows you're a woman. Because it's absolutely critical to understand that femmes are *women* to women and *dykes* to men in the straight world. You and I are talkin' girl to girl. We're not talking what I was in straight life.

I was ruthless with men, sexually, around what I felt. It was only with women I couldn't avoid opening up my need to have something more than an orgasm. With a woman, I can't refuse to know that the possibility is just there that she'll reach me some place very deeply each time we make love. That's part of my fear of being a lesbian. I can't refuse that possibility with a woman.

You see, I want you as a woman, not as a man; but I want you in the way you need to be, which may not be traditionally female but which is the area that you express as butch. Here is where in the other world you have suffered the most damage. My feeling is, part of the reason I love to be with butches is because I feel I repair that damage. I make it right to want me that hard. Butches have not been allowed to feel their own desire because that part of butch can be perceived by the straight world as male. I feel I get back my femaleness and give a different definition of femaleness to a butch as a femme. That's what I mean about one of those unexplored territories that goes beyond roles, but goes through roles to get there.

CM: How I fantasize sex roles has been really different for me with different women. I do usually enter into an erotic encounter with a woman from the kind of butch place you described, but I have also felt very ripped off there, finding myself taking all the sexual responsibility. I am seriously attracted to butches sometimes. It's a different dynamic, where the sexuality may not seem as fluid or comprehensible, but I know there's a huge part of me that wants to be handled in the way I described I can handle another woman. I am very compelled toward that "lover" posture. I have never totally reckoned with being the "beloved," and, frankly, I don't know if it takes a butch or a femme or what to get me there. I know that it's a struggle within me and it scares the shit out of me to look at it so directly. I've done this kind of searching emotionally, but to combine sex with it seems like very dangerous stuff.

AH: Well, I think everybody has aspects of roles in their relationships, but I feel pretty out there on the extreme end. I think what feminism did, in its fear of heterosexual control of fantasy, was to say that there was almost no fantasy safe to have where you weren't going to have to give up power or take it. There's no sexual fantasy I can think of that doesn't include some aspect of that. But I feel like I have been forced to give up some of my richest potential sexually in the way feminism has defined what is, and what's not, "politically correct" in the sexual sphere.

CM: Oh, of course, when most feminists talk about sexuality, including lesbianism, they're not talking about *desire.* It is significant to me that I came out only when I met a good feminist, although I knew I was queer since eight or nine. That's only when I'd risk it because I wouldn't have to say it's because I want her. I didn't have to say that when she travels by me, my whole body starts throbbing.

AH: Yes, it's just correct.

CM: It was OK to be with her because we all knew men were really fuckers and there were a lot of "OK" women acknowledging that. Read: white and educated. But that's not why I "came out." How could I say that I wanted women so bad I was gonna die if I didn't get me one soon! You know, I just felt the pull in the hips, right?

AH: Yes, really. Well, the first discussion I ever heard of lesbianism among feminists was: "We've been sex objects to men, and where did it get us? And here when we're just learning how to be friends with other women, you got to go and sexualize it." That's what they said! "Fuck you. Now I have to worry about you looking down my blouse." That's exactly what they meant. It horrified me. "No, no, no," I wanted to say, "that's not me. I promise I'll only look at the sky. Please let me come to a meeting. I'm really OK. I just go to the bars and fuck like a rabbit with women who want me. You know?"

Now, from the onset, how come feminism was so invested in that? They would not examine sexual need with each other except as oppressor-oppressee. Whatever your experience was, you were always the victim. Even if you were the aggressor. So how do dykes fit into that? Dykes who wanted tits, you know?

Now a lot of women have been sexually terrorized, and this makes sense, their needing not to have to deal with explicit sexuality, but they made men out of every sexual dyke. "Oh my God, she wants me, too!"

So it became this really repressive movement where you didn't talk dirty and you didn't want dirty. It really became a bore. So, after meetings, we ran to the bars. You couldn't talk about wanting a woman except very loftily. You couldn't say it hurt at night wanting a woman to touch you. I remember at one meeting breaking down after everybody was talking about being a lesbian very delicately. I began crying. I remember saying, "I can't help it. I just . . . want her. I want to feel her." And everybody forgiving me. It was this atmosphere of me exorcising this crude sexual need for women.

CM: Shit, Amber. I remember being fourteen years old, and there was this girl, a few years older than me, who I had this crush on. And, on the last day of school, I knew I wasn't going to see her for months! We had hugged good-bye, and I went straight home. Going into my bedroom, I got into my unmade bed, and I remember getting the sheets, winding them into a kind of rope, and pulling them up between my legs, and just holding them there under my chin. I just sobbed and sobbed because I knew I couldn't have her, maybe never have a woman to touch. It's just pure need, and it's whole. It's like using sexuality to describe how deeply you need/want intimacy, passion, love.

Most women are not immune from experiencing pain in relation to their sexuality, but certainly lesbians experience a particular pain and oppression. Let us not forget, although feminism would sometimes like us to, that lesbians are oppressed in this world. Possibly, there are some of us who came out through the movement who feel immune to "queer attack," but not the majority of us (no matter when we came out), particularly if you have no economic buffer in this society. If you have enough money and privilege, you can separate yourself from heterosexist oppression. You can be sapphic or something, but you don't have to be queer. It's easier to clean up your act and avoid feeling like a freak if you have a margin in this society because you've got bucks.

The point I am trying to make is that I believe most of us harbor plenty of demons and old hurts inside ourselves around sexuality. I know, for me, that each time I choose to touch another woman, to make love with her, I feel I risk opening up that secret, harbored, vulnerable place. I think that why feminism has been particularly attractive to many "queer" lesbians is that it kept us in a place where we wouldn't have to look at our pain around sexuality any more. Our sisters would just sweep us up into a movement.

AH: Yes, we're not just accusing feminism of silence, but our own participation in that silence has stemmed from our absolute terror of facing that profound sexual need. Period.

There is no doubt in my mind that the feminist movement has radically changed, in an important way, everybody's concept of lesbianism. Everybody across the board. There's not a dyke in the world today (in or out of the bars) who can have the same conversation that she could have had ten years ago. It seeps through the water system or something, you know? Lesbianism is certainly accepted in feminism, but more as a political or intellectual concept. It seems feminism is the last rock of conservatism. It will not be sexualized. It's prudish in that way.

Well, I won't give my sexuality up, and I won't not be a feminist. So I'll build a different movement, but I won't live without either one.

Sometimes, I don't know how to handle how angry I feel about feminism. We may disagree on this. We have been treated in some similar ways, but our relationship to feminism has been different. Mine is a lot longer. I really have taken a lot more shit than you have, specifically around being femme. I have a personal fury. The more I got in touch with how I felt about women, what made me desire and desirable, the more I felt outside the feminist community, and that was just terrifying because, on the one hand, it had given me so much. I loved it. And then I couldn't be who I was. I felt that about class, too. I could describe my feelings about being a woman, but if I described it from my own class, using that language, my experience wasn't valid. I don't know what to do with my anger, particularly around sexuality.

CM: Well, you've gotta be angry. I mean, what you were gonna do is turn off the tape, so we'd have no record of your being mad. What comes out of anger—if you, one woman, can say I have been a sister all these years and you have not helped me, that speaks more to the failure of all that theory and rhetoric than more theory and rhetoric.

AH: Yeah. Remember that night you and me and M. were at the bar and we were talking about roles? She told you later that the reason she had checked out of the conversation was because she knew how much it was hurting me to talk about it. You know, I can't tell you what it meant to me for her to know that. The desperation we all felt at that table talking about sexuality was so great, wanting to be able to understand why we are the way we are sexually.

CM: I know. I remember how at that forum on S/M that happened last spring how that Samois woman came to the front of the room and spoke very plainly and clearly about feeling that through S/M she was really coping with power struggles in a tangible way with her lover. That this time, for once, she wasn't leaving the relationship. I can't write her off. I believed her. I believed she was a woman in struggle. And as feminists, Amber, you and I are interested in struggle.

The Challenge
We would like to suggest that, in terms of dealing with sexual issues both personally and politically, women go back to consciousness-raising groups. We believe that women must create sexual theory in the same way we created feminist theory. We need to simply get together

in places where people agree to suspend their sexual values so that all of us can feel free to say what we do sexually or what we want to do or have done to us. We do have fear of using feelings as theory. We do not mean to imply that feelings are everything. They can, however, be used as the beginning to form a movement which can politically deal with sexuality in a broad-based, cross-cultural way.

We believe our racial and class backgrounds have a huge effect in determining how we perceive ourselves sexually. Since we are not a movement that is working-class-dominated or a movement that is Third World, we both hold serious reservations as to how this new consciousness raising will be conceived. In our involvement in a movement largely controlled by white middle-class women, we feel that the values of their cultures (which may be more closely tied to an American-assimilated puritanism) have been pushed down our throats. The question arises then, Whose feelings and whose values will still be considered normative in these consciousness-raising groups? If there is no room for criticism in sexual discussion around race and class issues, we foresee ourselves being gut-checked from the beginning.

We also believe our class and racial backgrounds have a huge effect in determining how we involve ourselves politically. For instance, why is it that it is largely white middle-class women who form the visible leadership in the antiporn movement? This is particularly true in the Bay Area, where the focus is less on actual violence against women and more on sexist ideology and imagery in the media. Why are women of color not particularly visible in this sex-related single-issue movement? It's certainly not because we are not victims of pornography. More working-class and Third World women can be seen actively engaged in sex-related issues that directly affect the life-and-death concerns of women (abortion, sterilization, abuse, health care, welfare, etc.). It's not like we choose this kind of activism because it's an ideologically correct position but because we are the ones pregnant at sixteen (straight and lesbian), whose daughters get pregnant at sixteen, who get left by men without child care, who are self-supporting lesbian mothers with no child care, and who sign forms to have our tubes tied because we can't read English. But these kinds of distinctions between classes and colors of women are seldom absorbed by the feminist movement as it stands to date.

Essentially, we are challenging other women and ourselves to look where we haven't gone (this includes through and beyond our class and color) in order to arrive at a synthesis of sexual thought that originates and develops from our varied backgrounds and experiences. We refuse to be debilitated one more time around sexuality, race, or class.

PART VI

Thinking About Sex

•••

At the heart of the sexual revolution of the sixties and seventies was an intellectual revolution. It was a profound shift in the way we think about sexuality and how we conceive of sexual repression, but also about the effect of social factors. On one level, the development of ideas proceeded from the tremendous strides in sex research—the Kinsey Reports, Masters and Johnson, and technological advances in birth control—on another level, the ideas grew out of the everyday lives of the men and women who had sex, who rejected codes of behavior that their parents had upheld, who resisted the etiquette that governed polite language, who discovered ways to express their sexual fantasies in magazines, books, photography and film, or who found ways to exploit sexual imagery to sell commodities. As the articles collected in this anthology show, the worlds of scientific research, political critique, pornographic enterprise, and the everyday lives of women and men with their enormous range of desires, were not easily separable.

The proliferation of sexualities and the creation of social forms to shelter and shape those sexualities led very quickly to the realization that there was tremendous power in social institutions to give shape to sexual lives. Several examples can illustrate that. One is the ability of feminist conscious-raising groups to dramatically modify its members' perceptions and interpretations of their male partners. Another was the creation of mate-swapping parties or open marriages to allow for sexual behavior not easily manageable in a monogamous marriage.

These developments were consistent with the widespread recognition that social actors could exercise a tremendous degree of control and power over everyday social interactions. This discovery of the social by the generations growing into adulthood underwrote the political activities and the belief in personal change that marked the sixties and the seventies.

In the fifties, most thinking about sexual behavior, sex roles, and psychological development was influenced by the Freudian intellectual tradition. That intellectual lineage had sought to map the relations between biological energies (libido) and capacities (oral, anal and genital sexualities) and the social forms established to regulate them: monogamous heterosexual marriage. The Freudian tradition focused on repression and sublimation (i.e. transforming sexual impulses into cultural energies) to control unruly libidinal energies. In some of his early work, Freud saw the costs of sexual repression, but he also believed that the libidinal energies were powerful and disruptive forces. Toward the end of his life, he came to believe that sexual repression and sublimation were necessary to the survival of modern society. Wilhelm Reich drew a more radical conclusion—that sexual expression (primarily, the orgasm) was natural and that social control of libidinal energies by the family, conservative sexual morality, and the state was destructive. Reich believed that sexual repression profoundly distorted psychological development and led to authoritarian behavior (fascism).

It is difficult to overestimate the impact of Wilhelm Reich's thinking about sexuality on intellectuals and more indirectly on the general culture. The sexual revolution of the sixties was initiated by people who shared many of Reich's beliefs (whether or not they got them from him directly) about the detrimental impact of sexual repression. This perspective was reinforced by Kinsey's research—which also shared Reich's assumption. In fact, many of the first people on the barricades of the sexual revolution were inspired by Reich.

However, as the sexual revolution increasingly succeeded, it increasingly undermined the credibility of Reich's narrow focus on repression and its naïve implications of the 'naturalness' and the 'goodness' of liberated sexuality. Though Marcuse remained within Freud and Reich's theory of repression, he moved beyond Reich's emphasis on the genital sexuality. Marcuse sought to broaden the view of erotic life. He had written *Eros and Civilization* as a synthesis of Freud and Marx. In his view, sexual repression encouraged working people to sublimate their energies into their jobs—thus contributing to economic productivity which increased corporate profits rather individual incomes. In *Eros and Civilization* Marcuse envisioned creating workplaces that did not rely upon the sublimation of sexual energies. Less than 10 years later, in *One-Dimensional Man* (1964), Marcuse was much more pessimistic about the ultimate effect of reducing the repression required for subli-mation. He was discouraged by the ability of the capitalist system to channel libidinal energies to increase productivity or use sexual imagery to sell consumer goods.

Many activists and intellectuals in the sixties and seventies turned to the Freudian tradition to explore the way that it had defined gender and sexuality and find ways of thinking about sex in the larger historical context. Simone de Beauvoir had critically examined Freud's work in *The Second Sex* (1952): later Shulamith Firestone (1970), Kate Millet (1970), and Juliet Mitchell (1974) followed de Beauvoir in emphasizing Freud and Reich's treatment of gender more than their work on female sexuality. Gay liberationists found in Marcuse and Brown thinkers who had identified the limits of heterosexual genitality.

The sexual revolution had shown how important changes in sexual behavior and mores had been shaped by social actions and social movements. John Gagnon and William Simon, in a series of scholarly articles and in their book *Sexual Conduct* (1973) portrayed sex as pro-foundly social—no one before them had written so thoroughgoing a social interpretation of sexuality. Both of them had been trained in the Chicago sociological tradition which had a long history of analyzing patterns of social interaction and how those patterns contributed to larger social institutions. Gagnon and Simon used the metaphor of a script to link everyday patterns of social interaction to larger cultural symbols and frameworks by seeing sexual conduct as a scripted activity—incorporating lines, cues, roles, cultural myths and symbols to guide and shape sexual interactions.

It was a French theorist and historian—Michel Foucault—who iden-tified the cultural and historical implications of the social construc-tionist theory (as it later came to be called) of sexuality. In his book, published in the US as *The History of Sexuality* (1978) Foucault launched an attack on what he called "the repressive hypothesis." The main point was that sexual conduct was not shaped only by repressive mechanisms—as Freud, Wilhelm Reich and others had argued—but also by a process of discourse and social interaction. Sexuality was not an "essential" characteristic of human nature or gender, but a thoroughly social-historical construction. Foucault's attack thus sought to remove the "hydraulic" model of sexuality as a theoretical framework. The "hydraulic" metaphor as used by Freud, Reich, or even Kinsey implied that sex was based on biological energies; Foucault's critique thus shifted attention to the discursive production of sexuality.

Foucault's understanding of sex shared much with that developed by Gagnon and Simon. Like them, Foucault argues that the self is socially constructed, and that sexuality is shaped through the bodily coordination and symbolic interaction of social subjects. Foucault and his followers concentrated their analysis on the deployment of sexuality on a broad historical terrain, while Gagnon and Simon focused on the individual's scripting of sexual behavior through a three way dialectic of cultural symbolic systems, an individual's fantasy life, and social interactional norms.

Thus the revolution that had begun under the sway of Wilhelm Reich and his ideas about sexual repression had through its very success shown the limitations of his way of thinking about sexuality, the function of orgasm and sexual repression. The sexual revolution was a success because sexuality was amenable to the actions of both social groups and of individuals in social contexts. The sexual revolution had wrought its enormous changes because of the social and discursive processes identified by Gagnon, Simon and Foucault. Thus as the sexual revolution both changed sexual conduct and mores, it also opened up a new way of thinking about sex.

"Civilized" Sexual Morality and Modern Nervousness

Sigmund Freud

from *Sexuality and the Psychology of Love*, 1963

This early essay is probably one of the first serious examinations of sexuality within a broad social historical process. Much like Max Weber's essay on religion and the rise of capitalism, Freud situated changing sexual mores in the rise of modern industrial society. Freud lays out the consequences for individuals and for society if sexual freedom is severely circumscribed and every sexual activity other than monogamous marriage is banned. Does sexual repression lead to rebellion and neurosis? In a sexually repressive society, is the alternative neurosis or perversion?

In his recently published book on sexual ethics, von Ehrenfels dwells on the difference between "natural" and "civilized" (cultural) sexual morality. By "natural" sexual morality he understands that system of control which enables a race to preserve its health and efficiency; by "civilized," that system which when followed spurs man to more intensive and productive cultural activity. According to him this contrast is best elucidated by comparing the innate character of a people with its cultural attainments. While referring to von Ehrenfels' paper for the better appreciation of this significant line of thought, I shall take from it only so much as I need to establish the connection with my own contribution to the subject.

It is natural to suppose that under the domination of a "civilized" morality the health and efficiency in life of the individuals may be impaired, and that ultimately this injury to the individual, caused by the sacrifices imposed upon him, may reach such a pitch that the "civilized" aim and end will itself be indirectly endangered. Indeed, von Ehrenfels points to a series of injurious effects, responsibility for which he attributes to the code of sexual morality at present prevailing in our Western society; and although he fully acknowledges its high value for the furtherance of civilization, he concludes by judging it to be in need of reform. Characteristic of present-day sexual morality is the extension of the demands made upon women on to the sexual life of the male, and the taboo on all sexual intercourse except in monogamous marriage. Even so, consideration of the natural difference in the sexes necessitates less condemnation of lapses in the male, and so in effect admission of a double code of morality for him. But a society which accepts this double code cannot attain to "love of truth, honesty, and humanity" except to a certain narrowly limited degree, and must incline its members to concealment of the truth, to euphemism, to self-deception, and to the deception of others. Civilized sexual morality does worse, indeed, than this, for by glorifying monogamy it cripples virile selection—the sole influence by which an improvement of the race can be attained, for among civilized peoples vital selection is reduced to a minimum by humane and hygienic considerations.

Among the injurious effects attributed to sexual morality the physician misses precisely the one whose significance we are now to consider. I refer to the way in which it promotes modern nervousness, which under our present social conditions is rapidly spreading. Occasionally a nervous patient will himself draw the physician's attention to the part played in the causation of his sufferings by the opposition between his constitution and the demands of civilization, and will remark: "We in our family have all become nervous because we wanted to be something better than what with our origin we were capable of being." The physician is also frequently given matter for thought by observing that neurosis attacks precisely those whose forefathers, after living in simple, healthy, country conditions, offshoots of rude but vigorous stocks, came to the great cities where they were successful and were able in a short space of time to raise their children to a high level of cultural attainment. But, most cogent of all, neurologists themselves have loudly proclaimed the connection between the "increasing nervousness" of the present day and modern civilized life. A few extracts from the opinions of eminent observers will show clearly upon what they base this connection.

W. Erb: "The original question may now be summarized thus: Are those causes of nervousness which have been put before you so markedly, on the increase under modern conditions of life as to declare those conditions responsible? This question can be answered without hesitation in the affirmative, as a cursory glance at our modern life and its character will show.

This is already clearly evidenced by an array of general facts: the extraordinary achievements of modern times, the discoveries and inventions in every field, the maintenance of progress in the face of increasing competition, have been gained and can be held only by great mental effort. The demands on the ability of the individual in the struggle for existence have enormously increased, and he can meet them only by putting forth all his mental powers; at the sane time the needs of the individual, and the demand for enjoyment, have increased in all circles; unprecedented luxury is displayed by classes hitherto wholly unaccustomed to any such thing; irreligion, discontent, and covetousness are spreading widely through every degree of society. The illimitable expansion of communication brought about by means of the network of telegraphs and telephones encircling the world has completely altered the conditions of business and travel. All is hurry and agitation: night is used for travel, day for business; even "holiday trips" keep the nervous system on the rack; important political, industrial, financial crises carry excitement into far wider circles than formerly; participation in political life has become quite general: political, religious, and social struggles, party-interests, electioneering, endless associations of every kind heat the imagination and force the mind to ever greater effort, encroaching on the hours for recreation, sleep and rest; life in large cities is constantly becoming more elaborate and more restless. The exhausted nerves seek recuperation in increased stimulation, in highly-seasoned pleasures, only thereby to become more exhausted than before; modern literature is concerned predominantly with the most questionable problems, those which stir all the passions—sensuality and the craving for pleasure, contempt of every fundamental ethical principle and every ideal demand; it brings pathological types, together with sexual psychopathic, revolutionary and other problems, before the mind of the reader. Our ears are excited and overstimulated by large doses of insistent and noisy music. The theatres captivate all the senses with their exciting modes of presentation; the creative arts turn also by preference to the repellent, ugly and suggestive, and do not hesitate to set before us in revolting realism the ugliest aspect offered by actuality.

"This merely general picture suffices to show a series of dangers in our modern cultural evolution, the details of which may be filled in by a few strokes!"

Binswanger: "Neurasthenia especially has been described as essentially a modem disorder, and Beard, to whom we are first indebted for a general description of it, believed that he had discovered a new nervous disease which had developed specifically in America. This assumption was of course erroneous; nevertheless the fact that an *American* physician was the first to perceive and maintain—as the fruit of great experience—the particular symptoms of this disorder cannot fail to point to a close connection between them and the modern way of life—the unbridled lust and haste for gold and possessions, those immense advances in technical spheres which have reduced to insignificance all limitations of time and space where communication is concerned."

Von Krafft-Ebing: "The mode of life of innumerable civilized peoples shows at the present time an abundance of anti-hygienic factors which make it easy to understand the deplorable increase of nervousness, for these harmful factors take effect first and foremost on the brain. Changes have taken place in the political and social, and particularly in the mercantile, industrial and agricultural conditions of civilized peoples, in the course of no more than the last decade, which have abruptly transformed professional life, citizenship and property at the direct cost of the nervous system; this is then called upon to meet the increased social and domestic demands by a greater expenditure of energy, unredressed by any satisfactory forms of recuperation."

Of these and many other similarly-worded opinions I have to observe, not that they are erroneous, but that they show themselves insufficient to explain in detail the manifestations of nervous disturbance, and that they leave out of account the most important aetiological factor. If one passes over the less definite forms of "nervousness" and considers the actual forms of nervous disease, the injurious influence of culture reduces itself in all essentials to the undue suppression of the sexual life in civilized peoples (or classes) as a result of the "civilized" sexual morality which prevails among them.

The proof of this statement I have attempted to establish in a series of technical papers. It cannot be repeated here; still I will at this point put forward the most important arguments arising from my researches.

Close clinical observation empowers us to distinguish two groups of nervous disorder, the true neuroses, and the psychoneuroses. In the former, the disturbances (symptoms), whether bodily or mental, appear to be of a toxic character. The phenomena are essentially, the same as those due to excess or deficiency of certain nerve-poisons. These neuroses, usually designated collectively as "neurasthenia," can be induced by certain injurious influences in the sexual life, without any hereditary taint being necessarily present; indeed, the form taken by the disease corresponds with the nature of these noxiae, so that not seldom the clinical picture can be directly employed as a key to the particular sexual aetiology. Any such regular correspondence between the form of nervous disorder present and the other injurious influences of civilization to which the writers quoted above attribute so much is, however, entirely absent. It may, therefore, be maintained that the sexual factor is the essential one in the causation of the true neuroses.

With the psychoneuroses, hereditary influence is more marked, and the causation less transparent. A peculiar method of investigation known as psychoanalysis has, however, enabled us to recognize that the symptoms of these disorders (hysteria, obsessional neurosis, etc.) are psychogenic, and depend upon the operation of unconscious (repressed) ideational complexes. This same method has taught us what these unconscious complexes are, and has shown us that, speaking quite generally, they have a sexual content. They originate in the sexual needs of unsatisfied people, and represent a kind of substitute for gratification of them. So that we must regard all factors which operate injuriously upon the sexual life and suppress its activity or distort its aims as likewise pathological factors in the psychoneuroses.

The value of the theoretical distinction between the toxic and the psychogenic neuroses is, of course, in no way lessened by the fact that disturbances arising in both sources are to be observed in most nervous people.

Anyone who is prepared to look with me for the aetiology of nervousness pre-eminently in influences which cripple the sexual life, will willingly give his attention to some further considerations, to be appended here, which are intended to review the question of increasing nervousness in a broader application.

Our civilization is, generally speaking, founded on the suppression of instincts. Each individual has contributed some renunciation—of his sense of dominating power, of the aggressive and vindictive tendencies of his personality. From these sources the common stock of the material and ideal wealth of civilization has been accumulated. Over and above the struggle for existence, it is chiefly family feeling, with its erotic roots, which has induced the individuals to make this renunciation. This renunciation has been a progressive one in the evolution of civilization; the single steps in it were sanctioned by religion. The modicum of instinctual satisfaction from which each one had abstained was offered to the divinity as a sacrifice; and the communal benefit thus won was declared "holy." The man who in consequence of his unyielding nature cannot comply with the required suppression of his instincts, becomes a criminal, an outlaw, unless his social position or striking abilities enable him to hold his own as a great man, a "hero."

The sexual instinct—or, more correctly, the sexual instincts, since analytic investigation teaches us that the sexual instinct consists of many single component impulses—is probably more strongly developed in man than in most of the higher animals; it is certainly more constant, since it has almost entirely overcome the periodicity belonging to it in animals. It places an extraordinary amount of energy at the disposal of "cultural" activities; and this because of a particularly marked characteristic that it possesses, namely, the ability to displace its aim without materially losing in intensity. This ability to exchange the originally sexual aim for another which is no longer sexual but is psychically related, is called the capacity for sublimation. In contrast with this ability for displacement in which lies its value for civilization, the sexual instinct may also show a particularly obstinate tendency to fixation, which prevents it from being turned to account in this way, and occasionally leads to its degenerating into the so-called abnormalities.

The original strength of the sexual instinct probably differs in each individual; certainly the capacity for sublimation is variable. We imagine that the original constitution pre-eminently decides how large a part of the sexual impulse of each individual can be sublimated and made use of. In addition to this, the forces of environment and of intellectual influence on the mental apparatus succeed in disposing of a further portion of it by sublimation. To extend this process of displacement inimitably is, however, certainly no more possible than with the transmutation of heat into mechanical power in the case of machines. A certain degree of direct sexual satisfaction appears to be absolutely necessary for by far the greater number of natures, and frustration of this variable individual need is avenged by manifestations which, on account of their injurious effect on functional activity and of their subjectively painful character, we must regard as illness.

Further aspects are opened up when we take into consideration the fact that the sexual instinct in man does not originally serve the purposes of procreation, but has as its aim the gain of particular kinds of pleasure. It manifests itself thus in infancy, when it attains its aim of pleasurable gratification not only in connection with the genitalia, but also in other parts of the body (erotogenic zones), and hence is in a position to disregard any other than these easily accessible objects. We call this stage that of auto-erotism, and assign to the child's training the task of circumscribing it, because its protracted continuance would render the sexual instinct later uncontrollable and unserviceable. In its development the sexual instinct passes on from auto-erotism to object-love and from the autonomy of the erotogenic zones to the subordination of these under the primacy of the genitals, which come into the service of procreation. During this development a part of the self-obtained sexual excitation is checked, as being useless for the reproductive functions, and in favourable cases is diverted to sublimation. The energies available for "cultural" development are thus in great part won through suppression of the so-called perverse elements of sexual excitation.

It would be possible to distinguish three stages in cultural development corresponding with this development in the sexual instinct: first, the stage in which the sexual impulse may be freely exercised in regard to aims which do not lead to procreation; a second stage, in which the whole of the sexual impulse is suppressed except that portion which subserves procreation; and a third stage, in which only *legitimate* procreation is allowed as a sexual aim. This third stage represents our current "civilized" sexual morality.

If we regard the second of these stages as our standard, we must acknowledge that a number of people, on account of their constitution, are not equal to its demands. With whole classes of individuals, the development of the sexual impulse referred to above, from auto-erotism to object-love, with its aim of union of the genitalia, has not been correctly and sufficiently completed. As a result of this disturbance of development mere arise two kinds of harmful deviation from normal or "civilized" sexuality; and these are related to one another almost as positive to negative. They are, first (disregarding altogether those persons with an over-powerful and uncontrollable sexual instinct in general), the different varieties of perverts, in whom an infantile fixation on a preliminary sexual aim has impeded the establishing of the primacy of the reproductive function; secondly, the homosexuals or inverts, in whom, in a way not yet quite understood, the sexual aim has been deflected from the opposite sex. If the injurious results of those two forms of disturbance in development are less than might have been expected, this can be directly ascribed to the complicated co-ordination within the sexual instinct, which makes it possible for the sexual life to express itself finally in some form or other, even if one or more components of the instinct have been excluded from development. The constitution of those suffering from inversion—the homosexuals—is indeed often distinguished by the sexual impulse lending itself to "cultural" sublimation in a special degree.

Stronger developments of the perversions and of homosexuality, especially if exclusive, do indeed make those who harbour them socially unadaptable and unhappy, so that even the cultural demands of the second stage must be recognized as a source of suffering for a certain proportion of human beings. The fate of those persons who differ constitutionally in this way from their fellows depends on whether they are endowed with comparatively stronger or weaker sexual impulses in an absolute sense. In the latter case, that of an impulse which is on the whole weaker, perverts succeed in completely suppressing those tendencies which bring them in conflict with the moral demands of their level of civilization. But this, from the ideal point of view, remains also their only achievement, because for this repression of their sexual instinct they make use of all those energies which otherwise they would employ in cultural activity. They are at once inwardly stunted, and outwardly crippled. What we shall presently say about the state of abstinence (of men and women) demanded by the third state of culture applies to these also.

Where the sexual instinct is very strong but yet perverted, there are two possible outcomes. In the first, which it is not necessary to consider further, the afflicted person remains perverted, and has to bear the consequences of his deviation from the prevailing level of culture. The second way is much more interesting. Here, under the pressure of education and social demands, a suppression of the perverse impulse is indeed attained, but it is of such a kind as not to be a true one, and can be better described as a miscarriage of suppression. The inhibited sexual impulses are not expressed as such—and to that extent the inhibition is successful—but they are expressed in other ways which are quite as injurious to the person concerned, and make him quite as useless to society as satisfaction of these suppressed impulses in their original form would have done; and in this lies the failure of the process, which in the long run far outweighs the success of the suppression. The substitute-manifestations which thus present themselves in consequence of suppression of the impulses constitute what we describe as neurosis, in particular the psychoneuroses. Neurotics are that class of people, naturally rebellious, with whom the pressure of cultural demands succeeds only in an apparent suppression of their instincts, one which becomes ever less and less effective. Consequently their co-operation in civilized life is maintained only by means of a great expenditure of energy, combined with inner impoverishment, and at times it has to be suspended altogether during periods of illness. I have, however, described the neuroses as the "negative" of the perversions, because in the neuroses the perverse tendencies come to expression from the unconscious part of the mind, after the repression, and because they contain the same tendencies in a state of repression that manifest perverts exhibit.

Experience teaches that for most people there is a limit beyond which their constitution cannot comply with the demands of civilization. All who wish to reach a higher standard than their constitution will allow, fall victims to neurosis. It would have been better for them if they could have remained less "perfect." The realization that perversion and neurosis stand to one another as positive and negative is often unambiguously confirmed by observations made on members of the same family. Quite often in one family the brother will be sexually perverted, while the sister, who as a woman is endowed with a weaker sexual instinct, becomes a neurotic—one whose symptoms, however, express the same tendencies as the perversion of the brother who has a more active sexual impulse. Accordingly in many families the men are healthy, but from the social point of view undesirably immoral: while the women are high-principled and over-refined, but highly neurotic. It is one of the obvious injustices of social life that the standard of culture should demand the same behaviour in sexual life from everyone—a course of conduct which, thanks to his nature, one person can attain without effort, whereas it imposes on another the severest mental sacrifices; though, indeed, the injustice is ordinarily nullified by disregard of the commands of morality.

These considerations have been confined so far to what applies to the second stage of cultural development, postulated as interdicting every "perverse" sexual activity, so-called, but allowing the free practice of "normal" sexual intercourse. We have found that even when the line between sexual freedom and restriction is drawn at this point, a number of persons have to be ruled out as perverse, while others who endeavour not to be perverse, and yet constitutionally should be so, are forced into neurosis. It is now easy to predict the result which will ensue if sexual freedom is still further circumscribed, and the standard demanded by civilization is raised to the level of the third stage, which taboos every sexual activity other than that in legitimate matrimony. Under these conditions the number of strong natures who openly rebel will be immensely increased: and likewise the number of weaker natures who take refuge in neurosis owing to their conflict between the double pressure from the influences of civilization and from their own rebellious constitutions.

We propose to answer time questions which now arise:

1. What is the task that is laid upon the individual as a result of the demands of the third cultural stage?

2. Whether the legitimate sexual satisfaction allowed may be said to offer reasonable compensation for the abstention in other directions?

3. In what relation the possible injurious effects of this abstention stand to the benefit accruing to culture?

The answer to the first question touches a problem which has often been discussed and cannot here be treated exhaustively, i.e., that of sexual abstinence. The third stage of our civilization demands from both sexes abstinence until marriage, and lifelong abstinence for all who do not enter into legal matrimony. The position sanctioned by every authority, that sexual abstinence is not harmful and not difficult to maintain, has also obtained a good deal of support from physicians. It may be said that the task of mastering such a mighty impulse as the sexual instinct is one which may well absorb all the energies of a human being. Mastery through sublimation, diverting the sexual energy away from its sexual goal to higher cultural aims, succeeds with a minority, and with them only intermittently; while the period of passionate youth is precisely that in which it is most difficult to achieve. Of the others, most become neurotic or otherwise come to grief. Experience shows that the majority of those who compose our society are constitutionally unfit for the task of abstinence. Those who would have fallen ill even under moderate sexual restrictions succumb to illness all the earlier and more severely under the demands of our present civilized sexual morality; for we know no better security against the menace to normal sexual life caused by defective predisposition and disturbances in development than sexual satisfaction itself. The greater the disposition to neurosis, the less can abstinence be tolerated. For in proportion as the component-impulses have been excluded from development (as described above) they become precisely thereby less controllable. But even those who would have retained their health while complying with the demands of the second stage of civilization will in many cases succumb to neurosis in the third stage; for the psychical value of sexual satisfaction increases under privation. The frustrated libido is now put in the position of spying out one or other of the weaker spots which are seldom wanting in the structure of the sexual life, so that it may break through at that point as a neurotic substitute-gratification in the form of a morbid symptom. Anyone who understands how to penetrate to the factors conditioning nervous illness will soon be convinced that its increase in our society originates in the greater stringency of sexual restraint.

We thus come closer to the question whether sexual intercourse in legitimate marriage can offer full compensation for the restraint before marriage. The abundance of the material supporting a reply in the negative is so overwhelming that we are obliged to make only the briefest summary of it. We must above all keep in mind that our civilized sexual morality also restricts sexual intercourse even in marriage itself, for it compels the married couple to be satisfied, as a rule, with a very small number of acts leading to conception. As a consequence of this, satisfying sexual intercourse occurs in marriage only over a period of a few years, allowing also, of course, for intervals of abstention on hygienic grounds required by the woman's state of health. After these three, four or five years, marriage ceases to furnish the satisfaction of the sexual needs that it promised, since all the contraceptives available hitherto impair sexual enjoyment, disturb the finer susceptibles of both partners, or even act as a direct cause of illness. Anxiety for the consequences of sexual intercourse first dissipates the physical tenderness of the married couple for each other, and usually, as a more remote result, also the mental affection between them which was destined to succeed the originally tempestuous passion. Under the spiritual disappointment, and physical deprivation which thus become the fate of most marriages, both partners find themselves reduced again to their pre-conjugal condition, but poorer by the loss of an illusion, and are once more driven back to their determination to restrain and "sidetrack" their sexual instinct. We will not inquire how far a man in mature years succeeds in this task; experience seems to show that he very frequently makes use of that amount of freedom which is allowed him even by the strictest sexual code, though but reluctantly and furtively. The "double" code of morality conceded to the male in our society is the plainest possible admission that society itself does not believe in the possibility of adherence to those precepts which it has enjoined on its members. But experience also shows that women, as the true guardians of the sexual interests of the race, are endowed with the power of sublimation only in a limited degree; as a substitute for the sexual object the suckling child may suffice, but not the growing child, and under the disappointments of matrimony women succumb to severe, lifelong neurosis affecting the whole course of their lives. Marriage under the present cultural standard has long ceased to be a panacea for the nervous sufferings of women; even if we physicians in such cases still advise matrimony, we are nevertheless aware that a girl must be very healthy to "stand" marriage, and we earnestly counsel our male inquirers not to marry a girl who has been neurotic. Marital unfaithfulness would, on the other hand, be a much more probable cure for the neurosis resulting from marriage; the more strictly a wife has been brought up, the more earnestly she has submitted to the demands of civilization, the more does she fear this way of escape, and in conflict between her desires and her sense of duty she again will seek refuge in a neurosis. Nothing protects her virtue so securely as illness. The conjugal state, which is held out to the youthful among civilized people as a refuge for the sexual instinct, thus proves inadequate even to the demands of the later period which it covers; beyond all question, it fails to compensate for the earlier abstention.

To our third question, even he who admits the injurious results thus attributable to civilized sexual morality may reply that the cultural gain derived from the sexual restraint so generally practised probably more than balances these evils, which after all, in their more striking manifestations, affect only a minority. I own myself unable to balance gain and loss precisely: nevertheless I could advance a good many considerations as regards the loss. Returning to the theme of abstinence, already touched on, I must insist that yet other injurious effects besides the neuroses result therefrom, and that the neuroses themselves are not usually appraised at their full significance.

The retardation of sexual development and sexual activity at which our education and culture aim is certainly not injurious to begin with; it is seen to be a necessity, when one reflects at what a late age young people of the educated classes attain independence and begin to earn a living. Incidentally, one is reminded here of the intimate relations existing between all our civilized institutions, and of the difficulty of altering any part of them irrespective of the whole. But the benefit, for a young man, of abstinence continued much beyond his twentieth year, cannot any longer be taken for granted; it may lead to other injuries even when it does not lead to neurosis. It is indeed said that the struggle with such powerful instincts and the consequent strengthening of all ethical and aesthetic tendencies "steels" the character, and this, for some specially constituted natures, is true. The view may also be accepted that the differentiation of individual character, now so much in evidence, only becomes possible with sexual restraint. But in the great majority of cases the fight against sexuality absorbs the available energy of the character, and this at the very time when the young man is in need of all his powers to gain his share of worldly foods and his position in the community. The relation between possible sublimation and indispensable sexual activity naturally varies very much in different persons, and indeed with the various kinds of occupation. An abstinent artist is scarcely conceivable: an abstinent young intellectual is by no means a rarity. The young intellectual can by abstinence enhance his powers of concentration, whereas the production of the artist is probably powerfully stimulated by his sexual experience. On the whole I have not gained the impression that sexual abstinence helps to shape energetic, self-reliant men of action, nor original thinkers, bold pioneers and reformers; for more often it produces "good" weaklings who later become lost in the crowd that tends to follow painfully the initiative of strong characters.

In the results produced by efforts towards abstinence the stubbornness and insubordination characteristic of the sexual instinct also come to expression. Civilized education attempts, in a sense, only a temporary suppression of it up to the period of matrimony, intending men to give it free rein in order to make use of it. Extreme measures, however, are more successful in effecting repression of the instinct than are moderate ones; but then suppression very often goes too far, with the unwished-for result that when the sexual instinct is set free it shows itself permanently impaired. For this reason complete abstinence during youth is often not the best preparation for marriage in a young man. Women dimly recognize this, and among their suitors prefer those who have already proved themselves men with other women. The injurious results which the strict demand for abstinence before marriage produces are quite particularly apparent where women are concerned. Clearly, education does not look lightly on the task of suppressing the sensuality of the girl until marriage, for it employs the most drastic measures. It not only forbids sexual intercourse and sets a high premium upon the preservation of sexual chastity, but it also protects the developing young woman from temptation by keeping her in ignorance of all the facts concerning the part she is ordained to play, and tolerates in her no love-impulse which cannot lead to marriage. The result is that when the girl is suddenly allowed by parental authority to fall in love, she cannot accomplish this mental operation and enters the state of marriage uncertain of her own feelings. As a result, the artificial retardation in the development of the love-function provides nothing but disappointments for the husband, who has treasured up all his desires for her. Psychically she is still attached to her parents, whose authority has brought about the suppression of the sexual feeling; and physically she shows herself frigid, which prevents her husband finding any great enjoyment in relations with her. I do not know whether the anaesthetic type of woman is also found outside the range of civilized education, but I consider it probable. In any case this type is directly cultivated by education, and these women who conceive without pleasure show later little willingness to endure frequent childbirths, accompanied as they are by pain: so that the training that precedes marriage directly frustrates the very aim of marriage. When later the retarded development of the wife becomes rectified, and during the climax of her womanly life the full power to love awakens in her, her relation to her husband has been long undermined. As a reward for her previous submission, there remains for her only the choice between unappeased desire, infidelity, or neurosis.

The behaviour of a human being in sexual matters is often a prototype for the whole of his other modes of reaction to life. A man who has shown determination in possessing himself of his love-object has our confidence in his success in regard to other aims as well. On the other hand, a man who abstains, for whatever reasons, from satisfying his strong sexual instinct, will also assume a conciliatory and resigned attitude in other paths of life, rather than a powerfully active one. A particular application of the general statement that the course of the sexual life is typical for the way in which other functions are exercised is easily demonstrable in the entire female sex. Their training excludes them from occupying themselves intellectually with sexual problems, in regard to which naturally they have the greatest thirst for knowledge, and terrifies them with the pronouncement that such curiosity is unwomanly and a sign of unmoral tendencies. And thus they are thoroughly intimidated from all mental effort, and knowledge in general is depreciated in their eyes. The prohibition of thought extends beyond the sexual sphere, partly through unavoidable associations, partly automatically, acting precisely in the same way as the prohibition of religious speculation among men, and the taboo of any thought out of harmony with loyalty in faithful subjects. I do not support Moebius in the view he has put forward, which has met with so much opposition, that the biological contrast between intellectual work and sexual activity explains the "physiological mental weakness" of women. On the contrary, I think that the undoubted fact of the intellectual inferiority of so many women can be traced to that inhibition of thought necessitated by sexual suppression.

In considering the question of abstinence, far too little distinction is made between two forms of it, namely, abstention from any kind of sexual activity at all, and abstention from heterosexual intercourse. Many who are proud of maintaining abstinence successfully have only been able to achieve it with the help of masturbation and other similar means of satisfaction, which are connected with the auto-erotic sexual activities of early childhood. But this very connection makes these substitutive measures of sexual satisfaction by no means harmless; they predispose to the numerous forms of neurosis and psychosis, which are conditional on a regression of the sexual life to its infantile form. Nor does masturbation at all correspond to the ideal demands of civilized sexual morality, and it therefore drives young people into the same conflicts with the ideals of education which they design to escape by abstinence. Further, the character is undermined in more ways than one by this indulgence; first, because it shows the way to attain important aims in an otiose manner, instead of by energetic effort, in line with the view that the attitude to sex is the prototype of the attitude to life; and secondly, because in the phantasies accompanying this gratification the sexual object is exalted to a degree which is seldom to be reproduced in reality. A witty writer, K. Kraus in the Vienna *Fackel*, has, as it were, expressed this truth paradoxically in the cynical saying: "Coitus is merely an unsatisfactory substitute for onanism!"

The severe standard demanded by civilization and the arduous task of abstinence have combined to make avoidance of the genital union of the sexes the main point of abstinence, whilst favouring other forms of sexual activity—two results which may be said to betoken obedience by halves. The so-called perverse forms of intercourse between the sexes, in which other parts of the body assume the role of the genitalia, have undoubtedly become of greater social significance since normal intercourse has been so remorselessly tabooed in the name of morality—and also on grounds of hygiene because of the possibility of infection. These activities, however, cannot be regarded as so harmless as irregularities of a similar kind interwoven with a normal love-intercourse: ethically they are reprehensible, for they degrade the love-relationship of two human beings from being a serious matter to an otiose diversion, attended neither by risk nor by spiritual participation. The spread of the homosexual means of gratification must be regarded as a further consequence of the difficulties placed in the way of normal sexual life; and in addition to those who are constitutionally homosexual, or who become so in childhood, must be reckoned the great number of those in whom, by reason of the check on the main stream of the libido, the lateral channel of homosexuality is forced open in maturer life.

All these unavoidable and unintended consequences of the insistence upon abstinence unite in one general result: they strike at the roots of the condition of preparation for marriage, which according to the intentions of civilized sexual morality should after all be the sole heir of all sexual tendencies. All those men whose libido, as the result of masturbatory or perverse sexual practices, has become habituated to situations and conditions of satisfaction other than the normal develop in marriage a diminished potency. And all those women who could preserve their virginity only by similar means show themselves anaesthetic to normal intercourse in marriage. A marriage begun with impaired capacity to love on both sides succumbs to the process of dissolution even more quickly than otherwise. As a result of the diminished potency of the man, the woman will not be satisfied and will remain anaesthetic, whereas a powerful sexual experience might have been the means of overcoming the disposition to frigidity that results from her education. The prevention of conception is also more difficult to such a couple than to a healthy pair, because the weakened potency of the man tolerates the use of contraceptives badly. In such perplexity, sexual intercourse comes to be regarded as the source of all difficulties and is soon abandoned, and with it the fundamental condition of married life.

I call upon all who have studied these matters to aver that I am not exaggerating, but am describing conditions glaringly evident to any observant eye. The uninitiated can hardly believe how rarely normal potency is to be found in the men, and how often frigidity in the women, among those married couples living under the sway of our civilized sexual morality; what a degree of renunciation, often for both partners, is associated with marriage, and of how little the marriage comes to consist, instead of bringing the happiness that was so ardently desired. I have already shown that neurosis is the most obvious way of escape from these conditions. I would, however, further point out how such a marriage will increasingly affect the only child— or the limited number of children—which spring from it. On appearance it looks as if we then had an inherited condition to deal with, but closer inspection shows the effect of powerful infantile impressions. As a mother, the neurotic woman who is unsatisfied by her husband is over-tender and over-anxious in regard to the child, to whom she transfers her need for love; thus awakening in it sexual precocity. The bad relations between the parents then stimulate the emotional life of the child, and cause it to experience intensities of love, hate and jealousy while yet in its infancy. The strict training which tolerates no sort of expression of this precocious sexual state lends support to the forces of suppression, and the conflict at this age contains all the elements needed to cause lifelong neurosis.

I return now to my earlier assertion that, in appraising the neuroses, their full significance is seldom reckoned with. I do not mean by this the insufficient appreciation of these states exhibited in the frivolous dismissal of them on the part of relatives, or in the magniloquent assurances on the part of physicians that a few weeks of cold-water cure or a few months of rest and convalescence will cure the condition— these are merely the opinions of ignorant physicians and laymen, and mostly nothing but forms of speech designed to afford the sufferer a short-lived consolation. Rather, it is established that a chronic neurosis, even if it does not completely paralyse existence, represents for the person concerned a heavy handicap in life, much the same as tuberculosis or a cardiac affection. We might in a measure compound with this if neurotic illness merely excluded from communal activity a number of individuals in any case infirm, and permitted the remainder to take their share at the cost of merely subjective disabilities; but I would rather draw attention to the point of view that the neuroses, as far as they extend and in whomever they occur, always succeed in frustrating the social purpose, and thereby actually do the work of the socially inimical mental forces which have been suppressed. So that in paying for compliance, with its own exorbitant prescriptions by increased neurosis, society cannot claim an advantage purchased by sacrifice—cannot indeed claim any advantage whatever. Let us examine, for example, the frequent case of a woman who does not love her husband, because, owing to the conditions of the consummation of her marriage and the experience of her married life, she has no cause to love him; but who ardently wishes to do so, because this alone corresponds to the ideal of marriage in which she has been brought up. She will then suppress in herself all impulses which seek to bring her true feelings to expression and contradict her ideal endeavours, and will take particular pains to play the part of a loving, tender and obedient wife. The result of this self-suppression will be a neurotic illness, and this neurosis will in a short time have taken revenge upon the unloved husband and have caused him precisely as much dissatisfaction and trouble as would have arisen merely from an acknowledgement of the true state of affairs. This example is literally typical of what neurosis can do. A similar miscarriage of compensation can be observed after suppression of other socially inimical impulses not directly sexual. A man, for example, who has become excessively "kind-hearted" as the result of powerful suppression of a constitutional tendency to harshness and cruelty, often loses by so doing so much energy that he does not achieve the full measure of his compensatory impulses, and on the whole does rather less good than he would have done without suppression.

Let us add that together with the restrictions on sexual activity in any nation there always goes an increase of anxiety concerning life and fear of death, which interfere with each individual's capacity for enjoyment, and do away with his willingness to incur risk of death in whatever cause—showing itself in a diminished inclination to beget offspring, thus excluding any people or group of such a type from participation in the future. We may thus well raise the question whether our "civilized" sexual morality is worth the sacrifice which it imposes upon us, the more so if we are still so insufficiently purged of hedonism as to include a certain degree of individual happiness among the aims of our cultural development. It is certainly not the physician's business to come forward with proposals for reform, but it seemed to me that, by pointing out what significance the injurious results of our sexual morality, enumerated by von Ehrenfels, have in connection with the increase in modern nervousness, I could supplement the account be gives of them, and could thus support the urgency of such reform.

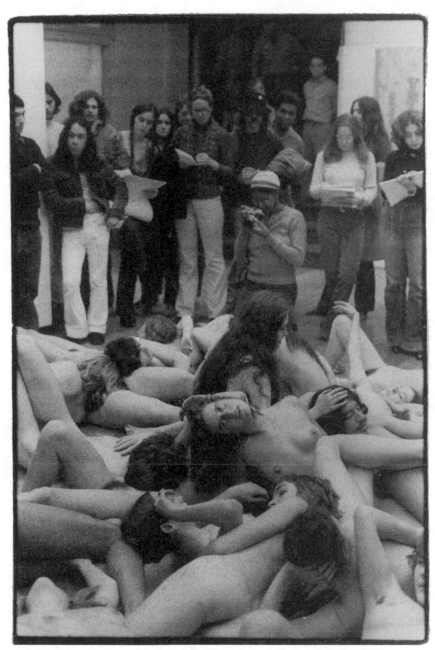

© Fred W. McDarrah

Sexual Repression, Instinctual Renunciation and Sexual Reform

Wilhelm Reich

from *The Sexual Revolution*, 1951

*In **The Sexual Revolution**, Wilhelm Reich elaborates on the relationship between social repression and sexual repression by examining how the family and conservative sexual morality stifle political freedom. In the second half of the book Reich illustrates his theory in a case study of how sexual conservatism in the Soviet Union contributed to the revolution's ultimate failure*

reud's cultural philosophical standpoint was always that culture owes its existence to instinctual repression and renunciation. The basic idea is that cultural achievements are the result of sublimated sexual energy; from this it follows logically that sexual suppression and repression are an indispensable factor in die cultural process. There is historical evidence of the incorrectness of this formulation; there are in existence highly cultured societies without any sexual suppression and a completely free sex life.

What is correct in this theory is only that sexual suppression forms the mass-psychological basis for a *certain* culture, namely, the *patriarchal authoritarian* one, in all of its forms. What is incorrect is the formulation that sexual suppression is the basis of culture in general. How did Freud arrive at this concept? Certainly not for conscious reasons of politics or Weltanschauung. On the contrary: early works such as that on "cultural sexual morals" ["civilized sexual morality"] point definitely in the direction of a criticism of culture in the sense of a sexual revolution. Freud never followed this path; on the contrary, he was adverse to any attempts in this direction and once called them "not being in the middle of the road of psychoanalysis." It was exactly my early attempts at a sex policy involving criticism of culture which led to the first serious differences of opinion between Freud and me.

In analyzing the psychic mechanisms, Freud found the unconscious filled with antisocial impulses. Everyone using the psychoanalytic method can confirm these findings. Every man has phantasies of murdering his father and of taking the father's place with his mother. In everyone, sadistic impulses, inhibited by more or less conscious guilt feelings, are found. In most women, violent impulses to castrate men, to acquire the penis, e.g., by swallowing it, can be found. The inhibition of such impulses, which continue to work in the unconscious, results not only in social adjustment, but also in all kinds of disturbances (as, for example, hysterical vomiting). The man's sadistic phantasies of hurting or piercing the woman in the sexual act lead to various kinds of impotence if they are inhibited by anxiety and guilt feelings; if they are not, they may lead to perverse activities or sex murder. Such unconscious desires as that of eating feces can be found in a great many individuals, regardless of their social class. Such psychoanalytic discoveries as that the over-solicitude of a mother for her child or of a woman for her husband corresponds to the intensity of her unconscious phantasies of murder were highly inconvenient for the ideological champions of "sacred mother love" or of the "sacrament of marriage"; nevertheless, they are correct. Such examples could be multiplied indefinitely; but let us return to our subject. These contents of the unconscious were shown to be remnants of infantile attitudes toward parents, siblings, etc. In order to exist and to fit into our culture, the children have to suppress these impulses. The price they pay for it is the acquisition of a neurosis, that is, a reduction of their ability to work and of their sexual potency.

The finding of the antisocial nature of the unconscious was correct; so was the finding of the necessity of instinctual renunciation for the purpose of adjustment to social existence. However, two facts are at variance: On the one hand, the child has to suppress its instincts in order to become capable of cultural adjustment. On the other hand, it

579

acquires, in this very process, a neurosis which in turn makes it incapable of cultural development and adjustment and in the end makes it antisocial. In order to make natural instinctual gratification possible, one has to eliminate the repression and to liberate the instincts. This is the prerequisite of cure, although not as yet the cure itself as Freud's early statements would have it. What, then, should take the place of instinctual repression? Certainly not the repressed instincts themselves, because, according to psychoanalytic theory, that would mean the impossibility of existing in this culture.

In many places in psychoanalytic literature we find the statement that the uncovering of the unconscious, that is, the affirmation of its existence, does by no means imply an affirmation of the corresponding action. The analyst lays down a law here which applies for life as well as for the treatment session: "You are allowed and supposed to *say* what you want; but that does not mean that you also can *do* what you want."

However, the responsible analyst was—and always is—confronted with the question as to what is to happen to the previously repressed and now liberated instincts. The psychoanalytic answer was: *sublimation* and *rejection*. Since, however, only the fewest patients prove capable of sublimation to a sufficient degree, the only other way out is renunciation through rejection of the instinct. Repression comes to be replaced by rejection. This demand was justified by the following formulation: The child faced its instincts with a weak, undeveloped ego and thus had no other choice but that of repression; the adult faces his instincts with a strong, adult ego which is capable of handling the instincts by way of rejection. Though this formulation contradicts clinical experience, it became—and still is—the accepted one. This point of view also dominates psychoanalytic pedagogy, as represented, for example, by Anna Freud.

Since, according to this concept, the individual becomes capable of culture as a result of instinctual renunciation instead of repression, and since society is regarded as behaving like the individual, it follows from this concept that culture is based on instinctual renunciation.

The whole construction seems unobjectionable and enjoys the approval not only of the majority of analysts but of the representatives of an abstract concept of culture in general. This substitution of renunciation and rejection for repression seems to banish the ghost which raised its threatening head when Freud confronted the world with his early findings. These findings showed unequivocally that sexual repression makes people not only sick but also incapable of work and cultural achievement. The whole world began to rage against Freud because of the threat to morals and ethics, and reproached Freud with preaching the "living out," with threatening culture, etc. Freud's alleged antimoralism was one of the most potent weapons of his early opponents. This ghost did not begin to vanish until the theory of rejection was propounded; Freud's earlier assurance that he was affirming "culture," that his discoveries constituted no threat to it, had made little impression. This was shown by the never-ending talk about "pansexualism." Then, after the new formulation of rejection, the previous enmity was replaced by partial acceptance. For just as long as the instincts were not lived out, it did not make any difference, from a "cultural point of view," whether it was the mechanism of instinctual rejection or that of repression which played the Cerberus keeping the shadows of the underworld from emerging to the surface. One was even able to register progress: that from the unconscious repression of evil to the voluntary renunciation of instinctual gratification. Since ethics does not consist in being asexual but, on the contrary, in resisting sexual temptations, everybody could now agree with everybody. Psychoanalysis, previously condemned, had now itself become capable of culture—unfortunately by way of "renunciation of the instinct," that is, the renunciation of its own theory of the instincts.

I regret to have to destroy some illusions. The whole system contains a miscalculation which is easily demonstrable. Not by any means in the sense that the psychoanalytic findings on which these conclusions are based are incorrect. On the contrary, they are quite correct; only, they are incomplete, and many of the formulations are abstract and thus distract from the real conclusions.

Instinctual gratification and instinctual renunciation.

Those German psychoanalysts who attempted a "Gleichschaltung" [to bring into line with the Nazi ideology] of psychoanalysis tried to justify their unscientific behavior by quotations from Freud's writings. They contain, in fact, formulations which nullify the revolutionary character of clinical psychoanalytic findings and which clearly demonstrate the contradiction between the scientist and the middle-class cultural philosopher in Freud. One such quotation runs:

> It is a bad misunderstanding, explained only by ignorance, if people say that psychoanalysis expects the cure of neurotic illness from the free "living out" of sexuality. On the contrary, the making conscious of the repressed sexual desires makes possible their *control* [italics mine. W.R.], a control which could not have been achieved by the repression. It would be more correct to say that the analysis liberates the neurotic from the shackles of his sexuality.
>
> (Ges. Schriften, Bd. XI, p. 217f.)

If, for example, the 17-year-old daughter of a National Socialist [the official name of the Nazi party] dignitary suffers from hysterical attacks as a result of a repressed desire for sexual intercourse, this desire, in the psychoanalytic treatment, will be recognized, to begin with, as an incestuous desire, and will be rejected as such. So far so good. But what happens to the sexual need? According to the above-quoted formulation, the girl is "liberated" from the shackles of her sexuality. Clinically, however, it looks like this: When the girl, with the aid of the analysis, frees herself from her father, she liberates herself only from the toils of her incest wish, *but not from her sexuality as such.* Freud's formulation neglects this basic fact. The scientific dispute about the role of genitality took its origin precisely from this clinical problem; it is the central point of divergence between the sex-economic and the revised psychoanalytic formulation. Freud's formulation postulates a renunciation on the part of the girl of all sexual life. In this form, psychoanalysis is acceptable even to the Nazi dignitary and becomes, in the hands of analysts like Müller-Braunschweig, an instrument for the "breeding of the heroic human." This form of psychoanalysis, however, has nothing in common with that psychoanalysis contained in the books which Hitler had burned. The latter kind of psychoanalysis, not hide-bound by reactionary prejudice, states unequivocally that the girl can get well only if she transfers the genital desires from the father to a friend with whom she satisfies them. But just this is at variance with the total Nazi ideology and inexorably brings up the whole question of

the social sexual order. Because, in order to be able to live sex-eco-
nomically, it is not sufficient that the girl have a free genital sexuality;
she needs, in addition, an undisturbed room, proper contraceptives, a
friend who is capable of love, that is, not a National Socialist with a
sex-negative structure; she needs understanding parents and a sex-
affirmative social atmosphere; these needs are all the greater the less
she is in a financial situation which would allow her to break through
the social barriers of adolescent sex life.

The replacement of sexual repression by renunciation or rejection
would be a simple matter were it not for the fact that these latter mechanisms are also dependent on the economy of instinctual life. Renunciation of the instinct is possible only under definite sex-economic
conditions. The same is true of sublimation. Character-analytic experience shows clearly that lasting renunciation of a pathological or antisocial impulse is possible only when the sexual economy is in order,
that is, if there is no sexual stasis which provides energy for the impulse
which is to be renounced. *An ordered sex-economy, however, is possible
only in the presence of such sexual gratification as corresponds to any given
age.* Which means that an adult can give up infantile and pathogenic
desires only if he experiences full genital gratification. The perverse and
neurotic modes of gratification against which society should be protected are in themselves only substitutes for genital gratification and
arise only if genital gratification is disturbed or made impossible. This
fact makes it clear that we cannot speak of instinctual gratification or
renunciation in general. We must ask concretely: the gratification of
what instinct, the renunciation of *what* instinct? If analytic therapy sees
its job in eliminating repressions and not in preaching morals, then it
can bring about the renunciation only of *one* kind of gratification: that
which does not correspond to the respective age or stage of development. Thus, it will bring a girl to the renunciation of her infantile fixation to her father by nothing else but making this fixation conscious.
But that does not imply a renunciation of sexual desires as such,
because the sexual energy continues to urge toward discharge. While it
is easy to make her give up her sexual desires for her father, she cannot
be brought to renounce her sexual gratification with a boy her age
except by moralistic arguments; to do this, however, is at variance with
therapeutic principles and possibilities of cure. On the other hand, she

can really dissolve her fixation to her father only under one condition: when her sexuality finds another, normal object and *actual gratification*. Unless this is the case, the infantile fixation is not dissolved, or there occurs a regression to other infantile instinctual goals, and the basic problem continues to exist.

The same is true of *any* case of neurotic disease. If a woman is dissatisfied in her marriage, she will unconsciously reactivate infantile sexual demands; these she can give up only if her sexuality finds another satisfactory outlet. True, the rejection of the infantile sexual desires is a prerequisite for the establishment of a normal sexuality; but the establishment of a normal sex life with actual gratification is also an indispensable prerequisite for the final relinquishing of the infantile instinctual goals. A sexual pervert or criminal, such as a sex murderer, can be cured of his pathological impulses only if he finds his way into a biologically normal sex life. The alternative, thus, is not instinctual renunciation or instinctual living out, but renunciation of *what* impulses, and gratification of *what* impulses?

In speaking abstractly of the evil nature of the repressed unconscious, one obscures the most fundamental facts not only of the therapy and prevention of the neuroses, but of education as well. Freud made the discovery that the unconscious of the neurotics—that is, the vast majority of people in our civilization—contains essentially infantile, cruel, antisocial impulses. This finding is correct. But it obscured another fact, the fact, namely, that the unconscious also contains many impulses which represent natural biological demands, such as the sexual desire of adolescents or of people tied down in an unhappy marriage. The intensity of the later infantile and antisocial impulses derives, historically and economically, from the non-gratification of these natural demands; the dammed-up libidinal energy partly reinforces primitive infantile impulses, partly creates entirely new ones, mostly of an antisocial nature, such as the desire for exhibitionism or impulses to sex murder. Ethnological research shows that such impulses are absent in primitive peoples up to a definite point of economic development and begin to make their appearance only after social repression of normal love life has become an established feature.

These antisocial impulses, which result from social repression of normal sexuality and which have to be repressed because society—

rightly—does not allow them to be satisfied, these impulses are considered *biological facts* by psychoanalysis. This concept is closely related to that of Hirschfeld that exhibitionism is due to special exhibitionistic hormones. This naive mechanistic biologism is so difficult to unmask because it serves a definite function in our society: that of shifting the problem from the sociological to the biological realm where nothing can be done about it.

There is such a thing as a *sociology of the unconscious* and of antisocial sexuality, that is, a social history of the unconscious impulses, with regard to their intensity as well as their contents. Not only is repression itself a sociological phenomenon, but also that which causes the repression. The study of the "partial impulses" will have to take pointers from ethnological findings such as the fact that in certain matriarchal societies there is little if any of the anal phase of libidinal development which in our society is considered a normal stage between the oral and the genital phase. This is so because in these societies the children are nursed until the third or fourth year when they immediately enter a phase of intensive genital play activities.

The psychoanalytic concept of antisocial impulses is an absolute one and thus leads to conclusions which are at variance with the facts. If, on the other hand, one realizes the *relative* character of the antisocial impulses, one arrives at basically different conclusions regarding not only psychotherapy but especially sociology and sex-economy. The anal activities of a child of one or two have nothing whatsoever to do with "social" or "antisocial." If, however, one adheres to the abstract view that these anal impulses are antisocial, one will institute a regime designed to make the child "capable of culture" as early as the sixth month of life; the later result is exactly the opposite, namely, incapacity for anal sublimation and the development of anal-neurotic disturbances. The mechanistic concept of the absolute antithesis between sexuality and culture makes even analytically trained parents take measures against infantile masturbation, at least in the form of "mild diversions." As far as I know, none of the writings of Anna Freud mention what in private conversation she admitted to be an inevitable conclusion from psychoanalytic findings: that infantile masturbation is a physiological manifestation and should *not* be inhibited. If one adheres to the concept that that which is repressed and unconscious is also antisocial, one will, for example, condemn the genital demands of the adolescent. This is substantiated by such phrases as that the "reality principle" requires the postponement of instinctual gratification.

The fact that this reality principle is *itself relative*, that it is determined by an authoritarian society and serves its purposes, this decisive fact goes carefully unmentioned; to mention this, they say, is "politics," and science has nothing to do with politics. They refuse to see the fact that not to mention it is also politics. Such attitudes have seriously endangered analytic progress; not only have they prevented the discovery of certain facts, but, more important, they have hindered the practical application of definitely established facts by misinterpreting them in terms of conservative cultural concepts. Since psychoanalysis constantly deals with the influences exerted upon the individual by society as well as with judgments as to what is healthy or sick, social or antisocial, and at the same time is unaware of the revolutionary character of its method and findings, it moves around in a tragic circle: it finds that sexual repression endangers culture and at the same time that it is a necessary prerequisite of culture.

Let us summarize the facts which psychoanalysis has overlooked and which are at variance with the psychoanalytic concept of culture:

The unconscious itself is—quantitatively as well as qualitatively—socially determined;

The giving up of infantile and antisocial impulses presupposes the gratification of the normal physiological sexual needs;

Sublimation, as the essential cultural achievement of the psychic apparatus, is possible only in the absence of sexual repression; in the adult, it applies only to the *pregenital*, but not to the *genital* impulses;

Genital gratification—the decisive sex-economic factor in the prevention of neuroses and establishment of social achievement—is at variance, in every respect, with present-day laws and with every patriarchal religion;

The elimination of sexual repression—introduced by psychoanalysis as a therapy as well as a sociologically important factor—is strictly at variance with all those cultural elements in our society which are based just on this repression.

To the extent to which psychoanalysis maintains its cultural standpoint, it does so at the expense of the very results of its own work. The conflict between the cultural concepts of the analytic investigators on the one hand and the scientific results which militate against this culture on the other hand is solved by them in favor of the patriarchal Weltanschauung. When psychoanalysis does not dare to accept the consequences of its findings, it points to the allegedly non-political (unpragmatic) character of science, while, in fact, every step of psycho-analytic theory and practice deals with political (pragmatic) issues.

If one investigates ecclesiastical, fascist and other reactionary ide-ologies for their unconscious content, one finds that they are essen-tially defense reactions. They are formed for fear of the unconscious inferno which everyone carries within himself. From this, one could deduce a justification of an ascetic morality only if the unconscious antisocial impulses were absolute and biologically given; if that were so, the political reaction would be correct, and any attempt to elimi-nate sexual misery would be senseless. Then, the conservative world could correctly point out that the destruction of "the higher qualities," "the central values," the "divine" and the "moral" in the human would lead to sexual and ethical chaos. This is what people mean uncon-sciously when they talk of "Kulturbolschewismus." The revolutionary movement—except for the sex-political wing—does not know this connection; in fact, it often finds itself on the same front with the polit-ical reaction when it comes to basic questions of sex-economy. True, it turns against sex-economic principles for different reasons than does the political reaction: it does not know these principles and their implications. It also believes in the biological and absolute nature of the antisocial impulses and consequently in the necessity of moral inhibition and regulation. It overlooks, like its opponents, the fact that the moral regulation of instinctual life creates exactly what it pretends to master: antisocial impulses.

Sex-economic investigation, on the other hand, shows that the anti-social unconscious impulses—as far as they are really antisocial and not just regarded as such by the moralists—are a result of moral regu-lation and will continue to exist as long as that regulation exists. Sex-economic regulation alone can eliminate the antithesis between culture and nature; with the elimination of sexual repression, the per-verse and antisocial impulses will also be eliminated.

Secondary Impulses and Moral Regulation

A very important contention in the struggle between so-called "Kultur-bolschewismus" and the fascist "antibolshevism" was that the social revolution completely destroyed morals and would lead to sexual chaos. This contention used to be countered by the argument that, quite on the contrary, capitalism had produced the social chaos and the social revolution would undoubtedly establish security in social living. In the Soviet Union, the attempt to replace the authoritarian moral principle by non-authoritarian self-regulation failed.

No more convincing was the attempt to compete with authoritarian society in pointing to one's own "morality." First of all, one has to learn to understand why it is that the average person is such a slave to the concept of morality, why to him the idea of a "social revolution" is inevitably synonymous with the idea of sexual and cultural chaos. This question has been already answered, in part, by our study of fascist ideology: to the unconscious of the average person, with his sex-nega-tive structure, "Kulturbolschewismus" means the "living out of sensual sexuality." To assume that it should be possible, in social revolution, to apply immediately, in a practical way, the findings of sex-economy which would eliminate moral regulation, would be completely to mis-understand sex-economic thinking.

As soon as a society assumes the ownership of the social means of production, it is inevitably confronted by the question as to how human living should be regulated: morally or "freely." Quite obvi-ously, an immediate liberation of sexuality or immediate elimination of moral norms and moral regulation is out of the question. We know that people, their structure being what it is today, are incapable of self-regulation; they may be able to establish economic democracy imme-diately, but not a rational, self-governing society. This is, after all, what Lenin meant when he said that the state could disappear only gradu-ally. If one wants to eliminate moral regulation and to replace it by self-regulation, one has to know to what extent the old, moral regulation was indispensable and to what extent it was harmful, individually and socially.

The compulsive moral point of view of the political reaction is that of an absolute antithesis between biological impulse and social interest. Based on this antithesis, the reaction points to the necessity of moral regulation; for, they say, were one to "eliminate morals," the "animal instincts" would gain the upper hand and this would "lead to chaos." It is evident that the formula of the threatening social chaos is nothing but the fear of human instincts. Are morals necessary, then? Yes, since antisocial impulses actually do endanger social living. This being so, how would it be possible to abolish compulsive moral regulation?

This question cannot be answered without first considering the following sex-economic findings. Moral regulation represses and keeps from gratification the *natural* biological needs. This results in *secondary, pathologically antisocial* impulses. These, in turn, have to be inhibited of necessity. Thus, morality does not owe its existence to the necessity of inhibiting antisocial tendencies. It developed, in primitive society, when a certain upper class with economic superiority began to attain power; for economic reasons, this class had an interest in suppressing the natural needs, though they, in themselves, *in no way* disturbed sociality. Compulsive moral regulation gained a reason for its existence the moment when that which it produced *actually* began to endanger social life. For example, the suppression of the natural gratification of hunger led to theft; this in turn necessitated the moral condemnation of theft.

Thus, in any discussion as to whether morals are necessary or should be abolished, whether one set of morals should be replaced by another, whether, finally, moral regulation should be replaced by self-regulation—in such a discussion we will not get one step farther unless we distinguish the *natural* biological impulses from the *secondary* antisocial impulses which owe their existence to compulsive morals. The unconscious of the human in an authoritarian society is filled with both kinds of impulses. If one suppresses—as one needs must—the antisocial impulses, the natural biological impulses suffer the same fate. While to the political reaction the concept of impulses and that of "antisocial" are one and the same thing, the differentiation just mentioned points a way out of the dilemma.

As long as the alteration of human structure has not succeeded to such an extent that the natural regulation of the biological energies automatically excludes any antisocial tendency, so long is it impossible to abolish moral regulation. This process of alteration of structure is bound to take a very long time. The elimination of moral regulation and its displacement by sex-economic regulation will be possible only to the degree to which the realm of the natural biological impulses is extended at the expense of the secondary antisocial impulses. That, and how, this takes place we know with certainty from character-analytic experience with the individual patient. Here, we see how the patient demobilizes his moral compulsions only to the extent to which he regains his natural sexuality. With the loss of moral regulation by his conscience he also loses his antisociality; he develops a natural morality, as contrasted with a compulsive one, to the same extent that he becomes genitally healthy.

Thus, the coming social evolution—if it knows what it is doing—will not suddenly abolish moral regulation. It will first alter the structure of people in such a manner that they become capable of social living and working without authority and moral pressure, out of their own independence and really voluntary discipline which cannot be imposed from outside. Moral regulation will apply only to the antisocial impulses. Such things as the punishment of the seduction of children by adults will not be abolished as long as the structure of the masses of adults contains the impulse to seduce children. To this extent, conditions after the revolution would seem to be identical with those in an authoritarian society. The difference—and it is an important one—between the two societies, however, would be that a free society would not put any obstacles in the path of the gratification of the *natural* needs. It would, for example, not only not prohibit a love relationship between adolescents; it would give its full protection and help. It would, for example, not only not prohibit infantile masturbation; it would deal severely with any adult who would prevent the child from developing its natural sexuality.

However, we should guard against an absolute and rigid concept of the "sexual impulse." The secondary impulse, too, is determined not only by its goal, but also by the period at which it develops and by the conditions under which it strives for gratification. One and the same manifestation may be natural in one case and at a certain period, antisocial and unnatural in another case or at another period. To illustrate: If a child of one or two wets the bed or plays with its feces, this is a natural phase in its pregenital development. At this period, punishing the child for these impulses is an action which itself deserves the most severe punishment. If, however, the same individual at the age of 14 were to eat its feces or play with them, this would be a secondary, antisocial, pathological impulse. The individual should not be punished but hospitalized for treatment. But in a free society, this would not be sufficient. Rather, the most important task of society would be that of changing education in such a manner that such pathological impulses would not develop at all.

To take another example. If a boy of 15 were to develop a love relationship with a girl of 13, a free society not only would not interfere, it would affirm and protect it. If, however, the boy of 15 tried to seduce little girls of 3 for sexual gains or tried to force a girl of his age into a sexual relationship, this would be considered antisocial. It would indicate that the boy's healthy impulse to establish a normal sex relationship with a girl his age was inhibited. In summary one would say that in the transition period from an authoritarian to a free society, the rule should be: Moral regulation for secondary, antisocial impulses, and sex-economic self-regulation for natural biological needs. The goal is that of increasingly putting out of function the secondary impulses and with them moral compulsion, and of replacing them completely by sex-economic self-regulation.

These formulations regarding the secondary impulses could easily be misinterpreted by moralists and other pathological people in such a way as to be made to serve their own purposes. But before long it should be possible to make so clear the difference between natural and secondary impulses that the authoritarian moral hypocrisy will find it impossible to sneak again into human sex life by a back door. The existence of severe moral tenets always proves, and always has, that the biological needs, particularly the sexual needs, are not being gratified. Every kind of moral regulation is *per se* sex-negative, condemns or denies the natural sexual needs. Any kind of moralism is life-negative, and the most important task of a free society is that of making possible for its members the satisfaction of their natural needs. Sex-economy has as its aim "moral behavior" no less than does moral regulation. Only, in sex-economy, "morality" means an altogether different thing: not something which is diametrically opposed to nature, but a complete harmony of nature and culture. Sex-economy fights compulsive moral regulation because moral regulation produces just what it attempts to fight: antisocial impulses. Sex-economy does not fight a morality which is life-affirmative.

Sex-Economic "Morality"

Everywhere in the world people are fighting for a new regulation of social life. In this fight they are hampered not only by the most difficult economic and social conditions; they are also inhibited, confused and endangered by their own biopsychic structure which is basically the same as that of the very people against whom they fight. The goal of a cultural revolution is the development of people with a character structure which would make them capable of self-regulation. Those who today fight for this goal often live according to principles which correspond to this goal; but, they are no more than "principles." We have to be quite clear about the fact that today there are no people with a solid, fully developed sex-affirmative structure, for all of us have gone through an authoritarian, religious, sex-negative educational machine. Nevertheless, in shaping our personal lives, we achieve an attitude which could be called sex-economic. Some succeed better in achieving this alteration of structure, others less well. If one has lived and worked for a long time with industrial workers, one knows that among them a bit of the future sex-economic regulation is occasionally anticipated.

A few examples may show what "sex-economic morality" is and how it anticipates the "morality of the future." The fact should be emphasized that, in living thus, we do not form an island by any means; what enables us to have such concepts and to live according to them is the fact that such modes of living and such new "moral principles" are part of a general developmental process in society, a process which takes place entirely independently of the views of this or that individual or political or cultural group.

Fifteen or twenty years ago, it was a disgrace for an unmarried girl *not* to be a virgin. Today the girls of all social circles and strata—some more, some less, some more clearly, some more vaguely—have begun to develop the view that it is a disgrace *still* to be a virgin at the age of 18, 20 or 22.

Not long ago, it was considered a moral crime, calling for drastic punishment, when a couple who intended to be married became sexually acquainted with each other beforehand. Today, quite spontaneously, and in spite of the influence of church, scholastic medicine and puritanical minds, the view becomes more and more general that it is unhygienic, imprudent and possibly disastrous if two people bind themselves without having first convinced themselves that they are matched in the basis of their life together, that is, in their sexual life.

Extramarital sexual intercourse, looked upon as a vice a few years ago and considered "moral turpitude" before the law, today (1936) has become a matter of course, and a vital necessity, for example with the youth among workers and the middle classes of Germany.

A few years ago, the idea that a girl of 15 or 16—though she be sexually mature—had a boy friend seemed absurd; today it has already become a matter for serious discussion; in a few more years it will be as much a matter of course as is today the right of the unmarried woman to have a sexual partner. A hundred years from now, such demands as that women teachers should have no sex life will provoke the same incredulous smile as does today mention of the times when men put chastity belts on their women. Just as ridiculous will appear what today still is an almost general ideology: that the man has to seduce a woman, while a woman is not supposed to seduce a man.

It is still far from being a matter of course that one does not engage in sexual intercourse if the sexual partner does not want to. The concept of "marital duty" has legal backing and legal consequences. Nevertheless, in our sex hygiene clinics and medical practice we see that a contrasting attitude makes itself felt: the attitude that, notwithstanding social and legal ideology, a man does not have intercourse with his partner when she does not wish it; more, when she is not genitally aroused. It still is generally considered a "natural" fact, however, that women suffer the sexual act without any inner participation. It is part of natural morality not to have sexual intercourse unless both are in full genital readiness; this eliminates the masculine ideology of rape and the attitude of the woman that she has to be seduced or mildly raped.

The attitude is still quite common that one should jealously watch over one's partner's fidelity. Newspaper stories and suicide statistics eloquently show how rotten our society is in this respect. Nevertheless, gradually the insight gains ground that nobody has the right to prohibit his or her partner from entering a temporary or lasting sexual relationship with somebody else. He has only the right either to withdraw or to win the partner back. This attitude, which is entirely in accordance with sex-economic findings, has nothing to do with the hyper-radical idea that one should not be jealous at all, that "it doesn't make any difference" if the partner enters another relationship. It is absolutely natural to suffer pain at the thought that a *beloved* partner embraces somebody else. This *natural jealousy* has to be strictly distinguished from *possessive jealousy*. It is natural not to want a beloved partner in somebody else's arms; but it is equally unnatural if—no longer having sexual intercourse oneself with one's partner, as in a marriage or other relationship of long duration—one were to forbid the partner another relationship.

These few examples may suffice. Complicated as the personal and particularly the sexual life of people is today, it would regulate itself with the greatest simplicity if they were able fully to appreciate the pleasure in life. The essence of sex-economic regulation lies in the avoidance of any absolute norms or precepts and in the recognition of the will to life and pleasure in living as the regulators of social life. The fact that today, due to the disordered human structure, this recognition is reduced to a minimum does not speak against the principle of self-regulation; on the contrary, it speaks against the moral regulation which has created this pathological structure.

There are *two* kinds of "morality," but only *one* kind of moral regulation. That kind of "morality" which everybody acknowledges and affirms as a matter of course (not to rape, not to murder, etc.) can be established only on the basis of full gratification of the natural needs. But the other kind of "morality" which we refute (sexual abstinence for children and adolescents, compulsory marital fidelity, etc.) is in itself pathological and creates the very chaos which it professes to control. It is the arch-enemy of natural morality.

There are people who say that sex-economic living will destroy the family. They babble about the "sexual chaos" which would result from a healthy love life, and the masses are impressed by them because they are professors or the authors of best-sellers. One has to know what one is talking about. It is a matter, first of all, of eliminating the *economic* enslavement of women and children. And their *authoritarian* enslavement. Not until that is done will the husband love his wife, the wife the husband, and will parents and children love each other. They will no longer have any reason to hate each other. What we want to destroy is not the family, but the *hatred* which the family creates, the coercion, though it may take on the outward appearance of "love." If familial love is that great human possession it is made out to be, it will have to prove itself. If a dog which is chained to the house does not run away, nobody will, for this reason, call him a faithful companion. No sensible person will talk of love when a man cohabits with a woman who is bound hand and foot. No half-way decent man will be proud of the love of a woman whom he buys by supporting her or by power. No decent man will take love which is not given freely. Compulsive morality as exemplified in marital duty and familial authority is the morality of cowardly and impotent individuals who are incapable of experiencing through natural love capacity what they try to obtain in vain with the aid of the police and marriage laws.

These people try to put all humanity into their own straitjacket because they are incapable of tolerating natural sexuality in others. It annoys them and fills them with envy, because they themselves would like to live that way and cannot. Far be it from us to force anybody to give up the familial life if he wants it; on the other hand, we do not want to let anybody force into it those who do not want it. Let him who can live in monogamy all his life and wants to, do so; he who cannot do it, who is going to be ruined by it, should have the opportunity to arrange his life differently. But if one wants to establish a "new kind of life" one has to know the contradictions inherent in the old one.

The Failure of Sexual Reform

Sexual reform aims to eliminate conditions in sexual life which, in the last analysis, are rooted in economic conditions and which express themselves in psychic illness. In authoritarian society, the conflict between a morality which is imposed on the total society by a minority in the interests of maintaining its power, on the one hand, and the sexual needs of the individual on the other, leads to a crisis which— within the existing social framework—is insoluble. Never in all the history of mankind, however, has this conflict led to such crass and cruel consequences as during the past three decades. Thus, there never was any other period during which sexual reform was so much discussed and written about. Nor any other during which all attempts at sexual reform failed as thoroughly as in this "age of technic and science." The contrast between the devitalizing sexual misery and the enormous progress in sexology is a corollary to that other contrast between the economic misery of the working masses and the enormous technical advances of our industrial age. Or another contrast—which is again only seemingly paradoxical—that in this age of aseptic operations and highly developed surgery about 20,000 women in Germany died annually from abortions between 1920 and 1932 and that 75,000 women annually were seriously ill from infections after abortions. Or that, with increasing rationalization of production, between 1930 and 1933 more and more industrial workers were unemployed, their families physically and morally ruined. This contrast, far from being senseless, is quite intelligible if one does not try to comprehend it apart from the economic and social structure which creates it. We will have to show that sexual misery as well as the impossibility of solving the sexual problem are both an integral part of the social order to which they owe their existence.

The sex-reform struggles are part of the cultural struggle in general. The Liberal, like Norman Haire, fights with his sexual reform against only one individual defect of this society, without wanting to criticize it otherwise. The Socialist, the "Reformist," attempts, by introducing sexual reforms, also to introduce a bit of socialism into the existing society. He tries to reverse the process of development by having the sexual reform take place before an alteration of the economic structure.

The moralist will never understand that sexual misery is an integral part of the social order which he defends. He sees its cause either in human sinfulness, in some supernatural will or a no less mysterious will to suffer, or he believes that sexual misery exists simply because people do not follow his ascetic and monogamous demands. He cannot be expected to admit that he is an accomplice in the very thing which he himself, piously though perhaps honestly, tries to abolish with his reforms. The consequences of such an admission—even to himself—might shake his economic basis, the very basis from which he undertakes his reforms. For he has not yet learned that the fascist, no matter what variety, does not joke about serious matters and will, if his existence is at stake, unceremoniously have the liberal pacifist replaced by the hangman.

Sexual reform has for decades been attempting to alleviate sexual misery. The problems of prostitution and venereal disease, of sexual misery, abortion and sexual murders, as well as the problem of the neuroses, are always in the center of public interest. Not one of the measures taken has so much as touched the prevailing sexual misery. More than that, what proposals for reform are made are always a few steps *behind* the actual changes which take place in the relations between the sexes. The decrease in marriages, the increase in divorces and adultery force a discussion of marriage reform; extramarital sexual relations become more and more a recognized fact, the views of ethically oriented sexologists notwithstanding; sexual intercourse among large sections of the youth between 15 and 18 is a general phenomenon; this at a time when the sexual reform movement still debates the question whether sexual abstinence of adolescents should be continued beyond the age of 20, or the question whether masturbation is to be considered a normal manifestation. "Criminal" abortion and the use of contraceptives become more and more widespread, while the sexual reform movement debates whether, in addition to medical reasons, social factors should also be considered as indication for abortion.

So we see that the concrete changes in sex life are always far ahead of the negligible efforts of the sex reformers. This lag in the reform movement indicates that there is something basically wrong with these reform efforts; there is an inner contradiction which works like a brake mechanism and dooms all effort to become fruitless.

We are confronted with the task of finding out the hidden meaning of this fiasco of sex reform. We will have to find out what links this kind of sex reform and its failure with the authoritarian social order. The connections are by no means simple. In particular, the problem of the formation of sexual ideologies is so complex as to require a special study. Here, only a sector of the whole problem will be treated. We find here an interlacing of the following factors:

1. The institution of marriage as the brake on sexual reform.
2. The compulsive family as the educational apparatus.
3. The demand for sexual abstinence of youth as the logical

measure—from an authoritarian standpoint—for education to lifelong, monogamous marriage and the patriarchal family.

4. The contradiction between sexual reform and conservative marriage ideology.

Many of these connections have gone unnoticed, mainly because the critics of sexual reform concentrated their attention on the external forms of sex life (housing, abortion, marriage laws, etc.) while the sexual needs, mechanisms and experiences were largely overlooked. Little is to be added to this sociological criticism which in Europe came from such men as Hodann, Hirschfeld, Brupbacher, Wolff and which was highlighted by the sexual revolution in Russia between 1918 and 1921.

However, an evaluation of the psychic and cultural results of the authoritarian sexual order for the sexual economy of the individual and of society presupposes a knowledge of the psychic and somatic mechanisms of sexuality.

The Transformation of Sexuality into Eros

Herbert Marcuse

from *Eros and Civilization*, 1955

After Paul Goodman, Herbert Marcuse was the only thinker to capture the intellectual and political spirit of the radical student movement in its struggle against the war in Vietnam and its dissatisfaction with consumer capitalism—especially in his book, **One-Dimensional Man** *(1964). In 1934, Marcuse emigrated from Germany where he had long been associated with the Frankfurt School of Marxist theorists. Even before the political and cultural movements of the sixties were a twinkle in anyone's eye, Marcuse had written* **Eros and Civilization** *in which he attempted to create a synthesis of Freud and Marx. Marcuse goes beyond Reich by stressing an erotic view of reality, in which sexual liberation is just one component.*

The vision of a non-repressive culture, which we have lifted from a marginal trend in mythology and philosophy, aims at a new relation between instincts and reason. The civilized morality is reversed by harmonizing instinctual freedom and order: liberated from the tyranny of repressive reason, the instincts tend toward free and lasting existential relations—they generate a *new* reality principle. In Schiller's idea of an " aesthetic state," the vision of a non-repressive culture is concretized at the level of mature civilization. At this level, the organization of the instincts becomes social problem (in Sehiller's terminology, *political*), as it does in Freud's pyschology. The processes that create the ego and superego also shape and perpetuate specific societal institutions and relations. Such psychoanalytical concepts as sublimation, identification, and introjection have not only a psychical but also a social content: they terminate in a system of institutions, laws, agencies, things, and customs that confront the individual as objective entities. Within this antagonistic system, the mental conflict between ego and superego, between ego and id, is at one ant the same time a conflict between the individual and his society. The latter embodies the rationality of the whole, and the individual's struggle against the repressive forces is a struggle against objective reason. Therefore, the emergence of a non-repressive reality principle involving instinctual liberation would *regress* behind the attained level of civilized rationality. This regression would be psychical as well as social : it would reactivate early stages of the libido which were surpassed in the development of the reality ego, and it would dissolve the institutions of society in which the reality ego exists. In terms of these institutions, instinctual liberation is relapse into barbarism. However, occurring at the height of civilization, as a consequence not of defeat but of victory in the struggle for existence, and supported by a free society, such liberation might have very different results. It would still be a reversal of the process of civilization, a subversion of culture—but *after* culture had done its work and created the mankind and the world that could be free. It would still be "regression"—but in the light of mature consciousness and guided by a new rationality. Under these conditions, the possibility of a non-repressive civilization is predicated not upon the arrest, but upon the liberation, of progress-so that man would order his life in accordance with his fully developed knowledge, so that he would ask again what is good and what is evil. If the guilt accumulated in the civilized domination of man by man can ever be redeemed by freedom, then the "original sin" must be committed again: "We must again eat from the tree of knowledge in order to fall back into the state of innocence."[1]

The notion of a non-repressive instinctual order must first be tested on the most "disorderly" of all instincts—namely, sexuality. Non-repressive order is possible only if the sex instincts can, by virtue of their own dynamic and under changed existential and societal conditions, generate lasting erotic relations among mature individuals. We have to ask whether the sex instincts, after the elimination of all surplus-repression, can develop a "libidinal rationality" which is not only compatible with but even promotes progress toward higher forms of civilized freedom. This possibility will be examined here in Freud's own terms.

1. "Wir müssen wieder vom Baum der Erkenntnis essen, um in den Stand der Unschuld zurückzufallen." Heinrich von Kleist, " Ueber de Marionettentheater," conclusion.

We have reiterated Freud's conclusion that any genuine decrease in the societal controls over the sex instincts would, even under optimum conditions, reverse the organization of sexuality toward precivilized stages. Such regression would break through the central fortifications of the performance principle: it would undo the channeling of sexuality into monogamic reproduction and the taboo on perversions. Under the rule of the performance principle, the libidinal cathexis of the individual body and libidinal relations with others are normally confined to leisure time and directed to the preparation and execution of genital intercourse; only in exceptional cases, and with a high degree of sublimation, are libidinal relations allowed to enter into the sphere of work. These constraints, enforced by the need for sustaining a large quantum of energy and time for non-gratifying labor, perpetuate the desexualization of the body in order to make the organism into a subject-object of socially useful performances. Conversely, if the work day and energy are reduced to a minimum, without a corresponding manipulation of the free time, the ground for these constraints would be undermined. Libido would be released and would overflow the institutionalized limits within which it is kept by the reality principle.

Freud repeatedly emphasized that the lasting interpersonal relations on which civilization depends presuppose that the sex instinct is inhibited in its aim.[2] Love, and the enduring and responsible relations which it demands, are founded on a union of sexuality with "affection," and this union is the historical result of a long and cruel process of domestication, in which the instinct's legitimate manifestation is made supreme and its component parts are arrested in their development.[3] This cultural refinement of sexuality, its sublimation to love, took place within a civilization which established possessive private relations apart from, and in a decisive aspect conflicting with, the possessive societal relations. While, outside the privacy of the family, men's existence was chiefly determined by the exchange value of their products and performances, their life in home and bed was to be permeated with the spirit of divine and moral law. Mankind was supposed to be an end in itself and never a mere means; but this ideology was effective

2. *Collected Papers* (London: Hogarth Press, 1950), IV, 203ff; *Group Psychology and the Analysis of the Ego* (New York: Liveright Publishing Corp., 1949), pp. 72, 78
3. *Collected Papers*, IV, 215.

in the private rather than in the societal functions of the individuals, in the sphere of libidinal satisfaction rather than in that of labor. The full force of civilized morality was mobilized against the use of the body as mere object, means, instrument of pleasure; such reification was tabooed and remained the ill-reputed privilege of whores, degenerates, and perverts. Precisely in his gratification, and especially in his sexual gratification, man was to be a higher being, committed to higher values; sexuality was to be dignified by love. With the emergence of a non-repressive reality principle, with the abolition of the surplus-repression necessitated by the performance principle, this process would be reversed. In the societal relations, reification would be reduced as the division of labor became reoriented on the gratification of freely developing individual needs; whereas, in the libidinal relations, the taboo on the reification of the body would be lessened. No longer used as a full-time instrument of labor, the body would be resexualized. The regression involved in this spread of the libido would first manifest itself in a reactivation of all erotogenic zones and, consequently, in a resurgence of pregenital polymorphous sexuality and in a decline of genital supremacy. The body in its entirety would become an object of cathexis, a thing to be enjoyed—an instrument of pleasure. This change in the value and scope of libidinal relations would lead to a disintegration of the institutions in which the private interpersonal relations have been organized, particularly the monogamic and patriarchal family.

These prospects seem to confirm the expectation that instinctual liberation can lead only to a society of sex maniacs—that is, to no society. However, the process just outlined involves not simply a release but a *transformation* of the libido: from sexuality constrained under genital supremacy to erotization of the entire personality. It is a spread rather than explosion of libido—a spread over private and societal relations which bridges the gap maintained between them by a repressive reality principle. This transformation of the libido would be the result of a societal transformation that released the free play of individual needs and faculties. By virtue of these conditions, the free development of transformed libido *beyond* the institutions of the performance principle differs essentially from the release of constrained sexuality *within* the dominion of these institutions. The latter process explodes *suppressed* sexuality; the libido continues to bear the mark of suppression and manifests itself in the hideous forms so well known in the history of civilization; in the sadistic and masochistic orgies of desperate masses, of "society elites," of starved bands of mercenaries, of prison and concentration-camp guards. Such release of sexuality provides a periodically necessary outlet for unbearable frustration; it strengthens rather than weakens the roots of instinctual constraint; consequently, it has been used time and again as a prop for suppressive regimes. In contrast, the free development of transformed libido within transformed institutions, while eroticizing previously tabooed zones, time, and relations, would *minimize* the manifestations of *mere* sexuality by integrating them into a far larger order, including the order of work. In this context, sexuality tends to its own sublimation: the libido would not simply reactivate precivilized and infantile stages, but would also transform the perverted content of these stages.

The term *perversions* covers sexual phenomena of essentially different origin. The same taboo is placed on instinctual manifestations incompatible with civilization and on those incompatible with repressive civilization, especially with monogamic genital supremacy. However, within the historical dynamic of the instinct, for example, coprophilia and homosexuality have a very different place and function.[4] A similar difference prevails within one and the same perversion: the function of sadism is not the same in a free libidinal relation and in the activities of SS Troops. The inhuman, compulsive, coercive, and destructive forms of these perversions seem to be linked with the general perversion of the human existence in a repressive culture, but the perversions have an instinctual substance distinct from these forms; and this substance may well express itself in other forms compatible with normality in high civilization. Not all component parts and stages of the instinct that have been suppressed have suffered this fate because they prevented the evolution of man and mankind. The purity, regularity, cleanliness, and reproduction required by the performance principle are not naturally those of any mature civilization. And the reactivation of prehistoric and childhood wishes and attitudes is not necessarily regression; it may well be the opposite—proximity to a happiness that has always been the repressed promise of a better future. In one of his most advanced formulations, Freud once defined happiness

4. See Chapter 2 *Eros and Civilization.*

as the "subsequent fulfillment of a prehistoric wish. That is why wealth brings so little happiness: money was not a wish in childhood."[5]

But if human happiness depends on the fulfillment of childhood wishes, civilization, according to Freud, depends on the suppression of the strongest of all childhood wishes: the Oedipus wish. Does the realization of happiness in a free civilization still necessitate this suppression? Or would the transformation of the libido also engulf the Oedipus situation? In the context of our hypothesis, such speculations are insignificant; the Oedipus complex, although the primary source and model of neurotic conflicts, is certainly not the central cause of the discontents in civilization, and not the central obstacle for their removal. The Oedipus complex "passes" even under the rule of a repressive reality principle. Freud advances two general interpretations of the "passing of the. Oedipus complex": it "becomes extinguished by its lack of success"; or it "must come to an end because the time has come for its dissolution, just as the milk-teeth fall out when the permanent ones begin to press forward."[6] The passing of the complex appears as "natural" event in both cases.

We have spoken of the *self-sublimation of sexuality*. The term implies that sexuality can, under specific conditions, create highly civilized human relations without being subjected to the repressive organization which the established civilization has imposed upon the instinct. Such self-sublimation presupposes historical progress beyond the institutions of the performance principle, which in turn would release instinctual regression. For the development of the instinct, this means regression from sexuality in the service of reproduction to sexuality in the "function of obtaining pleasure from zones of the body."[7] With this restoration of the primary structure of sexuality, the primacy of the genital function is broken—as is the desexualization of the body which has accompanied this primacy. The organism in its entirety becomes the substratum of sexuality, while at the same time the instinct's objective is no longer absorbed by a specialized function-namely, that of bringing "one's own genitals into contact with those of someone of the

5. Ernest Jones, *The Life and Work of Sigmund Freud*, Vol. I (New York: Basic Books, 1953), P. 330
6. *Collected Papers*, II, 269.
7. *An Outline of Psychoanalysis* (New York: W. W. Norton, 1949), p. 26..

opposite sex."[8] Thus enlarged, the field and objective of the instinct becomes the life of the organism itself. This process almost naturally, by its inner logic, suggests the conceptual transformation of sexuality into Eros.

The introduction of the term Eros in Freud's later writings was certainly motivated by different reasons: Eros, as life instinct, denotes a larger biological instinct rather than a larger scope of sexuality.[9] However, it may not be accidental that Freud does not rigidly distinguish between Eros and sexuality, and his usage of the term *Eros* (especially in *The Ego and the Id, Civilization and Its Discontents*, and in *An Outline of Psychoanalysis*) implies an enlargement of the meaning of sexuality itself. Even without Freud's explicit reference to Plato the change in emphasis is clear: Eros signifies a quantitative and qualitative aggrandizement of sexuality. And the aggrandized concept seems to demand a correspondingly modified concept of sublimation. The modifications of sexuality are not the same as the modifications of Eros. Freud's concept of sublimation refers to the fate of sexuality under a repressive reality principle. Thus, sublimation means a change in the aim and object of the instinct "with regard to which our social values come into the picture."[10] The term is applied to a group of unconscious processes which have in common that

> . . . as the result of inner or outer deprivation, the aim of object libido undergoes a more or less complete deflection, modification, or inhibition. In the great majority of instances, the new aim is, one distinct or remote from sexual satisfaction, i.e., is an asexual or non-sexual aim.[11]

This mode of sublimation is to a high degree dictated by specific societal requirements and cannot be automatically extended to other and less repressive forms of civilization with different "social

8. Ibid., p.. 25
9. See the papers of Siegfried Bernfeld and Edward Bibring in *Imago*, Vols. XXI, XXII (1935, 1936).
10. Freud, *New Introductory Lectures on Psychoanalysis* (New York: W. W. Norton, 1933), p.133.
11. Edward Glover, "Sublimation, Substitution and Social Anxiety," on *International Journal of Psychoanalysis*, Vol. xiii No. 3. (1931) p. 264.

values." Under the performance principle, the diversion of libido into useful cultural activities takes place after the period of early-childhood. Sublimation then operates on a preconditioned instinctual structure, which includes the functional and temporal restraints of sexuality, its channeling into monogamic reproduction, and the desexualization of most of the body. Sublimation works with the thus preconditioned libido and its possessive, exploitative, aggressive force. The repressive "modification" of the pleasure principle precedes the actual sublimation, and the latter carries the repressive elements over into the socially useful activities.

However, there are other modes of sublimation. Freud speaks of aim-inhibited sexual impulses which need not be described as sublimated although they are "closely related" to sublimated impulses. They have not abandoned their directly sexual aims, but they are held back by internal resistances from attaining them; they rest content with certain approximations to satisfaction."[12] Freud calls them "social instincts" and mentions as examples "the affectionate relations between parents and children, feelings of friendship, and the emotional ties in marriage which had their origin in sexual attraction." Moreover, in *Group Psychology and the Analysis of the Ego*, Freud has emphasized the extent to which societal relations (" community " in civilization) are founded on unsublimated as well as sublimated libidinous ties: "sexual love for women" as well as "desexualized, sublimated, homosexual love for other men" here appear as instinctual sources of an enduring and expanding culture.[13] This conception suggests, in Freud's own work, an idea of civilization very different from that derived from repressive sublimation, namely, civilization evolving from and sustained by free libidinal relations. Géza Róheim used Ferenczi's notion of a "genitofugal libido"[14] to support his theory of the

12. Encyclopedia article "The Libido Theory ' reprinted in *Collected Papers*, V, 134
13. *Versuch einer Genitaltheorie* (Leipzig: Internationaler Psychoanalytischer Verlag, 1924), pp. 51-52. This book has appeared in English as *Thalassa*, transl. H. A. Bunker (Albany: Psychoanalytic Quarterly, Inc., 938).
14 Róheim, *The Origin and Function of Culture*, (New York: Nervous and Mental Disease Monograph No. 69, 1943), p. 74. In his article "Sublimation" in the *Yearbook of Psychoanalysis*, Vol. I (1945), Róheim stresses that in sublimation "id strivings reconquer the ground in a disguised form." Thus, "in contrast to the prevailing view, in sub. limation we have no ground wrested from the id by the super-ego, but quite to the contrary, what we have is super ego territory inundated by the id" (p. 177). Here, too, the emphasis is on the ascendancy of libido in sublimation.

libidinous origin of culture. With the relief of extreme tension, libido flows back from the object to the body, and this "recathecting of the whole organism with libido results in a feeling of happiness in which the organs find their reward for. work and stimulation to further activity." The concept assumes a genitofugal " libido trend to the development of culture"—in other words, an inherent trend in the libido itself toward "cultural" expression, without external repressive modification. And this "cultural" trend in the libido seems to be genitofugal, that is to say, away from genital supremacy toward the erotization of the entire organism.

Sexuality and Psychoanalysis

Simone de Beauvoir

from *The Second Sex*, 1952

Simone de Beauvoir's **The Second Sex** *is one of the great classics of feminist theory. De Beauvoir, a novelist, playwright, memoirist, and philosopher, was one of the most influential intellectuals in the world during the 40 years after World War II. She and her partner Jean-Paul Sartre were the voices of existentialist philosophy.* **The Second Sex** *is an application of existentialist philosophy to the situation of women. In this excerpt, she undertakes a critical discussion of psychoanalytic thinking about sex and gender.*

Sexuality most certainly plays a considerable role in human life; it can be said to pervade life throughout. We have already learned from physiology that the living activity of the testes and the ovaries is integrated with that of the body in general. The existent is a sexual, a sexuate body, and in his relations with other existents who are also sexuate bodies, sexuality is in consequence always involved. But if body and sexuality are concrete expressions of existence, it is with reference to this that their significance can be discovered. Lacking this perspective, psychoanalysis takes for granted unexplained facts. For instance, we are told that the little girl is *ashamed* of urinating in a squatting position with her bottom uncovered—but whence comes this shame? And likewise, before asking whether the male is proud of having a penis or whether his pride is expressed in his penis, it is necessary to know what pride is and how the aspirations of the subject can be incarnated in an object. There is no need of taking sexuality as an irreducible datum, for there is in the existent a more original "quest of being," of which sexuality is only one of the aspects. Sartre demonstrates this truth in *L'Être et le néant,* as does Bachelard in his works on Earth, Air, and Water. The psychoanalysts hold that the primary truth regarding man is his relation with his own body and with the bodies of his fellows in the group; but man has a primordial interest in the substance of the natural world which surrounds him and which he tries to discover in work, in play, and in all the experiences of the "dynamic imagination." Man aspires to be at one concretely with the whole world, apprehended in all possible ways. To work the earth, to dig a hole, are activities as original as the embrace, as coition, and they deceive themselves who see here no more than sexual symbols. The hole, the ooze, the gash, hardness, integrity are primary realities; and the interest they have for man is not dictated by the libido, but rather the libido will be colored by the manner in which he becomes aware of them. It is not because it symbolizes feminine virginity that integrity fascinates man; but it is his admiration for integrity that renders virginity precious. Work, war, play, art signify ways of being concerned with the world which cannot be reduced to any others; they disclose qualities that interfere with those which sexuality reveals. It is at once in their light and in the light of these erotic experiences that the individual exercises his power of choice. But only an ontological point of view, a comprehension of being in general, permits us to restore the unity of this choice.

It is this concept of choice, indeed, that psycholanalysis most vehemently rejects in the name of determinism and the "collective unconscious"; and it is this unconscious that is supposed to supply man with prefabricated imagery and a universal symbolism. Thus it would explain the observed analogies of dreams, of purposeless actions, of visions of delirium, of allegories, and of human destinies. To speak of liberty would be to deny oneself the possibility of explaining these disturbing conformities. But the idea of liberty is not incompatible with the existence of certain constants. If the psychoanalytic method is frequently rewarding in spite of the errors in its theory, that is because there are in every individual case certain factors of undeniable generality: situations and behavior patterns constantly recur, and the moment of decision flashes from a cloud of generality and repetition. "Anatomy is destiny," said Freud; and this phrase is echoed by that of

Merleau-Ponty: "The body is generality." Existence is all one, bridging the gaps between individual existents; it makes itself manifest in analogous organisms, and therefore constant factors will be found in the bonds between the ontological and the sexual. At a given epoch of history the techniques, the economic and social structure of a society, will reveal to all its members an identical world, and there a constant relation of sexuality to social patterns will exist; analogous individuals, placed in analogous conditions, will see analogous points of significance in the given circumstances. This analogy does not establish a rigorous universality, but it accounts for the fact that general types may be recognized in individual case histories.

The symbol does not seem to me to be an allegory elaborated by a mysterious unconscious; it is rather the perception of a certain significance through the analogue of the significant object. Symbolic significance is manifested in the same way to numerous individuals, because of the identical existential situation connecting all the individual existents and the identical set of artificial conditions that all must confront. Symbolism did not come down from heaven nor rise up from subterranean depths—it has been elaborated, like language, by that human reality which is at once *Mitsein* and separation; and this explains why individual invention also has its place, as in practice psychoanalysis has to admit, regardless of doctrine. Our perspective allows us, for example, to understand the value widely accorded to the penis. It is impossible to account for it without taking our departure from an existential fact: the tendency of the subject toward *alienation*. The anxiety that his liberty induces in the subject leads him to search for himself in things, which is a kind of flight from himself. This tendency is so fundamental that immediately after weaning, when he is separated from the Whole, the infant is compelled to lay hold upon his alienated existence in mirrors and in the gaze of his parents. Primitive people are alienated in mana, in the totem; civilized people in their individual souls, in their egos, their names, their property, their work. Here is to be found the primary temptation to inauthenticity, to failure to be genuinely oneself. The penis is singularly adapted for playing this role of "double" for the little boy—it is for him at once a foreign object and himself; it is a plaything, a doll, and yet his own flesh; relatives and nurse-girls behave toward it as if it were a little person. It is easy to see, then, how it becomes for the child "an *alter ego* ordinarily more artful, more intelligent, and more clever than the individual."[1] The penis is regarded by the subject as at once himself and other than himself, because the functions of urination and later of erection are processes midway between the voluntary and the involuntary, and because it is a capricious and as it were a foreign source of pleasure that is felt subjectively. The individual's specific transcendence takes concrete form in the penis and it is a source of pride. Because the phallus is thus set apart, man can bring into integration with his subjective individuality the life that overflows from it. It is easy to see, then, that the length of the penis, the force of the urinary jet, the strength of erection and ejaculation become for him the measure of his own worth.[2]

Thus the incarnation of transcendence in the phallus is a constant; and since it is also a constant for the child to feel himself transcended— that is to say, frustrated in his own transcendence by the father—we therefore continually come upon the Freudian idea of the "castration complex." Not having that *alter ego*, the little girl is not alienated in a material thing and cannot retrieve her integrity. On this account she is led to make an object of her whole self, to set up herself as the Other. Whether she knows that she is or is not comparable with boys is secondary; the important point is that, even if she is unaware of it, the absence of the penis prevents her from being conscious of herself as a sexual being. From this flow many consequences. But the constants I have referred to do not for all that establish a fixed destiny—the phallus assumes such worth as it does because it symbolizes a dominance that is exercised in other domains. If woman should succeed in establishing herself as subject, she would invent equivalents of the phallus; in fact, the doll, incarnating the promise of the baby that is to come in the future, can become a possession more precious than the penis.[3] There

1. Alice Balint: *La Vie intime de l'enfant*, p. 101.
2. I have been told of peasant children amusing themselves in excremental competition; the one who produced the most copious and solid feces enjoyed a prestige unmatched by any other form of success, whether in games or even in fighting. The fecal mass here plays the same part as the penis—there is alienation in both cases. [Pride in this peculiar type of eminence is by no means confined to European peasant children; it has been observed in young Americans and is doubtless well-nigh universal.—TR.]

3. We shall return to these ideas in the second part; I note them here only as a matter of method.

are matrilineal societies in which the women keep in their possession the *masks* in which the group finds alienation; in such societies the penis loses much of its glory. The fact is that a true human privilege is based upon the anatomical privilege only in virtue of the total situation. Psychoanalysis can establish its truths only in the historical context.

Woman can be defined by her consciousness of her own femininity no more satisfactorily than by saying that she is a female, for she acquires this consciousness under circumstances dependent upon the society of which she is a member. Interiorizing the unconscious and the whole psychic life, the very language of psychoanalysis suggests that the drama of the individual unfolds within him—such words as *complex, tendency*, and so on make that implication. But a life is a relation to the world, and the individual defines himself by making his own choices through the world about him. We must therefore turn toward the world to find answers for the questions we are concerned with. In particular psychoanalysis fails to explain why woman is the *Other*. For Freud himself admits that the prestige of the penis is explained by the sovereignty of the father, and, as we have seen, he confesses that he is ignorant regarding the origin of male supremacy.

We therefore decline to accept the method of psychoanalysis, without rejecting *en bloc* the contributions of the science or denying the fertility of some of its insights. In the first place, we do not limit ourselves to regarding sexuality as something given. The insufficiency of this view is shown by the poverty of the resulting descriptions of the feminine libido; as I have already said, the psychoanalysts have never studied it directly, but only in taking the male libido as their point of departure. They seem to ignore the fundamental ambivalence of the attraction exerted on the female by the male. Freudians and Adlerians explain the anxiety felt by the female confronted by the masculine sex as being the inversion of a frustrated desire. Stekel saw more clearly that an original reaction was concerned, but he accounts for it in a superficial manner. Woman, he says, would fear defloration, penetration, pregnancy, and pain, and such fear would restrain her desire—but this explanation is too rational. Instead of holding that her desire is disguised in anxiety or is contested by fear, we should regard as an original fact this blending of urgency and apprehension which is female desire: it is the indissoluble synthesis of attraction and repulsion that characterizes it. We may note that many female animals avoid copulation even as they are soliciting it, and we are tempted to accuse them of coquetry or hypocrisy, but it is absurd to pretend to explain primitive behavior patterns by asserting their similarity to complex modes of conduct. On the contrary, the former are in truth at the source of the attitudes that in woman are called coquetry and hypocrisy. The notion of a "passive libido" is baffling, since the libido has been defined, on the basis of the male, as a drive, an energy; but one would do no better to hold the opinion that a light could be at once yellow and blue—what is needed is the intuition of green. We would more fully encompass reality if instead of defining the libido in vague terms of "energy" we brought the significance of sexuality into relation with that of other human attitudes—taking, capturing, eating, making, submitting, and so forth; for it is one of the various modes of apprehending an object. We should study also the qualities of the erotic object as it presents itself not only in the sexual act but also to observation in general. Such an investigation extends beyond the frame of psychoanalysis, which assumes eroticism as irreducible.

Furthermore, I shall pose the problem of feminine destiny quite otherwise: I shall place woman in a world of values and give her behavior a dimension of liberty. I believe that she has the power to choose between the assertion of her transcendence and her alienation as object; she is not the plaything of contradictory drives; she devises solutions of diverse ranking in the ethical scale. Replacing value with authority, choice with drive, psychoanalysis offers an *Ersatz*, a substitute, for morality—the concept of normality. This concept is certainly most useful in therapeutics, but it has spread through psychoanalysis in general to a disquieting extent. The descriptive schema is proposed as a law; and most assuredly a mechanistic psychology cannot accept the notion of moral invention; it can in strictness render an account of the *less* and never of the more; in strictness it can admit of checks, never of creations. If a subject does not show in his totality the development considered as normal, it will be said that his development has been arrested, and this arrest will be interpreted as a lack, a negation, but never as a positive decision. This it is, among other things, that makes the psychoanalysis of great men so shocking: we are told that such and such a transference, this or that sublimation, has not taken place in them; it is not suggested that perhaps they have refused to undergo the process, perhaps for good reasons of their own; it is not thought desirable to regard their behavior as possibly motivated by purposes freely envisaged; the individual is always explained through ties with his past and not in respect to a future toward which he projects his aims. Thus the psychoanalysts never give us more than an inauthentic picture, and for the inauthentic there can hardly be found any other criterion than normality. Their statement of the feminine destiny is absolutely to the point in this connection. In the sense in which the psychoanalysts understand the term, "to identify oneself" with the mother or with the father is to *alienate oneself* in a model, it is to prefer a foreign image to the spontaneous manifestation of one's own existence, it is to play at being. Woman is shown to us as enticed by two modes of alienation. Evidently to play at being a man will be for her a source of frustration; but to play at being a woman is also a delusion: to be a woman would mean to be the object, the *Other*—and the Other nevertheless remains subject in the midst of her resignation.

The true problem for woman is to reject these flights from reality and seek self-fulfillment in transcendence. The thing to do, then, is to see what possibilities are opened up for her through what are called the virile and the feminine attitudes. When a child takes the road indicated by one or the other of its parents, it may be because the child freely takes up their projects; its behavior may be the result of a choice motivated by ends and aims. Even with Adler the will to power is only an absurd kind of energy; he denominates as "masculine protest" every project involving transcendence. When a little girl climbs trees it is, according to Adler, just to show her equality with boys; it does not occur to him that she likes to climb trees. For the mother her child is something quite other than an "equivalent of the penis." To paint, to write, to engage in politics—these are not merely "sublimations"; here we have aims that are willed for their own sakes. To deny it is to falsify all human history.

The reader will note a certain parallelism between this account and that of the psychoanalysts. The fact is that from the male point of view—which is adopted by both male and female psychoanalysts—behavior involving alienation is regarded as feminine, that in which the subject asserts his transcendence as virile. Donaldson, a historian of woman, remarked that the definitions: "man is a male human being, woman is a female human being," have been asymmetrically distorted;

and it is among the psychoanalysts in particular that man is defined as a human being and woman as a female—whenever she behaves as a human being she is said to imitate the male. The psychoanalyst describes the female child, the young girl, as incited to identification with the mother and the father, torn between "viriloid" and "feminine" tendencies; whereas I conceive her as hesitating between the role of *object, Other* which is offered her, and the assertion of her liberty. Thus it is that we shall agree on a certain number of facts, especially when we take up the avenues of inauthentic flight open to women. But we accord them by no means the same significance as does the Freudian or the Adlerian. For us woman is defined as a human being in quest of values in a world of values, a world of which it is indispensable to know the economic and social structure. We shall study woman in an existential perspective with due regard to her total situation.

Liberation: Toward the Polymorphous

Dennis Altman

from *Homosexual: Oppression and Liberation*, 1971

Homosexual: Oppression and Liberation is literally the first book to emerge from the gay liberation movement that discussed the political and theoretical issues raised by a sexual liberation movement created by homosexuals. At the time, Dennis Altman, a native of Australia, was a young faculty member at New York University when he participated in the heady excitement of gay liberation. He is also the author of **The Homosexualization of America/The Americanization of Homosexuality** *(1982), and* **AIDS in the Mind of America** *(1986). In the early days of gay liberation, identity had not yet become the focus of gay and lesbian politics, the emphasis was on sexual liberation—and on polymorphous sexuality (sexual desire that went beyond sexual orientation) as Herbert Marcuse and Norman O. Brown had envisioned.*

Liberation implies more than the mere absence of oppression. Obviously there is a need to end laws that discriminate against homosexuals, to proscribe police harassment, to break down the psychiatric ideologies that see us as sick and maladjusted. Yet to remove the obvious forms of oppression is only a necessary rather than a sufficient step toward liberation. To achieve liberation, as Marcuse has pointed out in another context, will demand a new morality and a revised notion of "human nature."

Thus to talk of gay liberation demands a broader examination of sexual mores than merely the attitudes towards homosexuality, for the liberation of the homosexual can only be achieved within the context of a much broader sexual liberation. What is needed in fact is a theory of sexuality and of the place sexuality occupies within human life. Inevitably any such theory will rely heavily on Freud. Indeed, despite the hostility of many in the sexual liberation movements to elements of Freudian—and particularly of neo-Freudian—-thought, these very movements are in fact part of a contemporary revival of Freudian thought, in particular its emphasis on the central and paramount role that sexuality plays in both social and individual life. (This revival, in which Herbert Marcuse and Norman O. Brown have played a leading role, belongs to a general contemporary attack on positivistic social science and a resurrection of metaphysical speculation.) In this discussion I am particularly indebted to Marcuse for his explorations of the concepts of repression and liberation.

Patterns of Sexual Repression

Western societies are remarkable for their strong repression of sexuality, a repression that has traditionally been expressed and legitimized in the Judaeo-Christian religious tradition. This repression is expressed in three closely related ways.

Above all, sex is linked with guilt. Despite theological refinement, the Fall of Adam and Eve is popularly viewed as being caused by their discovery of sex. Sex becomes a sin, and this equation gives rise to strong feelings of guilt about enjoying sexual pleasure. Today this concept of sin has been modified, but it is by no means dead. Indeed one may still find traces of an Elmer Gantry concept of sin, as in the decision of the Tennessee Baptist Convention in 1970 to ban dancing in its colleges. One preacher, it was reported, was cheered for his comment that: "Any man who says he can dance and keep his thoughts pure is less than a man or he is a liar." Women's thoughts were not mentioned.

America has a particularly strong fundamentalist tradition in which sex is viewed as sin, and probably the current boom in pornography and "permissiveness" feeds on the feelings of guilt so imbued into the American consciousness, reinforcing, as such permissiveness does, the whole feeling that sex is dirty and secretive. But guilt about sex is expressed in far broader terms. It may be profitable to regard the whole Western mystique about love as a means of resolving guilt feelings about sex (an argument that Germaine Greer hints at in her attacks on romantic love in *The Female Eunuch*). Nor is it only in the United States that politicians find it more profitable to talk about pornography than poverty, or tolerate unwanted births, bungled abortions and syphilis epidemics rather than provide proper education about contraception and venereal disease. Attitudes towards sex in prisons and hospitals—where authorities prefer to deny sexual feelings exist rather than provide proper facilities and opportunities for sexual activity—underline just how far general repression of sexuality remains in the so-called permissive society.

Secondly, sex has been firmly linked, and nowhere more clearly than in Christian theology, with the institution of the family and with childbearing. Sex is thus legitimized for its utilitarian principles, rather than as an end in itself, and marriage becomes a "sacred partnership" entered into for the purpose of begetting children. Even where sexual pleasure is accepted as a complementary goal, the connection between marriage and sex still remains, and is reinforced by countless television advertisements and magazine articles. It is from this particular form of sexual repression—and the nature of the resulting family institution—Wilhelm Reich has argued, that stems the repressive nature of modern society.

How strongly this particular view of sex is held to be true is suggested by the fact, already mentioned, that many homosexuals mold their behavior essentially on that of heterosexual couples, even, in some cases, playing out socially prescribed roles of husband and wife. Indeed Dotson Rader, a journalist and novelist with a strong interest in homosexuality, has claimed that many homosexuals have a desire for pregnancy. Comparably, those who have sought to explain *Who's Afraid of Virginia Woolf?* as a homosexual play manqué make much of the imaginary child that Martha and George have created. I think that Rader makes the point far too strongly, but inasmuch as he is correct, it suggests how strongly the view of sex-as-procreation has permeated.

Thirdly, and as a consequence of the utilitarian view of sex, there is an extremely strong negative attitude toward all sexual urges other than those that are genital and heterosexual. Counter to this is Freud's belief that the infant is polymorphous perverse at birth, that is, that the infant enjoys an undifferentiated ability to take sexual pleasure from all parts of the body. As part of this view Freud also believed in the essential bisexual nature of our original sex drive. (This is a view supported by considerable historical and anthropological evidence. "The Greeks," wrote the British anthropologist Rattray Taylor "recognized that the sexual nature of every human being contains both homosexual and heterosexual elements.") Yet, while positing the bisexual character of the sex drive, Freud also linked it to a linear concept of sexual development that made heterosexuality more mature than homosexuality. One of his more sophisticated followers, Sandor Ferenczi, whose paper "The Nosology of Male Homosexuality" introduces a subtle, if unconvincing distinction between "subjective" and "objective" homosexuality, took another view: "The extension of object homoerotism is an abnormal reaction to the disproportionately exaggerated repression of the homoerotic instinct component by civilized man, that is, a failure of this repression." He goes on to argue: "It is thinkable that the sense of cleanliness, which has been so specially reinforced in the past few centuries, that is, the repression of anal eroticism, has provided the strongest motive in this direction, for homoeroticism, even the most sublimated, stands in a more or less unconscious associative connection with pederastia, that is, anal-erotic activity." Which brings to mind Rattray Taylor's comment that "the Greeks distributed their sexuality and were as interested in bosom and buttocks as in genitals," a polymorphousness that declined with the development of guilt and the justification of sex-as-procreation.

Now, the traditional libertarian view of sexual repression has tended to stress and sought to change the first two attitudes that help generate it, while ignoring the last. The traditional position is most clearly expressed in Reich's concept of sexual liberation as demanding a perfect orgasm, which could be achieved only through genital heterosexual coupling by individuals within the same generation. It is from Reich's views that Norman Mailer has derived his cult of the orgasm, and hence his suspicion of homosexuality and of contraception which are seen as preventing full sexual "freedom." The importance of Marcuse and Brown is that they have stressed the third of the major forms of repression, and have reminded us—correctly, I believe—that any real theory of sexual liberation must take into account the essentially polymorphous and bisexual needs of the human being.

There exist a number of explanations of how sexual repression of the sort I have discussed came into being. The simplest review will help clarify the issues involved. The simplest explanation is a theory that attributes sexual repression to a need, developed early in the history of humankind, to beget large numbers of children for both economic and defense purposes. This would explain why homosexuality and non-genital sexuality came to be subordinated to heterosexual coupling organized in the patriarchal family. Women for biological reasons were seen primarily as bearers of children, and by extension as their rearers as well. In this view both repression of our polymorphous instincts and the creation of the patriarchal family can be linked to the importance attributed to procreation.

Freud himself advanced a partly anthropological argument, in which repression stems from the assertion of domination of one individual over others, that individual being the father. Through such domination, the patriarchal form of society is established, based both on the inferiority of women and on the strong repression of sexuality channeled into socially approved forms. Freud argued that even when the sons banded together to overthrow the father, thus ushering in a new period in which women played an increasingly important role, they were unable to escape fully from the domination of the father, and patriarchal authority came to reassert itself. Marcuse quotes Otto Rank's version of this argument: "The development of the paternal domination into an increasingly powerful state system administered by man is thus a continuance of the primal repression, which has its purpose the ever wider exclusion of woman."

Freud linked his theory of patriarchal authority with the rise of religion, and in particular the triumph in the Western World of monotheism. Support for this connection is found in Rattray Taylor's argument that "a remarkable psychological change" emerged in the classical world after 500 B.C. This change, he claims, led to an increasing repression of sexuality and the development of a sense of guilt, both of which factors facilitated the triumph of the more repressive Jewish view of sex over that of the early Greek view.

A related explanation of sexual repression sees its cause in just this fact, the dominance of the Western Judaeo-Christian tradition. Unlike Freud's view, this explanation stresses the particular as against the universal forms of sexual repression, seeing religion as not merely a rationalization and legitimization of sexual repression but as a major cause. Certainly there is considerable evidence that the Western religious tradition has placed great stress on sexual repression. At times indeed, especially during the Middle Ages, to repress sexual desire totally was considered a mark of virtue, and the resulting hysteria, masochism and persecution set the tone of much of the underside of life in Medieval Europe. Continence for all was hardly a practical policy for an entire society, leading as it does to its own self-annihilation, but the next best thing was the development of the view that sex exists merely as a means of procreation—hence continuing Catholic opposition to birth-control and masturbation, and the institution of clerical celibacy. To the best of my knowledge the church has advanced beyond its teachings that made sex illegal three days each week and eleven weeks each year; yet the rhythm method, when followed conscientiously, has a similar effect.

Religion may well have been a particularly important influence on the repression of bisexuality, for as the Jewish view of sex came to supplant the Greek in the Western World, homosexuality was more and more frowned upon, and Biblical evidence was produced to show its inherent sinfulness. Thus the story of Sodom and Gomorrah has long been used (probably inaccurately) as proof of the homosexual's sin; in Leviticus 20 we read that: "If a man also lie with mankind as he lieth with a woman, both of them have committed an abomination; they shall surely be put to death; their blood shall be upon them." To which Paul, never one to encourage sexuality, added his condemnation in the Epistle to the Romans.

To the Jewish heritage, so much bound up with the whole history of the patriarchal family, was added the Christian theology of "natural law," whence a long line of Popes (denied, one assumes, any first-hand experience) have derived the Catholic views on sex. The linkage of sexuality exclusively with procreation made homosexuality (plus a considerable number of heterosexual acts) unnatural and hence sinful. The concept of "natural" sex has affected even those who are not practicing Christians, and indeed provides the argument most often advanced against homosexuality. But there is no necessity to link sex exclusively with procreation, and few societies have applied this ideology as rigidly as the Western Judaeo-Christian. Even the most repressed admit the dual function of the (male) sex organ: sex and bodily evacuation. It is, theoretically, no more difficult to admit that the sexual act itself has more than one function, and that sensual gratification is as much its purpose as is procreation.

There has also been an attempt to link Marx to Freud and relate sexual repression to a theory of economic development. In this view Freud's theory of the origin of patriarchal authority is taken as having symbolic rather than anthropological reality, and is related to the organization of society around certain forms of productive relationships. Something of this approach is expressed—faultily, in my opinion—in an article by Roxanne Dunbar in a collection of women's liberation articles, *Notes from the Second Year*: "The patriarchal family is economically and historically tied to private property, and under Western capitalism with the development of the national state. The masculine ideology most strongly asserts home and country as primary values, with wealth and power an individual's greatest goal. The same upper class of men who created private property and founded nation-states also created the family." Yet the patriarchal family long preceded Western concepts of property and nation-states, and is indeed very much in evidence in societies that are in no real sense capitalist. Furthermore, most civilizations of which we have any knowledge have defined "male" and "female" as sharply differentiated categories, and one might in fact argue that the subordination of women under Western capitalism, while certainly real, has been less than in, say, pre-capitalist Chinese or Arab society. The eagerness to wed Marx to Freud has too often ignored the realities of both history and anthropology.

Nonetheless it is undoubtedly true that sexual repression was highly functional for the rise of capitalism and later industrialization which, at least in the early stages, demanded considerable repression in the interests of economic development. One can make connections between, for example, the rapid industrial growth of nineteenth-century England and the ideology of the Victorian era toward sex. Similarly, it is hardly surprising that countries seeking rapid industrialization, from Russia under Stalin to much of the Third World today, adopt rigid puritanical codes similar to those now being rejected in the West.

Marcuse has argued that the sexual repression that is brought about under the primal dictatorship is linked to economic subordination—through this dictatorship the sons come to channel their energies into unpleasant but necessary activity. However, as Paul Robinson has pointed out in his book *The Freudian Left*, Marcuse neither makes clear whether sexual repression causes economic subordination or vice versa, nor, most important for our purposes, does he connect his use of Freud's notion of the primal crime with his own ideas about the repression of non-genital and homosexual drives. This last point is important because one of the primary differences between Freud and Marcuse is the latter's belief in the desirability of overcoming the repression of polymorphous perversity.

For Marcuse the homosexual occupies a particular role—Robinson interprets some of his writings as suggesting that "in a certain sense, then, the social function of the homosexual was analogous to that of the critical philosopher"—and it is perhaps surprising that Marcuse's works, and in particular *Eros and Civilization* to which Robinson is referring, are rarely if ever referred to in gay liberation literature. Marcuse seems to suggest that the homosexual represents a constant reminder of the repressed part of human sexuality, not only in his/her interest in the same sex, but also in the variety of non-conventional sexual behavior that homosexuality implies. Sodomy, of course, recalls repressed feeling of anal eroticism, as Ferenczi suggests—not that sodomy is restricted to homosexuals, as Rozjak in Mailer's *American Dream* should remind us. Even more do female homosexuals disturb the myth that sex need be phallus-centered, a belief that underlies what Mailer has called the "peculiar difficulty" of lesbianism. "Man we can do without it and keep it going longer too!" wrote Martha Shelley in the gay liberation newspaper *Come Out!*

Anatomy has forced the homosexual to explore the realities of polymorphous eroticism beyond the experiences of most heterosexuals, for we are denied the apparently "natural" navel-to-navel coupling of men/women. There is among most homosexuals, I suspect, an awareness of their body, a knowledge of human sensuality, that is one of their strengths, although this is easily distorted in the body-building cult among men or the disregard of physical appearance among women.

Because homosexuality cannot find its justification in procreation nor in religiously sanctioned marriage, it represents an assertion of sexuality as an expression of hedonism/love free of any utilitarian social ends, and it is this very fact that may help explain the horror with which homosexuality is regarded. Marcuse has observed in *Eros and*

Civilization that: "Against a society which employs sexuality as a means for a useful end, the perversions uphold sexuality as an end in itself; they thus place themselves outside the domination of the performance principle [Marcuse's term for the particular variety of repression necessary for the organization of capitalism] and challenge its very foundations." This is spelled out by Marcuse in detail in the case of Orpheus, traditionally associated with the introduction of homosexuality, who "like Narcissus . . . protests against the repressive order of procreative sexuality. The Orphic and Narcissistic Eros is to the end the negation of this order—the Great Refusal." In the context of a society based on rigorous repression of polymorphous and bisexual urges, the homosexual thus comes to represent a challenge to the conventional norms. This challenge makes him/her a revolutionary.

Still, even in the Marcusian variation of Freudian thought, exclusive homosexuality represents a repression that is as great as exclusive heterosexuality, despite the fact that, because of the legitimization of sex-as-procreation, it places the homosexual outside society in a way that is not true for the heterosexual. Homosexuals who like to point out that "everyone is queer"—"either latent or blatant" as one girl put it—rarely concede that "everyone" is equally "straight," and that to repress the one is as damaging as to repress the other. It may be the historic function of the homosexual to overcome this particular form of repression—to accept his/her heterosexuality as well—and bring to its logical conclusion the Freudian belief in our inherent bisexuality.

Sex Roles and Repression

The repression of polymorphous perversity in Western societies has two major components: the removal of the erotic from all areas of life other than the explicitly sexual, and the denial of our inherent bisexuality. The latter in particular is bound up with the development of very clear-cut concepts of "masculine" and "feminine" that dominate our consciousness—and help maintain male supremacy. It is awareness of the socially imposed masculine/feminine dichotomy that especially characterizes the analyses associated with women's liberation. The de-erotization of our lives is the primary concern of Norman O. Brown, who ascribes the grand neuroses that he associates with organized civilization to the subordination of the generally erotic to specifically genital urges. This view is argued too by Marcuse, though he is less willing to move to the ultimate conclusion extolled by Brown. Marcuse sees modern industrial society as being particularly repressive of our non-specific erotic instincts; thus in *One Dimensional Man*, his major critique of modern society, he writes of the "reduction of erotic to sexual experience and satisfaction."

> For example, compare love-making in a meadow and in an auto-mobile, on a lover's walk outside the town walls and on a Man-hattan street. In the former cases, the environment partakes of and invites libidinal cathexis and tends to be eroticized. Libido transcends beyond the immediate erotogenic zones—a process of nonrepressive sublimation. In contrast, a mechanized envi-ronment seems to block such self-transcendence of libido. Impelled in the struggle to extend the field of erotic gratifica-tion, libido becomes less 'polymorphous,' less capable of eroti-cism beyond localized sexuality, and the *latter* is intensified.

One might note that there is a strong romanticism to Marcuse's views, which is echoed in the moves to establish rural communes that have become so marked in the United States in recent years.

As the whole structure of socialization acts so as to channel our polymorphous perverse instincts into narrow but socially approved norms, there is not only a repression of general eroticism but also of bisexuality. There is a marked connection in our society between the repression of bisexuality and the development of clearly demarcated sex roles. Now this is not a necessary connection. There are few soci-eties which have not held up models of masculine and feminine into which recalcitrants were to be forced, but a sharp distinction between the two roles does not of itself produce repression of homosexual urges. The ancient Greeks extolled both bisexuality *and* the supremacy of men, and homoeroticism thrives, in fact, where men and women are kept apart and sharply differentiated (as for example in the Arab custom of addressing love songs to boys because women are regarded as too inferior to be objects of such praise). Unlike Greek society, how-ever, ours is one that defines masculinity and femininity very much in heterosexual terms, so that the social stereotype—and often indeed the

self-image—of the homosexual is someone who rejects his/her mas-
culinity/femininity. Thus, as already suggested, one finds the two
extremes of male homosexual role playing: the drag queen who tends
to accentuate the image of the homosexual as a man-who-would-be-a-
woman, and the "leather" type who seeks to overcome it. To a lesser
extent comparable stereotypes exist among lesbians.

It is in fact probably true that individuals are often forced into exclusive homosexuality because of both the way in which society brands
those who deny its roles and the penalties meted out to those who are
unwilling to accept them.

Whether it be the educational system—boys are naturally good at
math and science, girls at languages and arts—or the Tiffany's notice—
"We do not, nor will we in future, carry earrings for men"—sex roles are
a first, and central, distinction made by society. Being male and female
is, above all, defined in terms of the other: men learn that their masculinity depends on being able to make it with women, women that
fulfillment can only be obtained through being bound to a man. In a
society based on the assumption that heterosexuality represents all that
is sexually normal, children are taught to view as natural and inevitable
that they in turn will become "mummies" and "daddies," and are
encouraged to rehearse for these roles in their games. In an article on
the importance of feminism, Theodore Roszak observes: "The woman
most desperately in need of liberation is the 'woman' every man has
locked up in the dungeons of his own psyche. *That* is the basic act of
oppression that still waits to be undone, though the undoing might
well produce the most cataclysmic reinterpretation of the sexual roles
and of sexual 'normalcy' in all human history." And equally there is
need to unlock the "man" every woman has in the dungeons of *her*
psyche.

The way in which our concepts of sex roles are bound up with
making it with the opposite sex illustrates how far our definitions of
these roles are influenced by the fears of homosexuality that most
straights have repressed. Proving one's man/womanhood is in the popular imagination bound up with the rejection of any fag or dyke characteristics. If this seems more obvious in the case of men, it is because
women have traditionally been defined as inferior, and whereas there
is some grudging respect accorded women with masculine qualities,

none is given to "womanly" men. Even among children "tomboys" are more acceptable than "sissies."

That lesbianism is stigmatized less than male homosexuality in one of the clichés about homosexuality, and to the extent that it is true it reflects the inferior position of women in our society. (Reports of group sex activities—see for example an article in *Newsweek*, June 21, 1971— suggest that sex between women is far more easily accepted by "middle Americans" than that between men.) Nor, even apart from apocryphal stories about Queen Victoria's disbelief in lesbianism, thereby exempting lesbians from legal sanction, is this lesser condemnation of lesbians restricted to modern times. Derrick Bailey, in his book *Homosexuality and the Western Christian Tradition*, points out that this difference was equally true of early and medieval Christianity, and argues it is due to the inferior position of women, in particular to the fact that male homosexual acts, and particularly sodomy, "involves the degradation, not so much of human nature itself as of the male, since in it he stimulates or encourages or compels another to simulate the coital function of the female—a 'perversion' intolerable in its implications to any society organized in accordance with the theory that woman is essentially subordinate to man." Indeed, female homosexuality may well touch on that deep-hidden fear of men, the suspicion that women are in fact more capable of sexual enjoyment than they, an attitude that helps explain the male-created ideology that for a long time denied sexual feelings to women.

Gay women are, after all, doubly oppressed, and suffer particularly from the social norms that expect women to repress not only their homosexual but even, to a considerable extent, their heterosexual urges. In some ways the equivalent of the compulsively promiscuous male who never dares know his partners may well be the woman who cannot admit the sexual component of her love for other women; both are victims of the sexual expectations of a society that perceives masculinity as "making it," femininity as preserving one's virtue. It is often claimed, for example, that men react more to physical stimuli than women. Yet if the media bombarded us constantly with pictures of pretty boys and semi-clad men who knows whether (heterosexual) women might not in fact objectify beautiful men with all the single mindedness of the *Playboy* male. And, by extension, whether lesbians might not behave more like men, both straight and gay, than like straight women.

The major way in which children are socialized into particular forms of sexual repression and concepts of sex roles is through the family, and indeed achieving this development may be the only major socialization task that the family retains in modern society. (Which may explain the strength of opposition to providing sex education in schools, thus usurping even this role of the family.) The patriarchal family as we know it in our time is essentially a nuclear family; indeed the transformation from the extended (or stem) to the nuclear family has been one of the major effects of industrialization, irrespective of whether industrialization is achieved through capitalist or non-capitalist means. As this change has occurred, most of the functions performed by the extended family necessarily have dropped away. Yet the family still retains one of them, albeit in a modified form, that is teaching children to make clear-cut role distinctions between the sexes.

Equally, the institution of the family as we know it contributes very importantly to the development of the repression of homosexuality and the stigma attached to it. As all parents are either fully heterosexual in behavior—or, except in special cases, will appear so to their children—it follows that children are exposed to models of sexual role playing that are fully heterosexual, and denied virtually all contact with homosexuals, for even friends or relatives who are gay will by and large conceal this in front of children. A social system that provided instead an opportunity for children to grow up regarding *both* homo- and heterosexuality as part of the human condition, a system perhaps approximated—for men—in ancient Greece, would be a far better one for enabling children to come to terms with their own diverse sexual impulses. As long as homosexuals are denied any role in child-rearing—in which numbers, of course, participate through their careers, but concealing in almost all cases their homosexuality— it is unlikely that children can grow up with other than a distorted view of what is natural.

The Effects of Sexual Repression

It is basic to the whole psychoanalytic approach that repressed desires find other ways of expressing themselves, and it is from the concept of repression or sublimation of sexual urges that Freud derived his theory of civilization and Brown, and to a lesser extent Marcuse, derive their explanations of human aggression. Here I am particularly concerned with the effects of repressing our non-genital and bisexual desires. Given the subject of this book I want to consider in some detail the social consequences of the repression of homosexuality, both emotional and sexual. This is not to deny the significance of the repression of heterosexuality, which I have already suggested is of comparable importance *for the individual*. But for a society based on the ideology that heterosexuality is the only normal form of sexual behavior, repression of homosexuality has particular social consequences. Largely because of the different ways in which society regards hetero- and homosexuality, the repression of the latter is much more widespread and has, I believe, much more considerable social implications.

This is a problem that few social theorists have been prepared to take seriously. Despite the undercurrent of jokes and comments about repressed homosexuality—which is held to account for a large variety of social phenomena, from behavior in British public schools through Australian "mate-ship" to sexual attitudes among American cowboys—there has been little exploration of the consequences for society of the enormous amount of libidinal energy devoted to repressing our inherent bisexuality. Yet Protestant Anglo-Saxon cultures are remarkable for the extent to which they seek to deny all and any homosexual urges; thus the embarrassment of Protestant Anglo-Saxon males when faced with the Mediterranean custom of men embracing. (Our societies are also noted for the prevalence of overt and exclusive homosexuality, nor is this coincidence accidental.) Men are so concerned to deny any homosexual feelings that they tend to adopt extreme postures of aggression so as to reject feelings of tenderness or love as well as sexual desire for each other. Lionel Tiger has observed:

> There are important inhibitions in much of Euro-American culture—if not elsewhere too—against expressing affection between men, and one result of this inhibition of tenderness and warmth is an insistence on corporate hardness and forcefulness which has contributed to a variety of tough-minded military, economic, political and police enterprises and engagements.

629

• • •

Ultimately what we conceive of as "human nature" is in large part the product of the nature and extent of sexual repression, and if one accepts the analyses of radical Freudians like Marcuse and Brown, one can also accept the thesis, implicit in much of the writings of gay and women's liberation, that human nature is mutable. Now this is ultimately a belief for which we do not yet have empirical evidence; just as we do not know how far there are inherent differences between men and women beyond the purely anatomical, so also we do not know how far repression of our sexual instincts is responsible for aggression and competitiveness. The theory of sexual liberation that I am moving toward in this argument rests on a belief that it is possible through the removal of at least some of the restraints on human eroticism to develop a greater sense of warmth, affection and community between people.

Toward Liberation

Any discussion of sexual liberation involves some concept of over-coming sexual repression, although there is considerable debate as to how far we can in fact dispense with any form of repression at all. Freud distinguished between repression and sublimation, and argued not only that the latter was a healthy variant of the former but that it was in fact essential for the maintenance of civilization. Norman O. Brown on the other hand appears to be arguing for a total end to repression and a return to the infantile state of "polymorphous perversity," a position that is more Utopian than programmatic. If one accepts the centrality of the sexual urge, it is difficult to argue for a total relaxation of repression without answering the claim that this would mean an end to all forms of socially necessary activity. Marcuse seeks to overcome this objection with his concept of "surplus repression," that part of sexual repression which acts so as to maintain the domination of the ruling class but which is not necessary for the maintenance of a genuinely co-operative human community. He also suggests the possibility of the eroticization of everyday life, including work. I would further argue that there are other basic human needs and urges apart from the erotic, and that because of these some forms of sexual repression would be freely accepted even by an individual totally untouched by social conditioning. At the very least I suspect one needs to accept the need for some form of postponed gratification.

Kate Millett in *Sexual Politics* defined a "sexual revolution" as follows:

> [It] would require, perhaps first of all, an end of traditional sexual inhibitions and taboos, particularly those that most threaten patriarchal monogamous marriage: homosexuality, "illegitimacy," adolescent, pre- and extramarital sexuality. The negative aura with which sexual activity has generally been surrounded would necessarily be eliminated, together with the double standard and prostitution. The goal of revolution would be a permissive single standard of sexual freedom, and one uncorrupted by the crass and exploitative economic bases of traditional sexual alliances.
>
> Primarily, however, a sexual revolution would bring the institution of patriarchy to an end, abolishing both the ideology of male supremacy and the traditional socialization by which it is upheld in matters of status, role and temperament. This would produce an integration of the separate sexual subcultures, an assimilation by both sides of previously segregated human experience . . .

Millet, like most women's liberationists, is primarily concerned here with sex roles, which she sees as underlying the nuclear family structure (which in turn, as Reich saw, "forms the mass psychological basis for a *certain* culture, namely the *patriarchal authoritarian one* in all of its forms"). I would not dispute Millett's aims. Yet it seems to me that liberation requires, as well, a general erotization of human life—by which I mean an acceptance of the sensuality that we all possess, and a willingness to let it imbue all personal contacts—and a move toward polymorphous perversity that includes more than reassessment of sex roles.

Let me make clear at once a point to which I shall have reason to return: liberation as a concept embraces far more than sexual liberation. Moreover, the concepts of liberation with which we shall be concerned relate almost entirely to affluent Western societies; as Susan Sontag and others have pointed out, to change consciousness in an underdeveloped and once neo-colonial state like Cuba must in some ways reverse the changes applicable to North America/Western

Europe/Australasia. (Though I am less willing than she, writing in *Ramparts* in 1969, to excuse Cuban treatment of homosexuals.) Were I concerned with broader conceptions of liberation I should, of course, need to concern myself as much with the nature of Western capitalism/imperialism/consumerism, etc., as with sexual repression and freedom.

How far sexual freedom can be conceived without coming to grips with the basic features of our society is a key ideological concern of both the women's and the gay movements. Yet there is a sense in which we should be suspicious of attempts to deny the centrality of sexuality in any discussion of liberation. "I do not believe in a nonerotic philosophy. I do not trust any desexualized idea," wrote the Pole Witold Gombrowicz in his diary. It is the desexualization of the concept of liberation that accounts for much of the abstruse intellectualism of sections of the left—and the common tendency of revolutionaries to become vicious and puritanical on winning power. As the song goes in *Marat/Sade*:

> What's the point of a revolution
> Without general copulation?

The more difficult question with which we have to come to grips is what's the *possibility* of a revolution without . . .

Liberation, then, in the restricted context with which we are primarily concerned implies freedom from the surplus repression that prevents us recognizing our essential androgynous and erotic natures. "Originally," wrote Marcuse in *Eros and Civilization*, "the sex instinct had no extraneous temporal and spatial limitations on its subject and object; sexuality is by nature 'polymorphous perverse.' " And as examples of "surplus repression" Marcuse notes not only our total concentration on genital coupling but phenomena such as the repression of smell/taste in sexual life. For both him and Brown liberation implies a return to original sexuality.

Yet this definition is perhaps too narrow. Liberation entails not just freedom from sexual restraint, but also freedom for the fulfillment of human potential, a large part of which has been unnecessarily restricted by tradition, prejudice and the requirements of social organization. If it is true that social needs still demand a certain degree of repression of sexuality, it is also true that affluent, post-industrial societies, such as those of the developed Western World, offer an unparalleled opportunity for freedom. Technology, which too often becomes restrictive, in fact allows the individual far greater liberty from toil and opens up the possibility that work might truly become play, not just for a small minority as at present but instead for the vast majority. Which in turn opens up the possibility for breaking down the rigid lines our society draws between art and life, or in other words the possibility of the eroticization of everyday living. Underdeveloped countries are not in this position, which is why they must define liberation differently; on the other hand, the degree of affluence in America, if properly distributed, is far greater than would be needed for an immediate and considerable decrease in personal restrictions. Liberation demands a renunciation of the traditional puritan ethic, so successfully imitated by Communist states, that sees hard work and expanding production as goods in themselves. Instead it requires a new examination of the basic erotic instincts that we have repressed in the name of morality and production:

> As human beings we are unique among animals in having a largely unspecified potential. Besides the basic biological needs for food, water and rest, we have needs which are specifically human and subject to conscious development: the need for relationship, the need to create and build. We are all erotic beings. We experience our lives as a striving for realization and satisfaction. We experience our lives sexually, as enlivened by beauty and feeling. At base we have a need for active envolvement [sic] and creation, the need to give form and meaning to our environment and ourselves. [From *Gay Liberation*, a pamphlet of the Red Butterfly movement, a group of revolutionary Socialists within gay liberation.]

One of the problems involved in discussing liberation is that we live in a time in which traditional sexual restraints are apparently collapsing, and the individual's freedom for sexual expression appears greater than ever before. As Abbie Hoffman put it, society is "simultaneously more repressive and more tolerant," a truth Marcuse attempts to explain through the concept of "repressive tolerance."

The present experience of the homosexual, in particular the liberal tolerance of which I have already written, seems to bear out all Marcuse's fears of "repressive desublimation," that is, greater apparent freedom but a freedom manipulated into acceptable channels. Thus most of the Western World has abolished legal restrictions against homosexuality while maintaining social prejudices. But to realize the falsity of the idea that existing bourgeois society has in fact permitted full personal liberation, it is instructive to examine the position of the homosexual in the Netherlands, a society often held up as a model of enlightenment.

In an article with the typical snideness of most that deal with homosexuality, *Newsweek* described Amsterdam in 1968 as the "mecca of homosexuals." What this means in practice however is that homosexuals are not bothered by the police and that they are allowed to meet freely in their own clubs and organizations. Men may dance with men and women with women—but only in certain specified places, and attempts to break this down have led to scuffles, for example at a dance in the Hague in May 1970. Some extremely progressive social measures, for example in regard to housing, have been achieved. Yet the entire bias of the media and of education remains heterosexual— Dutch schools, for example, do not teach the equal validity of homosexual and heterosexual love—and the prevailing social climate is one of tolerance rather than acceptance. Opinion polls have shown that dislike of homosexuality remains strong, and it is thus not surprising that other studies have revealed that Dutch homosexuals, particularly teenagers, are oppressed by the same feelings of guilt and social outcasteness as are American.

"Repressive tolerance" underlies contemporary permissiveness. Sex in our time has become increasingly used as a commodity, and the first principle of advertising appears to be to imply that your product enhances sex-appeal. It takes little imagination to see how this helps maintain the capitalist need for continuing production. "If you work hard and earn lots of money then you too can have a beautiful man/woman" is the barely concealed message. Indeed we are so programmed into accepting fashionable standards of beauty that the more "permissive" the society becomes—meaning the more that pleasant but standardized bodies are displayed—the more discontented we become with the inevitable flaws of our own, and our lovers', bodies, and the more unable to perceive the beauty that lies in those unlike the current stereotype.

But the gap between sexual freedom and repressed eroticism goes deeper. "In America," Kate Millett has said, "you can either fuck or shake hands," and this sums up the situation. The ability to feel, to hold, to embrace, to take comfort from the warmth of other human beings is sadly lacking; we look for it in the artificial situations of encounter groups rather than accepting it in our total lives. From the rock-musical *Salvation:*

> If you let me make love to you
> Then why can't I touch you . . .

Perhaps there lies the difference between sex and eroticism.

The cartoonist Jules Feiffer is reported to have said that "the love ethic went to Chicago, was polarized and came out as the fuck ethic," and it is certainly true that the permissive society with its high component of voyeurism, sexual objectification and "dildo journalism" is hardly a liberated one. Nonetheless I am less sure than Marcuse that growing sexual freedom is all illusionary. Without it movements like women's and gay liberation could hardly have come into being. But it is necessary now to transform sexuality into eroticism. As Marcuse writes in *Eros and Civilization,* there must be "not simply a release but a *transformation* of the libido: from sexuality constrained under genital supremacy to erotization of the entire personality. It is a spread rather than an explosion of libido—a spread over private and societal relations which bridges the gap maintained between them by a repressive reality principle."

Liberation would involve a resurrection of our original impulse to take enjoyment from the total body, and indeed to accept the seeking of sensual enjoyment as an end in itself, free from procreation or status-enhancement. To quote Marcuse again: "The full force of civilized morality was mobilized against the use of the body as mere object, means, instrument of pleasure: such reification was tabooed and remained the ill-reputed privilege of whores, degenerates and perverts." Which is why "whores, degenerates and perverts" become the new anti-hero(in)es of books such as *Last Exit to Brooklyn.*

But there are, I think, some reservations to Marcuse's argument which he partly avoids by the sheer abstractness of his writing. For one, if there were in fact an erotization of the entire personality, this would act *against* the use of the body "as mere object, means, instrument of pleasure." A concept of liberation that involves a transformation of the libido would not include, I would argue, sex based solely on the objectification of the body (the clearest example of which is necrophilia—though such objectification is evident in much of the depersonalized sex of the permissive society), for sex would be seen as a means of expanding contact and creating community with other persons, and would demand some reciprocity other than the purely physical. Sex as much as everyday life would be eroticized and would become a means of human communication rather than purely physical gratification or consumation of a sacred union. One of the implications of this, of course, is that sexual activity among children would be encouraged rather than, as is now the case, hindered.

Affirmation of the total body involves, as Brown puts it in *Life Against Death*, "a union with others and with the world around us based not on anxiety and aggression but on narcissism and erotic exuberance." It involves, too, an acceptance of the funkiness of the body, a rejection of the plastic, odorless, hairless and blemishless creations of *Playboy* and its homosexual equivalents, and a new sense of play and spontaneity, a move towards what Brown, perhaps unfortunately, called "a science of enjoyment rather than a science of accumulation." "The Underground," claims Richard Neville in *Playpower*, "is turning sex back into play."

Paul Goodman has suggested that the homosexual has, in fact, already partly achieved this:

A happy property of sexual acts, and perhaps especially of homosexual acts, is that they are dirty, like life: as Augustine said, "Inter urinas et feces nascitur." In a society as middle-class, orderly and technological as ours, it is essential to break down squeamishness, which is an important factor in what is called racism, as well as in cruelty to children and the sterile putting away of the sick and aged. Also, the illegal and catch-as-catch-can nature of many homosexual acts at present breaks down other conventional attitudes. Although I wish I could have had many a party with less apprehension and more unhurriedly— we would have enjoyed them more—yet it has been an advantage to learn that the ends of docks, the backs of trucks, back alleys, behind the stairs, abandoned bunkers on the beach and the washrooms of trains are all adequate samples of all the space there is. For both good and bad, homosexual behavior retains some of the alarm and excitement of childish sexuality. [From "Memoirs of an Ancient Activist."]

With Goodman's formulation I would agree and disagree. Undoubtedly there is a positive side to the sordidness of traditional gay life, in that it represents an acceptance of sexuality in a way that perhaps fewer heterosexuals have experienced. *Some* one-night stands can be rewarding, just as *some* lasting relations can be disastrous. In arguing for the erotization of everyday life, I am certainly not extolling some new form of puritanism that would deny the possibility of transitory sexual encounters nor would I want to uphold monogamy as either necessary or, indeed, desirable. Casual sex can be a good way of getting to know people.

But it is hardly sufficient. Goodman was attacked in *Come Out!* by the poet Milani for advocating "lust without the rhythms of Eros," and the accusation, though I think overdone, has its point. Promiscuity, even selective, hardly equals liberation, nor is the ability to appreciate the varieties of human eroticism—unlike Reich, I am a firm believer in non-orgasmic sex in certain situations, and the extension of sexual play to large areas of life appears to me a necessary part of liberation—a substitute for the creation of real relationships.

Nonetheless we need to move towards a full acceptance of the erotic qualities of humankind and of the many different kinds and levels of sexual encounters that are possible. As part of this there is required an acceptance of our basic androgyny. To turn again to Brown: "The 'magical' body which the poet seeks is the 'subtle' or 'spiritual' or 'translucent' body of occidental mysticism, and the 'diamond' body of oriental mysticism, and in psychoanalysis the polymorphous perverse body of childhood. Thus, for example, psychoanalysis declares the fundamentally bisexual nature of human nature; Boehme insists on the androgynous character of human perfection; Taoist mysticism invokes feminine passivity to counteract masculine aggressivity; and Rilke's poetic quest is a quest for a hermaphroditic body." There is a danger in Brown of the realities of the body dissolving into metaphysical flights, so that his concept of polymorphous perversity becomes ultimately an asexual one and he seems to envision not a move to expand sexuality from its obsessive genitality but rather the total supplanting of that genitality. It is often, indeed, difficult to relate Brown's writings to the real world of sexuality in which bodies tend to impose on us in more than "spiritual" or "translucent" ways. Nor am I as concerned as he to break down all differences between the sexes, beyond of course ending the false dichotomies imposed by social roles.

With liberation, homosexuality and heterosexuality would cease to be viewed as separate conditions, the former being a perversion of the latter, but would be seen rather as components of us all. Liberation would also, as women's liberation theorists have pointed out, mean an end to the nuclear family as the central organizing principle of our society. It would not, emphatically, mean an end to the importance of human relationships, although it would suggest an end to legalizing them, to compulsory monogamy and possessiveness, to the assumption, often echoed by homosexuals, that it is "natural" to divide up into couples who live isolated by and large from other couples. Perhaps it is our cult of acquisitiveness that makes us feel that love need be rationed. I suspect, in contrast to such a view, that the more one gives the more one is replenished, and that humans are capable of many more love-relationships, both sexual and non-sexual, than social norms prescribe. (It is this realization among young people that underlies the considerable experimentation with communal living that is already occurring.)

In a situation of liberation there would develop radical changes in the attitude towards bearing and rearing children, changes related— but only in part—to the fact that for the first time in human history it is technologically possible to control the rate of childbirth.

Brown, relying largely on Nietzsche, argues that the desire for children is often a product of suffering, of a need to reject oneself. "Joy," he quotes Nietzsche assaying, "does not want heirs or children—joy wants itself, wants eternity, wants recurrence, wants everything eternally the same." Free from a sense of guilt and of the social pressures towards pro-creation, with a decline too in the institution of the patriarchal and monogamous family structure, one might expect both a substantial number of women to consciously decide against having children and, conversely, an increase in communal child-rearing which would involve non-parent adults, including homosexuals. Both for society—which faces the specter of overpopulation—and for individual children who hardly benefit from the smothering effect of the present family—"being sole focus of attention for an adult who has little to worry about but your psyche is too much burden for an adult, let alone a small child" Marge Piercy argued in the first issue of the radical quarterly *Defiance*—the changes would be an improvement. There are great advantages for children in communal living, representing as it does a compromise between the tyranny of overpossessive parents and the repression of the typical educational system. It is also probably the only really effective way to break down the sex-role stereotypes into which the family structure tends to force us. The idea that a child "belongs" to his parents is a logical extension of the cult of property, only exceeded in horror by the concept that the child "belongs" to the state.

Ultimately, as Marcuse insists, liberation implies a new biological person, one "no longer capable of tolerating the aggressiveness, bru-tality and ugliness of the established way of life." Speaking to the 1967 Congress of the Dialectics of Liberation, Marcuse argued that this new person would be "a man [one assumes also a woman] who rejects the performance principles governing the established societies; a type of man who has rid himself of the aggressiveness and brutality that are inherent in the organization of established society, and in their hypo-critical, puritan morality; a type of man who is biologically incapable of fighting wars and creating suffering; a type of man who has a good conscience of joy and pleasure, and who works collectively and indi-vidually for a social and natural environment in which such an exis-tence becomes possible." And elaborating on this in *An Essay on Liberation* he argues that as such new men (women) appear, they will redefine the objectives and the strategy of the political structure.

Those who seek to relate sexual to total liberation tend often to argue that the two are interdependent in some chicken-and-egg manner. This has been put strongly by the gay revolutionary Socialist

639

group, the Red Butterfly, who claim: "To break our chains and become free we are going to have to work for fundamental changes in the institutions which oppress us, such as the existing family system with its web of supports: male chauvinism, sex typing of personality traits and arbitrary labels such as 'gay' and 'straight.' But to change any one basic institution will require changes in related ones. Change in family patterns would mean changes in education, in the economy, in laws, etc. This will mean coming up against vested interests, those who gain at the expense of our oppression. It will mean a struggle to free ourselves." From the Red Butterfly perspective, the upshot would be some genuine form of socialism.

It seems to me that the connection between sexual liberation and total liberation should be made somewhat differently. Liberation is a process that individuals strive toward, and part of this striving involves a recognition of the way in which oppression is implanted in the very structures of our society. To overcome the stigma society places on homosexuality, for example, does mean radical alterations in the way in which we order the socialization process. More than this, as individuals come to a greater acceptance of their erotic/sexual being they tend spontaneously to reject the "performance principle" that underlies the dominant ethos of property, competition and aggression. Thus, between individual and social liberation there is a dialectic relationship, and as Marcuse puts it in his *Essay on Liberation*, "radical change in consciousness is the beginning, the first step in changing social existence: emergence of the new Subject." (Brown's views on the other hand seem to me less acceptable, for he seems to posit a personal liberation within a social vacuum.) Only a socialism highly flavored by anarchism would seem to me consistent with sexual liberation, for conventional notions of socialism do not contain sufficient protection for the individual vis-à-vis the collective. One might note, however, that individual rights are not the same as property rights, and that those who most ardently extoll the latter are often those most willing to impinge on the former.

One of the most important statements of the gay movement is Carl Wittman's "The Gay Manifesto," where he argues—a position with which I would basically agree—that a change in individual consciousness is a basic requirement for any qualitative social change. Until we have come to grips with the meaning of liberation for ourselves, to talk of liberation for others (that is, society) is meaningless. In terms of social actuality I find most persuasive the argument of the American anti-psychiatrist Jo Berke in *Counter-culture* that: "As more and more groups associate with each other we shall see the large-scale creation of 'liberated zones' within bourgeois society, who will have the same relationship to themselves and established institutions as 'liberated areas' of Mozambique and Vietnam have to each other and to the Portuguese or Americans." Such "liberated zones" will be defined, however, more by a shared consciousness than a geographic base, although the commune movement attempts to combine the two.

I argued at the beginning of this chapter that gay liberation as a concept makes sense only within a broader context. Yet my concern is basically with the homosexual, and the move from tolerance to acceptance. While one would expect a liberated society to regard bisexuality as the norm, this view would not mean that all persons would behave bisexually—or at least not in the symmetrical way suggested by Gore Vidal when he wrote "that it is possible to have a mature sexual relationship with a woman on Monday, and a mature sexual relationship with a man on Tuesday, and perhaps on Wednesday have both together. . . ." The non-repressed person recognizes his bisexual potential; he is not some ideal person midway along the Kinsey behavioral scale. People would still fall in love and form relationships, and those relationships would be homosexual as well as heterosexual. What would be different is that the social difference between the two would vanish, and once this happened, we would lose the feeling of being limited, of having to choose between an exclusively straight or exclusively gay world. The lack of any available sense of identity for the bisexual in present society, and the pressures on him/her from both sides—for bisexuality threatens the exclusive homo- as much as heterosexual—probably explain why it is relatively uncommon. Given a change in social repression we would all be less uptight about the whole thing—and probably accept some experimentation with each sex as natural.

Liberation would mean the end of the gayworld as we now know it, with its high premium on momentary and furtive contacts. It would involve a breakdown of the barriers between male and female homosexuals, and between gays and straights. Masculinity and femininity would cease to be sharply differentiated categories, and one would expect an end to the homosexual parodies of role playing in the cult of leather and of drag. The nuclear family would come to be seen as only one form of possible social organization, not as the norm from which everything seems a deviation. This would mean an end not only to the oppression of gays, but major changes in general consciousness. Sexuality, once it became fully accepted, would be joyful, spontaneous and erotic, and with that one could hope for a withering away of both *Playboy* and the League of Decency. Above all, liberation implies a new diversity, an acceptance of the vast possibilities of human experience and an end to the attempt to channel these possibilities into ends sanctioned by religious and economic guidelines.

If the homosexual cannot achieve full sexual liberation within society as it exists—for this can only be achieved through a revolutionary change in both social attitudes and structures—he/she can however achieve liberation from at least much of the internal oppression imposed by social stereotypes and roles. To overcome this is not sufficient for liberation, but it is an essential step toward it for those who have been deeply stigmatized. And by overcoming this part of her/his stigma, the homosexual is also able to move toward liberation from the restraints of sex roles and the repression of eroticism.

One cannot prescribe liberation, for it arises out of the individual consciousness and demands a greater sense both of autonomy and of community than at present exists. Above all, there is need for a new sense of sister/brother-hood, a willingness to fully accept one's own erotic and sexual being, and a search to construct new sorts of human relationships. It may indeed be profitable to regard liberation as a process rather than an attainable goal, to regard the writings of men like Marcuse and Brown as providing us with aims for which we strive. Liberation does not mean an end to struggle, but it does alter the ends for and the means by which we struggle.

The Social Origins of Sexual Development

John H. Gagnon and William Simon

From *Sexual Conduct: The Social Sources of Human Sexuality*, 1972

Sociologists John Gagnon and William Simon were both on the staff of the Kinsey Institute for Sex Research in the late sixties when they began to develop the social constructionist theory of sexuality. Ironically, it was an approach not at all compatible with Kinsey's empirical naturalism. Their approach was built around a theory of sex as a scripted activity. **Sexual Conduct** *was the first comprehensive formulation of sexual activity as a form of social behavior*

Introduction

Underlying all human activity, regardless of the field or its stage of development, there exist metaphors or informing imageries—commonly unnamed until they lose their potency—that shape thought, experiment, and the directions of research. In the earliest days of the development of what is now modern physics, the metaphorical content of Newtonian mechanics could be found not only in the sciences, but in religion, philosophy and the widest range of activities of educated men.[1] The Newtonian (or Descartian) metaphor of the universe as a large clock running its immutable course after having been designed and wound up by the creator was widely and easily accepted far beyond the narrow domain of physics. The content of the mental life of educated men, whether in the sciences or not, for that brief moment overlapped and the metaphors of the larger society and the paradigms of the sciences interpenetrated.

1. Murray Turbayne, *The Myth of Metaphor* (New Haven: Yale University Press, 1962).

Once that central and organizing paradigm had been selected, as Kuhn points out, there began the separation of physics and then the other natural sciences from an immediate accessibility to even educated men.[2] The content of the sciences has become increasingly limited to scientists and the generation of useful metaphors from scientific formulations has declined as the sciences separate from the society at large. Most recently it is argued that with the increased difficulty of translating the mathematical formulations of modern physics into usable social coinage, the field of physics has ceased to have any serious effect on the way most men think about the world.[3]

Such unrecognized conceptions and metaphors are still characteristic of modern studies of man, however, and these continue to draw upon conventional historical thought and upon folk wisdom to develop their modes of thought. In this important sense the study of man and society is close to pre-paradigmatic; that is, there is no organizing scheme which directs our activities. Thus, central to the study of social life is a commonly unspoken belief in the existence of natural man, a man who has innate transhistorical and transcultural attributes and needs. A dependence on the constancy of the human seems to be a necessary element in our desire to understand the past and in our belief in our capacity to control the future. A commitment to a fixed psychological (in some cases, physiological) nature of man allows us to see all of the actors of history as operating with our motives, concerns, and goals, so that Moses and Luther, Michelangelo and Manet, Dante and Joyce, are equivalent figures removed from each other only by the exterior accidents of time and culture. At the higher cultural levels this tyranny of the present over the past is represented most vividly in Marxist and Freudian reinterpretations of history which involve profound assumptions not only about the past, but the present as well; in its more vulgar form it is in those cinematic personifications that allow Charlton Heston to be Moses, Michelangelo, and Ben Hur and serve as the crucial condensate of our cultural heritage. Taken together, the high and low cultural responses are variants of two historical fallacies pointed out by David Fischer, the idealist

2. Thomas Kuhn, *The Structure of Scientific Revolutions* (Chicago: University of Chicago Press, 1962).
3. Hannah Arendt, *The Human Condition* (Chicago: University of Chicago Press, 1958).

fallacy (resting upon a narrow and exclusive concept of homo sapiens), and the fallacy of universal man. As Fischer argues:

> People, in various places and times, have not merely thought different things. They have thought them differently. It is probable that their most fundamental cerebral processes have changed through time. Their deepest emotional drives and desires may themselves have been transformed. Significant elements of continuity cannot be understood without the discontinuities, too. . . . There is accumulating evidence of expressions of thought and feeling that make no sense unless we allow a wide latitude for change in the nature of cerebral activity through space and time. The range of this change is as obscure as its nature. But its existence is, in my opinion a historical fact which is established beyond a reasonable doubt.[4]

This rummaging through the past for useful arguments and ideologies to introduce cultural and social innovation in the present has been a characteristic of modern societies, and the impulse to connect ourselves no matter how tenuously with the past is in part an attempt to cast wider the net of a common humanity. However, it is in quest for (motivational) immortality that the modern impulse to use the past is converted into an attempt to psychologically colonize the future. High culture and low again combine in Committees on the Year 2000, Institutes for the Future, movies such as *2001 A .D.*, and television shows such as *Star Trek*.

At no point in human history has the historical-cultural specificity of the human personality and the concept of what is human been more evident, and at the same time there are extraordinary pressures against such a changed conception of the human. Committing the ethological fallacy, wherein we are warned that our hunting-gathering natures are the central themes around which modern man must organize his marriage and reproductive life or in which we are instructed to consider our common attributes with other primates, is an example of an unwillingness to live with the existential and changing nature of man at an individual and

4. David H. Fischer, *Historical Fallacies* (New York: Harper Torch Books, Harper & Row, 1970), pp. 203–24.

collective level. Continuity is sought with all living things until one has an urge to plead for the theory of special creation.[5]

At no point is the belief in the natural and universal human more entrenched than in the study of sexuality. The critical significance of reproduction in species survival is made central to a model of man and woman in which biological arrangements are translated into sociocultural imperatives. In consequence it is not surprising that it is in the study of the sexual that there exists a prepotent concern with the power of biology and nature as opposed to an understanding of the capacities of social life.

Naturalness and the Body

In an important sense our concern with the natural in sexual conduct is ambiguous. At one level our view of sex insists that it is a natural function, growing out of biological or evolutionary or species needs or imperatives. It is this view that supplies us a belief in cultural, historical, and transpecies comparisons. At another level, however, the natural also exists in opposition to the unnatural; of the wide variety of sexual expressions there are those that are natural (i.e., contribute to species survival, virtuous in the eyes of God, or mental-health enhancing) and those that are unnatural (i.e., reduce species survival, are sinful or vicious, or involve mental pathologies). There is a linkage between these two levels, but more often we move from one to the other confusing our ideological inheritances about the sexual (as well as our ideologies about evolution, species survival, virtue, and mental health) in order to conserve one or another of our cultural-historical values.

In large measure our distinctions between the *natural* and the *unnatural* in sex behavior is directly based on the physical activities in which people engage when they are doing what are conventionally described as sexual acts. For most persons (even the most liberated of the post-Freudians) most of the time, it is the assembly of bodies in time and space that is the primary defining characteristic of normalcy or perversion, health or sickness, virtue or vice, conformity or deviance. Our laws embody our felt margin between those acts that are natural and those that are crimes against nature, delineating a narrow domain of *de jure* legitimacy by constraining the age, gender, legal,

5. Lionel Tiger, *Men in Groups* (New York: Random House, 1969).

and kin relationships between sexual actors, as well as setting limits on the sites of behavior and the connections between organs. Even if one leaves aside the legal allowances for the married, a status which clearly normalizes many aspects of sexual activity, coitus in the "missionary position" (the male above prone, the female below supine) is the physical arrangement of bodies that calls forth our greatest sense of comfort in thinking about the physical aspects of sex. To move beyond this arrangement of bodies either in fantasy or fact is to move into a more shadowy realm where anxiety, guilt, and eroticism await. Indeed, to think about sex in terms of what bodies do is to begin to perform a sexual act—an act with its own norms and constraints, but at the same time an act that provokes the physiological beginnings of what Masters and Johnson have classified as sexual excitement.

It is perhaps startling to consider that when we think about the sexual, nearly our entire imagery is drawn from the physical activities of bodies. Our sense of normalcy derives from organs being placed in legitimate orifices. We have allowed the organs, the orifices, and the gender of the actors to personify or embody or exhaust nearly all of the meanings that exist in the sexual situation. Rarely do we turn from a consideration of the organs themselves to the sources of the meanings that are attached to them, the ways in which the physical activities of sex are learned, and the ways in which these activities are integrated into larger social scripts and social arrangements where meaning and sexual behavior come together to create sexual conduct.[6]

It is this assembly of the reality of the body and the social and cultural sources of attributed meaning that is missing in the two greatest modern students of sexuality in the West. In Freud we find a world dominated by the search for motivation, a world in which the body never seems to be very problematic since it is both the source of naturalness (anatomy becomes destiny) and the passive recipient of meanings attributed to it. At no point in psychoanalytic theory is there an extended consideration of the physical activities of sexual behavior and the ways in which these physical activities themselves require systematic linkage to social roles and social meanings. Sexual arousal lies in

6. Ernest W. Burgess, "The Sociologic Theory of Psychosexual Behavior," in *Psychosexual Development in Health and Disease*, eds. Paul H. Hoch and Joseph Zubin (New York: Grune and Stratton, 1949) pp. 227-43.

647

nature; the social world responds and shapes but does not initiate. In Freud sex itself seems disembodied and we are left with a world full of ideas and psychic structures only tangentially related to the bodies that are performing the acts.[7]

In the work of Kinsey we see the opposite thrust. Here we have sexual man in the decorticated state; the bodies arrange themselves, orgasm occurs, one counts it seeking a continuum of rates where normalcy is a function of location on a distribution scale. Once again in our search for the natural sources of behavior, the meanings that actors attribute to their own behavior and that the society collectively organizes are left out. In the Kinsey reports sexual activity among primates and primitive societies, in the historical past and the present, are functional equivalents because the arrangement of organs and orifices appear similar. Thus, each instance of the presence or absence of homosexuality in various cultures is counted as an identical manifestation of evolutionary principles rather than being examined within the complex of meanings that a physical sexual relationship between persons of the same gender may have in various circumstances, at various moments in history, and in various subgroupings in a society. The physical sexual activity of two males when one of them is defined as *berdache* among the Western Plains Indians is identical with the sexual activity of two men in ancient Greece or in a modern Western society; but the meanings attached to the behavior and its functions for the society are so disparate in these cases that seeing them as aspects of the same phenomena except in the most superficial way is to vitiate all we know about social analysis.

Of the two figures, Freud has surely been of greater influence in shaping theoretical models of development and in the penetration of his ideas into the cultural ambiance. It is in the work of Kinsey, however, that we find the largest body of empirical data about sexual behavior. Despite the predominance of these two men in the discussion of the sexual, there is, from the point of view of the history of science, a curiously nonconsequential quality about their work. While the status of their ideas as cultural events has been substantial, there has been a painful lack of scientific follow-up of either their concepts or

7. Sigmund Freud, "Three Essays on Sexuality," *Complete Psychological Works*, vol. 7 (London: Hogarth Press, 1953) pp. 135-245.

their data. This is not to say that there is not a substantial literature that has developed out of the psychoanalytic tradition, but in the largest part it has been narrowly concerned with the Talmudic imposition of Freud's original models on clinical case histories or the reading of collective and sociocultural events.[8]

Kinsey's scientific fate has perhaps been ruder than Freud's, since very little research of any sort has followed upon the publication of his two major works, perhaps no more than two to three papers of merit each year. His two large volumes continue to be for the most part undigested lumps in the craw of the research community. While Kinsey's work had serious consequences in changing and creating cultural attitude, in bringing the language of sex into general public discussion (as Freud had done among intellectuals a generation before), there has been only a minimal increase in activity at the level of science, most of that preoccupied with the burdens of social bookkeeping, at the most significant points providing a context of cultural journalism.[9]

To some degree this failure to develop a research concern for sexual matters in the conventional disciplines can be laid at the door of scientific and cultural prudery, but it is equally a function of two other forces: the historical (and perhaps reactive) self-insulation of "sexological" researches and researchers from the mainstream disciplines, and the continued commitment—shared by both Freud and Kinsey—to a belief in "biological knowingness" or to the wisdom of nature in the explanation of sexual behavior and development.

The very idea of "sexology" tends to insulate those interested in sexual behavior from theoretical and methodological developments that occur on a broad front within the human sciences. Because sex is culturally isolated in general, researchers often claim exemption from normal methodological strictures and become deeply and defensively invested in the substantive content of sexuality while remaining indifferent to the rest of social life. The very specialness of sex makes

8. While the deeply beleaguered condition of psychoanalysis as a movement accounts for at least some of the sectarian politics of its earlier days, the adherence to doctrinal purity on the part of younger analysts may be equally attributed to the ambiguous conditions under which therapy is practiced. See John H. Gagnon, "Beyond Freud," *Partisan Review* 34 (Summer 1967): 400–14.

9. The publication of the two volumes by Masters and Johnson appear at some level to be as noncumulative as Kinsey's and to be similar kinds of cultural rather than scientific events.

its students special, both to themselves and others, and their posses-sion of secret cultural knowledge is in itself sometimes intellectually disabling, since it often is used as a device to disarm criticism.

It is the most suspect of the expository literature about sex that attempts in a limited way to bring together feelings about sex with descriptions of sexual activity. Though most written pornography may appear to be (in the words of Steven Marcus) "organ grinding," it does indicate a crude psychology and set of motivations for those who are performing the sexual acts.[10] As we argue elsewhere, there is more social life in literary pornography than those who wish to contrast it to "lit-erature" are wont to notice. In order for the sexual activity described or observed to have erotic stimulus value for the reader, the actors involved must be playing out some sociosexual script that has signifi-cance for the reader. The capacity for arousal itself (including physical tumescense) depends on the presence of culturally appropriate elic-iting stimuli composed of persons, motives, and activities combined to produce significant sexual actors in sexual situations. For all practical purposes, until the 1960s it was only pornography that made available descriptions of some of the physical aspects of sexual behavior. While limited in complexity and with a limited sensibility, the characters in pornography actually felt skin, smelled each other's odors, tasted bodily fluids, and did sexual things.

Only recently in the scientific literature and only now in "higher" art is a significant component of physicality present in the descriptions of sexual activity. Because we possess theories of sexual behavior based on the immediate connection between explicit sexual descriptions and overt behavior, our analysis of the erotic does not come to terms with the fact that these descriptions are received into already existing com-plex cognitive and emotional structures. As a result of our commitment to nature and to the sexual organs as the primary sources of meaning, we fail to observe that the doing of sex (even when alone) requires elaborated and sequential learning that is largely taken from other domains of life and a resultant etiquette that allows for the coordina-tion of bodies and meanings in a wide variety of circumstances.

The complex outcome which is marital coitus, the most common form of sexual conduct in our society, involves a vast array of human

10. Steven Marcus, *The Other Victorians* (New York: Basic Books, 1966), pp. 292ff.

learning and the coordination of physiological, psychological, and social elements, practically none of which can be attributed to nature writ large as evolution or nature writ small as a morality play based on glandular secretions. Our concern here is to understand sexual activities of all kinds (however defined, good or evil, deviant or conforming, normal or pathological, criminal or noncriminal) as the outcome of a complex psychosocial process of development, and it is only because they are embedded in social scripts that the physical acts themselves become possible. This combination of various periods of development into the articulate behavioral sequence that leads to orgasm is not fated or ordained at any level; it is neither fixed by nature or by the organs themselves. The very experience of sexual excitement that seems to originate from hidden internal sources is in fact a learned process and it is only our insistence on the myth of naturalness that hides these social components from us.

The Sexual Tradition

The most important set of images for sex or eroticism in the modern West, either for scientists or in conventional educated speech, derives from the language of psychoanalysis. It would be difficult to overstate the coercive power of Freud's innovative verbal reformulations of a whole range of early conceptualizations about the role of sexuality in its biological, personal, and societal contexts. In an important sense Freud remains the superego of nearly all researchers into the sexual, since we must in some measure either conform to or rebel against his body of ideas. As with most great innovators, Freud began with the available set of contemporary ideas that were part of the heritage of the eighteenth and nineteenth centuries. It is difficult for those in the 1970s, for whom Freud is received wisdom and whose conservative postures are now most evident and emphasized, to recognize his role as a radical theorist of sexuality as well as representing a force for sociopolitical liberalism. The emphasis on the instinctual basis for the experience of the sexual and the universality of man's sexual experience, though possibly wrong in fact and theory, served to introduce a great change in sexual values at the turn of the century. Perhaps more important, by asserting the universality of the human experience, Freud significantly helped erode the dubious anthropology that imperial Europe used to describe its colonial subjects.

The Freudian codification provided for modern, educated, Western man a set of verbal categories through which he might describe his internal states, explain the origins of his sexual proclivities, describe his own and others' motives, and ultimately reanalyze literature, histories, and societies as well as individual lives. The cultural assimilation of much of psychoanalytic theory, especially on a popular level, resides in its essential continuity with popular wisdom about the instinctive nature of sexuality. This version of sexuality as an innate and dangerous instinct is shared not only by the man in the street, but also by psychological theorists deeply opposed to Freudian thought, as well as by sociologists whose rejection of analytic theory is nearly total. Hence the language of Kingsley Davis:

> The development and maintenance of a stable competitive order with respect to sex is extremely difficult because sexual desire itself is inherently unstable and anarchic. Erotic relations are subject to constant danger—a change of whim, a loss of interest, a third party, a misunderstanding. Competition for the same sexual object inflames passions, and stirs conflicts; failure injures ones self-esteem. The intertwining of sex and society is a fertile ground for paranoia, for homicide and suicide.[11]

The seventeenth-century political image of the individual against the state is translated by the Romantic tradition into a contest between the individual and his culture. The Hobbesian contest between natural instinct and imposed constraint was moved by Freud (as well as many other post-Romantic innovators) from the arena of the state, power conflicts, and the social contract to the arena of the mind, sexuality, and the parent-child contract. The sexual instinct presses against cultural controls, pleasure contests with reality, as the sociocultural forces in the form of parents (Leviathan writ small) block, shape, and organize the sexual drive and convert it from lust to love, from societal destruction to social service.

This tradition is surely present in Freud with his emphasis on a drive model of development, a libidinal thrust that sequentially organizes

11. Kingsley Davis, "Sexual Behavior," in *Contemporary Social Problems* eds. R. K. Merton and R. Nisbet (New York: Harcourt Brace Jovanovich, 1971), p. 317.

intra- and extra-psychic life as well as the very meaning of the parts of the body. This direct relation between the external signs of physiological events and necessary motivational and cognitive states is a given for nearly all students of sexual behavior, whose frequent error is to confuse the outcomes of sexual learning with their apparent origins.

The Freudian or Kinseyian traditions share the prevailing image of the sexual drive as a basic biological mandate that presses against and must be controlled by the cultural and social matrix. This drive reduction model of sexual behavior as mediated by cultural and social controls is preeminent in "sexological" literature. Explanations of sexual behavior that flow from this model are relatively simple. The sex drive is thought to exist at some constant level in any cohort of the population, with rising and falling levels in the individual's life cycle. It presses for expression, and in the absence of controls, which exist either in laws and mores or in appropriate internalized repressions learned in early socialization, there will be outbreaks of "abnormal sexual activity." In the more primitive versions of this drive theory, there is a remarkable congruence between the potentiating mechanisms for specifically sexual and generally sinful behavior. The organism is inherently sexual (sinful) and its behavior is controlled by the presence of inhibitory training and channeling, internalized injunctions, and the absence of temptation. If these mechanisms fail, there will certainly be sexual misconduct (sin). More sophisticated models can be found in functional theories in sociology or in revisionist psychoanalytic models, but fundamental to each is a drive reduction notion that sees sex as having necessary collective and individual consequences because of its biological origins.

What is truly innovative about Freud's thought, is not his utilization of prior constructs about sexuality and the nature of man, but his placement of these ideas about sexuality at the center of human concerns, beginning in infancy, an essential to normal human development. As Erik Erikson has observed, prior to Freud, "sexology" tended to see sexuality as suddenly appearing with the onset of adolescence.[12] From Erikson's point of view, Freud's discovery of infantile and childhood expressions of sexuality was a crucial part of his contribution. Libido—the generation of psychosexual energies—was viewed after

12. E. H. Erikson, *Childhood and Society*, 2nd ed. (New York: Norton, 1963).

Freud as a fundamental element of the human experience from its very inception, beginning at the latest with birth and possibly prior to birth. Libido was conceived as something essential to the organism, representing a kind of constitutional factor with which forms of social life at all levels of sociocultural organization and development, as well as personality structure at each point in the individual life cycle, had to cope.

In Freud's view the human infant and child behaved in ways that were intrinsically sexual and these early behaviors remained in effective and influential continuity with later forms of psychosexual development.[13] Implicit in this view was the assumption that the relations between available sexual energies and emergent motives and attachments would be complex but direct. In some aspects of psychoanalytic thinking, both adolescent and adult sexuality were viewed as being in some measure a reenactment of sexual commitments developed, learned, or acquired during infancy and childhood.[14]

From the vantage point of the late twentieth century, it is apparent that this point of view presents both an epistemological and a sociolinguistic problem. Freud's descriptive language for sexuality was the language of adults describing their current and childhood "sexual" experience (as transmuted through psychoanalytic interviews), which was then imposed upon the "apparent" behavior and "assumed" responses, feelings, and cognitions of infants and children. Acts and feelings are described as sexual, not because of the child's sense of the experience, but because of the meanings attached to those acts by adult observers or interpreters whose only available language is that of adult sexual experience.

It is important to note here the extraordinary difficulties of all developmental research in getting accurate data and also that research on infancy and childhood through adulthood faces a problem which most of the psychoanalytic literature obscures. Part of the problem is faulty recall, some of which is locatable in the problem of inaccurate

13. Sigmund Freud, "Three Essays on Sexuality," *Complete Psychological Works*, vol. 7 (London: Hogarth, 1953), pp. 135-245. Also, E. Jones, "Freud's Conception of Libido," in *Human Sexual Behavior: A Book of Readings*, ed. Bernhardt Lieberman (New York: John Wiley & Sons, Inc., 1971), pp. 42-60; P. Chodoff, "Critique of Freud's Theory of Infantile Sexuality," *American Journal of Psychiatry* 123 (1966): 507-18.
14. Sigmund Freud. *A General Introduction to Psychoanalysis* (New York: Liveright, 1935), pp. 283-84.

memories, but another source of error is located in the existentalist insight that instead of the past determining the character of the present, the present significantly reshapes the past as we reconstruct our biographies in an effort to bring them into greater congruence with our current identities, roles, situations, and available vocabularies. Indeed, the role of the analyst in providing an alternative self-conception for patients by creating a new vocabulary of motives is central to the therapeutic impulse and opposed to the gathering of accurate information about the past.

The other major problem of data quality control results from attempting to gather data either from children who are, because of their stage of development, ill-equipped to report on their internal states or from adults who were asked to report about periods in their life when complex vocabularies for internal states did not exist for them.[15] How can the researcher determine what is being felt or thought when the researcher is confronted with organisms whose restricted language skills may preclude certain feelings and thoughts? The child in this situation possesses internal states that in a verbal sense are meaningless and that will begin to be named and organized only during later development. The adult loses access to that inchoate period of his own experience by learning new ways of attributing meaning to experiences. The organism cannot hold onto both sets of experiences at once. Indeed, this may be the central meaning of development, that the acquisition of new categories for experience erase the past. Opie and Opie report that adolescents quickly forget childhood games. How much more quickly do we forget earlier and more diffuse experiences?[16]

The assumption of an identity between perception is based upon a adult terminology for the description of a child's behavior and the meaning of that behavior for the child must be treated with extreme caution. The dilemma is in distinguishing between the sources of

15. E. Schachtel, *Metamorphosis* (New York: Basic Books, 1959).
16. There is a body of evidence that among young children there is a large amount of game and folklore material that is rapidly forgotten after puberty. A certain amount of this material is sexual, but the folklorists who work with children usually fail to keep records of this, or if they do so, do not publish it. An interesting aspect of this material is its eternal character—that is, it is passed on from generation to generation. For example, children in England are currently singing a recognizable variant of a song about Bonaparte popular in the early nineteenth century. See Iona Opie and Peter Opie. *The Lore and Language of School Children* (London: Oxford Press, 1959). pp. 98-99.

specific actions, gestures, and bodily movements and the ways in which they are labeled as sexual at various stages of development. For the infant touching his penis, the activity cannot be sexual in the same sense as adult masturbation but is merely a diffusely pleasurable activity, like many other activities. Only through maturing and learning these adult labels for his experience and activity can the child come to masturbate in the adult sense of that word. The complexity of adult masturbation as an act is enormous, requiring the close coordination of physical, psychological, and social resources, all of which change dynamically after puberty. It is through the developmental process of converting external labels into internal capacities for naming that activities become more precisely defined and linked to a structure of sociocultural expectations and needs that define what is sexual. The naive external observer of this behavior often imputes to the child the complex set of motivational states that are generally associated (often wrongly) with physically homologous adult activities.

In the Freudian schema, this gap between observer and observed, between the language of adult experience and the lived experience of the child is bridged by locating an instinctual sexual energy source within the infant. The child is seen as possessed of certain emergent sexual characteristics that express themselves regardless of parental action systems. These actions of the child are viewed as being rooted in the constitutional nature of the organism. Consequent upon this primitive Freudian position is an over generalized presumption that all contacts with or stimulation of the end organs of the infant have a protosexual or completely sexual meaning.

To suggest that infant or childhood experience, even that which is identified as genital, is prototypical of or determines adult patterns is to credit the biological organism with more wisdom than we normally do in other areas where the biological and sociocultural intersect. Undeniably, what we conventionally describe as sexual behavior is rooted in biological capacities and processes, but no more than other forms of behavior. Admitting the existence of a biological substrate for sex in no way allows a greater degree of biological determinism than is true of other areas of corresponding intersection. Indeed, the reverse is more likely to be true: the sexual area may be precisely that realm wherein the superordinate position of the sociocultural over the biological level is most complete.[17]

The unproven assumption in psychoanalytic theory (and much conventional wisdom) of the "power" of the psychosexual drive as a fixed biological attribute may prove to be the major obstacle to the understanding of psychosexual development. In its more specific psychoanalytic formulation, we find little evidence to suggest that such a "drive" need find expression in specific sexual acts or categories of sexual acts.[18] Similarly, we must call into question the even more dubious assumption that there are innate sexual capacities or specific experiences that tend to translate immediately into a kind of universal wisdom, that sexuality possesses a magical ability allowing biological drives to seek direct expression in psychosocial and social ways that we do not expect in ether biologically rooted behaviors. This assumption can be seen in the psychoanalytic literature, for example, in which the child who views the "primal scene" is seen on some primitive level as intuiting its sexual character. Also, the term *latency*, in its usage by psychoanalytic theorists, suggests a period of integration by the child of prior intrinsically sexual experiences and reactions; on this level, adolescence is reduced to little more than the management or organization on a manifest level of the commitments and styles already prefigured, if not preformed, in infancy and childhood experience.

In contradistinction to this tradition, we have adopted the view that the point at which the individual begins to respond in intrinsically sexual ways, particularly in terms of socially available or defined outlets and objects, reflects a discontinuity with previous "sexual experience" (however that might be defined). Further, at this point in the developmental process, both seemingly sexual and

17. Even on the level of organismic needs and gratification, the linking of these to the sexual or protosexual may be too limited, too simple. Robert White has argued cogently that during infancy and early childhood an emergent commitment to "competence" may rival sensual expressions of the pleasure principle in organizing the young organism's activities, as the child "sacrifices" immediate sensual gratification in order to develop and experience his or her own competence. See "Psychosexual Development and Competence," *The Nebraska Symposium on Motivation* (Lincoln, University of Nebraska Press, 1960).

18. Frank A. Beach, "Characteristics of Masculine 'Sex Drive'," *The Nebraska Symposium on Motivation* (Lincoin: University of Nebraska Press, 1956).

seemingly nonsexual elements "contend" for influence in complex ways that in no respect assure priority for experiences that are apparently sexual in character and occur earlier in the life cycle.

Essential to our perspective is the assumption that with the beginnings of adolescence—and with the increasing acknowledgement by the surrounding social world of an individual's sexual capacity—many novel factors come into play, and an overemphasis upon a search for continuity with infant and childhood experiences may be dangerously misleading. In particular, it may be a costly mistake to be overimpressed with preadolescent behaviors that appear to be manifestly sexual. In general, it is possible that much of the power of sexuality may be a function of the fact that it has been defined as powerful or dangerous. But this overenriched conception of sexual behavior (to the degree that it is possessed by any individual) must largely follow upon considerable training in an adult language that includes an overdetermined conception of sexuality. Thus it does not necessarily follow that the untrained infant or child will respond as powerfully or as complexly to his own seemingly sexual behaviors as an adult observer.

We must also question the prevailing image of the sexual component in human experience as that of an intense drive stemming from the biological substratum that constrains the individual to seek sexual gratification either directly or indirectly. This is clearly present in the Freudian tradition. A similar position is observable in more sociological writings. This is apparent, for example, in the thinking of sociologists for whom sex is also a high intensity, societal constant that must be properly channeled lest it find expression in behaviors which threaten the maintenance of collective life.[19]

Our sense of the available data suggests a somewhat different picture of human sexuality, one of generally lower levels of intensity or, at least, greater variability in intensity. There are numerous social situations in which the reduction and even elimination of sexual activity is managed by greatly disparate populations of biologically normal males and females with little evidence of corollary or compensatory intensification in other spheres of life.[20] It is possible that, given the

19. E. Durkheim, *Suicide* (Glencoe, Ill. The Free Press, 1951).
20. J. H. Gagnon and W. Simon, "The Social Meaning of Prison Homosexuality," *Federal Probation*, 1968.

historical nature of human societies, we are victim to the needs of earlier social orders. For earlier societies it may not have been a need to constrain severely the powerful sexual impulse in order to maintain social stability or limit inherently antisocial force, but rather a matter of having to invent an importance for sexuality. This would not only assure a high level of reproductive activity but also provide socially available rewards unlimited by natural resources, rewards that promote conforming behavior in sectors of social life far more important than the sexual. Part of the legacy of Freud is that we have all become adept at seeking out the sexual ingredient in many forms of nonsexual behavior and symbolism. We are suggesting what is in essence the insight of Kenneth Burke: it is just as plausible to examine sexual behavior for its capacity to express and serve nonsexual motives as the reverse.[21]

A major flaw in the psychoanalytic tradition is that psychosexual development, while a universal component in the human experience, certainly does not occur with universal modalities. Even ignoring the striking forms of cross-cultural variability, we can observe striking differences within our own population, differences that appear to require not a unitary description of psychosexual development but descriptions of different developmental processes characterizing different segments of the population.[22] The most evident of these are the large number of important differences between observable male and female patterns of sexual behavior.[23] This particular difference may in some respects be partly attributable to the role played by the biological substratum. We have to account not only for the gross physiological differences and the different roles in the reproductive process that follow from these physiological differences, but must also consider differences in hormone functions at particular ages.[24] However, while our knowledge of many of the salient physiological and physiochemical processes involved is far from complete, there is still little immediate justification for asserting a direct casual link between these processes

21. K. Burke, *Permanence and Change* (New York: New Republic, Inc., 1935).
22. C. F. Ford and F. A. Beach, *Patterns of Sexual Behavior* (New York: Harper, 1951).
23. E. Maccoby, ed., *The Development of Sex Differences* (Stanford: Stanford University Press, 1966).
24. D. A. Hamburg and D. T. Lunde, "Sex Hormones in the Development of Sex Differences in Human Behavior," in Maccoby, *The Development of Sex Differences*, pp. 1-24; W. R. Young, R. Goy, and C. Phoenix, "Hormones and Sexual Behavior," *Science* 143 (1964): 212-18.

and specific differential patterns of sexual development observed in our society. The work of Masters and Johnson, for example, clearly points to far greater orgasmic capacities on the part of females than males; however, their concept of orgasm as a physiological process would hardly be a basis for accurately predicting rates of sexual behavior.[25] Similarly, within each sex, important distinctions must be made for various socioeconomic status groups whose patterns of sexual development will vary considerably, more impressively for males than for females.[26] And with reference to socioeconomic status differences, the link to the biological level appears even more tenuous, unless one is willing to invoke the relatively unfashionable conceptual equipment of Social Darwinism. These differences, then, not only suggest the importance of sociocultural elements and social structure, but also stand as a warning against too uncritical an acceptance of unqualified generalizations about psychosexual development.

Scripts and the Attribution of Meaning

The term *script* might properly be invoked to describe virtually all human behavior in the sense that there is very little that can in a full measure be called spontaneous. Ironically, the current vogue of using "encounter groups" to facilitate "spontaneous" behavior can be defined as learning the appropriate script for spontaneous behavior. Indeed, the sense of the *internal rehearsal* consistent with both psychoanalytic and symbolic interactionist theory suggests just such scripting of all but the most routinized behavior.

It is the result of our collective blindness to or ineptitude in locating and defining these scripts that has allowed the prepotence of a biological mandate in the explanation of sexual behavior. (This possibly occurs precisely because the notion of such a biological mandate is a common element within the sexual scripts of Western societies.) Without the proper elements of a script that defines the situation, names the actors, and plots the behavior, nothing sexual is likely to happen. One can easily conceive of numerous social situations in which all or almost all of the ingredients of a sexual event are present

25. W. H. Masters and V. E. Johnson, *Human Sexual Response* (Boston: Little, Brown and Co., 1966).
26. A. C. Kinsey et al., *Sexual Behavior in the Human Male* (Philadelphia: W. B. Saunders Co., 1948).

but that remain nonsexual in that not even sexual arousal occurs. Thus, combining such elements as desire, privacy, and a physically attractive person of the appropriate sex, the probability of something sexual happening will, under normal circumstances, remain exceedingly small until either one or both actors organize these behaviors into an appropriate script.

Elements of such scripting occur across many aspects of the sexual situation. Scripts are involved in learning the meaning of internal states, organizing the sequences of specifically sexual acts, decoding novel situations, setting the limits on sexual responses, and linking meanings from nonsexual aspects of life to specifically sexual experience. These would at first seem only to be versions of the old sociological saw that nothing occurs internally that does not occur in the external social world. But it is more than this in two ways. Using this model the process of sexual learning can be specified without depending on nonbehavioral elements, and doing this reorders the sources of meaning for phenomena and the ways in which we think about the sexual experience.

This can be exemplified even more dramatically. Take an ordinary middle-class male, detach him from his regular social location, and place him for some business or professional reason in a large, relatively anonymous hotel. One might even endow him with an interest in sexual adventure. Upon returning to the hotel at night, he opens his hotel door and there in the shaft of light from the hallway, he observes a nearly nude, extremely attractive female. One may assume that his initial reaction will *not* be one of sexual arousal. A few men—the slightly more paranoid—might begin to cast about for signs of their wife's lawyer or a private detective. Most, however, would simply beat a hasty and profoundly embarrassed retreat. Even back in the hall and with a moment's reflection to establish the correctness of the room number, the next impulse would still *not* be one of sexual arousal or activity but most probably a trip to the lobby to seek clarification—via the affectively neutral telephone. What is lacking in this situation is an effective sexual script that would allow him to define the female as a potentially erotic actor (the mere fact of her being attractive or nearly nude is not sufficient) and the situation as potentially sexual. If these two definitional elements did exist, much of what might follow can be predicted with fair accuracy. But without such a script, little by way of sexual activity or even sexual arousal will transpire.

Our use of the term *script* with reference to the sexual has two major dimensions. One deals with the external, the interpersonal—the script as the organization of mutually shared conventions that allows two or more actors to participate in a complex act involving mutual dependence. The second deals with the internal, the intrapsychic, the motivational elements that produce arousal or at least a commitment to the activity.

At the level of convention is that large class of gestures, both verbal and nonverbal, that are mutually accessible. Routinized language, the sequence of petting behaviors among adolescents and adults, the conventional styles establishing sexual willingness are all parts of culturally shared, external routines. These are the strategies involved in the "doing" of sex, concrete and continuous elements of what a culture agrees is sexual. They are assembled, learned over time, reflecting—as will be clear in subsequent chapters—general patterns of stages of development. This relatively stylized behavior, however, tells us little of the meaning it has for its participants. The same sequence of acts may have different meanings for both different pairs of actors or the participants in the same act. This is the world where sexual activity can be expressive of love or rage, the will to power or the will to self-degradation, where the behavioral is experienced through the symbolic.

On the level of internal experience, it is apparent from the work of Schachter and others that the meaning attributed to many states of physiological arousal depends upon the situation in which they are experienced.[27] In this way, meaning is attributed to the interior of the body by many of the same rules as it is to an exterior experience, depending on a vocabulary of motives that makes the biological into a meaningful psychological experience. This phenomena is well understood in research in drug effects, with the meaning of the drug experience being dependent on mood, situation of use, prior history of the user, and the

27. Stanley Schachter, "The Interaction of Cognitive and Emotional Determinants of Emotional State," in *Advances in Experimental Social Psychology*, vol. 1, ed. Leonard Berkowitz (New York: Academic Press, 1964), pp. 49–80. That similar processes of control over the autonomic nervous system also exist and can be operantly conditioned is demonstrated by Neal Miller, "Learning of Visceral and Glandular Responses," *Science* 163 (January 31, 1969): 434–45. Work on increasing "voluntary" control of sexual responses (e.g., penile erection) is beginning only at the present moment.

like, rather than what is spuriously referred to as the drug effect. This is apparent in the effects of all of the so-called mind-altering drugs including marijuana. The differing reports on the internal effects of LSD—25 lysergic acid (good trips, psychomimetic experiences, paranoid trips, art nouveau hallucinations, meetings with God) seem more attributable to the person-situation effect than to the drug. This is observable in young adolescents when they are required to learn what the feelings they have with reference to early post-pubertal sexual arousal "mean." Events variously categorized as anxiety, nausea, fear are reported which are later finally categorized as (or dismissed, even though they still occur) sexual excitement. A vast number of physiological events get reported to the central nervous system, but of this number only a small proportion are attended to in any single moment. (How many persons, for instance, experience their toes curl or the anal sphincter twitch at the moment of orgasm?) It is this small proportion that is recognized as the internal correlates or internal "meanings" of the experience. In this case, the meaning is a consensual experience with various elements brought together to be the appropriate behaviors that will elicit the internal correlates or consequences of the external behaviors.

Scripting also occurs not only in the making of meaningful interior states, but in providing the ordering of bodily activities that will release these internal biological states. Here scripts are the mechanisms through which biological events can be potentiated. An example from the adult world is most apt in revealing this process. If one examines the assembly of events that are the physical elements of the current script in the United States for adolescent or adult heterosexual behavior that leads to coitus, it is clear that there is a progression from hugging and kissing, to petting above the waist, to hand-genital contacts (sometimes mouth-genital contacts) and finally to coitus. There is some variation about these acts in timing (both in order and duration), but roughly this is—at the physical level—what normal heterosexual activity is. Prior to or in the course of this sequence of physical acts, sexual arousal occurs, and in some cases orgasm results for one or both of the two persons involved. What is misleading in this physical description is that it sounds as if one were rubbing two sticks together to produce fire; that is, if only enough body heat is generated, orgasm occurs. However, orgasm is not only a physical event, but also the outcome of a combination of both biological and, more importantly, social psychological factors. Unless the two people involved recognize that the physical events outlined are sexual and are embedded in a sexual situation, there will not be the potentiation of the physiological concomitants that Masters and Johnson have demonstrated as necessary in the production of sexual excitement and the orgasmic cycle.[28] The social meaning given to the physical acts releases biological events. Most of the physical acts described in the foregoing sexual sequence occur in many other situations—the palpation of the breast for cancer, the gynecological examination, the insertion of tampons, mouth-to-mouth resuscitation—all involve homologous physical events. But the social situation and the actors are not defined as sexual or potentially sexual, and the introduction of a sexual element is seen as a violation of the expected social arrangements. The social-psychological meaning of sexual events must be learned because they supply the channels through which biology is expressed. In some cases, the system of naming must exist for the event to occur; in others, portions of the event that are biologically necessary are never observed in the psychological field of the participating persons.

The term *script* (or *scripted behavior*) immediately suggests the dramatic, which is appropriate; but it also suggests the conventional dramatic narrative form, which more often than not is inappropriate. The latter tendency is reinforced by our most general conception of the sex act itself, which is seen as a dramatic event with continuous cumulative action. This is suggested, for example, by the language of Masters and Johnson—"arousal, plateau, climax, and resolution"—a conception resembling somewhat an Aristotelian notion of the dramatic or the design for a nineteenth-century symphony. However, the sources of arousal, passion or excitement (the recognition of a sexual possibility), as well as the way the event is experienced (if, indeed, an event follows), derive from a complicated set of layered symbolic meanings that are not only difficult to comprehend from the observed behavior, but also may not be shared by the participants. Even where there is minimal sharing of elements of a script by persons acting toward each other (which, while not necessary, clearly facilitates execution of the

28. Masters and Johnson, *Human Sexual Response.*

acts with mutual satisfaction), they may be organized in different ways and invoked at different times.

The same overt gesture may have both a different meaning and/or play a different role in organizing the sexual "performance." The identical gesture undertaken during sexual activity may be read by one participant with a content that might resemble that of Sade or Sacher-Mosoch, while the other participant reads content from *Love Story*.

Elements entering into the performance may be both relatively remote to the erotic (or what is conventionally defined as remote to the erotic), as well as the immediately and intrinsically erotic. Moreover, the logic of organization may more closely follow the nonnarrative qualities of modern poetry, the surrealistic tradition, or the theater of the absurd than conventional narrative modes. The sexual provides us with a situation where the mere invocation of some powerfully organizing metaphor links behavior to whole universes of meaning; a situation where the power of a metaphorically enriched gesture, act, characteristic, object, or posture cannot be determined by the relative frequency with which it occurs; such organizing metaphors need only be suggested for their effects to be realized.

An example of this may be seen in Jerzy N. Kosinski's novel *Steps*,[29] where our nameless hero finds himself looking down upon a fellow office worker (female) whom he has long desired sexually and who is in a posture of unrestrained sexual accessibility. Though it is a moment he has long desired, he finds himself unable to become aroused. He then recalls the moment of his initial sexual interest; a moment in which, while watching her in the act of filing papers with uplifted arms, he catches a fleeing glimpse of her bra. This trivial image, originally arousing, remains arousing and our hero goes on to complete the act. It is that image (and what it links to) that both names her as an erotic object in terms of his sense of the erotic and names also what he is about to do to her. Though the image need only be briefly suggested (both in its origins and subsequent utilization), and though it may remain unknown to the behaviorist observer, it becomes critical to the performance. Its meanings could be multiple. For example, that the sexual becomes erotically enriched when it is hidden, latent, denied, or

29. Jerzy N. Kosinski, *Steps* (New York: Random House, 1968).

when it is essentially violative (deriving from unintended exposure). It also legitimates the appropriate name for the behavior. Consider the possible "labels" our hero could have invoked that could have been applied to the behavior, each with its own powerful and powerfully distinct associations—making love, making out, fucking, screwing, humping, doing, raping.

The erotic component we can assume is minimally necessary if sexual activity is to occur; that is its very importance. (A dramatic exception, of course, are many women whose participation in sexual activity has often—historically, possibly more often than not—had little to do with their own sense of the erotic.) On the other hand, a preoccupation with the erotic may reach obsessive proportions without overt sexual behavior necessarily following. Thus, like the biological component, it can be described as simultaneously being of critical importance and also insufficient by itself to be either fully descriptive or predictive of actual sexual careers.

While the importance of the erotic can be asserted, it may be the most difficult to elaborate, as a concern for the erotic—the acquisition of sexual culture—is possibly the least well understood or attended aspect of sexual behavior. We know very little about how it is acquired or, for that matter, the ways in which it influences both our sexual and nonsexual lives. Persistence of concepts such as libido or the sex drive obviate need for this knowledge. For those who hold these or comparable positions, the body is frequently seen as being both wise and articulate; recognizing and speaking a compelling language. Still others have assumed, in too unexamined a way, a direct link between collective sexual cultures and private sexual cultures, despite the fact that for many what is collectively defined as erotic may not be associated with sexual response or that much that the collectivity defines as non- or even anti-erotic may become part of the private sexual culture of a given individual; for example, various kinds of full and partial fetishisms. As a result, much of the research on responses to erotic materials often begins with the dubious assumption that experimental stimuli are recognizable in terms of a conventional social definition.[30]

One thing that is clear is that for contemporary society erotic imagery or metaphors are for the most part discontinuously or only

30. Masters and Johnson, *Human Sexual Response.*

latently a part of the images or metaphors of nonsexual identity or social life. (The exceptions are those social roles that are specifically assumed to have a "known" erotic aspect, such as the prostitute, the homosexual, the stewardess, or the divorcee, all of whom we tend to see as either fully erotic or unusually erotic to the point where we have difficulty seeing them in anything but erotic terms.) Thus, for conventional actors in relatively conventional settings, the invocation of the erotic, necessary for sexual arousal, frequently requires a series of rituals of transformation before the participants or the setting license (as it were) the sexual moment. For example, much of precoital petting or foreplay may serve less as facilitators of a physiological process, than as elements in a ritual drama that allow one or both actors to rename themselves, their partners, as well as various parts of the body in terms of the "special" purpose. The intrusion of nonerotic, manifest meanings to images—that is, parts of the body or other role commitments of one or another of the actors is experienced as disruptive of sexual interest or capacity, if only because such commitments are rarely predictive of sexual role needs. For most, as a consequence, the sexual flourishes best in a sheltered and, in some sense, isolated universe, a landscape denuded of all but the most relevant aspects of identity.

At the same time, the larger part of identity and sense of the rest of social life frequently intrude in an indirect way. The elaboration of the erotic or its direct expression is often constrained by an anticipation of an anticipated return to that larger social role, that more continuous sense of self. For some this may involve merely the insulation of silence; for others, symbolic reinterpretation and condensation—for example, an intensity of pressure that allows the actor to represent by that gesture either passion (or the message that uncharacteristic behavior is thereby explained), or love and affection (that the actor is the same as he or she is in their more conventional mode of relating), or sadistic aggression (illuminating a complicated fantasy rehearsed and experienced sufficiently that the gesture successfully evokes most of the emotional density generated by a long and frequently complicated scenario).

Beyond the very general level however, little can be said. Important questions dealing not only with origins but careers have yet to be even examined provisionally. Where do such images come from? In terms of what sexual and nonsexual experiences do their meaning change? Is there need for elaboration? These, and many more, are the questions that we may have to examine before sexual activity, which all too often can be described as a "dumb-show" for its participants, becomes something other than a dumb-show for behavioral science.

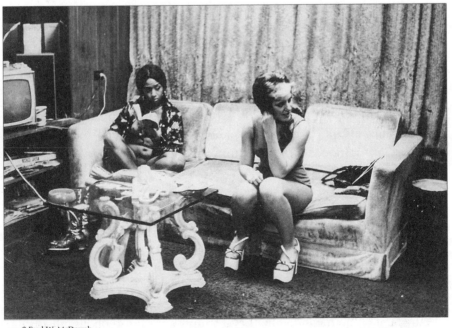

© Fred W. McDarrah

Power and Sex:
Interview with Michel Foucault

Bernard-Henri Levy

from *Telos*, 1977

*In 1976, Michel Foucault published the first volume of what was to be a multi-volume history of sexuality (**The History of Sexuality: An Introduction**, 1978 in the US). The book begins with a meditation on Steven Marcus' "Other Victorians" and ends with a long and devastating critique of Wilhelm Reich ("The Repressive Hypothesis"). In between, Foucault demonstrates how the discussion of sex by psychiatrists, social scientists, and educators, instead of eliminating sexual repression is, in fact, an integral aspect of the pervasive construction of sexuality. Foucault's work was a culmination of many strains of thought developed during the sexual revolution. In the late eighties and nineties, Foucault's work was influential in the development of a new wave of social constructionist thinking about sex. This interview by the well-known French intellectual Bernard-Henry Levy discusses the themes of **The History of Sexuality**.*

B.-H.L.: Your book *La Volonté de savoir* (The Will to Know) marks the beginning of a "history of sexuality" of monumental proportions. What justification is there today for you, Michel Foucault, to undertake so huge an enterprise?

FOUCAULT: So *huge*? No, no, say rather, so *needed*. I do not intend to write the chronicle of sexual behavior over the ages and civilizations. I want to follow a narrower thread: the one that through so many centuries has linked sex and the search for truth in our societies.

B.-H.L.: In precisely what sense?

FOUCAULT: In fact, the problem is this: how is it that in a society like ours, sexuality is not simply a means of reproducing the species, the family, and the individual? Not simply a means to obtain pleasure and enjoyment? How has sexuality come to be considered the privileged place where our deepest "truth" is read and expressed? For that is the essential fact: Since Christianity, the Western world has never ceased saying: "To know who you are, know what your sexuality is." Sex has always been the forum where both the future of our species and our "truth" as human subjects are decided.

Confession, the examination of conscience, all the insistence on the important secrets of the flesh, has not been simply a means of prohibiting sex or of repressing it as far as possible from consciousness, but was a means of placing sexuality at the heart of existence and of connecting salvation with the mastery of these obscure movements. In Christian societies, sex has been the central object of examination, surveillance, avowal and transformation into discourse.

B.-H.L.: Hence the paradoxical theme underlying this first volume: far from making sexuality taboo or bringing strong sanctions against it, our societies have never ceased speaking of sex, and making it speak.

FOUCAULT: They could speak very well—and very much—of sexuality, but only to prohibit it.

But I wanted to stress two important facts. First, that the bringing to light, the "clarification" of sexuality occurred not only in discussions but also in the reality of institutions and practices.

Secondly, that numerous, strict prohibitions exist. But they are part of a complex economy along with incitements, manifestations, and evaluations. We always stress the prohibitions. I would like to change the perspective somewhat, grasping in every case the entire complex of apparatuses.

And, as you well know, I have been given the image of a melancholic historian of prohibitions and repressive power, a teller of tales with only two categories: insanity and its incarceration, the anomaly and its exclusion, delinquency and its imprisonment. But my problem has always been on the side of another term: truth. How did the power exerted in insanity produce psychiatry's "true" discourse? The same applies to sexuality: to revive the will to know the source of the power exerted upon sex. My aim is not to write the social history of a prohibition but the political history of the production of "truth."

B.-H.L.: A new revolution in the concept of history? The dawn of another "new history?"

FOUCAULT: A few years ago, historians were very proud to discover that they could write not only the history of battles, of kings and institutions but also of the economy, now they are all amazed because the shrewdest among them have learned that it was also possible to write the history of feelings, behavior and the body. Soon, they will understand that the history of the West cannot be disassociated from the way its "truth" is produced and produces its effects.

We are living in a society that, to a great extent, is marching "toward the truth"—I mean, that produces and circulates discourse having truth as its function, passing itself off as such and thus attaining specific powers. The achievement of "true" discourses (which are incessantly changing, however) is one of the fundamental problems of the West. The history as true—is still virgin territory.

What are the positive mechanisms which, producing sexuality in this or that fashion, result in misery?

In any case, what I would like to study, as far as I'm concerned, is the sum total of these mechanisms which, in our society, invite, incite and force one to speak of sex.

B.-H.L.: Still, despite such discourse, you believe that repression, sexual misery also exist . . .

FOUCAULT: Yes, I've heard that objection. You are right: we are all living more or less in a state of sexual misery.

B.-H.L.: Why? Is that a deliberate choice?

FOUCAULT: In subsequent volumes, concrete studies—on women, children, the perverted—I will try to analyze the forms and conditions of this misery. But, for the moment, it is a question of establishing method. The problem is to know whether the misery should be explained negatively by a fundamental interdiction, or positively by a prohibition relative to an economic situation ("Work, don't make love"): or whether it is not the effect of much more complex and much more positive procedures.

B.-H.L.: What could be a "positive" explanation in this case?

FOUCAULT: I will make a presumptuous comparison. What did Marx do when in his analysis of capital he came across the problem of the workers' misery? He refused the customary explanation which regarded this misery as the effect of a naturally rare cause of a concerted theft. And he said substantially: given what capitalist production is, in its fundamental laws, it cannot help but cause misery. Capitalism's raison d'être is not to starve the workers but it cannot develop without starving them. Marx replaced the denunciation of theft by the analysis of production.

Other things being equal, that is approximately what I wanted to say. It is not a matter of denying sexual misery, nor is it however one of explaining it negatively by a repression. The entire problem is to grasp the positive mechanism which, producing sexuality in this or that fashion, results in misery.

Here is one example that I will deal with in a future volume: at the beginning of the 18th century tremendous importance was suddenly ascribed to childhood masturbation, which then was persecuted everywhere like a sudden epidemic, terrible and capable of compromising the whole human race.

Must one conclude from this that childhood masturbation had suddenly become unacceptable for capitalist society in the process of development? This is the position of certain "Reichians," but it does not seem at all satisfactory to me.

On the contrary, what was important at that time was the reorganization of the relations between children and adults, parents, educators; it was an intensification of the intra-family relations; it was childhood as a common area of interest for parents, the educational institutions, the public health authorities; it was childhood as the training-ground for future generations. At the crossroads of body and soul, of health and morality, of education and training, children's sex became both a target and an instrument of power. A specific "sexuality of children" was constituted—precautions, dangerous, constantly in need of supervision.

This resulted in a sexual misery of childhood and adolescence from which our own generations still have not recovered, but the objective was not to forbid, but to use childhood sexuality, suddenly become important and mysterious, as a network of power over children.

B.-H.L.: This idea that sexual misery stems from repression, and that, to be happy, we must have sexual liberation, is held basically by sexologists, doctors, and vice squads . . .

FOUCAULT: Yes, and that is why they present to us a formidable trap. What they are saying, roughly, is this: "You have a sexuality; this sexuality is both frustrated and mute; hypocritical prohibitions are repressing it. So, come to us, tell us, show us all that, confide in us your unhappy secrets . . ."

This type of discourse is, indeed, a formidable tool of control and power. As always, it uses what people say, feel, and hope for. It exploits their temptation to believe that to be happy, it is enough to cross the threshold of discourse and to remove a few prohibitions. But in fact it ends up repressing and dispersing movements of revolt and liberation . . .

B.-H.L.: Hence the misunderstanding of certain commentators: "According to Foucault, the repression or the liberation of sex amounts to the same thing." Or again: groups such as "The MLAC [a radical pro-abortion movement] and Laissez-les vivre [a pro-life movement], employ basically the same discourse . . ."

FOUCAULT: Yes! Matters still have to be cleared up on that point. I was quoted as saying in effect that there is no real difference between the language of condemnation and that against condemnation, between the discourse of prudish moralists and that of sexual liberation. They claimed that I was putting them all in one bag to drown them like a litter of kittens. Diametrically false: that is not what I meant to say. But the important thing is, I didn't say it at all.

FOUCAULT: But a statement is one thing, discourse another. They share common tactics even though they have conflicting strategies.

B.-H.L.: For example?

FOUCAULT: I believe that the movements labeled "sexual liberation" ought to be understood as movements of affirmation "starting with" sexuality. Which means two things: they are movements that start with sexuality, with the apparatus of sexuality in the midst of which we're caught, and which make it function to the limit; but, at the same time, they are in motion relative to it, disengaging themselves and surmounting it.

B.-H.L.: What do these surmountings look like?

FOUCAULT: Take the case of homosexuality. Psychiatrists began a medical analysis of it in the 1870s: a point of departure certainly for a whole series of new interventions and controls.

They began either to incarcerate homosexuals in asylums or to try to cure them. Sometimes they were looked upon as libertines and sometimes as delinquents (hence condemnations—which could be very severe, with burnings at the stake still occurring even in the eighteenth century—were necessarily rare). In the future we will *all* see them as manifesting forms of insanity, sickness of the sexual instinct. But taking such discourses literally, and thereby turning them around, we see responses arising in the form of defiance: "All right, we are the same as you, by nature sick or perverse, whichever you want. And so if we are, let us be so, and if you want to know what we are, we can tell you better than you can." The entire literature of homosexuality, very differently from libertine narratives, appears at the end of the 19th century: recall Wilde and Gide. It is the strategic return of one "same" desire for truth.

B.-H.L.: That indeed is what is happening with all minorities today, women, youth, the blacks in America . . .

FOUCAULT: Yes, of course. For a long time they tried to pin women to their sex. For centuries they were told: "You are nothing but your sex." And this sex, doctors added, is fragile, almost always sick and always inducing illness. "You are man's sickness." And towards the 18th century this ancient movement ran wild, ending in a pathologization of woman: the female body became a medical object *par excellence.* I will try later to write the history of this immense "gynecology" in the broad sense of the term.

But the feminist movements responded defiantly. Are we sex by nature? Well then, let us be so but in its singularity, in its irreducible specificity. Let us draw the consequences and reinvent our own type of existence, political, economic and cultural . . . Always the same movement: to use this sexuality as the starting point in an attempt to colonize them and to cross beyond it toward other affirmations.

B.-H.L.: This strategy which you are describing, this strategy of a double *détente,* is it still a strategy of liberation in the classical sense? Or must one not rather say that to liberate sex, one must from now on hate and surmount it?

FOUCAULT: A movement is taking shape today which seems to me to be reversing the trend of "always more sex," and "always more truth in sex," which has enthralled us for centuries: it is a matter—I don't say of "rediscovering"—but rather of inventing other forms of pleasures, of relationships, coexistences, attachments, loves, intensities. I have the impression of currently hearing an "anti-sex" grumbling (I am not a prophet, at most a diagnostician), as if an effort were being made, in depth, to shake this great "sexography" which makes us try to decipher sex as the universal secret.

B.-H.L.: What are some symptoms for this diagnosis?

FOUCAULT: Only an anecdote. A young writer, Herve Guibert, had written some children's stories: no editor wanted them. He wrote another book, certainly very remarkable and apparently very "sexy." It was the condition for being heard and published. And, presto, he was published (the book is *La Mort Propagande*). Read it: it seems to me the opposite of the sexographic writing that has been the rule in pornography and sometimes in good literature: to move progressively toward naming what is most unmentionable in sex. Herve Guibert opens with the worst extreme—"You want us to speak of it, well, let's go, and you will hear more than ever before"—and with this infamous material he builds bodies, mirages, castles, fusions, acts of tenderness, races, intoxications; the entire heavy coefficient of sex has been volatilized. But this is only one example of the "anti-sex" challenge, of which many other symptoms can be found. It is perhaps the end of this dreary desert of sexuality, the end of the monarchy of sex.

B.-H.L.: Unless we are pledged and chained to sex like an inevitable destiny. And since childhood, as they say . . .

FOUCAULT: Exactly, just look at what is happening where children are concerned. Some say that the child's life is sexual. From the milk-bottle to puberty, that is all it is. Behind the desire to learn to read or the taste for comic strips, from first to last, everything is sexuality. Well, are you sure that this type of discourse is effectively liberating? Are you sure that it will not lock children into a sort of sexual insularity? And what if, after all, they didn't give a hoot? If the liberty of not being an adult consisted just in not being a slave of the law, the principle, the *locus communis* of sexuality, would that be so boring after all? If it were possible to have polymorphic relationships with things, people and the body, would that not be childhood? This polymorphism is called perversity by the adults, to reassure themselves, thus coloring it with the monotonous monochrome of their own sex.

B.-H.L.: Children are oppressed by the very ones who pretend to liberate them?

FOUCAULT: Read the book by Schérer and Hocquenghem. It shows very well that the child has an assortment of pleasure for which the "sex" grid is a veritable prison.

B.-H.L.: Is this a paradox?

FOUCAULT: This stems from the idea that sexuality is not feared by power, and instead, is far more a means through which power is exercised.

B.-H.L.: But consider authoritarian states: can it be said that power is exercised not against but through sexuality?

FOUCAULT: Two recent events, apparently contradictory: About ten months ago, China launched a campaign against childhood masturbation, along exactly the same lines that defined this campaign in 18th century Europe (masturbation hampers work, causes deafness, brings about the degeneration of the species). On the other hand, before the year is out, the Soviet Union will, for the first time, host a congress of psychoanalysts (they have to come from abroad since there are none in Russia). Liberalization? A thaw on the part of the subconscious? The springtime of the Soviet libido against the moral bourgeoisificiation of the Chinese?

In Peking's archaic stupidities and the quaint Soviet novelties I see mainly a double recognition of the fact that, formulated *and* prohibited, expressed [*dite*] *and* forbidden [*interdite*], sexuality is a recourse which no modern system of power can do without. We should deeply fear socialism with a sexual physiognomy.

B.-H.L.: In other words, power is no longer necessarily what condemns and encloses?

FOUCAULT: In general terms, I would say that the interdiction, the refusal, the prohibition, far from being essential forms of power, are only its limits, power in its frustrated or extreme forms. The relations of power are, above all, productive.

B.-H.L.: This is a new idea compared with your previous books.

FOUCAULT: If I wanted to pose and drape myself in a slightly fictional style, I would say that this has always been my problem: the effects of power and the production of "truth." I have always felt uncomfortable with this ideological notion which has been used in recent years. It has been used to explain errors or illusions, or to analyze presentations—in short, everything that impedes the formation of true discourse. It has also been used to show the relation between what goes on in people's heads and their place in the conditions of production. In sum, the economics of untruth. My problem is the politics of truth. I have spent a lot of time dealing with it.

B.-H.L.: Why?

FOUCAULT: For several reasons. First, power in the West is what displays itself the most, and thus what hides itself the best: what we have called "political life" since the 19th century is the manner in which power presents its image (a little like the court in the monarchic era). Power is neither there, nor is that how it functions. The relations of power are perhaps among the best hidden things in the social body.

On the other hand, since the 19th century, the critique of society has essentially started with the nature of the economy, which is effectively determining. A valid reduction of "politics," certainly, but a tendency also to neglect the relations of elementary power that could be constitutive of economic relations.

The third reason is the tendency, itself common to institutions, parties, an entire current of revolutionary thought and action, not to see power in any form other than the state aparatus.

All of which leads, when we turn to individuals, to finding power nowhere except in the mind (under the form of representation, acceptance, or interiorization).

B.-H.L.: And faced with this, what did you want to do?

FOUCAULT: Four things: to investigate what might be most hidden in the relations of power; to anchor them in the economic infrastructures; to trace them not only in their governmental forms but also in the infra-governmental or para-governmental ones; to discover them in the material play.

B.-H.L.: What factor did you start with?

FOUCAULT: If you want a bibliographical reference, it was in *Surveiller et Punir* [published in the U.S. as *Discipline and Punish*]. But I would rather say that it started with a series of events and experiences since 1968 involving psychiatry, delinquency, the schools, etc. These events themselves could never have taken their direction and intensity without the two gigantic shadows of fascism and Stalinism looming in the background. If the workers' misery—this subexistence—caused the political thinking of the 19th century to revolve around the economy, then fascism and Stalinism—these superpowers—induce political anxiety in our current societies.

Hence two problems: power, how does it work? Is it enough for it to issue strong prohibitions in order to really function? And does it always move from above to below and from the center to the periphery?

B.-H.L.: I saw this movement—this sliding—in *La Volonté de Savoir*:

this time you made a clean break with the diffuse naturalism that haunts your previous books . . .

FOUCAULT: What you call naturalism refers, I believe, to two things. A certain theory, the idea that under power with its acts of violence and its artifice, we should be able to rediscover the things themselves in their primitive vivacity: behind the asylum walls, the spontaneity of madness; through the penal system, the generous fever of delinquency; under the sexual interdict, the freshness of desire. And also a certain aesthetic and moral choice: power is bad, ugly, poor, sterile, monotonous and dead; and what power is exercised upon is right, good and rich.

B.-H.L.: Yes. Finally, the theme common to orthodox Marxism and the New Left: "Under the cobblestones lies the beach."

FOUCAULT: If you like. At times, such simplifications are necessary. Such a dualism can be provisionally useful, to change the perspective from time to time and move from *pro* to *contra*.

B.-H.L.: Then comes the time to stop, the moment of reflection and regaining of equilibrium?

FOUCAULT: On the contrary. What should follow is the moment of new mobility and new displacement, for these reversals of *pro* and *contra* are quickly blocked, being unable to do anything except repeat themselves and forming what Jacques Rancière calls the "Leftist *doxa*." As soon as we repeat indefinitely the same refrain of the anti-repressive anthem, things remain in place; anyone can sing the tune, and no one pays attention. This reversal of values and truths, of which I was speaking a while ago, has been important to the extent that it does not stop with simple cheers (long live insanity, delinquency, sex) but allows for new strategies. You see, what often embarrasses me today— in fact, what I regret—is that all this work done in the past fifteen years or so—often under hardship and in solitude—functions for some only as a sign of belonging: to be on the "good side," on the side of madness, children, delinquency, sex.

B.-H.L.: There is no good side?

FOUCAULT: One must pass to the other side—the good side—but by trying to turn off these mechanisms which cause the appearance of two separate sides, by dissolving the false unity, the illusory "nature" of this other side with which we have taken sides. This is where the real work begins, that of the present-day historian.

B.-H.L.: Several times already you have defined yourself as an historian. What does that mean? Why "historian'" and not "philosopher"?

FOUCAULT: Under as naive a form as a child's fable, I will say that the question of philosophy for a long time has been: "In this world where everything dies, what does not pass away?" It seems to me that since the 19th century, philosophy has never stopped raising the same question: "What is happening right now, and what are we, we who are perhaps nothing more than what is happening at this moment?" Philosophy's question therefore is the question as to what we ourselves are. That is why contemporary philosophy is entirely political and entirely historical. It is the politics immanent in history and the history indispensable for politics.

B.-H.L.: But isn't a return to the most classical, metaphysical kind of philosophy taking place today?

FOUCAULT: I don't believe in any form of return. I would say only this, and only half seriously: The thinking of the first Christian centuries would have had to answer the question: "What is actually going on today? What is this time which we are living in? When and how will this promised return of God take place? What can we do with this intervening time, which is superfluous? And what are we, we who are in this transition?"

We could say that on this incline of history, when the revolution is supposed to hold back and has not yet come, we can ask the same question: "What are we, are we superfluous in this age when what should be happening is not happening?" The question of the revolution has dominated all modern thought, like all politics.

B.-H.L.: Are you, on your part, continuing to pose the question and to reflect on it? Does it, in your eyes, remain the question par excellence?

FOUCAULT: If politics has existed since the 19th century, it is because the revolution took place. The current one is not a variant or a sector of that one. Politics always takes a stand on the revolution. When Napoleon said "the modern form of destiny is politics," he was merely drawing the logical conclusions from this truth, for he came after the revolution and before the return of another one.

The return of the revolution—that is surely what our problem is. It is certainly that without it, the question of Stalinism would be purely academic—a mere problem of the organization of societies or of the validity of the Marxist scheme of things. But something quite different is at stake in Stalinism. You know very well what it is: the very desirability of the revolution is the problem today . . .

B.-H.L.: Do you want the revolution? Do you want anything more than the simple ethical duty to struggle here and now, at the side of one or another oppressed and miserable group, such as fools or prisoners?

FOUCAULT: I have no answer. But I believe that to engage in politics—aside from just party-politics—is to try to know with the greatest possible honesty whether the revolution is desirable. It is in exploring this terrible mole-hill that politics runs the danger of caving in.

B.-H.L.: If the revolution were not desirable, would politics remain what you say it is?

FOUCAULT: No, I believe not. It would be necessary to invent another one or something else as a substitute for it. We are perhaps experiencing the end of politics. For politics is a field that has been opened by the existence of the revolution, and if the question of the revolution can no longer be posed in these terms, then politics is in danger of disappearing.

B.-H.L.: Let us return to your politics in *La Volonté de Savoir.* You say: "Where there is power, there is resistance." Are you not thus bringing back nature, which a while back you wanted to dismiss?

FOUCAULT: I think not. This resistance I am speaking of is not a substance. It does not predate the power which it opposes. It is coextensive with it and absolutely its contemporary.

B.-H.L.: The inverse image of power? That would come to the same thing. The cobblestones under the beach always appear . . .

FOUCAULT: Absolutely. I am not positing a substance of resistance versus a substance of power. I am just saying: as soon as there is a power relation, there *is* a possibility of resistance. We can never be ensnared by power: we can always modify its grip in determinate conditions and according to a precise strategy.

B.-H.L.: Power and resistance, tactics and strategy . . . Why this stock of military metaphors? Do you think that power from now on must be visualized in the form of war?

FOUCAULT: I have no idea at the present time. One thing seems certain to me; it is that for the moment we have, for analyzing the relations of power, only two models: a) the one proposed by law (power as law, interdiction, institutions) and b) the military or strategic model in terms of power relations. The first one has been much used and its inadequacy has, I believe, been demonstrated: we know very well that law does not describe power.

The other model is also much discussed, I know. But we stop with words; we use ready-made ideas or metaphors ("the war of all against all," "the struggle for life"), or again formal schemata (strategies are very much in vogue among certain sociologists and economists, especially Americans). I think that this analysis of the power relations would have to be tightened up.

B.-H.L.: But this military conception of the power relations was already used by the Marxists?

FOUCAULT: What strikes me in the Marxist analyses is that they always contain the question of "class struggle" but that they pay little attention to one word in the phrase, namely, "struggle." Here again distinctions must be made. The greatest of the Marxists (starting with Marx himself) insisted sharply on the "military" problems (the army as an instrument of the state, armed insurrection, revolutionary war). But when they speak of the "class struggle" as the mainspring of history, they focus mainly on defining class, its boundaries, its membership, but never concretely on the nature of the struggle. One exception comes to mind: Marx's own non-theoretical, historical texts, which are better and different in this regard.

B.-H.L.: Do you think that your book can fill this gap?

FOUCAULT: I don't make any such claim. In a general way, I think that intellectuals—if this category exists, which is not certain nor perhaps even desirable—are abandoning their old prophetic function.

And by that I don't mean only their claim to predict what will happen, but also the legislative function that they so long aspired for: "See what must be done, see what is good, follow me. In the turmoil that engulfs you all, here is the pivotal point, here is where I am." The Greek wise man, the Jewish prophet, the Roman legislator are still models that haunt those who, today, practice the profession of speaking and writing. I dream of the intellectual who destroys evidence and generalities, the one who, in the inertias and constraints of the present time, locates and marks the weak points, the openings, the lines of force, who is incessantly on the move, doesn't know exactly where he is heading nor what he will think tomorrow for he is too attentive to the present; who, wherever he moves, contributes to posing the question of knowing whether the revolution is worth the trouble, and what kind (I mean, what revolution and what trouble), it being understood that the question can be answered only by those who are willing to risk their lives to bring it about.

As for all the questions of classification and program that are asked of us: "Are you a Marxist?" "What would you do if you had the power?" "Who are your allies and what are your resources?"—these are truly secondary questions compared with the one I have just indicated: it is the question of today.

Bibliography

Allyn, David. (2000) *Make Love. Not War: The Sexual Revolution. An Unfettered History*. Boston: Little Brown and Company.

Altman, Dennis (1971) *Homosexual Oppression and Liberation*. New York: Outerbridge & Dienstrey.

Altman, Dennis (1979) *Coming Out in the Seventies*. Sydney: Wild & Woolley.

Bailey, Beth. (1999) *Sex in the Heartland*. Cambridge. MA: Harvard University Press.

Baldwin, James (1961) "The Black Boy Looks at the White Boy," in *Nobody Knows My Name*. New York: Dial Press.

Berlant, Lauren and Lisa Duggan. (2001) Eds., *Our Monica, Ourselves: The Clinton Affair and the National Interest*. New York: New York University Press.

Brown, Helen Gurley (1962) *Sex and the Single Girl*. New York: Bernard Geis Associates.

Brown, Norman O. (1959) *Life Against Death: The Psychoanalytic Meaning of History*. Middletown. CT: Wesleyan University Press.

Bruce, Lenny. (1992) *How to Talk Dirty and Influence People*. New York: Fireside.

Burke, Tom. (1969) "The New Homosexuality" *Esquire*. December.

Cleaver, Eldridge (1968) *Soul on Ice*. New York: McGraw-Hill.

Clendinen, Dudley and Adam Nagourney (1999) *Out for Good: The Struggle to Build a Gay Rights Movement in America*. New York: Simon & Schuster.

Charters, Ann. (1992) Ed., *The Portable Beat Reader*. New York: Viking Penguin.

Collins, K.L. Ronald and David M. Skover. (2002) *The Trials of Lenny Bruce: The Fall and Rise of an American Icon*. Naperville. IL: SourceBooks Media-Fusion.

Comfort, Alex (1972) *The Joy of Sex: A Gourmet Guide to Love Making*. New York: Crown Publishers.

Comfort, Alex (1973) Ed., *More Joy: A Lovemaking Companion to the Joy of Sex*. New York: Crown Publishers.

Cory, Donald Webster (1951) *The Homosexual in America*. New York: Castle Books.

De Beauvoir, Simone (1952) *The Second Sex*. New York: Alfred A. Knopf.

Dell Olio, Anselma (1972). "The Sexual Revolution Isn't Our War." *Ms*.

D'Emilio, John (1980) *Sexual Politics. Sexual Communities: The Making of a*

Homosexual Minority in the United States. 1940-1970. Chicago: University of Chicago Press.

D'Emilio, John and Estelle Freedman (1988) *Intimate Matters: A History of Sexuality in America.* New York: Harper & Row.

Dollimore, Jonathan. (1991) *Sexual Dissidence: Augustine to Wilde. Freud to Foucault.* Oxford: Oxford University Press.

Duberman, Martin (1993) *Stonewall.* New York: Dutton

Duggan, Lisa and Nan D. Hunter. (1995) *Sex Wars: Sexual Dissent and Political Culture.* New York: Routledge.

Dyer, Richard (1992). "Coming to Terms: Gay Pornography." *Only Entertainment.* London: Routledge.

Echols, Alice. (1989) *Daring to Be Bad: Radical Feminism in America. 1967-1975.* Minneapolis: University of Minnesota.

Echols, Alice (2002) *Shaky Ground: The Sixties and Its Aftershocks.* New York: Columbia University Press.

Ehrenreich, Barbara. *The Hearts of Men: American Dreams and the Flight from Commitment* (Garden City: Anchor Press/Doubleday. 1984)

Ehrenreich Barbara, Elizabeth Hess and Gloria Jacobs. *Re-Making Love: The Feminization of Sex* (Garden City: Anchor Press/Doubleday. 1986)

Erickson, Julia A. (1999) *Kiss and Tell: Surveying Sex in the Twentieth-Century.* Cambridge: Harvard University Press

Escoffier, Jeffrey (1998) *American Homo: Perversity and Community.* Berkley. CA: University of California Press. 1998

Escoffier, Jeffrey (1999) "The Invention of Safer Sex: Vernacular Knowledge, Gay Politics and HIV Prevention." *Berkeley Journal of Sociology* (Spring).

Escoffier, Jeffrey (2003) "Fabulous Politics: Queer, Lesbian and Gay Movements, 1969-1999" in Van Gosse and Dick Moser. Eds. *The World the Sixties Made: Post-Sixties Culture and Politics.* Philadelphia: Temple University Press.

Escoffier, Jeffrey (2004) "Foreword" in John Gagnon, *An Interpretation of Desire* (Chicago: University of Chicago Press. 2004).

Fanon, Frantz (1967) *Black Skin. White Masks.* New York: Grove Press

Foucault, Michel. (1978) *The History of Sexuality: An Introduction.* New York: Pantheon.

Firestone, Shulamith. (1970) *The Dialectic of Sex: The Case for Feminist Revolution.* New York: William Morrow.

Frappier-Mazur, Lucienne (1993) "Truth and the Obscene Word in Eighteenth-Century Pornography" in Hunt. Lynn (1996) Ed., *The Invention of Pornography: Obscenity and the Origins of Modernity. 1500-1800.* New York: Zone Books.

Freud, Sigmund. (1930 [1960]) *Civilization and Its Discontents,* translation by James Strachey. New York: W.W. Norton.

Freud, Sigmund. (1905 [1962]) *Three Essays on the Theory of Sexuality,* translation by James Strachey. New York: Basic Books.

Freud, Sigmund (1908 [1963]) "'Civilized' Sexual Morality and Modern Nervousness"

Freud, Sigmund. (1930 [1960]) *Jokes and Their Relation to the Unconscious.* New York: W. W. Norton.

Friday, Nancy (1973) *My Secret Garden: Women's Sexual Fantasies.* New York: Trident Press.

Friedan, Betty (1963) *The Feminine Mystique.* New York: W.W. Norton.

Gagnon, John H. and William Simon (1973) Sexual Conduct: The Social Sources of Human Sexuality. Chicago: Aldine Publishing.

Gitlin, Todd (1987) *The Sixties: Years of Hope, Days of Rage.* New York: Bantam

Godbeer, Richard. (2002) *Sexual Revolution in Early America.* Baltimore: The Johns Hopkins University Press.

Gooch, Brad. (1996) *The Golden Age of Promiscuity.* New York: Alfred A. Knopf.

Goodman, Paul (1977) *Nature Heals: Psychological Essays.* Ed., Taylor Stroehr. New York: Free Life Editions.

Gornick, Vivian and Barbara K. Moran. Eds. (1971) *Woman in a Sexist Society: Studies in Power and Powerlessness.* New York: Basic Books.

Greene, Gerald and Caroline (1973) *S-M: The Last Taboo.* New York: Grove Press.

Hatfield, Tom (1975) *Sandstone Experience.* New York: Crown Publishers.

Heidenery, John. (1997) *What Wild Ecstasy: The Rise and Fall of the Sexual Revolution.* New York: Simon & Schuster.

Hollander, Xavier (1972) *The Happy Hooker: My Own Story.* New York: Dell Publishing

Horkheimer, Max and Theodor W. Adorno. (2002) *Dialectic of Enlightenment.* Stanford. CA: Stanford University Press.

Hunt, Lynn (1996) Ed. *The Invention of Pornography: Obscenity and the Origins of Modernity. 1500-1800.* New York: Zone Books.

Irvine. Janice M. (1990) *Disorders of Desire: Sex and Gender in Modern American Sexology.* Philadelphia: Temple University Press.

J. (1969) *The Sensuous Woman.* New York: Lyle Stuart.

Jay, Karla and Allan Young (1972) *Out of the Closets: Voices of Gay Liberation.* New York: Douglas/Links.

Jay, Karla and Allan Young (1979) Eds., *The Gay Report: Lesbians and Gay Men Speak Out About Sexual Experience and Lifestyles.* New York: Summit Books.

Johnston, Jill (1973) *The Lesbian Nation: The Feminist Solution.* New York: Simon & Schuster.

Jong, Erica (1974) *Fear of Flying.* New York: Signet Books.

Katz, Jonathan Ned (1995) *The Invention of Heterosexuality.* New York: Dutton.

Kendrick, Walter (1987) *The Secret Museum: Pornography in Modern Culture.* New York: Viking Penguin.

King, Richard (1972) *The Party of Eros: Radical Social Thought and the Realm of Freedom.* Chapel Hill: University of North Carolina Press.

Kinsey, Alfred C. et al. (1948) *Sexual Behavior in the Human Male.* Philadelphia: W.B. Saunders Co.

Kinsey, Alfred C. et al. (1953) *Sexual Behavior in the Human Female.* Philadelphia: W.B. Saunders Co.

Kipnis, Laura. (1996) *Bound and Gagged: Pornography and the Politics of Fantasy in America.* New York: Grove Press.

Lewis, Jon (2002) *Hollywood vs. Hardcore: How the Struggle over Censorship Saved the Modern Film Industry.* New York: New York University Press.

Lipton, Lawrence (1959) *The Holy Barbarians.* New York: Julian Messner.

Loftus, David. (2002) *Watching Sex: How Men Really Respond to Pornography.* New York: Thunder's Mouth Press.

M. (1971) *The Sensuous Man.* New York: Lyle Stuart.

Mailer, Norman (1963) Advertisements for Myself. New York: G.P. Putnam.

Marcus, Steven (1966) *The Other Victorians: A Study of Sexuality and Pornography in Mid-Nineteenth-Century England.* New York: Basic Books.

Marcuse, Herbert (1955) *Eros and Civilization: A Philosophical Inquiry into Freud.* Boston: Beacon Press.

Marcuse, Herbert (1964) *One-Dimensional Man: Studies in Advanced Industrial Society.* Boston: Beacon Press.

Marwick, Arthur (1998) *The Sixties.* Oxford: Oxford University Press

Masters, William and Virginia Johnson (1966) *Human Sexual Response.* Boston: Little. Brown.

Meyerowitz, Joanne (2002) *How Sex Changed: A History of Transsexuality in the United States.* Cambridge: Harvard University Press.

Millet, Kate. (1970) *Sexual Politics.* New York: Simon & Schuster.

Mitchell, Juliet. (1975) *Psychoanalysis and Feminism: Freud. Reich. Laing and Women.* New York: Vintage Books.

Morgan, Robin. Ed. *Sisterhood is Powerful: An Anthology of Writings from the Women's Liberation Movement.* New York: Vintage Books.

Mumford, Kevin. (1997) *Interzones: Black/White Sex Districts in Chicago and New York in the Early Twentieth-Century.* New York: Columbia University Press.

Reich, Wilhelm. (1933 [1970]) *The Mass Psychology of Fascism,* new translation. New York: Farrar, Straus & Giroux..

Reich, Wilhelm. (1935. [1951]) *The Sexual Revolution: Toward a Self-Governing Character Structure.* New York: Farrar, Straus & Giroux.

Reich, Wilhelm (1942) *The Function of the Orgasm.* New York: Farrar, Straus & Giroux.

Reich, Wilhelm (1972) *Sex-Pol: Essays. 1929-1934.* Ed. Lee Baxandall. New York: Vintage Books.

Rimmer, Robert (1967) *The Harrad Experiment.* New York: Bantam.

Rimmer, Robert (1975) "Introduction" to Tom Hatfield. *Sandstone Experience.* New York: Crown Publishers.

Robinson, Paul A. (1969) *The Freudian Left: Wilhelm Reich, Geza Roheim, Herbert Marcuse*. New York: Harper & Row.

Robinson, Paul A. (1976) *The Modernization of Sex. Havelock Ellis, Alfred Kinsey, William Masters and Virginia Johnson*. New York: Harper & Row.

Rubin. Gayle. (1984) "Thinking Sex: Notes for a Radical Theory of the Politics of Sexuality." In *Pleasure and Danger: Exploring Female Sexuality*. edited by Carole S. Vance. New York: Routledge.

Smith, Daniel Scott. (1978) "The Dating of the American Sexual Revolution: Evidence and Interpretation." In *The American Family in Social-Historical Perspective* (Second Edition) edited by Michael Gordon. New York: St Martin's.

Talese, Gay (1980) *Thy Neighbor's Wife*. New York: Doubleday.

Vance, Carole S. (1984) ed. *Pleasure and Danger: Exploring Female Sexuality*. Boston: Routledge Kegan & Paul

Weinberg, Martin and Colin Williams (1975) "Gay Baths and the Social Organization of Impersonal Sex." Social Problems. Vol. 23.

White, Kevin. (1993) *The First Sexual Revolution: The Emergence of Male Heterosexuality in Modern America*. New York: New York University Press.

White, Kevin. (2000) *Sexual Liberation or Sexual License?: The American Revolt Against Victorianism*. Chicago: Ivan R. Dee

Permissions